SPECIALTY GRAINS FOR FOOD AND FEED

Edited by

Elsayed Abdel-Aal and Peter Wood

Agriculture and Agri-Food Canada
Food Research Program
Guelph, Ontario, Canada

Published by the
American Association of Cereal Chemists, Inc.
St. Paul, Minnesota, U.S.A.

Library of Congress Catalog Card Number: 2004110510
International Standard Book Number: 1-891127-41-1

Printed in the United States of America on acid-free paper

American Association of Cereal Chemists
3340 Pilot Knob Road
St. Paul, Minnesota 55121-2097 U.S.A.

Contributors

E-S. M. Abdel-Aal, Agriculture and Agri-Food Canada, Food Research Program, Guelph, ON, Canada N1G 5C9

Joseph M. Awika, Cereal Quality Lab, Soil and Crop Sciences Department, Texas A&M University, College Station, TX 77843-2474

Samuel Bonti-Ankomah, Research and Analysis Directorate, Agriculture and Agri-Food Canada, Ottawa, ON, Canada K1A 0C6

Vernon D. Burrows, Agriculture and Agri-Food Canada, Eastern Cereal and Oilseed Research Centre, Ottawa, Canada K1A 0C6

Monisha Chakraborty, Department of Plant Sciences, College of Agriculture, North Dakota State University, Fargo, ND 58105

Ravindra N. Chibbar, Department of Plant Sciences, College of Agriculture, University of Saskatchewan, Saskatoon, SK, Canada S7N 5A8

Raimondo Cubadda, Department of Food Science Technology and Microbiology, University of Molise, Via De Sanctis, 86100 Campobasso, Italy

Christophe David, ISARA Lyon, Department of Agrosystems, Environment and Production, Cedex 02, France 69288

J. Frégeau-Reid, Agriculture and Agri-Food Canada, Eastern Cereal and Oilseed Research Centre, Ottawa, ON, Canada K1A 0C6

L. Gao, PEI Food Technology Centre, Charlottetown, PEI, Canada C1A 7N8

Pierre Gélinas, Food Research and Development Centre, Agriculture and Agri-Food Canada, Saint-Hyacinthe, QC, Canada J2S 8E3

John Henning, McGill University, Department of Agricultural Economics, Sainte-Anne de Bellevue, QC, Canada H9X 3V9

P. Hucl, Crop Development Centre, Department of Plant Sciences, University of Saskatchewan, Saskatoon, SK, Canada N7S 5A8

Massimo F. Marcone, Department of Food Science, Ontario Agricultural College, University of Guelph, Guelph, ON, Canada N1G 2W1

Emanuele Marconi, Department of Food Science Technology and Microbiology, University of Molise, Via De Sanctis, 86100 Campobasso, Italy

G. Mazza, Agriculture and Agri-Food Canada, Pacific Agri-Food Research Centre, Summerland, BC, Canada V0H 1Z0

C. W. Newman, Newman Associates Inc., Bozeman, MT 59715

R. K. Newman, Newman Associates Inc., Bozeman, MT 59715

B. Dave Oomah, Agriculture and Agri-Food Canada, Pacific Agri-Food Research Centre, Summerland, BC, Canada V0H 1Z0

Sanaa Ragaee, Department of Food Sciences, College of Food Systems, United Arab Emirates University, Al Maqam Campus, Al-Ain, United Arab Emirates

Lloyd W. Rooney, Cereal Quality Lab, Soil and Crop Sciences Department, Texas A&M University, College Station, TX 77843-2474

Graham Scoles, Department of Plant Sciences, College of Agriculture, University of Saskatchewan, Saskatoon, SK, Canada, S7N 5A8

P. J. Wood, Agriculture and Agri-Food Canada, Food Research Program, Guelph, ON, Canada N1G 5C9

Preface

This book has been designed to provide a single source of information on the numerous specialty or alternative grains that have been finding new niche markets in recent years. The increasing interest in specialty/organic/natural grain products from both consumers and industry and the increasing attention being paid to relationships between diet and health prompted us to plan this book, appropriately perhaps, around the start of the new millenium. The book compiles information on a wide range of ancient and recently developed grains, including einkorn, emmer, spelt, waxy wheat, hulless barley, hairless canary seed, hulless oats, specialty rye, specialty sorghum, blue and purple grains, amaranth, buckwheat, and organic grains. There are 15 chapters, each written by an expert in the field.

The grains are described in terms of history, genetic background, agronomic needs, uses, health aspects, and marketability. The roles of specialty grain production in maintaining agricultural diversity, protecting the environment, and contributing to the safety and nutritional value of our food supply are discussed. As an example, one chapter looks at fact and fiction about cereal grains and celiac disease. Grain consumption, health, and health claims are addressed in a separate chapter but also are frequently considered in individual chapters. The production of many of the specialty grains described in this book is related to the rapidly increasing interest in organically grown produce, which, in turn, is at least partly associated with public concern about, first, the safety and nutritional quality of the food supply and, second, the relationships between modern agronomic practices and the environment and agricultural diversity. This motivated us to include a chapter on organic grains and their products. Although, as experts involved with a subject, we are also enthusiasts, we and the authors have tried to treat the subjects rationally and objectively, and we hope this will allow the reader to reach informed conclusions about the issues involved. The compendium is fully referenced, allowing those interested to follow up on the information provided. This will be particularly important for the cereal and baking industry, as pressures continue to develop to produce food perceived as healthier, safer, and more environmentally friendly. The book should be a useful resource (and guide to references) for all involved in the grain industry, from the farmer to the informed consumer. We hope it contributes to the continuing development of markets for specialty grains, although we know it will continue to be a major challenge to develop and introduce new grains to the food and nonfood industries and adequately evaluate the impact of the issues discussed in this book on human health and the environment.

Last but not least, we would like to thank all the people who have helped bring this publication into print. Obviously, the greatest appreciation is due to the commitment of the authors who devoted their time and expertise to writing the articles and delivering the manuscripts on time. We are also most grateful to the reviewers for constructive and thorough reviews. Finally, a special thanks to the splendid staff at AACC headquarters for the production of this book and assistance in the preparation. We are also thankful to Agriculture and Agri-Food Canada for support and for providing the facilities that allowed us to produce the book.

Elsayed Abdel-Aal
Peter Wood

Contents

CHAPTER 1

Introduction to Specialty Grains

E-S. M. Abdel-Aal and P. J. Wood

Agriculture and Agri-Food Canada,[1] Food Research Program, Guelph, ON, Canada N1G 5C9

Cultivation of cereals and cereal-like grains extends well back into prehistory. Wheat is one of the oldest cultivated crops, grown for food at least as long ago as 8000–10,000 BC (Toussaint-Samat 1992). Barley also seems to have a very ancient history of use, dating back to 8000 BC, with suggestions of use back 17,000 years. Rice also has a long history, with early cultivation mentioned in about 3000 BC, apart from the prehistoric use. Indeed, evidence suggests that the ancient Egyptian, Babylonian, Greek, Cretan, and Roman civilizations were highly dependent on wheat and barley as the principal food. Nowadays, cereals remain the principal food for most of the world's population, with consumption of about 425 g/day/capita compared with 89 g/day/capita for potatoes and 14 g/day/capita for pulses (FAO 2000). Cereals provide approximately 1,339 calories/day/capita, 32.4 g protein/day/capita and 5.6 g fat/day/capita, which represent about 48, 43, and 7% of the totals, respectively. Thus, nearly one-half of the energy and more than two-fifths of the world's protein intake comes from the consumption of cereal foods. The total annual world production of cereals is estimated at about 1,900 million metric tons (tonnes, t) in which about 50% is used for food and 35% in animal feed, with the balance distributed between industrial processing, seeding, other uses, and waste (FAO 2000). The present global population growth is about 85–90 million per year, 50% of which is in Asia. This world population increase translates into a cultivation requirement to provide 14–15 million tonnes annual increase in cereal consumption. The actual per capita consumption is likely to continue to increase in developing countries. In North America, following a drastic decline during the first three-quarters of the twentieth century, cereal consumption has been steadily increasing. The per capita consumption in the United States has increased by almost 50% since 1970 (USDA Economic Research Service 2004), although the percentage of energy directly obtained from cereal grains has increased significantly less (19–25%

[1] For the Department of Agriculture and Agri-Food Canada, Food Research Program, Government of Canada. Publication number S175.

between 1970 and 1996). The current trend is toward greater whole grain consumption in North America, possibly as part of a move to healthier lifestyle and diet, which requires a change in both caloric intake and sources of energy.

Thus, cereals are a major source of starch and dietary fiber (complex carbohydrate) in our diets, and they convey health benefits. The availability of a diverse array of grain types and properties for each cereal has allowed the production of a seemingly limitless number of food products, resulting in considerable market diversification and expansion; cereals provide the major staples of the world—namely bread, pasta, and rice.

Cereal grains have evolved over the centuries, primarily to enhance yield, disease resistance, and quality both through traditional breeding programs and more recently through genetic manipulations. With regard to composition and quality, the emphasis has been to improve the key components, protein and starch; much less attention has been paid to secondary substances such as phenolics and dietary fiber, partly because of lack of knowledge regarding their function in plant protection and in promoting human health. Indeed, some of the secondary constituents, such as polyphenolics, phytate, carotenoids, and "ash" (i.e., minerals) have been targets for reduction or elimination because of adverse effects on quality. But recently, as documented in several chapters of this book, studies have accumulated to show a role of such secondary substances in promoting human health, reducing the risk of chronic diseases, and protecting plants against pests and disease. Accordingly, research programs are in progress to identify plant sources such as ancient grains that contain high levels of components that are biologically active and may provide health benefits.

Numerous claims have been made over the years for therapeutic properties of ancient grains, and they are used in alternative and folk medicine for the treatment of a wide range of problems such as ulcerous colitis, elevated serum cholesterol, hypertension, diabetes, rheumatoid arthritis, depression, and cancer. Little or no scientific evidence, at least of the kind acceptable in most modern clinical evaluations, exists to support these claims. Nevertheless, the beneficial health properties of whole grain foods are accepted widely and recognized and, in the United States, are supported by health claims (see Chapter 15). The primary candidate components for the health-promoting and disease-risk-reducing properties of whole grain products are antioxidants and dietary fiber (including slowly digested and resistant starch), although many researchers would suggest that this issue cannot be looked at on a simplistic component basis.

The planning of this book included a debate about whether the title should use the adjective *alternative* rather than *specialty*, with the latter winning out. Obviously we believe we have chosen the correct term, since *alternative* implies "replacement," whereas *specialty* simply means "for a special purpose." However, the issue is not clear-cut, and, for some consumers and suppliers, the intention certainly is replacement, with an "alternative" lifestyle that does not include consumption of any mainstream agrifood business produce.

The chapter on organic grains specifically addresses this definitely alternative food supply system. Many of the other chapters deal with grains that supply this rapidly growing organic market for various reasons, and overall the grains covered in this book owe much of their popularity to the belief that they are superior to mainstream modern agricultural produce. The consumer's motivation seems to be partly an altruistic, environmental concern and partly a question of personal health and well-being, but a simple organoleptic preference also plays a role.

The designation *specialty grains* is usually applied to grains (primitive or recently developed) that exhibit some unique characteristic and are currently produced on a marginal scale for a particular end use or market. However, this is not the entire story. Specialty grains, if chosen simply in reference to end use, encompass many aspects, including grains grown very much as part of mainstream agriculture and food supply, and, of course, all grain is grown for special end uses (e.g., durum wheat, waxy corn). Our selection in this book was for grains that serve the more unusual niche markets or those that may have special health benefits but whose properties and value are not well known. The selection is not exhaustive, and we apologize for any omissions.

The book compiles reviews of a wide range of grains that hold promise for specialty food markets, particularly organic, functional foods for health and nutraceuticals; however, chapters on more recently developed grains with unique or special properties, such as waxy wheat and canary seed, are also included. The other specialty grains included are spelt, einkorn, emmer, blue and purple grains, hulless oat, hulless barley, low- and high-viscosity rye, amaranth, buckwheat, and organic grains. The special features of each grain in terms of genetic background, composition, and structure are emphasized and discussed in relation to both current and potential end uses. Health aspects and market value are also highlighted.

The size of the specialty grain market is small but has the potential to grow, and this is driven, at least in part, by consumer perception that the products answer the demand for safer and healthier foods. Further expansion of the market depends strongly on availability of product, consistency of quality, and price, since despite specialty appeal, these grains must in the end compete with mainstream commercial grains. Some of the markets already indicated as appropriate for specialty crops are growing rapidly. The Canadian organic food market is expanding rapidly and is expected to rise from a retail value of $0.7 billion in 1997 to $3.1 billion in 2005, an average growth rate of about 20% (AAFC 2001). Organic food sales in the United States are estimated at $6.95 billion and are expected to reach $21.9 billion by 2010 (Sloan 2002). Most consumers believe that organic foods contribute to their overall health but do not relate this to a specific health condition (Sloan 2002). "Natural" food products, which are not well defined but certainly include organic, are perceived to reduce exposure to harmful chemicals and contribute to a healthier environment. Consumers have become more health conscious and more concerned about safety and quality of food. This may lead to positive changes in the food-production chain, particularly with regard to the extensive use of synthetic chemicals, high-yield farming, and aspects of milling and processing. Sustainable food-production practices are essential for a healthy environment and improved quality of life. It should not be forgotten, however, that these comments and considerations apply almost entirely to the concerns of developed, wealthy nations and consumers. For vast numbers, the only concern is staving off starvation. Starvation is less a problem of research and development and more one of economics, world trade, and agricultural subsidies.

The developing market for foods to which specific health benefits are attributed (functional foods for health) is also being driven by consumer demand and interest in foods that, besides providing pleasure and basic nutrition, may also improve health and prevent disease. In the United States, the functional food market was estimated at approximately $86 billion in 1997, with a growth rate of about 7.5% (Anonymous 1997). Cereal foods are perceived as healthy foods, forming the base of the food pyramid, and are sources of biologically active components such as dietary fiber, tocopherols, and carotenoids. However, these components are significantly depleted in refined cereals, as in white bread. This may in part be driving the promotion and the developing belief of the public in so-called low-carbohydrate or low-carb diets. Unfortunately, this promotion does not adequately discriminate between different sources and types of carbohydrate. Certainly this trend has the potential to reduce consumption of whole as well as refined grain products, and to interfere in the development of the market in both mainstream and specialty grains.

The mainstream pursuit in flours and ingredients, except for pasta, has been whiteness; however, a large group of cereals may possess health functionality because of their content of anthocyanins and antioxidants. These are the blue, purple, and red grains such as black and red rice, blue barley, purple corn, and blue wheat. These grains are potential sources of natural colorants, nutraceuticals, and pharmaceuticals, but they have not been much exploited or developed. As an example, lutein, the major yellow pigment in wheat and durum, was incorporated into ready-to-eat cereal (0.5 mg/30 g serving) and cereal bar (1.25 mg/50 g serving) recipes as a functional component with potential benefits in maintaining healthy vision and skin (Fullmer and Shao 2001). The development of high-lutein wheat-based products could more than double the daily per capita intake in North America on the basis of the recommended daily consumption of six servings of grains (i.e., six servings provide 2.1 mg lutein based on 86% dry matter) (Abdel-Aal et al 2002). This could have a favorable impact on macroreticular degeneration, the primary cause of blindness in the aging population. The development of genotypes of grains with increased levels of such functional components will benefit producers, processors, and consumers, an all-win situation if levels are sufficient and products are efficacious and appealing.

In the United States, 78% of supermarket shoppers used fortified food for health benefit, whereas 55% chose additive- and preservative-free foods, and 37% chose organic foods (Sloan 2002). These percentages compare favorably with the 86% for over-the-counter medicine, reported in the same study. Thus today's consumer believes in food as medicine, as has long been the case. Specialty grains can partially serve these niche markets, but improvements in agronomic performance, specific characteristics, and uses will determine whether the market will continue to grow. Some danger exists in any drive to improve agronomic performance, since this was the path to today's mainstream grains, so this would defeat the purpose unless a different improvement strategy were adopted.

The mechanism by which whole grain foods reduce the risk of degenerative chronic diseases is poorly understood, but correlations between diet and diet components and specific health benefits have been documented, some from long ago. In about the fifth century BC, Hippocrates,[2] the great Greek physician, advised eating liver as a remedy for night blindness, without knowing the basis for the treatment. Much later, in 1913, the active component was identified as vitamin A and its chemical formula was disclosed (Anonymous 2001). Cereal grains are obvious likely sources of dietary components that may improve physiological functions, reduce risk of disease, and possibly even act therapeutically to mitigate or cure illness. Some of these health benefits have been documented to the satisfaction of the FDA in the United States, and others are under investigation. Hippocrates was sufficiently satisfied as to the benefit of whole grain or bran to state that "to the human body it makes a great difference whether the bread be made of fine flour or coarse, whither of wheat with or without the bran" (Burkitt 1995). Health claims (see Chapter 15) should encourage increased consumption of grain-based food products.

Both primary and secondary metabolites of grains serve as food and feed ingredients and have many industrial uses based on diverse physicochemical characteristics and functional properties. The fractionation by milling of corn and wheat into anatomical fractions and isolated chemical components is a good example. Recently developed grains such as waxy wheat and hairless canary seed may have particular value for the grain-fractionation industry because of their specific composition and properties. Hairless canary seed's three main components—starch, protein, and oil—exhibit potentially valuable specialty traits. Waxy wheat might be a source of gluten and high-amylopectin starch. These two grains and their potential are highlighted and discussed in separate chapters.

We view this book as an initiative that should assist in the development or renaissance of a variety of ancient and newly released cereal and cereal-like grains. The chapters document promise for the grain and food-production and manufacturing industries in aspects such as biodiversity, genetic resources, unique properties, organic production, functional foods, and other niche markets. Developing and introducing new grains for both food and nonfood uses

2 Now regularly quoted in articles on functional foods and nutraceuticals as having said "Let food be your medicine and medicine your food."

will be a major challenge, and evaluating their impact on human health and environment will require a multidisciplinary approach. While the chapters in this book attempt to introduce and promote selected grains, several other grains that may have unique properties of potential value for food production and human health are not covered. By providing an examination of the food-production chain from field to table in terms of safety, quality, health and disease, environment, and genetic biodiversity, we hope the book emphasizes the message that the food-production and processing system must be socially, ecologically, and economically sustainable.

References

Abdel-Aal, E.-S. M., Young, J. C., Wood, P. J, Rabalski, I., Hucl, P., Falk, D., and Frégeau-Reid, J. 2002. Einkorn: A potential candidate for developing high lutein wheat. Cereal Chem. 79:458-464.

Agriculture and Agri-Food Canada (AAFC). 2001. Canada's organic industry. Online: http://ats-sea.agr.gc.ca/supply/3313_e.pdf

Anonymous 1997. Nutraceutical trend takes root despite definitional challenges. Nutr. Bus. J. 11:1-3, 15.

Anonymous 2001. Diet and health research needs. Food Technol. 55:189-191.

Burkitt, D. 1995. Historical aspects. Pages 3-10 in: Dietary Fiber in Health and Disease. D. Kritchevsky and C. Bonfield, Eds. American Association of Cereal Chemists, St. Paul, MN.

Fullmer, L. A., and Shao, A. 2001. The role of lutein in eye health and nutrition. Cereal Foods World 46:408-413.

Food and Agriculture Organization (FAO). 2000. FAOSTAT website: http://faostat.fao.org/faostat/collections?subset=agriculture

Sloan, A. E. 2002. The natural and organic foods marketplace. Food Technol. 56:27-37.

Toussaint-Samat, M. A. 1992. History of Food. (In French, translated by A. Bell.) Blackwell Publishers, Cambridge, MA.

USDA, Economic Research Service, 2004. Website: http://www.ers.usda.gov/data/foodconsumption/

CHAPTER 2

Organic Grains and Products

Christophe David,[1] Pierre Gélinas,[2] Samuel Bonti-Ankomah,[3] and John Henning[4]

[1]ISARA Lyon, Department of Agrosystems, Environment and Production, Cedex 02, France 69288; [2]Food Research and Development Centre, Agriculture and Agri-Food Canada, Saint-Hyacinthe, QC, Canada J2S 8E3; [3]Research and Analysis Directorate, Agriculture and Agri-Food Canada, Ottawa, ON, Canada K1A 0C6; [4]McGill University, Department of Agricultural Economics, Sainte-Anne de Bellevue, QC, Canada H9X 3V9

Organic farming is receiving increasing attention from consumers, citizen groups, the media, market players, and governments. Although the growth in popularity of organic foods has not met the expectations its promoters anticipated during the 1970s, the organic sector is now firmly established in the majority of developed countries and provides the basis of a creative tension with the evolution of the conventional agri-food system. We focus here on developments in the European Union and North American organic grains sectors through a review of production and quality assurance systems, market conditions, and technical considerations. However, analyzing and tracking the development of the structure of this sector remains challenging, since the rates of growth and development vary widely among countries and there is little systematic data collection.

In the next section, we briefly introduce the concept of organic agriculture and describe the increasingly sophisticated regulatory framework that now exists in the European Union, North America, and internationally. We move on to basic information on the scale of organic food and grain production, based on recently published data. Management systems and the profitability of organic grain production are discussed next, followed by a report on the size and structure of the organic grain market. The next section addresses the issues of safety, technical quality, and the nutritional value of organic grains as compared to conventional. The latter issues are at the heart of consumer interest in organic food products, and although environmental and social concerns have been identified as motivating factors, these are clearly of secondary importance to consumers and so we have given them little attention here. Finally, the last section quickly examines consumer perceptions and attitudes in terms of their willingness to pay more for organic foods than for conventional. Although the growth of the organic sector has been spectacular during the past decade, there is evidence of price resistance among consumers that may place limits on its potential for future growth at the same rate.

Definition of Organic Agriculture and Regulation

Definition

In the past decade, the definition of organic farming has become formally codified at subnational, national, and international levels (Codex Alimentarius 2001; EC Commission 1991, 1999; USDA 2001). It is an evolving and increasingly sophisticated technology that is informed by the past but continues to develop as quickly as the capacity of scientists and practitioners to respond to the challenge of understanding the complex processes of farming systems that are imbedded in a healthy, functioning ecosystem. The term *organic* is also used interchangeably with terms such as *ecological, biodynamic,* and *biological*, although these are not always synonymous.

In defining the meaning of organic, it is important to point out that this is not an anachronistic system based on "farming by neglect," without the use of fertilizers and methods of pest control, in spite of the fact that organic methods draw on the farming systems of the distant past. Although the genesis of organic farming dates back over a century, as a farming system that is identifiable with modern organic farming it did not appear in the literature until 1924, in a series of lectures given by Rudolf Steiner. The notion was further developed during the 1930s and 1940s by others, including Britain's Howard (1940) and Balfour (1975), the United States' Rodale (1945), and Japan's Fukuoka (1985a,b) and Mokichi Okada's Nature Farming (www.pan-american-moa.org). It was probably during the 1940s that the term *organic* was first used to describe an agricultural system by Northbourne (1940). This author used the term to describe farming systems that focus on the farm as a dynamic, living, balanced, organic whole: an organism. With the same intent, the term was also widely used and popularized in the United States during the 1950s by Rodale. By the early 1970s, *organic farming* had been popularized throughout Europe and North America.

Organic farming can be defined as a holistic system of agricultural production with the general objective optimizing a broadly based concept of ecosystem productivity that includes the well-being of diverse communities within agro-ecosystems: microorganisms, plants, animals, and human populations. The result should be agro-ecosystems that are socially and ecologically sustainable.

Modern Principles of Organic Farming

Concerning aids to production, processing, and distribution, organic methods avoid the use of synthetic inputs at the farm level (specifically, fertilizer, pesticides, herbicides, fungicides, antibiotics, growth hormones), and synthetic preservatives, additives, and irradiation beyond the farm. These limits on inputs have been the foundation of consumer expectations that organic foods are safer and more healthful than conventional foods (see the last section).

A fundamental strategy of organic farming is the prevention of problems through the careful design and management of the farming system, rather than the reliance of off-farm interventions to solve problems. Hill and Henning (1992) refer to the process a farmer must go through to learn this strategy within what is called an Efficiency, Substitution, Redesign (ESR) paradigm. When confronted with a problem, the farmer needs to first consider how to use inputs more efficiently, then seek more benign substitutes, and finally consider how to redesign the system to remove the niche that the problem occupies. Although organic farming does allow for the use of some approved chemicals to deal with problems, the routine use of any such chemical is not considered to be appropriate and points to a design failure in the system. A successful design should work with natural ecological processes, taking advantage of soil nutrient and water cycles, energy flows, beneficial organisms, and natural pest controls.

Long-term soil fertility is central to this approach and is maintained by promoting soil biological activity and diversity, recycling of plant and animal wastes, and the use of renewable resources. The soil is conserved through the use of minimal tillage, ground covers, and green manures. A key element is the reliance on farm resources within a relatively closed farming system, rather than dependence on inputs imported from outside the farm.

Beyond this, organic farming has embraced a philosophy that draws on a set of values that reflect an awareness of both ecological and social realities (MacRae et al 1990). Particularly in recent years, social and ethical goals for organic farming are gaining more attention (Blowfield 2001), now that the biophysical aspects have been fairly well established and the market for organics has clearly taken off. During the next decade, there will be a movement to formally incorporate measures of the social performance of organic agriculture into the standards that currently define what an organic system represents.

Standards, Certification, and Accreditation

Organic is somewhat unique in that production must also conform to prescribed standards under the supervision of an inspection agency that certifies the product as organic. When a product is labeled organic, this indicates it has been produced in accordance with a standard throughout production, handling, processing, and marketing. Thus, the label is a "process" claim rather than a product claim, since product testing is not a part of the system. There is no explicit claim that it is better than some other product; rather, it simply indicates that the product conforms to the process. A certification body uses the inspection report to certify the farm and its products as organic. Finally, an accreditation agency is responsible for ensuring that the certification body is competent to carry out the process of certification.

In the early years of organic farming, trade in organic products between farmers and consumers was relatively direct. The exchange was based primarily on trust by the consumer that the product was "organic," or direct knowledge of the farm and how the food was produced. But, as the market expanded, it became more likely that products would not pass directly from farmer to consumer, and so the potential for fraud increased. The market became one in which there were significant information asymmetries; the farmer knew whether the product was organic, but the consumer did not. Such markets and their problems are well known in the economics literature (Carlton and Perloff 1989), and the development of standards has been a common approach to addressing these problems in other parts of the agriculture and food sector.

For this purpose, standards and certification systems began to emerge in the late 1960s and 1970s. In 1967, the Soil Association (UK) was the first to develop organic standards, followed by legislated standards in Oregon and California in the 1970s. During the 1980s, many private organizations and government agencies developed these systems, and there emerged a plethora of certification bodies that used these standards as a basis to inspect farms and certify them as producers of organic foods.

The first transnational standard did not emerge until 1980, when the International Federation of Organic Agriculture Movements (IFOAM) published its standard. IFOAM is the worldwide umbrella organization for organic agriculture, with membership of more than 700 organizations from more than 100 countries. The intent of IFOAM's standard was to be a global guideline that could be used as a template by countries to develop their own standards, and to promote harmonization, in opposition to the trend of an increasing array of standards of varying requirements. For the same reason, many governments began to develop standards during the 1980s. The European Union was able to adopt an organic regulation in 1991 (Reg. EC 2092/91). Some countries took many years for standards to be completed, such as Canada in 1999 and the United States in 2000.

With international trade in organic products starting to accelerate, in 1993 the Codex Alimentarius Commission began to develop an international guideline for organic foods within its food-labeling committee. Codex is a forum in which member countries and international nongovernment organizations discuss food trade and safety issues to facilitate trade and to encourage consumer protection through the development of food production, processing, and labeling standards. Although the Codex organic guideline was published in 1999 (Codex Alimentarius 2001), it is still under development and will continue to evolve toward the status of a standard as countries become more experienced with organic farming and with managing certification and accreditation systems. Eventually, it will gain more official status as the basis for trade decisions at the level of the World Trade Organization and for harmonizing the systems being used by member countries. The need for harmonization is clear, considering that there are 54 countries with either fully implemented regulations or at least regulations in the process of elaboration (Commins and Wai 2002).

Already there has been significant progress towards harmonization through the process of developing the Codex guideline, together with the widespread adoption of the guidelines for quality assurance systems of the International Organization for Standardization (ISO). ISO Guide 65:1996, "General Requirements for Bodies Operating Product Certification Systems" (http://www.iso.org), provides the minimum requirements that certification bodies must meet to demonstrate that they are operating a competent third-party certification system. ISO Guide 61:1996, "General Requirements for Assessment and Accreditation of Certification/Registration Bodies," likewise lays out the requirements for accreditation organizations. The use of these guidelines also facilitates the harmonization of systems between countries since most organic control systems now are based on ISO guidelines and managed by professional staff.

In the United States, Canada, and the European Union, there are many certification bodies. Primarily run as private businesses, some of the best-known bodies are Quality Assurance International, Ecocert, OCIA, and Demeter. On the other hand, there are relatively few accreditation bodies, and these tend to be closely associated with government. In the United States, accreditation is the responsibility of the U.S. Department of Agriculture (USDA), while in Canada it is the Standards Council of Canada. In the European Union, member countries have their own accreditation bodies in addition to the European Commission. With a control program now in place in these countries, only a certification body that has been accredited by the importing country may certify imports of organic products. Since the systems across countries have not yet been harmonized, this means that a certification body might be required to be accredited in each country to which products it has certified are exported. This certainly adds to the cost of organic products that trade across national boundaries, since the costs of accreditation and certification have to be passed on through the marketing chain. Accreditation costs vary widely, from about $US 2,000 by the USDA to $US 28,000 through the Standards Council of Canada.

Organic Foods and Cereals Production

Worldwide, more than 23 million hectares are managed organically (Yussefi and Willer 2003), or less than 1% of the total agricultural land base. In the European Union, there are almost 5 million hectares and more than 150,000 farms (including accession countries) representing 2% of the total agriculture sector, while in North America there are more than 1.5 million hectares and 45,000 farms for 0.25% of the total.

Especially since the 1990s, the organic land base has grown tremendously, particularly in Europe, North America, and Latin America (FAO 2002). The growing market (Kortbech-Olsen 2003) and the existence of common regulations (EC Commission 1991, 1999; USDA 2001) linked with policy support have been instrumental in supporting the development of organic production. Consequently, since the early 1990s, organic farming has been growing by 25% per year in almost all European countries (Lampkin et al 1999) and North America (Klonsky and Tourte 1998).

In the European Union, about 44% of organic crop production is organic cereals, with over 1.6 million tonnes in 2000 (Hamm et al 2002). Nonetheless, this represents only 0.8% of total cereal output. Organic grains and root crops represent almost 1 million hectares, composed of 83% cereals, 7% pulses, 7% oilseeds, and 3% root crops (EC Commission 1999).

In North America, organic cereal production is proportionally small (under 0.4%) compared to total cereal production. Nonetheless, organic cereals represent a growing sector in the western prairies (Saskatchewan, Manitoba, Montana, the Dakotas, and Minnesota) (Entz et al 1998), but the development is slower in the eastern, southern, and Atlantic regions. In the United States, the proportion of farm area devoted to cropland as opposed to range and pastureland is higher for organic agriculture than for agriculture as a whole (Klonsky and Tourte 1998).

Managing Crop Production in Organic Farming Systems

Principles of Organic Crop Production

vCentral to organic crop production is the design of a system that enhances the prevention of diseases and weeds and self-supplies nitrogen through the use of N-fixing crops and cover crops (Askegaard et al 1999). Crop diversification can deliver many simultaneous agronomic benefits (e.g., reduced weed pressure) (Bond and Grundy 2001) and ecological benefits (e.g., reduced pest incidence) (Finckh and Wolfe 1998), while maintaining or enhancing production efficiency. In organic cereal production, the challenge is to develop a long-term sustainable cropping system that combines N-fixing crops, which may not have a market value, with high-N-demanding crops. Although, various authors (Bulson et al 1996, Younie et al 1996) have shown that a forage legume (e.g., clover) can enhance yield and gross margin of the following crop, nonetheless, the use of more than 25% legumes over the rotational area tends to limit the overall profitability of the rotation (Hogh-Jensen 1999, Olesen et al 2002). Consequently, several strategies have been developed that combine cereals and forage legumes to increase N nutrition, control weeds and diseases, and improve grain yield and quality without compromising the performance of the crop rotation (Bulson et al 1997, Holle and Untiedt 1999, Germeier 2000, Liebman and Davis 2000, Kankanen et al 2001, Mueller and Thorup-Kristensen 2001). Examples include intercropping (Theunissen 1997), undersowing, and mixed cropping systems.

Weed control and nutrient management are recognized as the most serious challenge to organic grain production (Barberi 2002). Nonetheless, Bond and Grundy (2001) confirmed that more weed-control options are becoming available to organic growers through crop rotation, soil cultivation, and mechanical weed control.

In organic agriculture, the fertility and biological activity of the soil should be maintained or increased by (1) the use of legumes, green manures, or deep-rooting plants in a multiannual rotation program or (2) the incorporation into the soil of plant and animal organic material. Mixed farming systems have the potential to supply a large amount of N to crops through crop residues, manures, and compost, resulting in positive N balances (Berry et al 2002). Nonetheless, matching the supply of N from the mineralization of organic materials with crop demand is difficult (Pang and Letey 2000). This can result in temporary N deficiencies that limit yield and grain protein content, or periods with excess N lost to the environment (Haraldsen et al 2000, Stopes et al 2002). Furthermore, the trend toward specialization on organic stockless farms requires the development of novel and suitable fertility-building strategies (Watson et al 2002). For this purpose, David et al (2004) have developed a decision-making tool to assist crop producers in selecting the optimal fertilization strategy for organic wheat.

Maintaining good growing conditions and avoiding stress enhances the natural tolerance of plants to plant competitors (Tamis and van den Brink 1999). Stimulating biodiversity in and above the soil, by amendments, good soil management, and rotation allows for the control of most soilborne pests and diseases (Altieri 1995). Finally, many foliar pests and diseases are effectively controlled by spatial crop diversification, including mixed cropping and variety mixtures (Finckh et al 2000), in combination with disease-resistance genotypes.

Currently, organic farmers depend largely on genotypes supplied by conventional plant breeders, who developed these for farming systems in which synthetic fertilizers and pesticides are widely used. According to Lammerts van Bueren et al (2002), there is a need to develop genotypes that are specifically adapted to low-input conditions with multiple constraints.

Portrait of Arable Farming Systems

In the 1980s, organic cereals were produced mainly by mixed livestock farms that operated a closed system for nutrients and organic matter (Köpke 1995). Early in the 1990s, the fast-growing market induced the development of specialized organic crop producers. These farms are characterized by an increased diversity of cropping patterns in time and space compared to conventional systems (Stockdale et al 2001). Considering the array of organic farms producing grains in Europe and North America, three major farming systems can be defined.

Mixed Farming Systems

Mixed farming systems are common in temperate and Atlantic climates (i.e., United Kingdom and Atlantic parts of North America). These systems are based on a large share (more than 40% of the area) of N-fixing crops such as grass/white clover leys or green manures (red clover and vetches) mulched and plowed in, associated with cereals within a long-term rotation (i.e., 8–10 years) (Younie et al 1996). To make maximum use of the large quantity of nitrogen released following the incorporation of leys, crops with high N-demand such as winter wheat or potatoes are usually grown at the start of the cropping phase. Since animal manure is abundant, even silage and root crops receive organic compost, although it would be more beneficial on cereals with a higher N-demand (Stein-Bachinger and Werner 1997). Weeds and diseases are controlled mainly by the crop diversity within the rotation.

Intensive Crop Production Systems

Mostly represented by farms in northern and central Europe, this farming system has followed the same path found in the intensification of conventional agriculture (Hogh-Jensen 1999), where there is a lack of grazing livestock. This specialization process has been possible because of the flexible norms for organic farming, particularly with regard to N-inputs (Baars 1998).

The poor profitability of forage crops has diminished their importance in the crop rotation while high market prices for grains, corn, and soybeans have encouraged their part. Consequently, there is a move toward high-profit crops (i.e., potatoes, sugar beets) and grains grown in relatively short rotations (i.e, three to four years). In some cases, the use of irrigation has permitted farmers to increase the rotation proportion of spring crops such as corn and soybean (Grignani et al 2001).

Considering nitrogen management, within four years of rotation, a frequent practice is the introduction of a one-year fallow that includes clover grass mixtures as green manure (Schmidt and von Fragstein 1999). These farms compensate for the loss of minerals and soil organic matter by importing manure from organic livestock farms. While expensive, other off-farm organic fertilizers (i.e., feather meal, guano) are used to some extent (David et al 2004).

Dry-Land Large-Scale Crop Production

Under dry conditions (rainfall under 700 mm), large-scale organic farms can be found in the prairie provinces of Canada, the plain states of the United States, and southern Europe. These farmers generally grow a diverse group of crops, including corn, soybeans, and other major grains and oilseeds, as well as crops such as spelt, buckwheat, and rye that are not grown on a large scale in conventional agriculture (Walz 1999). Moreover, niche market crops such as amaranth and alternative grains (e.g., triticale, kamut, and millet), can be found on these farms as a means of increasing diversity even though it requires management flexibility and presents marketing challenges. Some farms have their own livestock (beef or milk production). Greene and Dobbs (2001) noted that the complexity of organic rotations may result in the need for much more family labor compared to conventional systems. More time is spent scouting fields for pest and weed problems.

The maintenance of adequate levels of yield and soil organic nitrogen depends largely on both "fertility building" by nitrogen-fixing leguminous crops (sweet clover, alfalfa), representing 20–30% of the crop rotation, and manure from their own livestock or from neighborhood livestock farms (Entz et al 1998, Porter et al 2003).

Profitability of Organic Foods and Grains

Price Premiums for Organic Foods

Whereas studies show that most consumers are reluctant to pay a price premium of more than 10%, analyses of organic food markets indicate the existence of significant price premiums above the same conventional products. In a study by Turco (2002), price premiums for organics were reported to range from 10% to as high as 100% across several countries. Turco (2002) concluded that price premiums were lowest in countries with a large organic food market share and a high percentage of distribution into the supermarket system. This was particularly typical of European markets. The fact that price premiums are highly variable over space and time is a reflection of the immature state of the organic sector. Production remains relatively small; distribution channels are not well integrated; and market information is scarce relative to that for conventional markets.

Price Premiums for Organic Cereals

Hamm et al (2002) collected data in several markets and reported high price premiums for organic grains. In the European Union, the average farmer price premium for organic cereals was 102% in 2000 and ranged from 30% in Greece to as high as 281% in Luxembourg. Furthermore, there were large variations among organic grains: a premium of 30% for feed corn compared to 300% for high-quality breadmaking wheat. Nine out of the 15 European Union countries reported higher farmers' price premiums than the EU average. Differences might be explained by transport costs, transactions costs, quality, and the level of self-sufficiency in each country. For the consumer, the price premium for organic cereals was approximately 60% and ranged from 41% for whole wheat to 75% for flour. Nonetheless, there are important differences in premiums across countries for the same cereal, which reveals that markets are not operating efficiently either inside or among EU member states.

In North America, market and price information is also scarce. Although some information is available, credible and systematic price collection is just beginning and being led by nongovernment organizations, unlike the situation in conventional markets, for which governments have been the traditional source of market information. Farmers are receiving premiums for organic grains. At times, these can be on the order of 100% above conventional prices for milling quality wheat. However, these premiums fluctuate considerably over time and should not be used as a prudent basis for farm planning. Local supply and demand conditions can change quickly, and being able to achieve milling quality standards may not be possible because of weather-related factors. The premiums for feed wheat can be much lower.

Although premiums can be large at the farm gate, these do not translate into the same percentage of premiums at the retail level. Organic cereals tend to be processed into manufactured products just like conventional cereals. The most recent data on farm to retail price spreads from the USDA (2003) can be used to understand why. During the period 1998–2000, the farm-gate share of consumer expenditures on wheat flour was about 19%. For bread, the share drops to 5%, and this is similar to the shares for related products such as corn flakes, oatmeal, and corn syrup. For example, suppose that the price of the wheat used to produce one standard loaf of bread is increased by 100%. Then, according to the USDA data, the retail price of the loaf of bread would increase from 88 cents to 92.4 cents, or 5%.

Table 1 indicates that the price premiums for corn, spring wheat, and oats in the United States in 2000 were 89, 103, and 71%, respectively. There was also a positive trend in premiums between 1995 and 2000. The trend can be attributed to increases in demand, which have not been matched by supply. Table 2 presents retail price information collected by the OACC (Organic Agricultural Centre of Canada 2003) for several major cities in Canada. In March 2003, consumer price premiums for organic cereals ranged from 14% for oats to 50% for whole wheat flour. However, the price premiums for oats and whole wheat pasta declined considerably between November 2002 and March 2003.

Premiums for organic products at the farm gate, coupled with the relatively lower premium most consumers are willing to pay for the final product, have implications for the future of the organic cereal market. Several studies indicate a high negative price response for organic foods (Hansen and Sørensen 1993, Lengyel 2000; M. Wolf, *unpblished data*). In an econometric analysis of the organic market in Denmark, Wier and Andersen (2001) found that the demand for organic foods had a high elastic price (–2.27). Lengyel

TABLE 1
Price Premiums for Some Organic Cereals in the United States (%)[a]

Year	Corn	Spring Wheat	Oats
1995	35	54	35
1996	43	59	59
1997	73	73	73
1998	88	78	83
1999	98	87	77
2000	89	103	71

[a] Source: Bertramsen and Dobbs (2001).

TABLE 2
Consumer Price Premiums for Some Selected Organic Cereals in Canada[a]

	Price Premium (%)	
Product	**November 2002**	**March 2003**
Oats (for cooking)	63	14
Pasta (whole wheat spaghetti)	62	49
Whole wheat flour	44	50

[a] Source: Organic Agricultural Centre of Canada (2003).

(2000) found a similar result for the United States. For conventional food products, it is well known that elasticity tends to be less than 1 in magnitude. The highly elastic nature of organic products means that small changes in prices of final products would lead to proportionally greater declines in demand. From a marketing perspective, this suggests that price premiums paid by consumers should not be set very high so as not to discourage consumers at the edge of the market for organic foods. For example, the recent decline in organic food consumption in Italy was blamed on the high price premiums (Compagnoni et al 2000). According to Turco (2002), the price premiums of organic food should have an upper limit of about 15% for widely distributed goods, and, if a product is available only through specialty stores, then the limit of this premium should not exceed 20–25%. In most cases, a large part of the extra price that consumers have to pay does not go to farmers, but to the processing and distribution chain. The costs of distributing organic products are normally higher than for nonorganic products because the amount sold in most shops is usually smaller, and distributors operate on a much smaller scale than their conventional counterparts. Hence, it is important to identify alternative distribution systems that can reduce the cost. One way of doing this is through direct delivery from the farmer to consumer to maintain high premiums for farmers.

Various studies have used consumer surveys to investigate willingness to pay a price premium for organic products (Table 3). Most consumers would be willing to pay price premiums of not more than 10–15%, and few may pay

TABLE 3
Summary of Consumer Studies on Willingness to Pay

Source	Country of Study	Findings
Hay (1989)	Canada	Consumers willing to pay a price premium of not more than 25%
Ekelund (1990)	Sweden	55% of respondents willing to pay 25% price premium and 26% of respondents willing to pay 50% price premium
Ott (1990)	USA	66% of respondents willing to pay 10–15% price premium
Goldman and Clancy (1991)	USA	Consumers willing to pay 100% price premium
Wandel and Bugge (1997)	Norway	70% of respondents willing to pay an extra 5%
Hutchins and Greenlagh (1997)	UK	Consumers willing to pay 30% price premium particularly for cereals, fruits, and vegetables
Cunningham (2002b)	Canada	68% of consumers willing to pay 10% price premium
O'Donovan and McCarthy (2002)	UK	About 70% of consumers were not willing to pay more than 10% price premium
M. Wolf, *unpublished data*	USA	30.2% of respondents willing to pay a 50% price premium for organic grapes

more than 15%. Most of these studies involved organic products in general; for the few studies on specific organic commodities, there are no clear patterns. Retailers are aware of these tendencies, and some are using them as a guide to their pricing strategies. In late 2001, President's Choice (Canada) began a significant introduction of new organic products into its product mix and set price targets for processed products at prices "comparable" to conventional, with produce at about a 30% premium (Henning 2002).

Profitability of Organic Grain Production

Financial viability is a key issue for established organic farmers and those considering transition from nonorganic agriculture. It is critical during transition, since this is a time when specific machinery must be acquired, mistakes are most likely, yields are depressed, and there is no price premium (MacRae et al 1990, Cobb et al 1999). Some countries do provide supports for farmers in transition. For established organic farmers, various studies report that the profitability of organic systems can be as high as or higher than conventional systems (Table 4), even if crop rotations include low-value crops and the occasional low yield. Welsh (1999) found that while the price premiums paid for organic products increase profitability, a higher price was not always necessary for organic systems to be competitive with conventional systems.

Profitability of grain production tends to vary widely, since both yield and price can vary markedly. In general, yields in organic agriculture are 20–30% lower, which is mainly due to lower N-input, but also to high pressure from weeds, pests, and diseases (Halberg and Kristensen 1997). However, it is not difficult to find established organic farmers with high cereal yields, as high as conventional. Yet profitability depends on both yield and yield stability. Some evidence suggests that yields for organic crops fluctuate more than in conventional systems, so this could be an important barrier to continued growth of supply and market share (Tamm 2000, Mader et al 2002).

Overall, there is strong market potential for organic cereals in both Europe and North America. However, the high price premiums relative to what most consumers are willing to pay may stifle continued growth of the market, and organic cereals in particular. Other hindrances are consumer knowledge and product availability. Many consumers do not purchase organic products because they do not understand what they are, or the products are not readily available to them. In the longer term, this problem can be dealt with by providing more public information and making more organic products available on the shelves.

Organic Foods and Cereal Foods Markets

Organic Foods Market

The global organic food industry is one of the fastest-growing segments in the food sector, estimated at $US 26 billion per year and growing at an annual rate of 20–50% (Australian Trade Commission 2003). Tracking the development of this sector is somewhat challenging, since the growth rates vary

TABLE 4
Organic Cereal Profitability

Crop or Farm	Yield (t/ha)	Price ($US/t)	Gross Margin ($US/ha)	Conventional Gross Margin ($US/ha)	Rate (%)	Country of Study	Source
Winter wheat	4.8		1,293			UK	Bulson et al (1996)
	1.9	124	618	476	129	Canada	Entz et al (1998)
	4.5	194	361			Italy	Malagoni (1999)
	4.7	237	1,305	735	177	UK	Taylor et al (2001)
Spring wheat	2.2	744	1,241	1,289	96	Finland	Poutala et al (1994)
	4.1	251	1,204	870	138	UK	Taylor et al (2001)
Soybean	2.8		620	307	201	USA	Mahoney et al (2001)
	2.6		1,844	500	368	USA	Delate (2002)
Entire farm			98	136	72	Canada	Paillat et al (1994)
			111	109	101	USA	Hanson et al (1997)
			1,102	1,039	106	Italy	Pacini et al (2003)

widely among countries and there is little systematic data collection by governments. The vast majority of market intelligence comes from private sources such as the Organic Trade Association (www.ota.com) in the United States and from Data Monitor in Europe.

In 2001, the organic market in the European Union was worth $US 13 billion and growing at 33% (Data Monitor 2001). Yussefi and Willer (2003) forecasted that sales of organic products in seven EU countries would double by 2006. Denmark has the largest per capita spending on organic products, while the largest growth rate of per capita spending, from 1997 to 2000, was found in Sweden (Yussefi and Willer 2003). Production growth of organic foods in the Scandinavian countries is faster than elsewhere in Europe (OrganicDenmark 2001).

Yussefi and Willer (2003) estimated total U.S. retail sales for organic foods at $US 8 billion in 2000 and growth of 20–25% per year. Retail sales are certainly in excess of $US 10 billion in 2003, and assuming steady growth at a conservative rate of 20%, U.S. retail sales should reach $25 billion by 2008.

Cunningham (2002a) reported the retail organic food market in Canada to be worth $US 451 million in 2001, with an expected growth rate of 10–20%. The Canadian market depends very much on U.S. supplies of fresh and processed organic products; consequently, any condition that will affect the U.S. market for organic foods will also affect both Canadian producers and consumers of organic foods. For example, Cunningham (2002b) argued that the implementation of the U.S. national organic program (www.ams.usda.gov/nop/indexIE.htm) in October 2002 would be expected to foster further growth of both production and consumption of organic foods in the United States. This will therefore affect the ability of Canadian and EU producers of organic foods to penetrate the U.S. market.

Organic Cereal Foods Markets

Meanwhile, the organic grain market has developed rapidly in Europe and North America since the mid-1990s, but the growth in supply has not been matched by the growth in demand. Thus, many countries are importing to meet domestic demand. Furthermore, as more livestock farmers have converted to organic systems, feed grains have been in short supply, placing more demands on the limited supply of cereals (Taylor et al 2001). This phenomenon implies continued high prices for organic cereals relative to conventional (Offerman and Nieberg 2000). Moreover, the lack of supply has induced intense competition for that supply among processors.

The European Union has been a significant importer of organic cereals and was a net importer in 2000 (FAO 2002). In 2000, about 900,000 tonnes of cereals were consumed in the European Union, accounting for only 2% of total cereal consumption. Imports amounted to about 700,000 tonnes, with exports totaling 500,000 tonnes (Hamm et al 2002). Although the European Union is a net importer of organic cereals, Italy is a net exporter and accounted for 58% of total organic cereal exports from the European Union.

According to Hamm et al (2002), most of the organic cereal production in Spain (90%) and Italy (69%) is exported. Italy, the United Kingdom, France, and Germany were the major importers, accounting for about 85% of total EU imports. The ratio of organic cereal imports to organic cereal consumption is high in EU countries such as the Netherlands (278%), France (86%), the United Kingdom (81%), and Belgium (79%). The high percentage for the Netherlands and Belgium can be attributed to the fact that they are major distribution hubs for organic products in the European Union (Hamm et al 2002).

Most imports by EU member states are from Australia, Canada, the United States, and Eastern Europe. Under current EU regulations, with regard to imports from third countries, there are only six (Argentina, Australia, the Czech Republic, Hungary, Israel, and Switzerland) that have unrestricted trade access to any EU member state. Nonetheless, there are more than 70 countries, including the United States and Canada, that can export to individual EU member states based on authorizations implemented by individual members such as the Netherlands and Belgium. In the future, the demand-supply imbalance in the European Union should be improved with the accession of Poland, the Czech Republic, and Hungary, since their capacity to export is increasing (Viaux et al 2000).

Little official information is available on trade in organic products in North America. This is because trade information is aggregated and not specifically reported for organic products. It has been estimated that the United States exports more than US$ 40 million in organic foods annually to the United Kingdom and another US$ 40–60 million to Japan (FAO 2002). The FAO (2002) also reported that exports of organic foods to Europe are growing by 15% per year, while exports to Japan have grown by 30–50%. However, the proportion of organic cereals is not available.

The most important cereals in the U.S. market include wheat, buckwheat, barley, corn, millet, oats, spelt, kamut, and rice. Companies have emerged in the United States to link organic grain farmers with food processors and other end users located in several states and in other countries. Organic grain pro-

TABLE 5
Bread and Grains Retail Market

Commodity	Total Food (%)	Organic Food (%)
Baked goods	43	25
In-store bakery	23	11
Dry breakfast foods	17	40
Frozen breads and grains	4	6
Baking needs	6	8
Dried breads and grains	3	6
Pasta	4	5
Total	100	100

[a] Data from Cunningham (2002a).

duction is often contracted prior to planting as a way to manage traceability and technical qualities. For example, companies offer contracts specifically for cereals under organic certification (Greene and Dobbs 2001).

Table 5 indicates the breakdown of the Canadian retail market for expenditures related to organic grains compared to total food expenditures in the same categories. It is clear that organic breakfast cereals are a much more dominant category than in the conventional market, whereas organic baked goods are less important. It is not hard to imagine why, considering the longer shelf life of dry breakfast cereals compared to baked goods.

Safety, Technical Quality, and Nutritional Value of Organic Grains

Safety

Pesticides

The use of pesticides has been identified as an issue in conventional agriculture (Hansen et al 2001), so it is not surprising that organic foods would be attractive to consumers (Williams and Hammitt 2001). While it is likely that organic foods contain lower levels of synthetic pesticides than conventional foods (Woese et al 1997, Bourn and Prescott 2002), there have been few reports to confirm this for grains and grain products. While residues in organic foods can be expected to be lower, it would not be prudent to claim that organic foods are "pesticide free," since there is a potential for contamination through airborne pesticides (Majewski and Capel 1995).

Heavy Metals

Is there reason to expect more or less heavy-metal contamination in organic grains? According to studies by Petr et al (1999) and Jorhem and Slanina (2000), the content of heavy metals in grains (wheat, barley, rye, millet, buckwheat) was identical regardless of cultivation system. Malmauret et al (2002) confirmed these results and reported similar levels of lead and cadmium in wheat, barley, and buckwheat, regardless of agricultural technique. Meanwhile, some sources have suggested the possibility that plants might take up more heavy metals (cadmium, lead, mercury) when major nutrients are lacking (AFSSA 2003).

Mycotoxins

The presence of mycotoxins, especially deoxynivalenol (DON), is a major concern for grain growers using any system. Mycotoxins have negative effects on human and animal health, such as a potential link to cancer of the esophagus (Rotter et al 1996). In conventional agriculture, fungicides applied at specific times during grain development may reduce the occurrence of *Fusarium* spp. In organic systems, specific control strategies include selection of variety for resistance and the use of variety mixes and staggered seeding dates so as to have variable flowering dates.

Organic grains might be expected to be more susceptible to mycotoxins because they are not treated with fungicides. However, Birzele et al (1998) found that the concentration of DON in organically produced wheat was not greater than the DON concentration in wheat produced by integrated management. Based on the collection of 237 commercial cereal foods (27% organic) and 60 samples of wheat flours (40% organic) from mills and food stores, Schollenberger et al (1999, 2002) found that commercial organic cereal foods and flours contained less DON than nonorganic products. However, the degree of toxin contamination of wheat flour increased with ash content, confirming the results of Young et al (1984) and Trigo-Stockli et al (1996) who showed that fungal infection was concentrated in the outer grain fractions.

On the whole, our review of the literature suggests that the mycotoxin content of cereals is highly variable, regardless of the agriculture system. According to Malmauret et al (2002), DON content in wheat (11 samples each) or barley (five samples each) was no different in organic samples than in nonorganic. In a companion simulation study, Leblanc et al (2002) reported that 10% of people consuming organic wheat-based foods could be at risk for exposure to DON, considering their tendency to consume more cereal foods than conventional consumers. Marx et al (1994, 1995) showed that, regardless of fertilizing conditions, wheat and rye contained an equivalent load of bacteria and fungi and were slightly more contaminated by DON when grown under organic conditions. Jørgensen and Jacobsen (2002) reported that organic rye, but not wheat, contained more ochratoxin A than conventional grain or flour, but organic cereal foods and flours contained less DON than nonorganic products. Birzele et al (2002) and Döll et al (2002) showed that in the absence of fungicides, organic wheat was more tolerant to *Fusarium* infection than conventional, a result that would support the hypothesis that organic plants are more tolerant to diseases and drought (Gooding and Davies 1997).

Quality Value

Breadmaking Quality of Organic Wheat

When comparing organic wheat with conventional, various authors have shown lower protein content (Gooding et al 1993, Poutala et al 1994, Woese et al 1997), gluten, dough mixing tolerance, and loaf volume (Dlouhy 1981, Feil and Stamp 1993). Haglund et al (1998) emphasized that, regardless of the cultivation system used, flour with a protein content lower than 12% required less mixing for optimum dough development. As a consequence, small-scale bakers are used to adapting their baking processes to organically grown flours with low protein content.

Although organic agricultural practices vary widely, careful genotype selection and management of organic fertilizers can yield wheat protein content similar to that obtained with synthetic fertilizers (Gooding et al 1993; Salomonsson et al 1994, 1995). For organically grown wheat, Salomonsson and Larsson-Raźnikiewicz (1985) attributed the decrease of acetic acid-insoluble glutenins to nitrogen shortages in the early period of growing. During this period, the mineralization of compost was low and resulted in lower-than-expected elastic properties and loaf volume for organic wheat. Late, organic fertilization with a low level of nitrogen gave more gluten and higher loaf volume (Wirries and Büning-Pfaue 1995). According to Fredriksson et al (1997), wheat genotype had a greater effect on baking properties than did fertilizer treatment. Response of wheat varieties to organic fertilizers was associated with their protein and starch characteristics—namely, their respective proportion of small starch granules (Fredriksson et al 1998). Whatever the fertilizer treatment, there would be an optimum amount of small granules beyond which bread volume decreases (Soulaka and Morrison 1985), but this would vary according to protein level (Lelievre et al 1987). Selection of wheat genotype and the use of organic fertilizer affected several grain constituents besides gluten, which might partly explain why flours with similar protein content have different breadmaking potential.

Besides protein and starch, other grain components can vary according to agricultural practices. For example, Strobel et al (2001) found that organic winter wheat contained less soluble arabinoxylans than conventional wheat. Antioxidant properties of wheat bran are known to vary according to growing location in conventional agriculture (Yu et al 2003), so this could be an issue, considering that whole-meal bread is generally more popular among consumers of organic foods. Haglund et al (1998) has shown that, for a specific organic wheat-growing system (no livestock manure, minimum tillage), whole-meal bread had a more intense aroma than did bread from other organic and conventional systems. The authors suggested that the smaller size of the grains probably gave more hulls, which contributed to flavor differences. The bread was made under high mixing conditions (two intensities using speeds of about 1,500–4,700 RPM) using a no-time dough system. The quality of bread made from the organic system without manure was inferior (lower volume, drier and less elastic crumb) because of its lower protein content (8.8–9.4%, compared to 10.8%), even though the volume of whole-meal bread from both organic and conventional samples was very low (2.2–2.6 mL/g) compared to commercial flour (5.3 mL/g).

While sourdough-preparation conditions varied slightly, Rosenquist and Hansen (2000) obtained similar results when comparing the microbial stability of sourdough prepared from organic and conventional whole-meal rye, suggesting that the microbiological load and their nature were similar for both flour types.

Malting Quality of Organic Barley

Petr et al (2000) have described the malting potential of barley according to cultivation system. For malting and brewing, a lower nitrogen content of barley (about 11%) is beneficial because it increases fermentable sugar extract yield. Thus, organic barley would be expected to be interesting for these applications, considering its relatively low protein content compared to conventional. Based on data presented in Petr et al (2000), the average protein content of tested barley varieties did not change significantly according to cultivation system (three-year assays). Extract content and amylase activity did not vary, and the effect of year was much more important than cultivation system. However, all six varieties of organic barley gave worts with lower β-glucan, a positive attribute for malting.

Nutritive Value

While organic grains generally contain less protein than conventional, a survey of the existing literature does not indicate whether or not there is a difference in the profile of basic nutrients, including vitamins, minerals, and essential amino acids (Woese et al 1997, Worthington 2001, Bourn and Prescott 2002). The impact of these nutrients on human and animal health is also not clear, so it would be difficult to determine the practical significance of differences in the first place. Whole grains, especially wheat and oats, are an excellent source of polysaccharides and various antioxidants (flavonoids, phenolic acids, phytic acid, selenium, and vitamin E) because these compounds are concentrated in the bran and germ (Decker et al 2002). Asami et al (2003) have reported that organically and sustainably grown corn contained higher levels of total phenolics than corn produced by conventional methods. Yu et al (2003) showed that it is possible to optimize the content of antioxidants in winter wheat bran through specific growing conditions.

For those who eat whole grains, these results suggest that a nutritional benefit of organic cereals could be associated with such plant defense components, in addition to protein composition. Small differences in micronutrient content in cereals are unlikely to have major health implications (Williams 2002), but for plant secondary metabolites, the situation may be different, since some micronutrients might be beneficial (Brandt and Mølgaard 2001). More research is needed to thoroughly evaluate the effect of protective phytochemicals that could potentially be obtained from organic cereals. On the other hand, Ames et al (1990) suggested that there are potential hazards from natural plant toxins (that is, as a protection against pests). However, there is a lack of knowledge of human health effects of these natural toxins (Tomatis et al 2001).

In several countries, consumption of bread made from organic wheat is linked to the consumption of whole-meal bread (100% flour yield from grain). The nutritive value of whole meal is generally considered much superior to that of refined flour. For many consumers, this means that consumption of bread made from organic cereals is a standard way to get whole-meal bread. Through an interesting turn of the wheel, stone milling is still very popular for processing organic grain. Artisan millers, who are traditional suppliers for artisan bakers, often practice stone milling. In return, the latter have been traditional promoters of whole wheat bakery products. This has revived the interest in stone milling as the best-adapted processing method for producing whole meal, instead of roller milling, which is based on the sophisticated removal of bran and germ constituents.

Consumers' Perceptions and Attitudes Toward Attributes of Organic Foods

Large-scale organic production has been motivated in part by consumer concerns for the environment. The belief that conventional agriculture will have long-term adverse effects on the environment led many consumers to shift from conventional to organic food. Apart from environmental concerns, consumers are also concerned about their health. Recent scares of *E. coli* contamination and other food contaminants, as well as bovine spongiform encephalopathy, have reinforced the consumer attraction for organic food (Gregory 2000).

Several studies have been undertaken to determine consumer perceptions about organic foods (Hay 1989, Ott 1990, Goldman and Clancy 1991, Baker and Crosbie 1993, Groff et al 1993, Huang 1993, Swanson and Lewis 1993, Byrne et al 1994, Hack 1997, Hutchins and Greenlagh 1997, Thompson and Kidwell 1998, Cunningham 2002a, Demeritt 2002). Generally, these studies concluded that many consumers purchase organic as opposed to conventional because of the perception that organic is safer, more healthful, and more environmentally friendly than conventional products. Most of the studies identified food safety and health as the top attributes of organic products and the concern for the environment as less important. The review did not find any specific differences across countries in consumer perceptions about the attributes of organic foods. And it is not possible to draw conclusions about whether differences exist among products, since most studies are very general and without reference to specific product groups.

Several studies have been made to evaluate the specific factors that influence consumer preferences (Hay 1989, Ekelund 1990, Jolly 1991, Huang 1996, Kyriakopoulos and Oude-Ophius 1997, Wandel and Bugge 1997, Schifferstein and Oude-Ophuis 1998, Loureiro et al 2001, Cunningham 2002a, Demeritt 2002; M. Wolf, *unpublished data*). Our review indicates that quality characteristics generally affect consumer preferences for organic food. The most important attributes are nutritive value, freshness, flavor or taste, and general appearance. All the studies also indicated that regular consumers of organic foods are mostly affected by quality characteristics, not by price premium. Although price is not a major factor influencing the decision of regular consumers of organic foods to purchase, price as well as availability and knowledge are the most important factors preventing conventional consumers from purchasing organic products (Davies et al 1995, Roddy et al 1996, Latacz-Lohman and Foster 1997, Demeritt 2002). Finally, some consumers consider that taste, quality, and other sensory attributes are more important than food safety and environmental issues; others believe the contrary.

Conclusion

Since the mid-1990s, the market for organic foods in Europe and North America has expanded so much that it is now easy to find organic cereal foods on supermarket shelves. The market for organic foods is dynamic and growing quickly, as reflected in the evolution of Whole Foods Market, Inc., the largest retailer of natural and organic foods in the world. The company has grown from one health food store in 1980, to a network of 143 shops with combined sales of $US 2.7 billion in 2002.

Despite the success of the past decade, many challenges face the organic sector, and how these are addressed will affect how the sector develops over the next decade (Allard et al 2000). At the farm level, more research is needed to develop new genotypes that are adapted to organic systems and can produce grains with good technical qualities. Farmers and other market participants must develop effective means to avoid the contamination of organic grains by those that have been genetically modified, and at the same time ensure that their farms are not a source of weed seeds to their conventional neighbors. Moreover, policy actors should enhance segregation practices (e.g., in certified seed production) to ensure the coexistence of genetic modified crops with organic farming (EC Commission 2003).

Historically, organic grains have been associated with artisan or small-scale millers. This has been an excellent way to popularize specialty grains such as spelt or Khorasan wheat, that are normally obtained from organic agriculture. Nonetheless, the organic foods sector is quickly being transformed by recent trends. Pressure to make organic foods conform to the dominant mass-distribution system for food is forcing farmers producing organic foods to become larger and more specialized. This pressure to industrialize could expose farmers to long-term ecological, technical, and economic vulnerability. To date, little attention has been paid to these potential effects. On the other hand, this phenomenon could have beneficial consequences on food quality and help expand the organic food system beyond the niche stage that it presently occupies.

Organic grains are produced and marketed through a sophisticated quality assurance system that is becoming codified at the international level. The system defines what qualifies as organic and is designed to protect the integrity of the product as it moves from the farm to final consumer. It has similarities with HACCP standards, which also recognize the importance of traceability as part of quality assurance. But the organic system is "process-based" rather than one that relies on sampling and laboratory testing. Thus, it does not respond directly to some of the questions related to consumers' perceptions of the benefits associated with organically grown food. Is eating organic food an effective strategy to avoid food safety risks, improve nutrition, and support family farms and the environment? More research and new research methods are needed to arrive at conclusive answers to these questions.

References

AFSSA. 2003. Évaluation des risques et bénéfices nutritionnels et sanitaires des aliments issus de l'agriculture biologique. Agence Française de Sécurité Sanitaire des Aliments, Maisons-Alfort.

Altieri, M. A. 1995. Toward sustainable agriculture. Pages 367-379 in: Agro-ecology. The Science of Sustainable Agriculture. Westview Press, Boulder, CO.

Allard, G., David, C., and Henning, J. 2000. Organic Agriculture Faces Its Development: The Future Issues. 95. Institut National de la Recherche Agronomique, Paris.

Ames, B. N., Profet, M., and Gold, L. S. 1990. Dietary pesticides (99.99% all natural). Proc. Natl. Acad. Sci. U.S.A. 87:7777-7781.

Asami, D. K., Hong, Y.-J., Barrett, D. M., and Mitchell, A. E. 2003. Comparison of the total phenolic and ascorbic acid content of freeze-dried and air-dried marionberry, strawberry, and corn grown using conventional, organic, and sustainable agricultural practices. J. Agric. Food Chem. 51:1237-1241.

Askegaard, M., Rasmussen, I. A., and Olesen, J. E. 1999. Agronomic considerations and dilemmas in the Danish crop rotation experiment. Pages 63-69 in: Designing and Testing Crop Rotations for Organic Farming. Rep. 1. J. E. Olesen, R. Eltun, M. J. Gooding, E. S. Jensen, and U. Köpke, Eds. Danish Research School for Organic Agriculture and Food Systems, Copenhagen.

Australian Trade Commission. 2003. Organic Food Trade Statistics. Online: www.austrade.gov.au/overseas/layout/0,,0_S3-1_-2_-3_PWB1407159-4_-5_-6_-7_,00.html

Baars, T. 1998. Modern solutions for mixed systems in organic farming. Pages 23-30 in: Mixed Farming Systems in Europe. Wageningen University, Dronten, The Netherlands.

Baker, G. A., and Crosbie, P. J. 1993. Measuring food safety preferences: Identifying consumer segments. J. Agric. Res. Econ. 18:277-287.

Balfour, E. G. 1975. The Living Soil and the Haughley Experiment. Faber and Faber, London.

Barberi, P. 2002. Weed management in organic agriculture. Are we addressing the right issues? Weed Res. 42:177-193.

Berry, P., Sylvester-Bradley, R., Philips, L., Hatch, D. J., Cuttle, S. P., Rayns, F. W., and Gosling, P. 2002. Is the productivity of organic farms restricted by the supply of available nitrogen? Soil Use Manage. 18:248-255.

Bertramsen, S. K., and Dobbs, T. L. 2001. Comparison of Prices of "Organic" and "Conventional" Grains and Soybeans in the Northern Great Plains and Upper Midwest: 1995-2000. Econ. Pamphlet 2001-2001. Economics Department, South Dakota State University, Brookings.

Birzele, B., Backes, F., Berleth, M., and Kramer, J. 1998. Mycoflora, DON and OTA contents of winter wheat in the years 1995 until 1997. Rev. Med. Vet.-Toulouse 149:527-535.

Birzele, B., Meier, A., Hindorf, H., Krämer, J., and Dehne, H.-W. 2002. Epidemiology of Fusarium infection and deoxynivalenol content in winter wheat in the Rhineland, Germany. Eur. J. Plant Pathol. 108:667-673.

Blowfield, M. 2001. Ethical trade and organic agriculture. Trop. Agric. Assoc. Newsl. 3:22-26.

Bond, W., and Grundy, A. C. 2001. Non-chemical weed management in organic farming systems. Weed Res. 41:383-405.

Bourn, D., and Prescott, J. 2002. A comparison of the nutritional value, sensory qualities, and food safety of organically and conventionally produced foods. Crit. Rev. Food Sci. Nutr. 42:1-34.

Brandt, K., and Mølgaard, J. P. 2001. Organic agriculture: Does it enhance or reduce the nutritional value of plant foods? J. Sci. Food Agric. 81:924-931.

Bulson, H. A. J., Snaydon, R. W., and Stopes, C. 1997. Effects of plant density on intercropped wheat and field beans in an organic farming system. J. Agric. Sci. 128:59-71.

Bulson, H. A. J., Welsh, J. P., Stopes, C., and Woodward, L. 1996. Agronomic viability and potential economic performance of three organic four year rotations without livestock, 1988-1995. Aspects Appl. Biol. 74:277-286.

Byrne, P. J., Bacon, J. R., and Toensmeyer, U. C. 1994. Pesticide residue concerns and shopping location likelihood. Agribusiness 10:491-501.

Carlton, D. W., and Perloff, J. M. 1989. The Economics of Information. Food Marketing and Policy Center. Res. Rep. 5. University of Connecticut, Stores.

Cobb, D., Feber, R., Hopkins, A., Stockdale, L., O'Riordan, T., Clements, B., Firbank, L., Goulding, K., Jarvis, S., and Macdonald, D. 1999. Integrating the environmental and economic consequences of converting to organic agriculture: Evidence from a case study. Land Use Policy 16:207-221.

Codex Alimentarius. 2001. Organically Produced Foods. Food and Agriculture Organization of the United Nations/World Health Organization, Rome.

Commins, K., and Wai, O. J. 2002. Status of national organic regulations. Pages 8-11 in: The Organic Guarantee System: The Need and Strategy for Harmonization and Equivalence. 2003. G. Rundgren and W. Lockeretz, Eds. International Federation of Organic Agriculture Movements, Tholey-Theley, Germany.

Compagnoni, A., Pinton, R., and Zanoli, R. 2000. Organic Farming in Italy. Online: www.organic-europe.net/country_reports/pdf/2000/italy.pdf

Cunningham, R. 2002a. Canadian Natural and Organic Retail Markets. Economics and Competitiveness Information. Alberta Agriculture, Food and Rural Development, Alberta, Canada.

Cunningham, R. 2002b. Organic Consumer Profile. Alberta Agriculture, Food and Rural Development, Alberta, Canada. Online: www1.agric.gov.ab.ca/$department/deptdocs.nsf/all/sis4930

Data Monitor. 2001. Next Generation Organics. Data Monitor, London.

David, C., Jeuffroy, M. H., Laurent, F., and Mangin, M. 2004. The assessment of a decision making tool for managing the nitrogen fertilization of organic winter wheat. Eur. J. Agron. In press.

Davies, A., Titterington, A. J., and Cochrane, C. 1995. Who buys organic food: A profile of the purchasers of organic in Northern Ireland. Br. Food J. 97:17-23.

Decker, E., Beecher, G., Slavin, J., Miller, H. E., and Marquart, L. 2002. Whole grains as a source of antioxidants. Cereal Foods World 47:370-373.

Delate, K. 2002. Using an agroecological approach to farming systems research. Hortechnology 12:345-354.

Demeritt, L. 2002. All Things Organic 2002: A Look at the Organic Consumer. The Hartman Group, Bellevue, WA.

Dlouhy, J. 1981. Alternative Forms of Agriculture-Quality of Plant Products from Conventional and Biodynamic Growing. Rep. 91. Swedish University of Agricultural Sciences, Uppsala.

Döll, S., Valenta, H., Dänicke, S., and Flachowsky, G. 2002. Fusarium mycotoxins in conventionally and organically grown grain from Thuringia/Germany. Landbauforsch Völkenrode 52:91-96.

EC Commission. 1991. Regulation 2092/91 on organic production of agricultural products and indications referring thereto on agricultural products and foodstuffs. Doc. 24 June 1991. Online: europa.eu.int/eur-lex/en/consleg/main/1991/en_1991R2092_index.html

EC Commission. 1999. Supplementing Regulation 2092/91 on organic production of agricultural products and indications referring thereto on agricultural products and foodstuffs. Doc. 19 July 1999. Online: europa.eu.int/eur-lex/pri/en/oj/dat/1999/l_222/1_22219990824en00010028.pdf

EC Commission. 2003. Guidelines for the development of national strategies and best practices to ensure the coexistence of genetic modified crops with conventional and organic crops Doc. 23 July 2003. Online: europa.eu.int/comm/agriculture/publi/reports/coexistence2/index_en.htm

Ekelund, L. 1990. Vegetable consumption and consumer attitudes towards organically grown vegetables—The case of Sweden. Acta Hortic. 259:163-172.

Entz, M., Guilford, R., and Gulden, R. 1998. Productivity of organic cropping in the Eastern Prairies: On-farm survey and database development. Ext. Bull. University of Manitoba, Winnipeg. Online: www.umanitoba.ca/afs/plant_science/extension/organic.html

FAO. 2002. World Agriculture: Towards 2015/2030. An FAO Perspective, Summary Report. Food and Agriculture Organization of the United Nations/World Health Organization, Rome.

Feil, B., and Stamp, P. 1993. Sustainable agriculture and product quality: A case study for selected crops. Food Rev. Int. 9:361-388.

Finckh, M. R., and Wolfe, M. 1998. Diversification strategies. Pages 231-259 in: The Epidemiology of Plant Diseases. D. G. Jones, Ed. Kluwer Academic Publishers, Dordrecht, The Netherlands.

Finckh, M. R., Gacek, E. S., Goyeau, H., Lannou, C., Mundt, C. C., Munk, L., Nadziak, J., Newton, A. C., Vallavieille-Pope, C., and Wolfe, M. 2000. Cereal variety and species mixtures in practice with emphasis on disease resistance. Agron. Paris 20:813-837.

Fredriksson, H., Salomonsson, L., and Salomonsson, A.-C. 1997. Wheat cultivated with organic fertilizers and urea: Baking performance and dough properties. Acta Agric. Scand. Sect. B. Soil Plant Sci. 47:35-42.

Fredriksson, H., Salomonsson, L., Andresson, R., and Salomonsson, A.-C. 1998. Effects of protein and starch characteristics on the baking properties of wheat cultivated by different strategies with organic fertilizers and urea. Acta Agric. Scand. Sect. B. Soil Plant Sci. 48:49-57.

Fukuoka, M. 1985a. The Natural Way of Farming: The Theory and Practice of Green Philosophy. Japan Publications, Tokyo.

Fukuoka, M. 1985b. The One-Straw Revolution. Bantam New Age Books, Rodale Press, Maxatawny, PA.

Germeier, C. U. 2000. Wide row spacing and living mulch: New strategies for producing high protein grains in organic cereal production. Biol. Agric. Hortic. 18:127-139.

Goldman B. J., and Clancy, K. L. 1991. A survey of organic produce purchases and related attitudes of food cooperative shoppers. Am. J. Altern. Agric. 6:89-96.

Gooding, M. J., and Davies, W. P. 1997. Wheat Production and Utilization. Systems, Quality and the Environment. CAB International, Oxon, UK.

Gooding, M. J., Davies, W. P., Thompson, A. J., and Smith, S. P. 1993. The challenge of achieving breadmaking quality in organic and low input wheat in the UK—A review. Aspects Appl. Biol. 36:189-198.

Greene, C., and Dobbs, T. 2001. Organic wheat production in the United States: Expanding markets and supplies. Pages 31-37 in: Wheat Yearbook. U.S. Dep. Agric., Washington, DC.

Gregory, N. G. 2000. Consumer concerns about food. Outlook Agric. 29:251-257.

Grignani, C., Bassignana, E., and Zavattaro, L. 2001. Organic agriculture for intensive cereal production. Inf. Agrar. 57:35-40.

Groff, A. J., Kreidor, C. R., and Toensmeyer, U. C. 1993. Analysis of the Delaware market for organically grown products. J. Food Distr. Res. 24:118-125

Hack, M. D. 1997. Organically grown products: Perception, preferences and motives of Dutch consumers. Acta Hortic. (Wageningen) 340:247-253.

Haglund, Å., Johansson, L., and Dahlsted, L. 1998. Sensory evaluation of wholemeal bread from ecologically and conventionally grown wheat. J. Cereal Sci. 27:199-207.

Halberg, N., and Kristensen, I. S. 1997. Expected crop yield loss when converting to organic dairy farming in Denmark. Biol. Agric. Hortic. 14:25-41.

Hamm, U., Gronefeld, F., and Halpin, D. 2002. Analysis of the European Market for Organic Food. Organic Market Initiatives and Rural Development. Vol. 1. School of Management and Business, University of Wales.

Hansen, B., Alrøe, H. J., and Kristensen, E. S. 2001. Approaches to assess the environmental impact of organic farming with particular regard to Denmark. Agric. Ecosyst. Environ. 83:11-26.

Hansen, J. K., and Sørensen, H. C. 1993. The Importance of Price for the Sale of Ecological Products. MAPP Working Paper 13. Aarhus School of Business, University of Aarhus, Denmark.

Hanson, J. C., Lichtenberg, E., and Peters, S. E. 1997. Organic versus conventional grain production in the mid-Atlantic: An economic and farming system review. Am. J. Altern. Agric. 12:2-9.

Haraldsen, T. K., Asdal, A., Grasdalen, C., Nesheim, L., and Ugland, T. N. 2000. Nutrient balances and yields during conversion from conventional to organic cropping systems on silt loam and clay soils in Norway. Biol. Agric. Hortic. 17:229-246.

Hay, J. 1989. The consumer's perspective on organic food. Can. Inst. Food Sci. Technol. J. 22:95-99.

Henning, J. 2002. Organics in the supermarket. Pages 111-112 in: Introduction to Certified Organic Farming. R. Jannasch, Ed. Canadian Farm Business Management Council, Ottawa.

Hill, S. B., and Henning, J. 1992. Competing green. CGA Mag. 26(10):36-40, 66. Online: www.eap.mcgill.ca/Publications/EAP37.html

Hogh-Jensen, H. 1999. The proportion of green fallow in stockless farming systems: Grain N yield, N leaching and soil organic N. Pages 223-224 in: Designing and Testing Crop Rotations for Organic Farming. Rep. 1. J. E. Olesen, R. Eltun, M. J. Gooding, E. S. Jensen, and U. Köpke, Eds. Danish Research School for Organic Agriculture and Food Systems, Copenhagen.

Holle, R., and Untiedt, H. 1999. Crop rotations on organic farms in Northern Germany and development of the wide row system. Pages 159-162 in: Designing and Testing Crop Rotations for Organic Farming. Rep. 1. J. E. Olesen, R. Eltun, M. J. Gooding, E. S. Jensen, and U. Köpke, Eds. Danish Research School for Organic Agriculture and Food Systems, Copenhagen.

Howard, A. 1940. An Agricultural Testament. Oxford University Press, Oxford.

Huang, C. L. 1993. Simultaneous equation model for estimating consumer risk perceptions, attitudes and willingness to pay for residue free produce. J. Cons. Affairs 27:377-396.

Huang, C. L. 1996. Consumer preferences and attitudes towards organically grown produce. Eur. Rev. Agric. Econ. 23:331-342.

Hutchins, R. K., and Greenlagh, L. A. 1997. Organic confusion: Sustaining competitive advantage. Br. Food J. 99:336-338.

Jolly, D. A. 1991. Determinants of organic horticultural products consumption based on a sample of California consumers. Acta Hortic. (Wageningen) 295:141-148.

Jørgensen, K., and Jacobsen, J. S. 2002. Occurrence of ochratoxin A in Danish wheat and rye, 1992-99. Food Addit. Contam. 19:1184-1189.

Jorhem, L., and Slanina, P. 2000. Does organic farming reduce the content of Cd and certain other trace metals in plant foods? A pilot study. J. Sci. Food Agric. 80:43-48.

Kankanen, H., Eriksson, C., Rakkolainen, M., and Vuorinen, M. 2001. Effect of annually repeated undersowing on cereal yields. Agric. Food Sci. Finland 10:197-208.

Klonsky, K., and Tourte, L. 1998. Organic agricultural production in the United States: Debate and directions. Am. J. Agric. Econ. 5:1119-1124.

Köpke, U. 1995. Nutrient management in organic farming systems: The case of nitrogen. Biol. Agric. Hortic. 11:29-39.

Kortbech-Olsen, R. 2003. Overview on World Trade in Organic Food Products. The U.S. Market and Recent Tends. Online: www.intracen.org.

Kyriakopoulos, K., and Oude-Ophius, A.M. 1997. A pre-purchase model of consumer choice of biological foodstuff. J. Int. Food Agribus. Mark. 8:37-53.

Lammerts van Bueren, E. T., Struik, P. C., and Jacobsen, E. 2002. Ecological concepts in organic farming and their consequences for an organic crop ideotype. Neth. J. Agric. Sci. 50:1-26.

Lampkin, N., Foster, C., Padel, S., and Midmore, P. 1999. Organic Farming in Europe: Economics and Policy. Vol. 1. Universität Hohenheim, Germany.

Latacz-Lohman, U., and Foster, C. 1997. From "niche" to "mainstream"—Strategies for marketing organic food in Germany and the UK. Br. Food J. 99:275-282.

Leblanc, J.-C., Malmauret, L., Delobel, D., and Verger, P. 2002. Simulation of the exposure to deoxynivalenol of French consumers of organic and conventional foodstuffs. Regul. Toxicol. Pharmacol. 36:149-154.

Lelievre, J., Lorenz, K., Meredith, P., and Baruch, D. W. 1987. Effects of starch particle size and protein concentration on breadmaking performance. Starch/Stärke 39:347-352.

Lengyel, A. 2000. The Demand for Organic Agriculture: A Study of the Frozen Pea Market. Mary Washington College. Online: www.elon.edu/ipe/lengyel.pdf

Liebman, M., and Davis, A. S. 2000. Integration of soil, crop and weed management in low-external input farming systems. Weed Res. 40:27-47.

Loureiro, M. J., McCluskey, J. J., and Mittelhammer, R. C. 2001. Assessing consumer preferences for organic, eco-labeled, and regular apples. J. Agric. Res. Econ. 26:404-416.

MacRae, R. J., Hill, S. B., Henning, J., and Bentley, A. 1990. Policies, programs and regulations to support the transition to sustainable agriculture in Canada. Am. J. Altern. Agric. 5:76-92.

Mader, P., Fliessbach, A., Dubois, D., Gunst, L., Fried, U., and Niggli, U. 2002. Soil fertility and biodiversity in organic farming. Science 296:1694-1697.

Mahoney, P. R., Olson, K. D., Porter, P. M., Huggins, D. R., Perrilo, C. A., and Crookston, K. 2001. Profitability of organic cropping systems in southwestern Minnesota. Renew. Agric. Food Syst. 19(1):35-46.

Majewski, M. S., and Capel, P. D. 1995. Pesticides in the Atmosphere: Distribution, Trends, and Governing Factors. Ann Arbor Press, Chelsea, MI.

Malagoni, C. 1999. I cereali biologici: quanto costa produrli. Inf. Agrar. 30:27-29.

Malmauret, L., Parent-Massin, D., Hardy, J.-L., and Verger, P. 2002. Contaminants in organic and conventional foodstuffs in France. Food Addit. Contam. 19:524-532.

Marx, H., Gedek, B., and Kollarczik, B. 1994. Vergleichende untersuchungen zum mykologischen status von ökologisch und konventionell angebautem getreide. Z. Ernährungswiss. 33:239-243.

Marx, H., Gedek, B., and Kollarczik, B. 1995. Vergleichende untersuchungen zum mykotoxikologischen status von ökologisch und konventionell angebautem getreide. Z. Lebensm. Unters. Forsch. 201:83-86.

Mueller, T., and Thorup-Kristensen, K. 2001. N-Fixation of selected green manure plants in an organic crop rotation. Biol. Agric. Hortic. 18:345-363.

Northbourne, W. E. 1940. Look to the Land. J.M. Dent & Sons, London.

O'Donovan, P., and McCarthy, M. 2002. Irish consumer preference for organic meat. Br. Food J. 104(3/4/5):353-370.

Offermann, F., and Nieberg, H. 2000. Organic Farming in Europe: Economics and Policy. Vol. 5. Economic Performance of Organic Farms in Europe. University of Hohenheim, Germany.

Olesen, J. E., Rasmussen, I. A., Askegaard, M., and Kristensen, K. 2002. Whole-rotation, dry matter and nitrogen yields from the first course of an organic farming crop rotation experiment. J. Agric. Sci. 139:361-370.

Organic Agricultural Centre of Canada. 2003. Organic Food Prices in Canada. Online: www.organicagcentre.ca/MarketReports/market_info_prices.html

OrganicDenmark. 2001. OrganicDenmark Launches in UK. Press release, November 2001. Online: www.waymaker.net/bitonline/2001/12/10/20011210BIT00230/bit0001.pdf

Ott, S. L. 1990. Supermarket shoppers' pesticide concerns and willingness to purchase certified pesticide residue-free fresh produce. Agribusiness 6:593-602.

Pacini, C., Wossink, A., Giesen, G., Vazzana, C., and Huirne, R. 2003. Evaluation of sustainability of organic, integrated and conventional farming systems: A farm and field-scale analysis. Agric. Ecosyst. Environ. 95:273-288.

Paillat, N., Pellerin, M. D., Perrier, J. P., and Levallois, R. 1994. Comparaison de la rentabilité des entreprises céréalières biologiques et en transition par rapport aux entreprises conventionnelles du Québec. Rev. Can. Econ. Rurale 42:343-354.

Pang, X. P., and Letey, J. 2000. Organic farming: Challenge of timing nitrogen availability to crop nitrogen requirements. Soil Sci. Soc. Am. J. 64:247–253.

Petr, J., Škeřík, J., and Dlouhý, J. 1999. Cadmium, lead and mercury contents in ecologically grown crops. Sci. Agric. Bohemica 30:285-299.

Petr, J., Škeřík, J., Psota, V., and Langer, I. 2000. Quality of malting barley grown under different cultivation systems. Monatsschr. Brauwiss. 53:90-94.

Porter, P. M., Huggins, D. R., Perillo, C. A., Quiring, S. R., Crookston, R. K. 2003. Organic and other management strategies with two and four-year crop rotations in Minnesota. Agron. J. 95:233-244.

Poutala, R. T., Kuoppamaki, O., Korva, J., and Varis, E. 1994. The performance of ecological, integrated and conventional nutrient management systems in cereal cropping in Finland. Field Crops Res. 37:3-10.

Rodale, J. I. 1945. Pay Dirt: Farming and Gardening with Composts. Devin-Adair Company, New York.

Roddy, G., Cowan, C., and Hutchinson, G. 1996. Consumer attitudes and behaviour to organic foods in Ireland. J. Int. Cons. Marketing 9:1-19.

Rosenquist, H., and Hansen, Å. 2000. The microbial stability of two bakery sourdoughs made from conventionally and organically grown rye. Food Microbiol. 17:241-250.

Rotter, B. A., Prelusky, D. B., and Pestka, J. J. 1996. Toxicology of deoxynivalenol (vomitoxin). J. Toxicol. Environ. Health 48:1-34.

Salomonsson, L., and Larsson-Raźnikiewicz, M. 1985. Quantitative and qualitative studies of proteins of wheat from different growing systems. Swed. J. Agric. Res. 15:133-138.

Salomonsson, L., Jonsson, A., Salomonsson, A.-C., and Nilsson, G. 1994. Effects of organic fertilizers and urea when applied to spring wheat. Acta Agric. Scand. Sect. B Soil Plant Sci. 44:170-178.

Salomonsson, L., Salomonsson, A.-C., Olofsson, S., and Jonsson, A. 1995. Effects of organic fertilizers and urea when applied to winter wheat. Acta Agric. Scand. Sect. B Soil Plant Sci. 45:171-180.

Schifferstein, H. N. J., and Oude-Ophuis, P. A. M. 1998. Health-related determinants of organic food consumption in The Netherlands. Food Qual. Pref. 9:119-133.

Schmidt, H., and von Fragstein, P. 1999. Importance of varying management and environment conditions in long-term crop rotation trial. Effects on plant development, crop yield and N dynamics. Pages 191-202 in: Designing and Testing Crop Rotations for Organic Farming. Rep. 1. J. E. Olesen, R. Eltun, M. J. Gooding, E. S. Jensen, and U. Köpke, Eds. Danish Research School for Organic Agriculture and Food Systems, Copenhagen.

Schollenberger, M., Suchy, S., Terry Jara, H., Drochner, W., and Müller, H.-M. 1999. A survey of Fusarium toxins in cereal-based foods marketed in an area of southwest Germany. Mycopathologia 147:49-57.

Schollenberger, M., Suchy, S., Terry Jara, H., Drochner, W., and Müller, H.-M. 2002. Fusarium toxins in wheat flour collected in an area in southwest Germany. Int. J. Food Microbiol. 72:85-89.

Soulaka, A. B., and Morrison, W. R. 1985. The bread baking quality of six wheat starches differing in composition and physical properties. J. Sci. Food Agric. 36:719-727.

Stein-Bachinger, K., and Werner, W. 1997. Effect of manure on crop yield and quality in an organic agricultural system. Biol. Agric. Hortic. 14:221-235.

Stockdale, E. A., Lampkin, N. H., Hovi, M., Keatinge, R., Lennartsson, E. K. M., Macdonald, D. W., Padel, S., Tattersall, F. H., Wolfe, M. S., and Watson, C. A. 2001. Agronomic and environmental implications of organic farming systems. Adv. Agron. 70:261-327.

Stopes, C., Lord, E. I., Philipps, L., and Woodward, L. 2002. Nitrate leaching from organic farms and conventional farms following best practices. Soil Use Manage. 18:256-263.

Strobel, E., Ahrens, P., Hartmann, G., Kluge, H., and Jeroch, H. 2001. Gehalt an inhaltsstoffen von weizen, roggen und hafer bei anbau unter konventionellen und den bedingungen des ökologischen landbaus. Bodenkultur 53:221-231.

Swanson, R. B., and Lewis, C. E. 1993. Alaskan direct-market consumers: Perceptions of organic produce. Home Econ. Res. J. 22:138-155.

Tamis, W. L. M., and van den Brink, W. J. 1999. Conventional, integrated and organic winter wheat production in The Netherlands in the period 1993-1997. Agric. Ecol. Environ. 76:47-59.

Tamm, L., 2000. The future challenge and prospects in organic crop protection. Pages 106-109 in: Proc. Intern. IFOAM Scientific Conference. The World Grows Organic. T. Alföldi, W. Lockeretz, U. Niggli, Eds. International Federation of Organic Agriculture Movements, Tholey-Theley, Germany.

Taylor, B. R., Watson, C. A., Stockdale, E. A., McKinlay, R. G., Younie, D., and Cranstoun, D. A. S. 2001. Current Practices and Future Prospects for Organic Cereal Production: Survey and Literature Review. Res. Ed. Rev. No. 45. Home-Grown Cereal Authority, London.

Theunissen, J. 1997. Application of intercropping in organic agriculture. Biol. Agric. Hortic. 15:251-259.

Thompson, G. D., and Kidwell, J. 1998. Explaining the choice of organic produce: cosmetic defects, prices, and consumer preferences. Am. J. Agric. Econ. 80:277-287.

Tomatis, L., Melnick, R. L., Haseman, J., Barrett, J. C., and Huff, J. 2001. Alleged "misconceptions" distort perceptions of environmental cancer risks. FASEB J. 15:195-203.

Trigo-Stockli, D. M., Deyoe, C. W., Satumbaga, R. F., and Pedersen, J. R. 1996. Distribution of deoxynivalenol and zearalenone in milled fractions of wheat. Cereal Chem. 73:388-391

Turco, G. 2002. Organic Food—An Opportunity, at Whose Expense? Industry Note, Food and Agribusiness Research. Rabobank International, Sydney. Online: www.rabobank.com. Online: www.rabobank.com/repository/far/farpublications.pdf

USDA. 2001. The National Organic Program. Online: www.ams.usda.gov/nop.

USDA. 2003. Food marketing and price spreads: Farm-to-retail price spreads for individual food items. Econ. Res. Serv., U.S. Dep. Agric., Washington, DC. Online: www.ers.usda.gov/Briefing/FoodPriceSpreads/spreads/table1a.html

Viaux, P., Guionnet, S., and Maisons, S. 2000. Des céréales hongroises sur le marché européen. Pages 53-58 in: Organic Agriculture Faces Its Development. G. Allard, C. David, and J. Henning, Eds. INRA Éditions, Paris.

Walz, E, 1999. Third Biennial National Organic Farmer's Survey. Organic Farming Research Foundation, Santa Cruz, CA.

Wandel, M., and Bugge, A. 1997. Environmental concern in consumer evaluation of food quality. Food Qual. Pref. 8:19-26.

Watson, C. A., Atkinson, D., Gosling, P., Jackson, L. R., and Rayns, F. W. 2002. Managing soil fertility in organic farming systems. Soil Use Manage. 18:239-247.

Welsh, R., 1999. The Economics of Organic Grain and Soybean Production in the Midwest United States. Policy Studies Rep. 13. Henry A. Wallace Institute for Alternative Agriculture, Greenbelt, MA.

Wier, M., and Andersen, L. M. 2001. Studies on Consumer Demand for Organic Foods—A Survey. Working paper 1. AKF, Danish Institute of Local Government Studies, Copenhagen.

Williams, C. M. 2002. Nutritional quality of organic food: Shades of grey or shades of green? Proc. Nutr. Soc. 61:19-24.

Williams, P. R. D., and Hammitt, J. K. 2001. Perceived risks of conventional and organic produce: Pesticides, pathogens, and natural toxins. Risk Anal. 21:319-330.

Wirries, F.-M., and Büning-Pfaue, H. 1995. Wheat from organic agriculture. An improved analytical description of gluten quality. Pages 527-530 in: Current Status and Future Trends in Analytical Food Chemistry. Proc. 8th Eur. Conf. on Food Chemistry (Euro Food Chem VIII), Vol. 2.. G. Sontag and W. Pfannhauser, Eds. Austrian Chemical Society, Vienna.

Woese, K., Lange, D., Boess, C., and Bögl, K. W. 1997. A comparison of organically and conventionally grown foods—Results of a review of the relevant literature. J. Sci. Food Agric. 74:281-293.

Worthington, V. 2001. Nutritional quality of organic versus conventional fruits, vegetables, and grains. J. Altern. Compl. Med. 7:161-173.

Young, J. C., Fulcher, R. G., Hayhoe, J. H., Scott, P. M., and Dexter, J. E. 1984. Effect of milling and baking on deoxynivalenol (vomitoxin) content of Eastern Canadian wheats. J. Agric. Food Chem. 32:659-664.

Younie, D., Watson, C. A., and Squire, G. R. 1996. A comparison of crop rotations in organic farming: Agronomic performance. Aspects Appl. Biol. 47:379-382.

Yu, L., Perret, J., Harris, M., Wilson, J., and Haley, S. 2003. Antioxidant properties of bran extracts from "Akron" wheat grown at different locations. J. Agric. Food Chem. 51:1566-1570.

Yussefi, M., and Willer, H. 2003. The World of Organic Agriculture 2003: Statistics and Future Prospects. International Federation of Organic Agriculture Movements, Theley, Germany.

CHAPTER 3

Einkorn: A Potential Functional Wheat and Genetic Resource

J. Frégeau-Reid[1] and E.-S. M. Abdel-Aal[2]

[1]Agriculture and Agri-Food Canada, Eastern Cereal and Oilseed Research Centre, Ottawa, ON, Canada K1A 0C6; [2]Agriculture and Agri-Food Canada, Food Research Program, Guelph, ON, Canada N1G 5C9

Einkorn, named after the German expression meaning "one-grain," was widely cultivated for thousands of years in Turkey as well as through the Balkans, Germany, France, Spain, and Caucasia. It is also known as *small spelt* in English, *petit épeautre* in French, and *farro* (along with emmer and spelt) in Italian. Einkorn and its cousin emmer were the first wheats domesticated 10–12 millennia ago. Both have genes that prevent the grains from falling to the ground when ripe. Instead they remain on the plant until harvest, the first step in the evolution from a wild to a cultivated cereal. For both emmer and einkorn, the seeds are not free-threshing but remained enclosed by the hulls as in covered oat. With its tough hull-like oat, einkorn was used as a livestock feed and for humans in soups and porridge while its straw may have been used for thatched roofs. It is now cultivated in only a few places and probably just sporadically. The rising demands for low-input and organic farming and for more varied whole grain foods for healthier living are the primary stimulus for a renewed interest in einkorn.

Origin and Genetics

Extensive materials have been written about the origin, domestication, and genetics of einkorn. For details, readers should refer to chapters in the monograph by Padulosi et al (1995). In addition, a good review of wild cereal domestication was published recently (Salamini et al 2002). Einkorn wheat, *Triticum monococcum* ssp. *monococcum* (*T. monococcum*) was the first cereal to be domesticated. Seeds of the wild form, *T. monococcum* ssp. *boeoticum* (*T. boeoticum*), have been found at several archeological sites across the Fertile Crescent, a region now occupied by Israel, Jordan,

[1] For the Department of Agriculture and Agri-Food Canada, Eastern Cereal and Oilseed Research Centre and Food Research Program, Government of Canada.

Lebanon, western Syria, southeast Turkey, and along the Tigris and Euphrates rivers, into Iraq and western Iran. This area of the Near East is thought to be the cradle of modern agriculture. Remains of larger and plumper einkorn kernels are found with wild einkorn in the central part of the Fertile Crescent at sites dated around 10,000 years ago, evidence of the beginning of domestication. A thousand years later, domesticated einkorn was much more abundant and, with time, spread to the Balkans, then to Yugoslavia, Bulgaria, and Hungary. Einkorn was cultivated extensively in central Europe around 7,000 years ago. Its importance declined during the Bronze Age in favor of emmer and bread wheat. It is now a relic crop in most of the countries just mentioned. In the late 1990s, molecular technologies were applied to a large group of wild and domesticated einkorn accessions. DNA fingerprinting was combined with a study of morphological traits (Heun et al 1997). Several wild einkorn lines were found that are more closely related to domesticated einkorn and probably its ancestor. These wild einkorns were all from a specific region in southern Turkey, the Karacadağ Mountains, now said to be the site of domestication of einkorn.

Wild and domesticated einkorns differ in seed size and ear morphology. Wild einkorn has small, slender seeds, whereas domesticated einkorn produces larger and plumper kernels. In wild einkorn, the ripe spikelets fall apart by shattering because of the brittle rachis. Domesticated einkorn has a tough rachis that allows the seeds to remain on the plant for harvest. Only at threshing do ears of domesticated einkorn break apart into intact spikelets, which usually contain a single seed. Both types of einkorn have seeds that also remain covered because the kernels do not thresh free of the glumes when harvested; hence, the term *hulled wheat.* Einkorn also has long, narrow glumes that are awned. In 1926, a Russian expedition discovered a new type of wild einkorn in Turkey. It had soft, papery hulls that allowed more than half the seeds to become hulless on threshing. This einkorn line is now a subspecies, *T. monococcum* ssp. *sinskajae.* Its discovery became known only in the 1970s, when the information was published. The soft hulls opened the potential of commercializing a free-threshing einkorn crop.

Einkorn is a diploid wheat ($2n = 14$). For a long time, it was believed to be the contributor of the A genome found in polyploid wheat. Recent evidence, however, indicates that the A genome of modern wheats came from another diploid wheat, *Triticum urartu.* The genome of einkorn is designated as A^m genome to recognize that some differentiation has occurred between the two genomes. The genetics of einkorn have been studied extensively. Several papers on variability and inheritance of plant or grain traits of *T. monococcum* have been published but are beyond the scope of this chapter. Readers are referred to Anker et al (2001), Bullrich et al (2002), and Shindo et al (2002) for recent references on specific trait analyses and articles by Dubcovsky et al (1996), Kojima et al (1998), and Taenzler et al (2002) for studies on genetic mapping of einkorn wheat.

Agronomy and Production

Percival (1921) attributed the decline of einkorn to its late maturity and low yield in comparison to other wheats. The absence of a free-threshing form can also be added to the reasons behind this decrease in cultivation, even though Percival (1921) lists awns and thick glumes as a good feature to protect the grains from attacks by birds. He added that einkorn had good frost resistance and rust resistance and could grow on poor sandy, chalky, and rocky soils where other wheats fail. Historically, einkorn was cultivated in cool environments on marginal land. The discovery of the hulless form in *T. sinskajae* prompted Vallega (1979) to evaluate the agronomic potential of einkorn in comparison to durum wheats and barley. Einkorn in the late 1970s had not benefited from any modern breeding work. Furthermore, according to Vallega (1995), most of the domesticated forms of *T. monococcum* found in seed banks were collected during the last 70 years from remote cultivation sites in mountainous regions, by which time the primitive cultivars formerly grown in more fertile areas had already disappeared. Agronomic results from locations in Italy and Germany (Vallega 1979, 1992, Castagna et al 1995, 1996) showed that various accessions of *T. monococcum* collected from different parts of Europe could be equal and sometimes higher in grain yields than some durum wheat varieties specifically bred for the regions where the tests were grown. The accessions could not, however, surpass barley in yield, and better climatic conditions did not improve their performance, while the modern durum wheats and barley would benefit. At one of these sites, yields of hexaploid wheats averaged 7,102 kg/ha (13% moisture), while yields of einkorn averaged 2,437 kg/ha (13% moisture) (Vallega 1992). Across various locations, biomass yield and grain protein content were significantly influenced by nitrogen applications without any effect on grain yield or plant height. Seeding rate influenced these last two traits along with heading time. The overall conclusion from these European field trials was that primitive einkorn cultivars have low yield potential and strong genotype-by-environment interactions. Additionally, from an agronomic point of view, the crop would benefit from breeding for better adaptation.

Yields recorded in Montana in 1995 with 25 accessions ranged between 720 and 2,400 kg/ha (Stallknecht et al 1996). The best five accessions produced higher yields than oats, and the best three had higher yields than barley and spring wheat in the study. These yields were not adjusted for hull content. Einkorn was late maturing in comparison to hard wheat. According to these authors, einkorn would be most suitable for cropping in lower-moisture environments like the northern Great Plains area of Montana. In Canada, 19 accessions were evaluated at three sites in Saskatchewan in 1994 (Hucl et al 1995), and yield ranged between 2,911 and 4,287 kg/ha, while einkorn TM23 yield was 4,417 kg/ha. This was similar to the yield of Katepwa, a hard red bread wheat, at 4,449 kg/ha. A major difference, however, is a hull content of about 28% in TM23. Müller (2002) mentioned that, depending on the lines, hull content for einkorn can be very high, in some samples up to 50%

hulls, and losses during dehulling of einkorn can be higher than with spelt because of the narrow seeds and smaller kernels, which are very soft and can break easily.

The past few years have seen several groups in different countries looking for good field performance in domesticated einkorn. Although some primitive cultivars of einkorn can perform agronomically as well as or only slightly less than other cereals when grown in an appropriate environment, very few are available commercially for farm production. A few breeding programs are working on improving einkorn for modern agriculture. Müller (2002) lists three einkorn varieties bred at the Cereal Breeding Research Station in Darzau (Germany) and available for production: Albini, Tiffi, and Terzino. These cultivars are hulled and have different maturities as well as different gluten strengths. Some breeders have tried to introduce the free-threshing *T. sinskajae* as a parent in their einkorn program. The soft glumes trait of *T. sinskajae* does carry negative aspects with it. The ear is more compact and can lead to partial sterility and loss of spikelets (Salamini et al 2002). Nevertheless, Vallega (1996) developed and released MONOC BULK #1 VV in 1994. He described this bulked population as improved agronomically, partially free-threshing with higher spike fertility than *T. sinskajae*, a first step toward an improved modern einkorn cultivar. Sampson (*personal communication*) developed AC Knowles, a free-threshing einkorn cultivar adapted to the province of Ontario (Canada) from a cross between a covered einkorn and a hulless line (received from J. G. Waines, University of California) derived from *T. sinskajae*. AC Knowles has a weak gluten and shows very good resistance to mildew and rust but still yields less than spring wheats.

Composition

The reputation of einkorn is traditionally that of a soft wheat with high protein content, yellow endosperm pigments, and poor rheological properties. Renewed interest in the crop for specialty markets has prompted various groups to look into the variability present in the crop for grain-quality traits with potential end uses. Only one study, however, covered a large number of compositional traits in the same experiment. Abdel-Aal et al (1995) analyzed several ancient wheats for various nutritional traits. Einkorn accession TM23 was included in their study. Table 1 lists some of the components measured by these researchers. Most of these traits are similar to those found in durum and common wheat. The authors speculated that the higher fat content of einkorn could be related to a higher proportion of germ.

A few groups have characterized one or several einkorn varieties for nutritionally important traits like amino acids, minerals, and dietary fibers, and for grain components that provide functionality in a food matrix, like starch and gluten proteins. Their main objective was to source new variability for the improvement of common wheat. These traits could also be useful in a renewal of einkorn as a crop of today in new food applications or as functional ingre-

TABLE 1
Composition of Einkorn TM23 in Relation to Two Modern Wheats, Kyle Durum and Katepwa Hard Red Bread Wheat[a]

Constituent (%db)	Einkorn TM23	Kyle Durum	Katepawa Common Wheat
Digestible carbohydrates			
Starch	61.8	64.9	62.4
Soluble sugars	2.7	2.0	3.3
Crude protein	16.5	15.1	15.3
Crude fat	2.5	2.1	2.1
Total ash	1.9	1.6	1.7
Dietary fiber			
Insoluble	6.9	9.5	10.8
Soluble	1.7	1.6	1.7
Total	8.7	11.1	12.5
B vitamins (mg/100g)			
Thiamine	0.5	...	0.57
Riboflavin	0.45	...	0.55
Niacin	3.1	...	2.3
Pyridoxine	0.49	...	0.36

[a] Data from Abdel-Aal et al (1995).

dients in traditional wheat-based products. The carotenoid pigments of einkorn will be covered more specifically in a later part of the chapter.

Starch

Starch is a primary functional component in cereal grains and usually represents more than 60% of the grain. The texture and quality of wheat-based and starch-containing food products are substantially influenced by the starch properties. Wheat, barley, and rye exhibit a unique bimodal size distribution in their starch granules, which affects efficiency of starch extraction as well as starch characteristics, whether isolated or in flour. Stoddard (1999) reported that the small granules affect processing quality in two ways: 1) they are believed to have a higher rate of water absorption than large granules, which affects mixing of dough and baking performance, and 2) they do not sediment as rapidly in aqueous suspension, where they may be carried away in the supernatant during extraction. Stoddard (1999) surveyed several accessions of *T. monococcum* from subspecies *boeticum*, *sinskajae,* and primitive monococcum for starch granule size distribution. In comparison to bread wheat, these accessions showed a different average particle-size distribution pattern. The large granules were smaller than those of bread wheat, while the size distribution of the small granules was much wider than in other wheat species. Small granule content was also much more variable than for commercial Australian wheat cultivars. Abdel-Aal et al (1999a) extracted and characterized starch from einkorn TM23, as well as from emmer, Khorasan, spelt, durum, and common wheat. Einkorn yielded the lowest amount of starch and had the lowest starch extraction efficiency in the group. The amount of small granules in TM23 was also the highest, which might explain its lower starch extraction.

Pasting properties of these same starches (Abdel-Aal et al 1999b) were measured with a Brabender viscoamylograph. Einkorn TM23 starch had the highest peak viscosity, averaging 520 BU compared to 260 BU for common wheat. There were also differences in net syneresis under cold storage. In general, wheat starch gels are more stable than corn starch gel when stored at 4 or –15°C. Einkorn TM23 starch gel was very stable either in cold or frozen storage for the test period of seven days. No water was released during storage. This high degree of gel stability could be favorable in certain food applications. In the same study, starch X-ray diffraction patterns were recorded to measure the type and degree of starch crystallinity. This property of starch is a reflection of the molecular structure of the granules, which has an effect on viscosity and texture of food products. Einkorn TM23 starch, along with starch from Khorasan wheat, had a lower degree of crystallinity than other wheats. Native ungelatinized starches from these primitive and modern wheats were also hydrolyzed by pancreatic α-amylase. The rate of α-amylase hydrolysis differed among wheat species. Einkorn TM23 starch hydrolyzed at an average rate of 107 mg released maltose/g starch/hr, similar to Khorasan and modern durum starches, while the rate for common bread wheat was 89 mg released maltose/g starch/hr.

Differences in physicochemical structure of starches can be linked to variation in amylose and amylopectin contents. This variability affects functionality and utilization of starches in food and industrial applications. Einkorn TM23 and soft spelt starches had a lower proportion of amylose—22.8% and 23.2%, respectively—than the other wheat starches, including common bread wheat with a value of 28.3% (Abdel-Aal et al 1999a). The same einkorn starch also demonstrated the highest swelling power at 90°C, which may be associated with its lower amylose content. Mohammadkhani et al (1998) developed a rapid method to survey starch amylose content, requiring only two to three cereal grains. They looked at 247 *T. monococcum* accessions and reported that their apparent amylose content ranged from 15 to 28%. Values reported for durum and hexaploid wheats tend to be narrower in range and slightly higher, between 21 and 30%. In a follow-up inheritance study (Mohammadkhani et al 1999), the amylose content of an F2 segregating population ranged from 1 to 30%. Individual lines with amylopectin content of the starch approaching that of waxy wheat or corn starch were therefore found. Their results indicate that genetic improvement toward particular amylose content to suit specific end uses could also be possible for einkorn.

Dietary Fiber

Einkorn TM23 was significantly lower in insoluble and total dietary fiber (DF) than modern wheats (Abdel-Aal et al 1995), but it had similar levels of soluble DF (Table 1). When expressed as a percentage of the total DF, soluble fibers represented 20% of the total fiber in TM23 whole meal. In a group of einkorn grown in Denmark, total DF ranged from 7.6 to 9.9% dry basis (db), while the water-soluble DF varied between 0.21 and 1.74% db (Løje et al 2003), confirming the values observed in TM23. β-Glucans, components of the cell walls of the endosperm and aleurone in wheat, are part of the soluble dietary fibers. Beresford and Stone (1983) measured total and 65°C water-insoluble β-glucans in grains of various species from an Australian wheat collection. Several commercial wheat cultivars and one monococcum, einkorn W10, were included. The hexaploid wheats averaged 0.75% (db) in whole grain, while einkorn W10 showed a level of 0.44% (db) for both total and water-insoluble β-glucans, in this case significantly lower than the modern wheats. Content of β-glucan in einkorn samples grown in Denmark averaged 0.4% (db), also much lower than the common wheat value in the same study at 0.8% (db) (Løje et al 2003).

Although several of the nutritional and organoleptic benefits claimed for ancient wheats have not yet been proven scientifically, D'Antuono et al (1998) speculated that many of the beneficial effects that were traditionally attributed to ancient wheats may be a result of their secondary components, referred to by the authors as structural polymers, gums, and mucilages. They used analytical pyrolysis to look at fiber quality in a comparative study of pericarp fragments from emmer and einkorn landraces along with modern durum wheat. This technique looks at thermal degradation products of lignins and polysaccharides. Discriminant analysis was able to clearly distinguish the three wheat types. The first function, an indication of lower polyphenolic content, allowed a very good separation of durum wheat with respect to emmer and einkorn. The second function was related to the structure of cellulose and hemicellulose, and it allowed discrimination between emmer and einkorn. The authors concluded that the variability observed in their study should be interpreted as an indication of differences in biochemical structure of dietary fiber between durum and the two ancient wheats. They suggested that the fiber components of ancient wheats could be valuable in the development of special dietary products. Conventional analysis of the nonstarch polysaccharide composition and nature of the lignin is needed to determine whether this suggestion is firmly based.

Minerals

Mineral composition of hulled wheats is mentioned as more favorable to the human diet than that of modern wheat cultivars. Common wheat often contains very low amounts of iron and zinc, and copper and manganese are also insufficient for any diet that is largely wheat dependent (Salunkhe et al 1991). Mineral levels in whole grain depend on many factors besides genotype. Climate, soil properties, and crop-management techniques all play a role, so valid comparisons between wheat types must be made on lines grown in the same environments. Two studies (Table 2) have looked at mineral composition of einkorn in relation to spelt and common wheat. Each study assessed different minerals, but the three wheat types within each study were grown in the same environment. Abdel-Aal et al (1995) showed a signi-

TABLE 2
Mineral Composition of Einkorn , Spelt and Common Wheat

Minerals (mg/100g)	Einkorn	Spelt	Common Wheat
Phosphorus[a]	415	355	360
Potassium[a]	390	375	305
Sulfur[a]	190	190	185
Manganese[a]	4.4	5.9	5.1
Copper[b]	0.6	1.1	0.9
Zinc[b]	3.7	3.6	3.7
Iron[b]	4.7	3.8	2.7
Calcium[b]	50.4	35.5	56.7
Magnesium[b]	141	133	115

[a] Data from Abdel-Aal et al (1995).
[b] Data from Bálint et al (2001).

ficantly higher level of phosphorus in einkorn as well as a higher potassium content in relation to common wheat. Bálint et al (2001) found that the iron content of einkorn accessions, as well as magnesium concentration, were significantly higher than in recently cultivated common wheat. They suggested that diploid genotypes with higher values in iron content could be used in breeding for improved nutritional value of common wheat.

Proteins

Wheat proteins are known to be low in some of the amino acids essential in the human diet, especially lysine, which is the most deficient amino acid in wheat. In cereals, variation in amino acid composition is limited and correlated with variation in grain protein content (Martin del Molino et al 1989). Einkorn has always been known as a cereal with high protein content, which prompted several groups to look at the amino acid composition of einkorn either as a source of genes for wheat improvement or for its own nutritional merit for food applications. Analyses of the amino acid profile of einkorn protein (Acquistucci et al 1995, Galterio et al 1998) showed that the average amino acid composition of *T. monococcum* proteins was analogous to that of modern wheats: basically deficient in lysine and threonine. Table 3 lists levels of some amino acids measured on the total protein for *T. monococcum*, *T. spelt,* and *T. aestivum* along with the values recommended by the Food and Agricultural Organization of the United Nations. Recently, immunochemical methods confirmed that some einkorn accessions can have higher levels of lysine than those found in common wheats. These accessions are nevertheless still deficient in terms of human nutrition (Singh et al 2000).

Nutritionally, like the other wheat species and despite its high protein content, einkorn is deficient in lysine and threonine. The variability encountered in einkorn germ plasm suggests that superior accessions may be useful in inheritance studies or for wheat improvement.

TABLE 3
Amino Acid Levels (mg/100 g protein) of Various Wheat Species and FAO Recommended Levels[a]

Amino Acids	Einkorn	Spelt	Common Wheat	FAO Pattern[b]
Essential amino acids				
Threonine	3.16	3.1	3.07	3.4
Valine	4.23	4.93	3.91	3.5
Methionine	1.68	1.8	1.39	2.5
Isoleucine	3.97	3.92	3.54	2.8
Leucine	7.26	7.49	6.98	6.6
Phenylalanine	8.31	7.59	7.84	6.3
Lysine	3.29	3	2.93	5.8
Tryptophan	1.22	1.59	1.5	1.1
Functional amino acids				
Glutamic acid	28.07	28.65	32.06	...
Proline	10.18	9.6	10	...
Protein %	17.8	8.4	10.6	...

[a] Data from Galterio et al (1998).
[b] Based on Food and Agriculture Organization of the United Nations (FAO) pattern for preschool child (2–5 years).

Gluten Protein Fractions

The traditional context for protein quality relates to the variability in gluten protein fractions, the high- and low-molecular-weight (HMW and LMW) glutenin subunits, and the gliadins. These three groups of proteins are known to affect dough functionality. They are characterized by the ability to form a cohesive viscoelastic network in dough, which relates to baking properties. Differences in baking potential are mainly the result of variations in structure, amount, and proportion of these different gluten proteins. Gliadins are mostly monomeric proteins and are responsible for gluten viscosity, while glutenins are aggregated proteins that participate in gluten strength and elasticity. Several research groups have looked at einkorn proteins as a genetic “diploid” tool providing a simpler model system to understand quality in the complex hexaploid wheats, or as a source for new genetic variation for altering cultivated polyploid wheats. Most of these analyses were done with sodium dodecyl sulfate-polyacrylamide gel electrophoresis (SDS-PAGE). Results in general show that *T. monococcum* has proteins migrating in the same regions as those of common wheat, but different banding patterns are found, indicating different proteins.

For HMW glutenins, bread wheats can usually code, from their A genome, either subunit 1 or 2* or show as null. HMW subunits are also described as *x*- or *y*-subunits, based on their mobility in the HMW region of the SDS-PAGE gel. In wheat, subunits 1 and 2* are *x*-subunits, and no HMW *y*-subunits are present. In bread wheats, the null alleles can have deleterious effects on breadmaking as the percentage of HMW subunits decreases in the total protein content. Hundreds of einkorn accessions have been analyzed for

HMW glutenin subunits (Waines and Payne 1987, Sapanaro et al 1995). In general, they displayed a major subunit of low mobility, an *x*-subunit, and a series of less prominent bands of faster mobility with one dominating *y*-subunit. The less prominent bands were described as probable breakdown products of the dominant *y*-subunit. Some accessions were null, while others had only *x*- or only *y*-subunits.

Two assessments of the genetic diversity of LMW glutenin subunits in diploid wheats (Rodríguez-Quijano et al 1997, Lee et al 1999a) indicated that domesticated einkorn was less polymorphic than the other diploid species. The authors attributed this to the fact that primitive cultivars may represent a relatively small number of genotypes fixed during cultivation. Nine LMW glutenin subunits of different mobility were found in one collcction (Rodríguez-Quijano et al 1997). Their migration was between the slowest- and the fastest-moving subunits of the bread and durum wheat cultivars in the study. Each *T. monococcum* accession had one or two subunits, and seven different combinations were detected. These einkorn proteins represent variation that could be sought to modulate wheat flour functionality for new end uses. Breadmaking quality in einkorn seems associated with LMW glutenin subunits, their banding patterns, and total amount. In two studies (Galterio et al 1998, Curioni et al 2000), profiles or amounts of HMW glutenins could not explain the variation in breadmaking quality between "good" and "poor" einkorn accessions, but LMW glutenins could. LMW glutenin polypeptides have been suggested as being responsible for the degree of polymerization of the glutenin complex in einkorn wheat. This last point was reaffirmed when genes encoding for two LMW glutenins from *T. monococcum* were expressed in bacteria, and the proteins obtained were incorporated into dough preparations (Lee et al 1999b). These LMW glutenins caused significant increases in peak resistance and mixing time (2-g mixograph) and also contributed positively to dough extensibility (microextension tester).

Gliadin patterns were looked at more closely in a comparative study of spelt, emmer, einkorn, durum, common wheat, and triticale (Wieser 2000), using reversed-phase high-performance liquid chromatography (RP-HPLC) separation and SDS-PAGE of gluten protein fractions. Results for HMW and LMW glutenins confirmed previous analyses. The author observed that the HPLC patterns of gliadin and glutenin subunits from species with the same genome composition (i.e., common wheat/spelt or durum wheat/emmer) were related, while the pattern displayed by einkorn was different. However, in the HPLC analysis of gliadins, einkorn differed the most from the other wheats. In einkorn, the pattern of α-gliadins, the dominant group in gliadins, was different from that in the other cereals, as was its pattern for γ-gliadins, where the most hydrophilic γ-subunit was absent. The ω-gliadins were also different, and in a follow-up study (Seilmeier et al 2001), these gliadins were further characterized for the same group of cereals. Einkorn, like emmer, displayed only the ω5-type of gliadins, but not the ω1,2-type, which were present in the other cereals of the study. These ω1,2-gliadins were, however, detected in an earlier study in a different einkorn cultivar (Kasarda et al 1983).

Gluten proteins in einkorn differ not only in types, but also in amounts from those present in modern hexaploid wheats. Using a separation based on solvent extraction and Kjeldahl analysis, Abdel-Aal et al (1995) determined the gliadin-to-glutenin (GLI/GLU) ratio in einkorn TM23 flour. The GLI/GLU ratio for this einkorn was 2:1, in contrast to the 1:1 ratio for the common wheat in their study.

Besides essential amino acid content, protein quality can encompass several aspects. Protein quality in any member of the genus *Triticum* can also be considered in terms of toxicity to celiac patients. Celiac disease is a gluten-induced enteropathy in which affected individuals must avoid food made from grains of wheat, barley, and rye. The alcohol-soluble storage proteins of these cereals are responsible for the toxicity and, in wheat, this encompasses all the major gliadin proteins. These proteins can be heated or digested into peptides without loss of toxicity. Small peptides arising from gastrointestinal enzyme activity are the triggering factors. Ancient wheats are often portrayed in the health food literature as less "toxic" to celiac patients. Few scientific reports have considered einkorn in this context. Vallega (1995) mentioned reports from the early 1980s suggesting that einkorn flours might be nontoxic or less toxic for celiacs than polyploid wheats. He also added, however, that the evidence collected before 1995 was far from conclusive. Vallega's remark seems validated by more recent research on the topic. A study in Hungary (Matuz et al 2000b) used rabbit antiwheat gliadin antibodies in immunoblot analysis following SDS-PAGE to determine which cereal grains should not be recommended for gluten-intolerant celiac patients. One einkorn line was included in the study, and it showed immunoreactive zones. Although they observed differences in the mobility and intensity of these zones between the various wheat species in the study, the authors concluded that none of them, including einkorn, could be recommended to gluten-sensitive patients. Wieser (2001) made a comparison of flours from various wheats, making a point of testing "old" wheat species, including one einkorn of unknown origin, to provide a more rigorous evaluation of their safety for celiac patients. Reverse-phase-HPLC was used to separate the proteins following flour extraction. The separated proteins were then compared by N-terminal amino acid sequence analysis. The α-gliadins from all wheat species investigated contained amino acid sequences that could activate the celiac condition. Wieser also concluded that einkorn is not safe for celiac individuals.

Processing Characteristics

One of the earliest studies on einkorn processing quality was done by LeClerc et al (1918). Their objective was to determine whether the "rarer" wheats like spelt, emmer, and einkorn could be successfully milled and baked into bread. Only one accession of einkorn was studied. They concluded that the bread made from einkorn was the least desirable in volume, color, elasticity, and flavor. Later, einkorn was described as a grain with high protein and yellow pigment, giving a sticky dough but an acceptable bread volume

(Yamashita et al 1957). In recent years, researchers in Italy, Germany, and North America have explored the potential of einkorn for food applications with the experimental milling, rheological tools, and official methods used to evaluate modern wheat cultivars. These investigations have opened new perspectives for einkorn wheat.

Grain Characteristics

Einkorn needs dehulling before conventional milling. Research methods include using a pearling machine or a rice debranner (Satake, Japan) or passing the grains between rubber-coated rolls. Dehulled einkorn grains have, on average, smaller kernel weight and lower test weight than common wheat, although individual accessions can show values similar to those in wheat. Average kernel weight values between 23.9 and 27.4 mg were measured in various experiments from Italy (D'Egidio et al 1993, Borghi et al 1996), or between 21.2 and 37.4 mg in lines grown in Denmark (Løje et al, 2003), while einkorn TM23 (Abdel-Aal et al 1997) was measured at 32.4 mg in comparison to bread wheat Katepwa at 33.0 mg.

Grain hardness is an important quality trait in cereals because it determines some of the end-use properties. Einkorn grain hardness has been measured in only a few experiments. Williams (1986) had two accessions in a large study that looked at hardness in different wheat species. Hardness was measured by the PSI test based on sieving of ground meals. Both einkorns were found to be very soft. Other researchers have used the single-kernel characterization system (SKCS 4100, Perten) to measure hardness index on several einkorn accessions. All samples had a very soft texture ranging from –14.8 to 4.0 (Corbellini et al 1999) and from –7.3 to 27.2 (Løje et al 2003), all values lower than the threshold value of 42 for soft wheats. Recent molecular experiments with *T. monococcum* have shown that chromosome $5A^m$ does have similar grain texture genes as chromosome 5D in hexaploid wheats, and these can modulate grain hardness to become softer (Tranquilli et al 1999, 2002).

Milling Characteristics

Following grain tempering, einkorn flour has been produced with a variety of mills. A commercial wheat cultivar has commonly been included, so although flour yield per se cannot be compared between experiments, the performance of einkorn can be compared in relation to wheat. D'Egidio et al (1993) examined the milling quality of 12 einkorn accessions. The average straight-grade flour-milling yield of these einkorn wheats was similar to that of commercial soft wheat: 70.8 and 72.7%, respectively. Yields of shorts and bran, however, were different from those of common wheat on a Buhler MLU-202 mill. There were more shorts than bran for einkorn. The authors suggested that these higher yields for flour and shorts indicate that the pericarp of einkorn may be loosely attached to the endosperm, giving it a friable texture. They also mentioned that the crease in einkorn grains was not as deep as in polyploid wheats, which would also favor higher flour yields.

Flour particle-size distribution showed a greater proportion of fine particles, confirming that einkorn grains are soft textured. In other experiments, flour yield of einkorn lines was also found to be similar to that of commercial soft wheat (Borghi et al 1996, Corbellini et al 1999). The percentage of fine flour particles was also similar to the soft wheat variety. Einkorn TM23, however, gave lower flour yield than the hard bread wheat Katepwa on a Brabender Quadrumat Jr. mill (Abdel-Aal et al 1997), while its flour particle-size distribution indicated finer particles than Katepwa, a reflection of the soft texture of its grain. Flour ash content was measured in only one instance, on straight-grade experimental Buhler mill flours (D'Egidio et al 1993), and was found to be notably higher than that of the soft wheat check: 0.74 and 0.47%, respectively. The ash content of the einkorn whole meal in this study was 2.18%, which prompted the authors to suggest that current low-ash polyploid wheat cultivars are the result of deliberate selection for low mineral content. Einkorn TM23, however, did not show markedly higher whole-meal ash content (Table 1).

Flour Characteristics

Assessment of einkorn's potential for a food end use is largely linked to the characteristics of its flour, and more specifically, to the strength of the gluten. Most researchers, especially if they were surveying large numbers of einkorn accessions for flour quality, have applied the SDS sedimentation test as a rapid method to estimate breadmaking potential. SDS sedimentation volume is generally correlated with gluten strength. D'Egidio et al (1993) found SDS-specific sedimentation volumes (volume/protein) ranging from 1.0 to 2.8 mL for einkorn flours, while bread wheats gave an average value of 5.3 mL. Researchers looking at other accessions (Borghi et al 1996, Corbellini et al 1999) obtained specific SDS sedimentation volumes ranging from 0.5 to 6.6 mL, with an average of 2.6 mL, while bread wheats measured at 6.5 mL. Einkorn TM23 gave a value of 0.7 mL, while the hard wheat Katepwa was measured at 4.3 mL (Abdel-Aal et al 1997). Borghi et al (1996) also mention testing more than 1,000 accessions of einkorns and identified 16% of them as showing SDS sedimentation volumes higher than the threshold for breadbaking potential. Based on the SDS test, einkorn germ plasm displays a wide range of values that could translate to a wide range of gluten strength.

Rheological measurements of gluten strength with a mixograph, a farinograph, or an alveograph provide the best assessment of the potential end use of a common wheat dough. Only a limited number of studies on einkorn have included these measurements. The stickiness of einkorn's dough made rheology much more difficult, with some accessions impossible. Approximately 50 different accessions have been analyzed for dough strength so far. Rheological quality, in general, was similar to that of the soft wheats used in the pastry, cracker, and biscuit industry. A few accessions showed good potential for breadmaking. the mixograph was used with only one accession, TM23 (Abdel-Aal et al 1997), confirming that its gluten was weak. Table 4 summarizes the average and range in values recorded for dough performance parameters from einkorn flours over years and locations.

TABLE 4
Average Dough Strength Measurements for Various European Einkorn Accessions Grown in Italy and Germany

Accessions	Alveograph[a]				Farinograph[b]			
	W ($Jx10^{-4}$)	*P* (mm)	*L* (mm)	Ratio *P/L*	Abs. (%)	PK (mm)	Stab. (min)	MTI (BU)
Einkorn								
A1[c]	68	43	76	0.9	57	1.6	1.4	186
	(14–137)	(23–54)	(10–205)	(0.21–2.39)	(53–60)	(0.8–2.0)	(0.8–4.5)	(90–260)
A2[c]	45	36	46	1.07	54	1.5	2.6	155
	(9–100)	(19–57)	(10–129)	(0.31–3.30)	(52–57)	(1.0–2.3)	(0.4–4.5)	(30–270)
B1[d]					56.1	2.0	1.9	177
					(53–63)	(1.1–3.3)	(0.5–4.5)	(50–300)
B2[d]					56	2.1	2.8	159
					(54–61)	(0.8–4.0)	(0.4–6.5)	(50–260)
Wheat								
Pandas (bread)					60	2.8	5.5	75
Veronese (pastry)					53	1.5	2	130

[a] *W*: deformation energy; *P*: maximum over pressure; *L*: abscissa at rupture; *P/L*: configuration ratio.
[b] Abs.: farinograph water absorption; PK: peak time; Stab.: stability; MTI: mixing tolerance index.
[c] A: Data from Borghi et al (1996); ($n = 25$) where 1 = Milan (Italy) 1993 and 2 = Cologne (Germany) 1993.
[d] B: Data from Corbellini et al (1999); ($n = 24$) where 1 = Milan (Italy) 1995 and 2 = Milan (Italy) 1996.

Experimental Baking Quality

Following rheological measurements, einkorn flours were baked into bread or made into cookies following microtesting procedures. A modified AACC method, 10-10B, was used for making experimental loaves with most of the European accessions, while einkorn TM23 bread was made following a remix baking test. Cookie quality was assessed with AACC method 10-52, (Corbellini et al 1999). Table 5 provides baking performance data for a few accessions along with local commercial wheats. Bread loaf volume of the European accessions correlated significantly with rheology results (deformation energy [*W*] = *r* 0.73** and stability = *r* 0.58*) (Borghi et al 1996). Accessions with high alveograph *W* factor or high farinograph stability gave good bread loaf volume. A weak einkorn flour, such as einkorn TM23, gave the lowest loaf volume in the remix baking test in comparison to the bread wheat Katepwa and a strong gluten spelt accession: 394 cc, 626 cc, and 580 cc, respectively (Abdel-Aal et al 1997). On average, einkorn cookies showed larger diameter and were thinner than those produced with a soft wheat flour. Variability between accessions was demonstrated across location and crop year for cookie diameter and bread loaf volume.

Following baking, the next level of quality assessment is linkage to some type of sensory evaluation. Crumb color was noted as distinctly yellowish in the early studies and again in more recent ones because of the high carotenoid pigments. Crumb score, a visual assessment of the porosity of the crumb on a scale of 1–8, was measured and some of the promising einkorn accessions showed bread crumb scores similar to those of bread wheat (Borghi et al 1996, Corbellini et al 1999).

Based on these experimental baking tests, when appropriate accessions are selected for a specific end use, einkorn flours can be made into bread and

TABLE 5
Experimental Baking Performance of Selected Einkorn Accessions Grown in Two Locations[a]

			Cookie			
	Bread Volume (cc)		Width (cm)		Height (cm)	
Sample	Milan	Cologne	Milan	Cologne	Milan	Cologne
140	818 (5)[b]	903 (5)	9.4	10	0.68	0.59
280	810 (7)	770 (5)	9.3	9.9	0.75	0.6
361	740 (4)	780 (6)	9.3	9.3	0.71	0.63
201	...	...	8.7	9.4	0.8	0.8
372	...	...	8.5	8.4	0.75	0.7
559	...	...	9.7	9.8	0.59	0.68
1331	690 (4)	840 (5)	8.4	9.4	0.79	0.75
Bread flour	875 (7)	875 (7)	...	...	...	...
Cookie flour	...	...	8.7	8.7	0.78	0.78

[a] Data from Corbellini et al (1999).
[b] Crumb score (1–8).

cookies. The wide variability in performance observed with einkorn is a direct reflection of the fact that einkorn accessions have never been selected for food applications.

Experimental Product Quality

Although the main focus of the end-use quality of einkorn has been baking and pastry quality, other applications have been investigated. Abdel-Aal et al (1998) made flaked breakfast cereals from einkorn TM23. Flour slurries were drum dried and the sheets crushed into coarse flakes. Sensory evaluation was not favorable to einkorn TM23 for both aroma and texture of the flakes when compared to spelt. The flakes were, however, similar to those prepared from hard wheat. The flakes and the flour were also analyzed for lysine content (Abdel-Aal and Hucl 2002). Flour milling reduced lysine content in einkorn, and processing into flakes reduced it slightly more, while the glutamic acid levels were increased in the flour and slightly reduced by flaking. The reduction in lysine levels by processing was, however, more pronounced with hard spelt and hard red spring wheat. Einkorn was traditionally used in soups or porridge or as cooked whole grains. This prompted Løje et al (2003) to investigate the sensory profile of three einkorn lines cooked as whole kernels in comparison to spelt and common wheat. Three groups of sensory attributes were analyzed: aroma, taste, and consistency. Einkorn was similar in aroma to the other wheat species in the study. In the taste category, it had a more intense "hot oatmeal porridge" taste than wheat and was sweeter than the other cooked grains. For consistency, einkorn was perceived as softer and less mealy, adhesive, and fibrous than spelt and wheat. The authors suggested that cooked kernels of einkorn could be used as a rice substitute since both its flavor and consistency were rated as pleasant.

Current Uses

According to Vallega (1995), einkorn is currently produced in Italy for local use as feed for animals in remote areas with low-input crop management. Peña-Chocarro (1995) described einkorn as an animal feed in the few places in Spain where it could be found in 1991. Einkorn was milled and mixed with water and fed to pigs and cattle. Einkorn spikelets on their own or mixed with barley were given to mules, goats, donkeys, and hens. People from these remote places in Spain remembered that einkorn would be made into bread in lean times. Karagöz (1995) reported that hulled wheats, einkorn, and emmer are still cultivated in parts of Turkey for farm feed. The acreage, however, was very low.

Recent market trends for a return to whole grain foods and organic crop-management practices resulted in a renewed interest in einkorn in the 1990s, but on a smaller scale than for the other ancient cereals. Einkorn was being grown in southern France for specialty whole grain foodstuffs such as precooked grains for soups, muesli, and salads. Bond (1989) mentioned that in France, bread made from einkorn had a light, rich taste, and the grains were used in dishes like soups, salads, and casseroles. A report from an Agri-Food Trade Show held in Avignon, France, in 1991, noted that one of the intriguing new foods unveiled was actually an old food or *céréale ancienne*, einkorn. The report (Anonymous 1991) continued, "It cooks in 45 minutes like whole grain brown rice. It has a mild taste, is a good source of dietary fiber, and can be added to salads or served hot like rice." Müller (2002) provides a list of small, artisan-type bakeries in Germany, Denmark, and Australia where commercial products from einkorn flour are currently offered to the public. He described some of the recipe adaptations implemented by a baker to deal with the weaker einkorn gluten; lemon juice is added, the dough needs 70 minutes of resting time to become stable, and most breads are made in baking pans. The resulting bread is described as having a good volume, light texture, yellowish color, and a nutty taste.

Although threshability may provide wider opportunities for einkorn, modern cultivars will need to be more competitive in yield potential even for niche market end use. Several resistance traits for biotic and abiotic stresses are already in einkorn. Results from research over the last 15 years clearly indicate that the potential for diverse wheat-type products also exists within einkorn germ plasm. New applications can probably be developed that take advantage of unique einkorn traits such as the high gel stability of its starch or the high lutein content of its grain and flour.

High-Lutein Einkorn as a Functional Wheat

Lutein, one of the most naturally occurring hydroxycarotenoids or xanthophylls, is the major yellow pigment in wheat (*Triticum aestivum* L.) (Lepage and Sims 1968). It is responsible for the desirable amber yellow color of the endosperm of durum wheat, which contributes to the quality of semolina and pasta products. Lutein and other pigments (e.g., tricin, β-carotene) exist in wheat grains at very low concentrations, but they substantially influence the quality of wheat grains and products, and hence they are used to distinguish the major market classes of wheat (e.g., red versus white wheats). Additionally, a large number of studies have shown that carotenoids and flavonoids are associated with reducing the risk of degenerative chronic diseases and promoting good health (Brown et al 1999, Fullmer and Shao 2001, Landrum and Bone 2001).

Lutein is a tetraterpenoid containing eight isoprenoid residues. It is an oxygenated carotenoid containing two hydroxyl groups in contrast to the hydrocarbon carotenoids (e.g., carotene and lycopene), which have no oxygen atoms. The hydroxyl groups make lutein more polar than hydrocarbon carotenoids and may contribute to its unique role in maintaining the health of ocular tissues along with zeaxanthin, a lutein isomer. Lutein and zeaxanthin are the main carotenoids found in the macular region of the retina (Fullmer and Shao 2001).

A number of epidemiological (Seddon et al 1994, Brown et al 1999, Chasan-Taber et al 1999) and clinical (Bone et al 2001, Landrum and Bone 2001) studies have shown that lutein intake is associated with reduced incidence of age-related macular degeneration (AMD), the leading cause of irreversible blindness in elderly people, and cataracts. It was reported that approximately 5–6 mg daily intake of lutein might reduce the risk of AMD by about 57% relative to an intake of 0.5 mg per day (Seddon et al 1994). In mice, dietary lutein was found to delay and inhibit mammary tumor growth and to enhance lymphocyte proliferation (Chew et al 1996). In addition, diets rich in carotenoids were associated with a reduced incidence of cancer (Hughes 2001) and better health (Handelman 2001). Furthermore, the presence of lutein and zeaxanthin in the macular region of the retina supports a protective role for lutein in AMD (Fullmer and Shao 2001).

Early in the past century, einkorn flour was reported to possess high protein and yellow color (LeClerc et al 1918). More recently, several studies have confirmed that einkorn wheats contain elevated levels of protein and yellow pigments (D'Egidio et al 1993, Abdel-Aal et al 1995, Borghi et al 1996, Corbellini et al 1999, Matuz et al 2000a, Løje et al, 2003). Additionally, Borghi et al (1996) reported that einkorn may hold promise for the production of bakery products rich in carotenoids and proteins. These results suggest that einkorn has the potential to be a good candidate for the development of high-carotenoid (lutein) wheats as grains for the functional food industry.

Separation of carotenoids and xanthophylls by RP-HPLC and subsequent photodiode array ultraviolet-visible and mass spectrometric detection indicated that lutein is the major xanthophyll in wheat grains and is differentially distributed in the kernel depending upon wheat species (Abdel-Aal et al

TABLE 6
Lutein Content (mg/kg, dry basis) of Einkorn and Other Ancient Alternative Wheats[a]

Wheat	Cultivar/ Accession	2*n* Chromosome No.	Product: Whole Meal	Flour	Bran	Semolina
Spring einkorn	TM23	14	1.78	1.61	2.16	...
	PI 418587	14	8.23	9.05	7.01	...
	AC Knowles	14	7.29	8.24	5.93	...
Spring emmer	Vernal	28	3.68	2.71	4.19	2.72
Spring khorasan	PI 211691	28	5.37	6.69	5.22	6.09
Kamut	Commercial	28	6.09	6.67	5.51	6.57
Durum	Kyle	28	5.93	7.42	5.67	6.65
Spring spelt	CDC Bavaria	42	1.03	0.73	1.92	...
	PGR8801	42	1.31	0.68	2.41	...
Winter spelt	Frankencorn	42	1.61	1.55	2.19	...
	Rotkorn	42	2.58	2.18	3.23	...
Soft wheat	AC Reed	42	2.39	3.49	3.06	...
HRS[b] wheat	Katepwa	42	2.09	1.54	3.22	...
LSD ($P<0.05$)			0.21	0.23	0.15	0.35

[a] Data from Abdel-Aal et al (2002).
[b] Hard red spring.

2002). Lutein levels in the whole meal flours vary from 1.0 mg/kg in a spelt cultivar to 8.2 mg/kg in one of the einkorn cultivars (Table 6). Beta-carotene was found at very low levels in all wheats, ranging from 0.02 to 0.12 mg/kg in whole meals. Several unknown compounds presumed to be carotenoids also were observed in einkorn on the basis of the characteristic triple-absorption maxima of carotenoids (*C* in Figure 1). Einkorn accessions were found to contain the highest levels of lutein among wheat species. One of the einkorn samples, TM23, contained relatively low levels of lutein, but it contained other types of carotenoids. The flour fraction of einkorn samples with high lutein contents (PI 418587 and AC Knowles) had higher levels of lutein compared with the bran fraction. The same trend was found in wheats exhibiting intermediate concentrations of lutein (5.4–6.1 mg/kg) such as Khorasan, Kamut, and durum. Einkorn flour fractions obtained from PI 418587 and AC

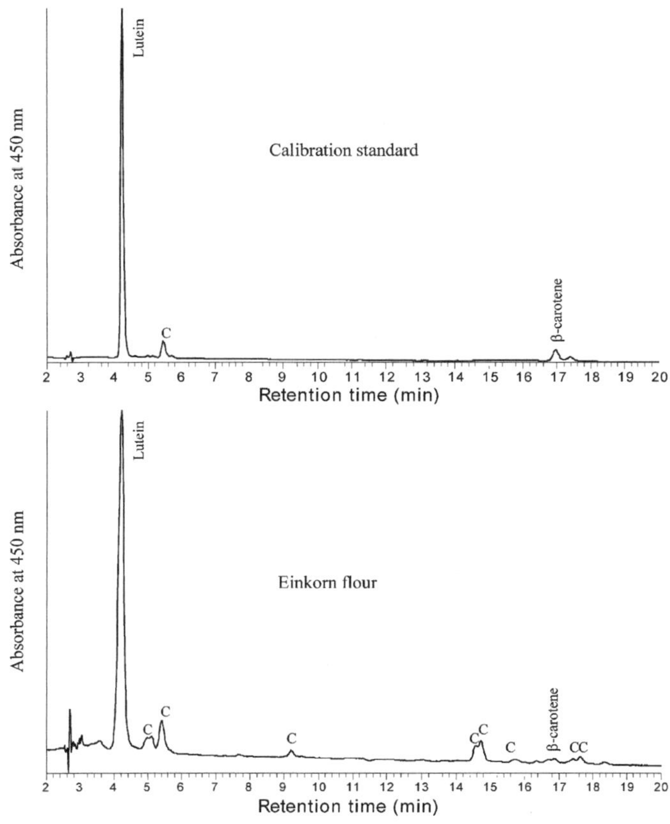

Fig. 1. Separation of lutein and β-carotene standard mixture and carotenoid extracts from einkorn using reverse-phase high performance liquid chromatography (HPLC). (Adapted from Abdel-Aal et al 2002)

Knowles were found to contain about sixfold more lutein than common wheat, averaging 8.6 mg/kg compared to 1.5 mg/kg. In another set of einkorn breeding lines, lutein content in whole meal flours averaged 8.1 mg/kg (Abdel-Aal et al 2002). Furthermore, lutein content in einkorn was also found to be consistently high when six crop years from 1996 to 2001 were evaluated for carotenoid composition (Abdel-Aal 2003 *unpublished data*).

Einkorn wheat cultivars with high levels of carotenoids, particularly lutein, may hold potential as high-lutein functional wheats. Examination of larger numbers of einkorn or monococcum germ plasm samples is still needed to explore carotenoid composition in einkorn wheats. The tetraploid wheats such as Khorasan, Kamut, and durum were found to contain somewhat high levels of lutein (i.e., 60–80% of lutein content in einkorn), which would make these wheats other potential sources for developing high-lutein wheats. A high-quality durum wheat cultivar, Kyle, which is a white-seeded tetraploid wheat bred over years for high content of yellow pigments, was relatively high in lutein, at levels of approximately 80% that in einkorn (Abdel-Aal et al 2002), offering a good choice for developing high-lutein pasta wheat.

Lutein intake in the United States ranges from 1.5 to 2.0 mg/day, which is only about 30% of the recommended daily intake (Fullmer and Shao 2001). Additionally, the level is declining because of a decrease in the consumption of dark green vegetables, the major dietary source of lutein. As a staple food, high-lutein wheat would enhance the daily intake of lutein by about 120% on the basis of the minimum recommended daily consumption of grain products, (e.g., six servings provide 2.1 mg of lutein based on 86% dry matter). This considers lutein alone. The total carotenoid contribution would be higher (e.g., contribution of lutein, zeaxanthin, and other carotenoid isomers). It is not known what level of lutein or total carotenoid would be required for a significant reduction in risk, but clearly the presently identified levels could significantly raise dietary intake. Also, new wheat genotypes with increased lutein levels could be developed.

Currently, several lutein products in the form of dietary supplements or lutein-fortified food and beverage products are being produced and marketed. Lutein has been added to a variety of foods, including ready-to-eat baked cereals, cereal bars, and fruit juices (Fullmer and Shao 2001). Sensory evaluation studies on lutein-containing foods indicate that lutein does not alter the flavor, odor, or texture of the finished products. Only the color of clear or white beverages may be affected. The stability of lutein during processing and handling of lutein-fortified foods was also investigated. When lutein was added to ready-to-eat cereal (0.5 mg/30 g serving) and cereal-bar (1.25 mg/50 g serving) products, it remained stable during processing and storage for 6 and 12 weeks (Fullmer and Shao 2001). Developing high-lutein wheat will provide the food industry with natural functional food ingredients (i.e., high-lutein flour fractions) at a modest price compared to using lutein as a food additive or a dietary supplement, which requires isolation and purification of lutein from its sources, resulting in increased processing cost.

Because the principal constraint in developing einkorn for commercial use is the low grain yield (Borghi et al 1996, Corbellini et al 1999), the development of high-yield genotypes needs to be emphasized in addition to the high lutein content. Several einkorn breeding programs are underway in Europe and North America. In such programs, screening for higher grain yield and lutein content (total yellow pigments) should be the primary criteria that will lead to the development of high-lutein wheats. Additionally, einkorn may offer a good genetic resource for lutein and other nutrients. The presence of adhering glumes in einkorn may help protect grains during development and storage against invasive insects and microorganisms and may not pose a problem in processing if efficient dehulling equipment is available. The higher grain yield of Khorasan, Kamut, and durum wheats make them good alternative choices for developing high-lutein wheat.

Conclusions

Compared to other ancient wheats, little in the primary composition of einkorn indicates specific health benefits, and certainly no clinical or observational studies have been done to suggest this. Nor do agronomic performance or functionality in the mainstream production of standard cereal foods indicate any rationale for expanded use, although this may be partly the result of neglect. As with other specialty crops described in this volume, the simple act of maintaining diversity in the food chain may be valuable enough to encourage maintenance of some acreage and use.

The primary potential niche end use for einkorn is probably to facilitate the development of high-lutein wheat grains whose products would be of interest to cereal producers and processors and consumers. As a staple food, wheat could provide a large proportion of lutein intake and significantly increase the present average daily intake. Additionally, developing high-lutein wheat as a food ingredient could offer a variety of functional food products at a reasonable cost compared with using lutein isolates as a food additive or supplement, which entails the costs of isolating, purifying, and mixing the lutein or preparing capsules. In the markets presently enjoyed by ancient wheats, and for a growing proportion of consumers, additives are less desirable than natural ingredients. The available data suggest that einkorn or monococcum wheats can be considered potential candidates for developing high-lutein functional wheats or a good genetic resource for lutein and other nutrients (e.g., proteins). Khorasan, Kamut, and durum wheats also hold promise for the development of high-lutein wheat products on the basis of their lutein content. More research is necessary to investigate genetic and environmental effects on lutein and to identify high-lutein wheat cultivars from diploid and tetraploid wheats and their potential end uses.

Acknowledgments

The authors are grateful to Janet Gale for gathering the reference materials.

This chapter is dedicated to the memory of Dexter Sampson, breeder with Agriculture and Agri-Food Canada, who developed the naked einkorn Canadian cultivar AC Knowles.

References

Abdel-Aal, E.-S. M., and Hucl, P. 2002. Amino acid composition and *in vitro* protein digestibility of selected ancient wheats and their end products. J. Food Comp. Anal. 15:737-747.

Abdel-Aal, E.-S. M., Hucl, P., and Sosulski, F. W. 1995. Compositional and nutritional characteristics of spring einkorn and spelt wheats. Cereal Chem. 72:621-624.

Abdel-Aal, E.-S. M., Hucl, P., Sosulski, F. W., and Bhirud, P. R. 1997. Kernel, milling and baking properties of spring-type spelt and einkorn wheats. J. Cereal Sci. 26:363-370.

Abdel-Aal, E.-S. M., Hucl, P., and Sosulski, F. W. 1998. Food uses for ancient wheats. Cereal Foods World 43:763-766.

Abdel-Aal, E.-S. M., Hucl, P., and Sosulski, F. W. 1999a. Starches from primitive wheats I. Extraction efficiency, granule size distribution and composition. Presented at Am. Assoc. Cereal Chem. Annual Meeting (online: www.aaccnet.org/meetings/).

Abdel-Aal, E.-S. M., Hucl, P., and Sosulski, F. W. 1999b. Starches from primitive wheats II. Thermal and structural properties. Presented at Am. Assoc. Cereal Chem. Annual Meeting (online: www.aaccnet.org/meetings/).

Abdel-Aal, E.-S. M., Young, J. C., Wood, P. J, Rabalski, I., Hucl, P., Falk, D., and Frégeau-Reid, J. 2002. Einkorn: A potential candidate for developing high lutein wheat. Cereal Chem. 79:458-464.

Acquistucci, R., D'Egidio, M. G., and Vallega, V. 1995. Amino acid composition of selected strains of diploid wheat, *Triticum monococcum* L. Cereal Chem. 72:213-216.

Anker, C. C., Buntjer, J. B., and Niks, R. E. 2001. Morphological and molecular chacterisation confirm that *Triticum monococcum* s.s. is resistant to wheat leaf rust. Theor. Appl. Genet. 103:1093-1098.

Anonymous. 1991. *Toronto Star*, January 15.

Bálint, A. F., Kovács, G., Erdei, L., and Sutka, J. 2001. Comparison of the Cu, Zn, Fe, Ca, and Mg contents of the grains of wild ancient and cultivated wheat species. Cereal Res. Comm. 29:375-382.

Beresford, G., and Stone, B. A. 1983. (1-3),(1-4)-β-D-Glucan content of *Triticum* grains. J. Cereal Sci. 1:111-114.

Bond, A. 1989. Discovering einkorn in Haute Provence, France. Cerealist 1:6-7.

Bone, R. A., Landrum, J. T., Mayne, S. T., Gomez, C. M., Tibor, S. E., and Twaroska, E. E. 2001. Macular pigment in donor eyes with and without AMD: A case-control study. IOVS 42:235-240.

Borghi, B., Castagna, R., Corbellini, M., Heun, M., and Salamini, F. 1996. Breadmaking quality of einkorn wheat (*Titicum monococcum* ssp. *monococcum*). Cereal Chem. 73:208-214.

Brown, L., Rimm, E. B., Seddon, J. M., Giovannucci, E. L., Chasan-Taber, L., Spiegelman, D., Willett, W. C., and Hankinson, S. E. 1999. A prospective study of carotenoid intake and risk of cataract extraction in U.S. men. Am. J. Clin. Nutr. 70:517-524.

Bullrich, L., Appendino, M. L., Tranquilli, G., Lewis, S., Dubcovsky, J. 2002. Mapping of a thermo-sensitive earliness *per se* gene in *Triticum monococcum* chromosome $1A^m$. J. Theor. Appl. Genet. 105:585-593.

Castagna, R., Borghi, B., Di Fonzo, N., Heun, M., and Salamini, F. 1995. Yield and related traits of einkorn (*T. monococcum* ssp. *monococcum*) in different environments. Eur. J. Agron. 4:371-378.

Castagna, R., Minoia, C., Porfiri, O., and Rocchetti, G. 1996. Nitrogen level and seeding rate effects on the performance of hulled wheats (*Triticum monococcum* L., *T. dicoccum* and *T. spelta* L.). Evaluated in contrasting agronomic environments. J. Agron. Crop Sci.176:173-181.

Chasan-Taber, L., Willett, W. C., Seddon, J. M., Stampfer, M. J., Rosner, B., Colditz, G. A., Speizer, F., and Hankinson, S. E. 1999. A prospective study of carotenoid and vitamin A intakes and risk of cataract extraction in U.S. women. Am. J. Clin. Nutr. 70:509-516.

Chew, B. P., Wong, M. W., and Wong, T. S. 1996. Effects of lutein from marigold extract on immuity and growth of mammary tumors in mice. Anticancer Res. 16:3689-3694.

Corbellini, M., Empilli, S., Vaccino, P., Brandolini, A., Borghi, B., Heun, M., and Salamini, F. 1999. Einkorn characterization for bread and cookie production in relation to protein subunit composition. Cereal Chem. 76:727-733.

Curioni, A., Pogna, N. E., Pasini, G., Spettoli, P., Voltarel, M., and Dal Belin Peruffo, A. 2000. Characterization of the glutenin fraction from einkorn wheat (*Triticum monococcum* ssp. *monococcum*) flours with different breadmaking quality. Ital. J. Food Sci. 12:91-102.

D'Antuono, L. F., Galletti, G. C., and Bocchini, P. 1998. Fiber quality of emmer (*Triticum dicoccum* Schubler) and einkorn wheat (*T. monococcum* L.) Landraces as determined by analytical pyrolysis. J. Sci. Food Agric.78:213-219.

D'Egidio, M. G., Nardi, S., and Vallega, V. 1993. Grain, flour and dough characteristics of selected strains of diploid wheat, *Triticum monococcum* L. Cereal Chem. 70:298-303.

Dubcovsky, J., Luo, M.-C., Zhong, G. Y., Bransteitter, R., Desai, A., Kilian, A., Kleinhofs, A., and Dvořák, J. 1996. Genetic map of diploid wheat, *Triticum monococcum* L., and its comparison with maps of *Hordeum vulgare* L. Genetics 143:983-999.

Fullmer, L. A., and Shao, A. 2001. The role of lutein in eye health and nutrition. Cereal Foods World 46:408-413.

Galterio, G., Borghi, B., Bucarelli, F., Cannella, C., and Salamini, F. 1998. Breadmaking quality, protein subunits and amino acid composition of einkorn (*Triticum monococcum*) compared with other wheat species. Pages 81-90 in: Cereals for Human Health and Preventive Nutrition (Proc. Int. Conf.). K. Vaculová and J. Ehrenbergerová, Eds. Food Research Institute, Prague.

Handelman, G. J. 2001. The evolving role of carotenoids in human biochemistry. Nutrition 17:818-822.

Heun, M., Schäfer-Pregl, R., Klawan, D., Castagna, R., Accerbi, M., Borghi, B., and Salamini, F. 1997. Site of einkorn domestication identified by DNA fingerprinting. Science 278:1312-1314.

Hucl, P., Abdel-Aal, E.-S. M., and Sosulski, F. W. 1995. Specialty wheats. Pages 40-47 in: Proc. "Cropportunities III" Conf. Extension Div., University of Saskatchewan, SK, Canada.

Hughes, D. A. 2001. Dietary carotenoids and human immune function. Nutrition 17:823-827.

Karagöz, A. 1995. Agronomic practices and socioeconomic aspects of emmer and einkorn cultivation in Turkey. Pages 172-177 in: Hulled Wheats: Proc. First Int. Workshop on Hulled Wheats. S. Padulosi, K. Hammer, and J. Heller, Eds. International Plant Genetic Resources Institute, Rome.

Kasarda, D. D., Autran, J.-C., Lew, E. J.-L., Nimmo, C. C., and Shewry, P. R. 1983. N-terminal amino acid sequences of ω-gliadins and ω-secalins. Implications for the evolution of prolamin genes. Biochim.Biophys. Acta 747:138-150.

Kojima, T., Nagaoka, T., Noda, K., and Ogihara, Y. 1998. Genetic linkage map of ISSR and RAPD markers in Einkorn wheat in relation to that of RFLP markers. Theor. Appl. Genet. 96:37-45.

Landrum, J. T., and Bone, R. A. 2001. Lutein, zeaxanthin and the macular pigment. Arch. Biochem. Biophys. 385:28-40.

LeClerc, J. A., Bailey, L. H., and Wessling, H. L. 1918. Milling and baking tests of einkorn, emmer, spelt and polish wheat. J. Am. Soc. Agron. 10:215-217.

Lee, Y.-K., Bekes, F., Gupta, R., Appels, R., and Morell, M. K. 1999a. The low molecular-weight glutenin subunit proteins of primitive wheats. I. Variation in A-genome species. Theor. Appl. Genet. 98:119-125.

Lee, Y.-K., Bekes, F., Gras, P., Ciaffi, M., Morell, M. K., and Appels, R. 1999b. The low molecular-weight glutenin subunit proteins of primitive wheats. IV. Functional properties of products from individual genes. Theor. Appl. Genet. 98:149-155.

Lepage, M., and Sims, R. P. A. 1968. Carotenoids of wheat flour: Their identification and composition. Cereal Chem. 45:600-604.

Løje, H., Møller, B., Laustsen, A. M., and Hansen, Å. 2003. Chemical composition, functional properties and sensory profiling of einkorn (*Triticum monococcum* L.). J. Cereal Sci. 37:231-240.

Martin Del Molino, I. M., Rojo, B., Martinez-Carrasco, R., and Perez, P. 1989. Varietal difference in amino acid composition of wheat (*Triticum aestivum* L.) grain. J. Sci. Food Agric. 48:177-188.

Matuz, J., Bartok, T., Morocz-Salamon, K., and Bona, L. 2000a. Structure and potential allergenic character of cereal proteins. I. Protein content and amino acid composition. Cereal Res. Comm. 28:263-270.

Matuz, J., Póka, R., Boldizsár, I., Szerdahelyi, E., and Hajós, G. 2000b. Structure and potential allergenic character of cereal proteins II: Potential allergens in cereal samples. Cereal Res. Comm. 28:433-442.

Mohammadkhani, A., Stoddard, F. L., and Marshall, D. R. 1998. Survey of amylose content in *Secale cereale*, *Triticum monococcum*, *T. turgidum* and *T. tauschii*. J. Cereal Sci. 28:273-280.

Mohammadkhani, A., Stoddard, F. L., and Marshall, D. R. 1999. Amylose content in segregating populations of einkorn, emmer and rye. Starch/Stärke 51:66-73.

Müller, K.-J. 2002. Einkorn—Cosmic Light from Oldest Grain. Cereal Breeding Research, Darzau, Germany. (www.einkorn.org.)

Padulosi, S., Hammer, K., and Heller, J., Eds. 1995. Hulled Wheats: Proc. First Int. Workshop on Hulled Wheats. International Plant Genetic Resources Institute, Rome.

Peña-Chocarro, L. 1995. *In situ* conservation of hulled wheat species: The case of Spain. Pages 129-146 in: Hulled Wheats: Proc. First Int. Workshop on Hulled Wheats. S. Padulosi, K. Hammer, and J. Heller, Eds. International Plant Genetic Resources Institute, Rome.

Percival, J. 1921. Small spelt. Pages 170-177 in: The Wheat Plant: A Monograph. Duckworth, London.

Rodríguez-Quijano, M., Nieto-Taladriz, M. T., and Carrillo, J. M. 1997. Variation in B-LMW glutenin subunits in Einkorn wheats. Genet. Res. Crop Evol. 44:539-543.

Salamini, F., Özkan, H., Brandolini, A., Schäfer-Pregl, R., and Martin, W. 2002. Genetics and geography of wild cereal domestication in the Near East. Nature Rev. Genet. 3:429-441.

Salunkhe, D. K., and Deshpande, S. S. 1991. Pages 1-501 in: Foods of Plant Origin: Production, Technology and Human Nutrition. Van Nostrand Reinhold, New York.

Saponaro, C., Pogna, N. E., Castagna, R., Pasquini, M., Cacciatori, P., and Redaelli, R. 1995. Allelic variation at the *Gli-A1*^{m}, *Gli-A2*^{m} and *Glu-A1*^{m} loci and breadmaking quality in diploid wheat *Triticum monococcum*. Genet. Res. Camb. 66:127-137.

Seddon, J. M., Ajani, U. A., Sperduto, R. D., Hiller, R., Blair, N., Burton, T. C., Farber, M. D., Gragoudas, E. S., Haller, J., Miller, D. T., Yannuzzi, L. A., and Willett, W. 1994. Dietary carotenoids, vitamins A, C, and E and advanced age-related macular degeneration. J. Am. Med. Assoc. 272:1413-1420.

Seilmeier, W., Valdez, I., Mendez, E., and Wieser, H. 2001. Comparative investigations of gluten proteins from different wheat species II. Characterization of ω-gliadins. Eur. Food Res. Technol. 212:355-363.

Shindo, C., Sasakuma, T., Watanabe, N., and Noda, K. 2002. Two-gene systems of vernalization requirement and narrow-sense earliness in einkorn wheat. Genome 45:563-569.

Singh, J., Sharp, P. J., and Skerritt, J. H. 2000. A new candidate protein for high lysine content in wheat grain. J. Sci. Food Agric. 81:216-226.

Stallknecht, G. F., Gilbertson, K. M., and Ranney, J. E. 1996. Alternative wheat cereals as food grains: Einkorn, emmer, spelt, kamut and triticale. Pages 156-170 in: Progress in New Crops, J. Janick, Ed. ASHS Press, Alexandria, VA.

Stoddard, F. L. 1999. Survey of starch particle-size distribution in wheat and related species. Cereal Chem. 76:145-149.

Taenzler, B., Esposti, R. F., Vaccino, P., Brandolini, A., Effgen, S., Heun, M., Schäfer-Pregl, R., Borghi, B., and Salamini, F. 2002. Molecular linkage map of Einkorn wheat: Mapping of storage-protein and soft-glume genes and bread-making QTLs. Genet. Res. 80:131-143.

Tranquilli, G., Lijavetzky, D., Muzzi, G., and Dubcovsky, J. 1999. Genetic and physical characterization of grain texture-related loci in diploid wheat. Mol. Gen. Genet. 262:846-850.

Tranquilli, G., Heaton, J., Chicaiza, O., and Dubcovsky, J. 2002. Substitutions and deletions of genes related to grain hardness in wheat and their effect on grain texture. Crop Sci. 42:1812-1817.

Vallega, V. 1979. Field performance of varieties of *Triticum monococcum*, *T. durum* and *Hordeum vulgare* grown at two locations. Genet. Agric. 33:363-370.

Vallega, V. 1992. Agronomical performance and breeding value of selected strains of diploid wheat, *Triticum monococcum*. Euphytica 61:13-23.

Vallega, V. 1995. The quality of *Triticum monococcum* L., in perspective. Pages 212-220 in: Hulled Wheats: Proc. First Int. Workshop on Hulled Wheats. S. Padulosi, K. Hammer, and J. Heller, Eds. International Plant Genetic Resources Institute, Rome.

Vallega, V. 1996. Registration of partially free threshing diploid wheat germ plasm. Crop Sci. 36:1717.

Waines, J. G., and Payne, P. I. 1987. Electrophoretic analysis of the high-molecular-weight glutenin subunits of *Triticum monococcum*, *T. urartu* and the A genome of bread wheat (*T. aestivum*). Theor. Appl. Genet. 74:71-76.

Wieser, H. 2000. Comparative investigations of gluten proteins from different wheat species I. Qualitative and quantitative composition of gluten protein types. Eur. Food Res. Technol. 211:262-268.

Wieser, H. 2001. Comparative investigations of gluten proteins from different wheat species. III. N-terminal amino acid sequences of α-gliadins potentially toxic for coeliac patients. Eur. Food Res. Technol. 213:183-186.

Williams, P. C. 1986. The influence of chromosome number and species on wheat hardness. Cereal Chem. 63:56-57.

Yamashita, K., Tanaka, M., and Koyama, M. 1957. Studies on the flour quality of *Triticum* and *Aegilops*. Seiken Ziho 11:20-26.

CHAPTER 4

Emmer Wheat

Emanuele Marconi and Raimondo Cubadda

Department of Food Science Technology and Microbiology, University of Molise, Via De Sanctis, 86100 Campobasso, Italy

The cultivated hulled wheats einkorn, emmer, and spelt, known in Italy under the common name of *farro*, are among the most ancient Triticeae cultivated in the world and have long represented a staple food. As early as Roman times, hulled wheats began to be replaced by higher-yielding, free-threshing wheats. However, the move in recent years toward more natural foods and sustainable agriculture and the rediscovery of ancient foods and flavors have brought about renewed interest in these neglected species.

For these reasons, research activities and selection programs are being conducted to assess the genetic, agronomic, and technological properties of emmer.

The main results of these studies and the knowledge acquired about the genetic, agronomic, and production aspects are reviewed in this chapter with particular emphasis on the technological and nutritional aspects.

Taxonomy and Phylogenesis

"Hulled wheat" (in the botanical sense) denotes any of the wild or cultivated *Triticum* populations that retain the hull during threshing. Their kernels are covered by tough paleas and spikelet glumes; thus, the threshing product is spikelets, not grains. Emmer is predominantly awned, with spikelets consisting of two well-developed kernels, and the emmer glumes are long and narrow with sharp beaks.

From a genetic point of view, hulled wheats represent a group of Triticeae in which hulledness is controlled by a single dominant gene, the Q factor (Szabò and Hammer 1996, Luo et al 2000).

Just as threshability is mostly a characteristic selected in cultivated crops, hulledness is primarily characteristic of ancient, obsolete, spontaneous, and wild wheats.

Hulled wheats comprise three cultivated species, made up of different levels of ploidy: einkorn (*Triticum monococcum* L., diploid: $2n = 2x = 14$ chromosomes, AA genome), emmer (*T. dicoccon* Schrank, tetraploid: $2n = 4x = 28$ chromosomes, AABB genome), and spelt (*T. spelta* L., hexaploid: $2n = 6x = 42$ chromosomes, AABBDD genome) (Szabò and Hammer 1996).

TABLE 1
Classification of Wild and Cultivated Species of *Triticum*

	Species	Genomic Formula	Wild (Brittle Spike) Hulled Grain	Hulled Grain	Cultivated (Non-brittle-Spike) Free-Threshing
Diploids ($2n = 14$)	*T. monococcum*	A^mA^m	subsp. *boeticum* (wild einkorn)	subsp. *monococcum* (cultivated einkorn)	...
Tetraploids ($2n = 28$)	*T. turgidum*	AABB	subsp. *dicoccoides* (wild emmer)	subsp. *dicoccum* (cultivated emmer)	subsp. *durum*
Hexaploids ($2n = 42$)	*T. aestivum*	AABBDD	...	subsp. *spelta*	subsp. *aestivum* (bread wheat)

T. dicoccon Schrank 1789 is generally accepted as the scientific denomination for emmer, although *T. dicoccum* Schubler 1819 (syn. *T. vulgare* subsp. *dicoccum* Korn. 1885, *T. sativum* subsp. *dicoccum* Aschers. et Graebn. 1901, and *T. turgidum* subsp. *dicoccum* (Schrank) Thell. 1918) are also often used.

The AA genomic constitution of emmer is thought to be derived from *T. monococcum*, while various sources for the BB genome have been suggested: *T. speltoides*, *T. searsii*, and *T. tripsacoides* (Morris and Sears 1967, Kimber and Sears 1987). *T. dicoccon,* derived from its wild progenitor *T. dicoccoides* has, in turn, originated different species of hulless tetraploid wheats (*T. turgidum durum*, etc.) (Table 1). Moreover, the genomes of both emmer (AABB) and *Aegilops tauschii* (DD) have been combined to give origin to *T. spelta* (AABBDD), which therefore does not have a wild hexaploid ancestor (Perrino et al 1996a, Porceddu and Lafiandra 1986, Hsam et al 2001).

Wild emmer, *T. dicoccoides*, like wild einkorn, *T. boeticum*, is distinguished by the brittleness of the rachis, which, when mature, disarticulates into individual spikelets in order to favor seed dissemination. The rachis of cultivated emmer is less fragile and tends to remain intact until threshed.

Origin and Diffusion

T. dicoccon Schrank (emmer) originated in the mountains of the Fertile Crescent, in Iran, Iraq, Jordan, Syria, and Palestine, where its wild progenitor (*T. dicoccoides*) still thrives. Therefore, the Middle East is regarded as its probable center of origin (Perrino et al 1996a).

Emmer is distributed over a vast area, extending from its center of origin to as far as India, Russia, Ethiopia, North Africa, the Iberian peninsula, Italy, and Turkey.

Emmer was cultivated from the beginnings of agriculture until Graeco-Roman times, when it was replaced by free-threshing wheats. Cultivated emmer emerged as the predominant wheat. It and barley were the chief cereals used in the late Mesolithic and early Neolithic periods around 10,000 B.C. (Zohary and Hopf 1993). Emmer was also the principal wheat cultivated throughout the Middle and Far East, Europe, and North Africa from the Stone Age (Neolithic period) through to the Bronze Age, 10,000–4,000 B.C. It continued to be grown throughout the Bronze Age 4,000–1,000 B.C., although it gradually began to be replaced by naked wheats, primarily the tetraploid species. Emmer was widely cultivated in Ancient Egypt where, together with barley, it was transformed into staples such as bread and beer (malt) (Samuel 1993, Nesbitt and Samuel 1996). It was also widely cultivated and used during Roman times for making *puls* (porridge), *alica* (groats/semolina), and breads (Braun 1995). The ancient Roman *puls* was a primitive meal made up of whole or coarsely crushed emmer grain boiled in water or milk. The Roman scholar Pliny specifically mentioned emmer in his *Naturalis Historia*, referring to it as *far/adoreum*: "It was the primary food of ancient Latium, and we have proof of this in the offering of the *adoria.*" (*Adorea* was the prize given to the soldiers who returned victorious from battle).

In Roman times, the popularity of emmer waned to such an extent that emmer bread was used only according to traditional custom to celebrate Roman marriages, known as *confarreatio*. As part of the ceremony, the young bride was to carry a loaf of emmer bread, the *farreum* (Papa 1996).

Later, emmer was superseded by high-yielding and free-threshing species and today is to be found only in a few pockets of land in Ethiopia, the Balkans, Italy, Spain, Anatolia, Iran, Turkey, Caucasia, and India.

Germ Plasm, Genetics, and Breeding

The world collection of emmer (>2,000 accessions) is stored in a few gene banks: in the United States (≈900 accessions at Fort Collins), Germany (≈450 accessions at the Gatersleben and Braunschweig gene banks), Russia (≈400 accessions at the Vavilov Institute, St Petersburg), Syria (≈350 accessions at the Genetic Resources Unit of ICARDA, Aleppo), and Italy (≈370 accessions at the Germplasm Institute of Bari) (Jaradat et al 1996, Perrino et al 1996a, Merezhko et al 1997).

Wild and cultivated emmer species were successfully used in breeding programs to improve the agronomic (abiotic and biotic stress resistance) and technological (color, gluten quality) properties of common and durum wheat in the United States, Russia, Canada, Italy, India, and other countries (Levy and Feldman 1987, Blanco et al 1990, Damania et al 1992, Hakim et al 1993, Feldman et al 1996, Merezhko et al 1997, Skovmand et al 1997, Sissons and Hare 2002, Schlichting et al 2003).

However, up to a few years ago, emmer had not been subject to genetic improvement, which enabled its original characteristics to be preserved. Prebreeding and breeding work (germ plasm assessment and the selection of better lines) were aimed exclusively at assessing yield stability and quality traits in order to select the best genotypes and register new cultivars (Perrino et al 1991, 1993; Laghetti et al 1999).

Only recently have rather controversial crosses between emmer and durum wheat been carried out to improve the agronomic and technological properties (gluten strength) of emmer. These crosses, however, run the risk of reproducing a hulled version of durum wheat.

Molecular Markers

Molecular markers are powerful tools for investigating and characterizing genetic variability, inter- and intraspecific relationships, and genetic resources of wheats. These techniques include restriction fragment length polymorphisms (RFLPs), random amplified polymorphic DNA (RAPD), and microsatellite loci of simple sequence repeats (SSRs). Figliuolo and Perrino (2004) assessed the genetic diversity of an emmer collection using 15 microsatellite loci SSRs and 19 RFLP probes. They found an average Dice's genetic distance (GD) of 0.22 when analyzing 38 emmer accessions by RFLPs and 0.38 when analyzing 194 emmer accessions by SSRs; these distances were higher than those for durum wheat (GD = 0.13; Figliuolo and Spagnoletti-Zeuli 2000), common wheat (GD = 0.09; Siedler et al 1994), and spelt (GD = 0.10; Bertin et al 2001). The Dice GD measures the number of unshared bands from multiple loci profiles for each genotypic pairwise comparison and for each class of genetic markers (Figliuolo and Perrino 2004). Genetic distances based on coancestry coefficients have brought to light the greater differentiation between the Italian and the Ethiopian germ plasm as opposed to the Spanish and Russian-Iranian germ plasm. In addition, the study showed that it is possible to identify each genotype with a minimum number of 10 loci per marker class.

Barcaccia et al (2002), when assessing the genetic diversity within and the relationships between 11 Italian local varieties of emmer by 17 RAPD marker loci, found that over half of the total genetic diversity (52%) was within populations, indicating that local emmer varieties are a mixture of a large number of distinct genotypes, despite the high level of selfing. The overall results confirm the great variability that can be found in landrace populations, underlining the values of landraces as an irreplaceable bank of genetically diversified and highly coadapted genotypes.

Therefore, this approach could be extremely useful in drawing basic conclusions about the genetic relationships between emmer genotypes, to fingerprint emmer cultivars and populations, to trace the genomes of newly released cultivars (true or hybrid emmers, *T. dicoccon* × *T. durum*), and to ensure the traceability of emmer chains (from the seed to the table), thus protecting both the breeder and farmer as well as the consumer.

Production and Importance

The renewed interest in traditional foods in agriculturally advanced countries has enabled hulled wheat to survive as a niche crop, whereas its low yields and difficulty in manipulation have led to a further decline in cultivation in countries where agricultural development is less advanced.

For these reasons, emmer is grown today only in limited areas in the Balkans, Italy, Spain, Anatolia, Iran, Turkey, Caucasia, and India. However, it had also spread to Ethiopia on the Abyssinian plateau, where it is still cultivated and appreciated (Perrino et al 1996a, Reddy et al 1998).

In Italy, renewed interest in emmer and research to characterize and improve quality (Perrino and Hammer 1982, 1984) have led to the selection and registration of a number of emmer populations and cultivars such as Basian, Farvento, Lucanica, Molise Colli, and Farro della Garfagnana (Bozzini et al 1994, Perrino et al 1996b). In 1996, the Farro della Garfagnana emmer was granted the designation of Protected Geographical Indication by the European Community (EEC 1996).

In Italy, around 1,500 ha of emmer are cultivated, primarily in the regions of Molise (≈350 ha), Basilicata (≈300 ha), and Tuscany (≈200 ha), as well as a few dozen hectares in each of the Abruzzo, Umbria, Apulia, Campania, and Lazio regions. Therefore, the average annual production amounts to around 2,500–3,000 t of dehulled grain.

In the rest of Europe, a few thousand hectares are still cultivated in marginal areas, and in Turkey there were about 10,000 ha in 1993 (Karagoz 1996). A few hectares are cultivated in the Asturias Region (Spain), in Russia, and in the Balkan areas (Pena-Chocarro 1996, Perrino et al 1996a, Merezhko et al 1997).

In India, emmer represents approximately 1% of the total wheat production (90% *T. aestivum* and 9% *T. durum*) and is cultivated on about 200,000 ha (Reddy et al 1998). In the United States, limited amounts of spring emmer are grown in small areas throughout Montana and North Dakota. In particular, two unidentified emmer selections are grown and available in limited amounts from a small number of seed grain dealers (Stallknecht et al 1996).

Agronomic Aspects

T. dicoccon comes into its own when cultivated in marginal areas and under conditions of sustainable agriculture, where modern wheats are unable to develop their full productive potentials because they have been genetically selected for favorable pedoclimatic and agronomic conditions. It is only under these conditions that emmer cultivation is justified and its agronomic performance (yield) becomes profitable with respect to modern free-threshing wheats.

Agronomic Practices

Cultivation Areas

Emmer is best cultivated on hillsides and in mountainous and marginal areas where no other crop can be grown economically, where its typical characteristics, such as the ability to adapt to poor and stony soils, resistance to low temperatures, considerable ability to control weeds, and resistance to diseases common to other cereals can be used to advantage (Corazza et al 1986, D'Antuono 1989, Hakim et al 1993, Castagna et al 1996, Merezhko et al 1997).

Sowing Aspects

Emmer genotypes are divided into winter types, which need a certain degree of vernalization, and spring types (D'Antuono and Pavoni 1993, Merezhko et al 1997). Spring types are sometimes planted very late in plots where more profitable crops could not be planted because of unexpected adverse weather conditions.

The Germplasm Institute of Bari (Italy) conducted a study specifically to investigate the growth habit of emmer and spelt germ plasm, comparing 312 emmer accessions and 311 spelt accessions in a two-year field trial covering both spring and winter sowings. The results showed wide genetic variability: of the emmer accessions, 10% (23% for spelt) were found to have a winter growth habit, and 30% were spring types (27% for spelt); the remaining 60% (50% for spelt) had a semiwinter growth habit. This type of screening could be valuable to breeders who want to obtain improved lines for this phenological trait (Skovmand et al 1997, Laghetti et al 2001).

The usual seeding rate adopted by farmers is 150 kg/ha (hulled grain), equivalent to approximately 200 kernels per square meter. However, some experimental trials have shown that a significant increase in yield can be obtained by increasing the rate of seeding to 400 germinating seeds per square meter (D'Antuono 1989, Mariani et al 1992, Castagna et al 1996).

Fertilizers and Weed Control

Low-input techniques (organic and sustainable agriculture) are mainly used to cultivate this species since it is resistant to abiotic and biotic stresses (Corazza et al 1986, D'Antuono 1989, Damania et al 1992). Organic manure is often the only fertilizer applied, and chemicals (including herbicides), are virtually not used. Emmer controls the weeds with its high tillering power and height. This species does not significantly benefit from the application of nitrogen-based fertilizers (in some cases, this results in reduced yields) since the very height of the plant (>100 cm) makes it prone to lodging. Experiments specifically carried out to test the plant's reaction to different nitrogen levels (0–150 kg/ha) showed, in fact, that high nitrogen levels did not increase grain yield, whereas modern wheats significantly responded with higher yield (Castagna et al 1996, D'Antuono 1989, Mariani et al 1992, Schiavone et al 2000). These findings illustrate the influence that prolonged genetic improvement activities have had on the ideotype of modern wheats compared with the still-primitive emmer. Therefore, it is possible to state that emmer is a crop best suited to agronomic practices that have low environmental impact.

Agronomic Performance

The results of evaluation tests on the germ plasm of hulled wheats conserved at the Germplasm Institute of Bari (Table 2) show that the emmer accessions are tall plants (plant height varying from 69 to 140 cm, the average height always over 100 cm) with low grain yields (0.6–4.9 t/ha, the averages ranging from 1.4 to 2.6 t/ha). Merezhko et al (1997) established an average plant height of 83.3 cm, ranging from 34 to 130.2 cm in 369 emmer accessions cultivated near St Petersbourg. Stallknecht et al (1996) reported yields

TABLE 2
Variability of Agronomic Characteristics of Different Emmer Accessions Cultivated in Experimental Field of Marginal Areas of Southern Italy

	Perrino et al (1991)[a]				Perrino et al (1993)[a]				Laghetti et al (1997)[b]			
	Emmer (141 accessions)			Spelt (248 accessions)	Emmer (50 accessions)			Spelt (50 accessions)	Emmer (500 accessions)			Spelt (250 accessions)
Character	Min	Max	Mean	Mean	Min	Max	Mean	Mean	Min	Max	Mean	Mean
Plant height (cm)	98.0	161.0	131.4	147.9	76.7	137.3	104.6	119.7	69.0	140.0	104.7	117.4
Hulled grain yield (t/ha)	1.5	7.3	3.9	4.7	2.1	5.3	3.9	3.8	0.8	3.9	2.0	2.4
Naked grain yield (t/ha)	0.6	4.9	2.6	2.9	1.1	3.7	2.6	2.5	0.6	3.1	1.4	1.9

[a] Cultivated in Molise.
[b] Cultivated in Basilicata.

from 0.2 to 3.7 t/ha in 350 U.S. emmer accessions, from the National Small Grain Germplasm Research Facility, Aberdeen, ID, cultivated in experimental fields at the Southern Agricultural Research Center, Huntley, MT. These authors also found that advanced selections of emmer produced dehulled kernel yields ranging from 1.5 to 2.5 t/ha (equivalent to 48–84% of spring wheat yields) under dryland cropping.

Advanced selections and local populations of emmer were also assessed over a four-year test period coordinated by the CERMIS Research Centre (Tolentino, Italy) and conducted in various Italian locations (Porfiri et al 1996, AAVV 1997, 1998, 1999). The dehulled grain yields, the dehulled/hulled grain ratio, the 1,000 kernel weight, and the plant height of seven emmer genotypes cultivated in different marginal areas in central and southern Italy over four years (Fig. 1) varied considerably both in regard to genotypes and cultivation year. With regard to productivity, the findings obtained for both emmer genotypes and spelt genotypes were similar. This is quite a controversial result, since some authors have found higher yields for emmer (Perrino et al 1993; Pisante et al 1996; Galterio et al 1999, 2003; Ferrante et al 2000; Schiavone et al 2000) whereas others have found higher yields for spelt (Perrino et al 1991; Castagna et al 1996; Laghetti et al 1997, 1999). Therefore, one may conclude that it is not the case of one species having absolute ascendancy over the other but rather that either one may become predominant depending on the genotype, growing conditions, production year, and relative interactions.

With regard to the dehulling yield, the dehulled/hulled grain ratio varied between 60 and 80%, with average values of 70–75%. Similar values were found by D'Antuono (1989) (72.8–75%), Castagna et al (1996) (75%), and Laghetti et al (1999) (64.1–72.8%).

A wide range of variability was found in 1,000-kernel weight (from 30 to 45 g), which was influenced by genotype and growing conditions, as highlighted in Figure 1.

The test weight of emmer, an important parameter for assessing the commercial value of the grain, is almost invariably lower than that of modern wheats, as shown by Schiavone et al (2000) (74.8 kg/hL for emmer, vs. 83.4 and 82.6 kg/hL for durum and soft wheat, respectively), Fares et al (2003) (65.4 kg/hL for emmer, vs. 79.8 kg/hL for durum wheat), Pisante et al (1996) (64.8 kg/hL vs. 79.6 kg/hL for soft wheat), and Schlichting et al (2003) (78.8 kg/hL vs. 82.5 for durum wheat).

To improve the agronomic characteristics of emmer (yield, plant height, and test weight), questionable genetic improvement programs have been undertaken, crossing it with durum wheat. This has resulted in the creation of three hybrid emmers, Davide, Padre Pio, and Mosè, which attain significantly higher yields than those obtained from true emmer (Codianni et al 1998, 2000; Galterio et al 1998, 2003). This approach seems the least appropriate for enhancing the qualities of emmer which, in order to become better established, should be further differentiated from modern wheats, especially from durum wheat.

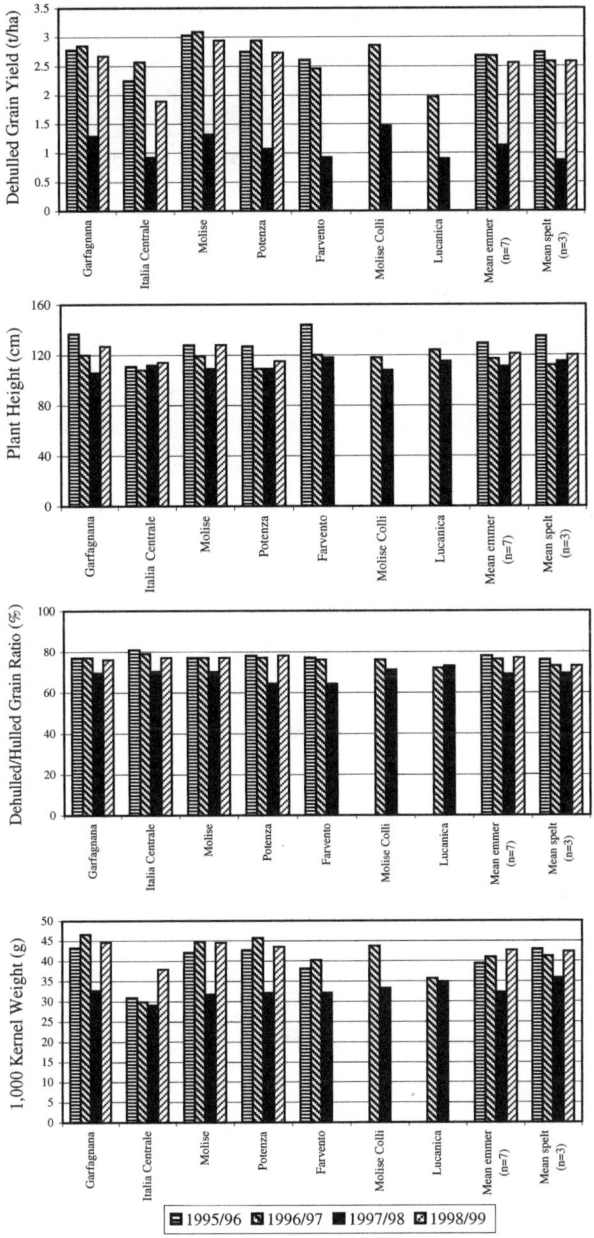

Fig. 1. Variability of agronomic characteristics of selected emmer populations cultivated in a multiyear test in different Italian locations. Spelt values are the means of three genotypes, Altgold Rotkorn, Rouquin, and Triventina. (Data from Porfiri et al, 1996; AAVV, 1997, 1998, 1999)

Chemical and Nutritional Composition

A study by the authors (Table 3) showed the proximate composition of the whole meal and the refined flour/semolina of three emmer genotypes. The proximate composition of emmer meal, when compared at the same level of refinement, is similar to that of spelt, durum, and bread wheats.

Therefore, the superior nutritional characteristics often claimed for emmer and hulled wheats in general, compared to free-threshing wheats, may be attributed to the following improper comparisons: (1) evaluation of meals characterized by different levels of refinement: whole meal for hulled wheat and refined meal (flour and semolina) for modern wheats; (2) evaluation of emmer-based end-products (pasta/bread, biscuits, etc.) made with whole meal or less-refined meal compared to end-products obtained with more-refined meals (white flour, semolina); and (3) smaller and weathered kernels (with low kernel weight and low test weight) for emmer, characterized by a higher surface-to-volume ratio and, consequently, more bran and aleurone layer per meal weight unit.

Protein Content

A selection of data available in the literature (Table 4) on the protein content and gluten quality of *T. dicoccum* shows significant variability. For example, Blanco et al (1990) found a protein range of 8.7–18.0% db (mean 12.5% db) in 50 accessions, whereas Perrino et al (1993) found a range of 14.2–20.2% db in another 50 accessions but a significantly higher average of 17.1% db. Others have confirmed this protein content variability with

TABLE 3
Energy and Proximate Composition of Whole Meal and Flour of Three Emmer Wheat Genotypes (per 100 g wb)[a,b]

	Farvento		Lucanica		Molise Colli	
	Whole Meal	Flour	Whole Meal	Flour	Whole Meal	Flour
Energy						
Kcal	307	330	303	327	311	329
kJ	1,303	1,399	1,283	1,388	1,320	1,396
Protein (g)	13.6	12.5	11.8	10.9	10.2	9.7
Lipid (g)	2.7	1.8	2.6	1.5	3.0	1.8
Ash (g)	1.88	0.70	1.84	0.82	1.79	0.88
Total dietary fiber (g)	10.4	4.6	11.3	4.8	9.6	4.6
Insoluble	8.3	3.2	9.0	3.0	7.3	2.7
Soluble	2.1	1.4	2.3	1.8	2.3	1.9
Soluble/total	0.20	0.30	0.20	0.38	0.24	0.41
Digestible carbohydrate (g)[c]	57.2	65.9	58.0	67.5	60.9	68.5

[a] Source: E. Marconi and R. Cubadda, *unpublished data*.
[b] Standardized at 14.5% moisture.
[c] Calculated by difference.

values ranging from 7.9% (Galterio et al 1994) to 19.9% db (Marconi and Schiavone 1997), depending on both the genotype and the cultivation environment (Galterio et al 1999, 2003; Schiavone et al 2000; Marconi et al 2004).

The protein content of hulled wheats (emmer and spelt) was consistently higher than those of modern wheats (*T. aestivum* and *T. durum*) cultivated under the same agronomic conditions (Castagna et al 1996, Reddy et al 1998, Marconi et al 1999b, Schiavone et al 2000). However, this does not justify the classification of emmer and hulled wheats in general as protein-rich crops since their high protein level (and high content of other nutrients) could be a consequence of low grain yield. In fact, on comparing the protein yields (g/m^2), the values for emmer are similar or lower than those for modern wheats (Piergiovanni et al 1996, Cubadda and Marconi 2001, Marconi et al 2004). For example, Piergiovanni et al (1996) found that protein yields of emmer (450 kg/ha) and spelt (460 kg/ha) were lower than that of the control wheats (mean 550 kg/ha), although the grain protein contents of the emmer (16.7% db) and spelt (17.1% db) were significantly higher than in durum wheats (15.3% db). When nitrogen fertilizer is used sparingly or not at all, hulled wheats can attain both higher protein content and protein yield since, under such conditions, modern wheats are unable to fully develop their potentials (E. Marconi, M. Carcea, G. Bassotti, L. Bartoli, and R. Cubadda, *unpublished data*).

TABLE 4
Protein Content and Gluten Quality (SDS[a] Sedimentation Test) of Emmer Wheat (Whole Meal) Reported by Different Authors

Reference	Samples (*n*)	Protein (% db; N × 5.70)		SDS Sedimentation Test (mL)	
		Range	Mean	Range	Mean
Blanco et al (1990)	50	8.7–18.0	12.5	25–53	34
Perrino et al (1993)	50	14.2–20.2	17.1	24–66	33
Galterio et al (1994)	9 (3 × 3)[b]	7.9–10.4	9.3	20–26	22
Piergiovanni et al (1996)	50	13.7–18.8	16.7	26–53	34
Marconi and Schiavone (1997)	3	12.5–19.9	17.1	18–19	19
Galterio et al (1999)	21 (7 × 3)[c]	10.0–12.0	11.0	13–18	15
Galterio et al (1999)	8	13.2–16.6	14.3	15–20	17
Schiavone et al (2001)	18 (3 × 3 × 2)[d]	11.4–19.1	15.4	13–27	20
Galterio et al (2003)	18 (3 × 6)[e]	11.6–18.5	16.1	20–38	27

[a] Sodium dodecyl sulfate.
[b] Three entries × three locations.
[c] Seven entries × three nitrogen levels.
[d] Three entries × three nitrogen levels × two locations.
[e] Three entries × six locations.

Protein Quality and Composition

Amino Acids

Data on the amino acid pattern of emmer wheat (in whole meal and refined flour) (Table 5) show a pattern similar to that of common, durum, and spelt wheats: the chief amino acids are glutamic acid (≈30 g/100 g protein) and proline (≈10 g/100 g protein), and the quantitatively minor amino acids are tryptophan (≈1.30 g/100 g protein) and methionine (≈1.5 g/100 g protein). From a nutritional point of view, the limiting amino acid, as expected, is lysine, with values ranging from 1.40 to 1.94 g/100 g of protein, resulting in chemical scores that vary between 0.36 and 0.52. The second limiting amino acid is, as in other wheat species, threonine (2.57–3.00 g/100 g protein). The essential amino acid showing the lowest percentage of the content of the same amino acid in the same quantity of a protein (real or hypothetical) selected as a reference protein is called the (first) limiting amino acid, and this percentage is the chemical score (FAO/WHO 1991).

It is interesting to note that the lysine content and the chemical score are higher in whole grain than in flour or semolina due to the presence of the aleurone layer, which is rich in albumins and globulins and characterized by a higher content of essential amino acids and lysine (Feillet 1988, Wrigley and Bietz 1988). This may have led to emmer and spelt being attributed a higher protein quality than modern wheats, simply because they are mainly used as whole meal or low-refined flour (meals) (Marconi et al 2000a). In fact, when the comparison is between whole meals or meals with the same level of refinement, the amino acid composition of emmer (hulled wheats) is equivalent to that of modern wheats (durum and soft).

Albumins and Globulins

The content of the albumin and globulin fractions in *T. dicoccon* is considerable, representing about 30–39% of total proteins (Galterio et al 1994, 1999) compared to 15–25% in durum and soft wheat (Feillet 1988, Pomeranz 1988). This finding could be attributed to the reduced production capacity of hulled wheats, which accumulate less starchy endosperm and, consequently, gliadin and glutenin. In fact, the albumins and globulins (functional proteins) are mainly found in the aleurone layer. For this reason, as protein yield increases, the percentage of albumins and globulins decreases, whereas that of gliadins increases (Gupta 1992; Galterio et al 1994, 1999).

Gliadins and Glutenins

The average percentages of gliadins and glutenins in whole-meal emmer are about 37% (range 33–39%) and 29% (range 27–33%) of total protein, respectively (Galterio et al 1994, 1999). The glutenin-gliadin ratio, which was found to be correlated with dough strength in modern wheats (Wasik and Bushuk 1975), was lower in emmer than in other wheat species (Galterio et al 1994, 1999; Wieser, 2000). Emmer, in particular, had very low proportions of total glutenins, the ratio of glutenins to gliadins being by far the lowest (Table 6).

Gliadins and glutenins can be fractionated into α, β, γ, and ω-gliadins and into high molecular weight (HMW) and low molecular weight (LMW) glu-

TABLE 5
Amino Acid Patterns (g/100 g protein) of Emmer and Reference Wheats According to Different Authors[a,b]

	Galterio et al (1994)		Cubadda and Marconi (1996)			Marconi and Cubadda (original data)			
	Emmer[c]	Durum Wheat	Emmer[d]		Soft Wheat	Emmer[e]		Durum Wheat	
Amino Acid	Whole Meal	Whole Meal	Whole Meal	Flour	Flour	Whole Meal	Flour	Whole Meal	Flour
Threonine	2.89	3.00	2.94	2.60	2.70	2.64	2.79	2.92	2.56
Valine	5.01	4.50	4.35	4.08	3.86	3.91	3.81	3.79	3.76
Methionine	1.94	1.67	1.40	1.42	1.48	1.57	1.52	1.53	1.47
Cysteine	2.60	2.17	2.24	2.19	2.30	2.08	2.18	2.18	2.30
Leucine	6.96	6.67	6.89	6.79	6.57	6.00	6.58	6.14	6.27
Isoleucine	3.86	4.00	3.65	3.44	3.17	2.88	3.23	3.01	2.77
Tyrosine	2.66	3.33	2.53	2.50	3.02	2.95	2.87	3.15	2.63
Phenylalanine	4.76	4.84	4.58	4.99	4.74	4.12	4.68	4.67	4.96
Lysine	2.95	2.83	2.46	2.11	2.06	2.80	2.32	2.94	2.30
Tryptophan	1.30	1.38	nd[f]	nd	nd	nd	nd	nd	nd
Aspartic acid	5.69	5.16	4.71	4.12	4.19	5.38	4.06	5.47	4.64
Serine	4.30	5.00	4.64	4.68	4.77	4.60	5.00	4.73	4.71
Glutamic acid	27.55	27.85	30.97	33.93	33.63	33.16	32.31	30.88	34.49
Proline	9.04	9.82	9.99	10.45	10.68	9.07	10.28	9.33	9.85
Glycine	3.99	4.00	3.29	2.92	3.24	3.36	3.11	3.52	2.83
Alanine	3.78	3.50	2.98	2.52	2.91	3.60	3.67	3.51	3.03
Arginine	4.68	4.50	4.91	4.06	3.72	4.30	3.96	4.42	4.05
Histidine	2.33	2.17	2.46	2.19	1.97	2.61	2.61	2.81	2.39
Essential amino acids	33.6	33.0	31.0	30.1	29.9	28.9	30.0	30.3	29.0
Chemical score[g]	0.51	0.49	0.42	0.36	0.36	0.48	0.40	0.51	0.40

[a] The sum of amino acids (without tryptophan) was normalized at 95% protein in order to allow a correct comparison between data.
[b] The first limiting amino acid is underlined.
[c] Mean of three genotypes.
[d] Mean of one genotype.
[e] Mean of three genotypes.
[f] Not determined.
[g] Based on the FAO 1985 pattern (threonine = 3.40; valine = 3.50; methionine + cysteine = 2.50; leucine = 6.60; isoleucine = 2.80; tyrosine + phenylalanine = 6.30; lysine = 5.80) (FAO/WHO, 1991).

TABLE 6
Proportion (%) of Gluten Protein Types in Flours from Different Wheat Species (Gluten = 100%)[a]

	Gliadins (GLI)				Glutenins (GLU)				
Wheat Species	α (α + β)	γ	ω	Total	HMW[b]	LMW[b]	ωb[c]	Total	GLU/GLI
Bread wheat (winter)	32.3	23.1	9.1	64.5	9.1	25.1	1.3	35.5	0.55
Bread wheat (spring)	28.0	30.4	13.2	71.6	9.3	18.3	0.8	28.4	0.40
Spelt	35.7	29.6	10.0	75.3	6.6	17.7	0.4	24.7	0.33
Durum wheat	39.0	30.0	6.4	75.4	5.0	19.3	0.3	24.6	0.33
Emmer	45.3	31.3	10.2	86.8	2.6	10.0	0.6	13.2	0.15
Einkorn	44.6	19.8	12.3	76.7	3.5	19.3	0.5	23.3	0.30

[a] Data from Wieser (2000).
[b] HMW = high molecular weight, LMW = low molecular weight.
[c] Glutenin-bound ω-gliadins.

tenins by polyacrylamide gel electrophoresis (acid-PAGE and SDS-PAGE), reversed-phase high-performance liquid chromatography (RP-HPLC), and capillary electrophoresis (CE).

Piergiovanni and Volpe (2003), using CE, found that β- and ω-gliadins were better for differentiating within a hulled wheat species (emmer or spelt), whereas γ- and ω-gliadins were more useful in discriminating emmer from spelt. In addition, considerable gliadin similarity was found between species with the same genome composition (durum wheat and emmer; common wheat and spelt). Quantitative characterization of the gliadin proteins of different wheat species by RP-HPLC (Wieser 2000) showed that the α (α+β) fractions dominated in hulled wheats (Table 6). Seilmeier et al (2001), in their study on the gliadins of emmer and spelt (one cultivar each) by RP-HPLC, observed that the proportion and pattern of ω-gliadins were strongly determined by the species and, within each species, by the genotype. The presence of the ω5-subgroup and the ω1,2-subgroup in emmer was reported by Kasarda et al (1983). The differences in the quantities of glutenin subunits between wheat species were even more pronounced than for the gliadins (Table 6). Hexaploid wheats (soft and spelt wheats) had significantly greater quantities of HMW glutenins than tetraploid and diploid wheats, whereas such a trend was not found for the LMW subunits (Wieser 2000). Emmer, in particular, had very low values for both the HMW and LMW subunits.

HMW and LMW subunits are of considerable interest because they affect bread and pasta quality (Payne et al 1984, Pena et al 1993). Nevertheless, those glutenin subunits linked to γ-45 gliadin seem to have a beneficial effect on pasta quality because of their strong aggregative properties. Durum wheat varieties that possess LMW-2 glutenin, which is associated with the ω-35 and γ-45 gliadin subunits, have a high gluten quality (gluten strength), whereas those that possess LMW-1 glutenin, associated with the ω-33, ω-38, and γ-42 gliadin subunits, have poor gluten quality (Payne et al 1984, Pogna et al 1990, Galterio et al 1998). With regard to the HMW glutenins, the 7+8 subunit affects pasta quality to a greater extent than the 20, 6+8, and 13+16 subunits (Boggini and Pogna 1989).

Galterio et al (1994, 1998, 2000, 2001), Mariani et al (2000), and Vallega and Waines (1987), using acid-PAGE and SDS-PAGE in all the emmer populations examined, identified the HMW subunit 1 (coded at locus *Glu-A1*, which is not usually found in durum wheat varieties) and the lack of γ-42, γ-45, and ω-35 gliadin subunits. Regarding HMW glutenins coded at locus *Glu-B1*, the emmer population showed the combinations 6+8 and 13+16 subunits. The 7+8 combination, found solely in some spikelets of the Molise Colli emmer population (Mariani et al 2000, 2001) is to be attributed more to spontaneous crosses than to intervention for quality improvement (Galterio et al 1998). Moreover, the lack of γ-45 and the related LMW-2 subunit, is responsible for the poor gluten characteristics detected in emmer wheats (Galterio et al 1994, 1998, 2001; Fares et al 2003).

On the contrary, Hakim et al (1993) found subunit 45 in some emmer accessions collected within the species' center of origin in the Fertile Crescent. These accessions could be used to improve the technological properties of emmer cultivars. Therefore, crosses between Molise Colli emmer and the Italian durum wheat variety Simeto, which has excellent gluten strength, were made. In this way, new genotypes (hybrid emmers) with good technological performances were obtained (Davide, Padre Pio, and Mosè). All of these genotypes had HMW 7+8 and LMW-2 glutenin, as well as ω-35 and γ-45 gliadin subunits that were not present in the emmer parent (Codianni et al 1998, 2000; Galterio et al 2001; Fares et al 2003).

The characterization of emmer gliadins and glutenins brings us to the problem of celiac disease. There have been anecdotal reports, not supported by any rigorous scientific evaluation, suggesting that hulled wheats are not toxic to celiac patients.

Species within the genus *Triticum* and the *turgidum* species are almost certainly harmful to people suffering from celiac disease. The very close affinity of emmer with bread and particularly with durum wheats, as attested by the considerable similarity of their α-, γ-, and ω-gliadins, which are responsible for celiac disease, means that emmer would be just as harmful to celiac patients as bread wheat, durum wheat, spelt, rye, barley, and triticale (Kasarda 2001). This was further confirmed in a specific study by Wieser (2001), in which emmer, bread, and spelt wheats had a high degree of sequence homology within the N-terminal region and considerable similarity of corresponding sequences of α-gliadin fractions. In particular, the potential celiac toxic sequences (PSQQQP, one-letter-code for amino acids, positions 13–18) occurred. In addition, on assaying two emmer and two spelt genotypes using the immunochemical test developed by Skerrit and Hill (1990) based on the detection of ω-gliadins by monoclonal antibodies, E. Marconi and R. Cubadda (*unpublished data*) found unmistakable immunoreactivity.

For all these reasons, emmer is assumed to be a toxic cereal for celiac patients and should therefore be avoided. Thus, emmer should be included by the EC Directive (EC 2003) in the list of allergenic foodstuffs (ingredients) containing gluten, together with wheat, rye, barley, oats, spelt, kamut, and their hybridized strains.

Digestible Carbohydrates (Starch)

Total starch is the main nutritional component of the emmer kernel (whole meal), with values ranging from 52.7 to 56.8% db (Galterio et al 2003). These values are similar to those of durum wheat, although the lowest values could be attributed to hulled wheats' minor capacity for starch accumulation compared to that of modern wheats. From a nutritional point of view, total starch can be divided into rapidly digestible starch (RDS), slowly digestible starch (SDS), and resistant starch (RS). The latter starch fraction is not susceptible to enzymatic hydrolysis and can be included in the dietary fiber. Galterio et al (2003) found that, in three emmer genotypes, the RDS, SDS, and RS amounted to around 30, 51, and 18% of total starch, respectively. The high SDS and RS values are typical of whole cereals that contain starch granules scarcely accessible to amylase (Colonna et al 1992, Behall and Hallfrish 2002,

Slavin 2002). High amylose concentration is one of the most relevant factors in determining starch resistance to digestion, since amylose is more slowly digested than amylopectin (Mohammadkhani et al 1998, Behall and Hallfrish 2002). Mohammadkhani et al (1998) found an amylose content ranging from 21.8 to 28.7% and from 19 to 31% in 96 accessions of emmer and 254 accessions of *T. dicoccoides*, respectively. These ranges are broad enough that it should be possible to select for high and low amylose content. In fact, Mohammadkhani et al (1999), by crossing the two highest-amylose and the two lowest-amylose emmer lines, obtained F2 populations characterized by a wider ranging amylose content (7–38%) and showed that amylose traits are genetically controlled.

Similar values of amylose were found by Galterio et al (2003) in three emmer populations (21.9–22.6% db, equivalent to about 40% of the total starch) and by Galterio et al (2001) in selected lines obtained from crossing emmer with durum wheat.

Dietary Fiber

Whole-meal emmer, like all whole-meal cereals, is a good source of dietary fiber and is characterized by a marked predominance of insoluble components, mostly cellulose and hemicellulose, over soluble components. The whole meal of three emmer genotypes had a total dietary fiber content of about 10–12% db, mainly insoluble fractions (85–88% of total fiber) (Table 3). Lower values of total dietary fiber were found by Galterio et al (1994) in three emmer populations (mean 7.11%), and by Galterio et al (1999) in another seven emmer populations (mean 8.4% db, range 8.04–8.94% db), where the soluble dietary fiber (mean 1.69% db, range 1.57–1.84% db) was about 20% of the total dietary fiber. In refined flour (ash 0.95% db), total dietary fiber content is significantly reduced, to around 5.0% db, and the ratio between soluble and total fiber (40%) is increased (Table 3).

β-Glucan, a soluble fiber component with hypocholesterolemic and hypoglycemic effects, is present in very small amounts in hulled wheats, similarly to free-threshing wheats (0.5–1.0% db) (Marconi et al 1999a). The whole meal of three Italian emmer varieties (Molise Colli, Farvento, and Lucanica) had a β-glucan content ranging from 0.6 to 0.8% db, similar to that of the durum wheat cultivar, Simeto (0.8% db) (E. Marconi and R. Cubadda, *unpublished data*).

D'Antuono et al (1998) and Galletti et al (1996) used pyrolysis/gas-chromatography/mass-spectrometry to analyze the pericarp fiber of 10 emmer samples. Pyrolysis fragments derived from the polysaccharide fraction were significantly more abundant in emmer than in durum wheat, whereas the highest percentage of lignin-derived pyrolysis fragments was detected in durum wheat. The pattern of furanic and pyranic compounds, derived from the polysaccharide fraction, and of the guaiacyl, *p*-hydroxyphenyl, and syringyl units, derived from lignin, showed significant differences between emmer and durum wheats. These data should be confirmed and investigated further by evaluation of a larger number of genotypes. The quantitative-qualitative composition of the pericarp fiber could be useful for discrimination of hulled and dehulled wheat species and to assess the susceptibility of hulled wheats to pests. Trematerra et al (1999) found that dehulled grain of emmer and spelt was more liable to be attacked by *Sitophilus oryzae* than durum and soft wheat grain, probably because of the greater release of volatile compounds from the pericarp layers.

Lipid

Lipids are relatively minor constituents in cereal grains. However, they must be taken into consideration when discussing nutrition, grain storage, and processing. The lipid fraction, particularly minor components such as phytosterols and tocochromanols, can contribute to the characterization of the botanical origin of grain and flour. Moreover, these substances may have an important role in human nutrition as they regulate serum cholesterol absorption and may reduce the risk of onset of certain tumors (Eldin and Appelqvist 1996, Piironen et al 2002).

Lipid Content

The lipid content of emmer has been reported in very few investigations. Marconi et al (2001) found an average lipid content of 2.8% db (range 2.4–3.0% db) in nine emmer genotypes, similar to that found in 12 spelt genotypes (mean 2.7% db, range 2.5–3.0% db) and in five varieties of durum wheat (2.8% db) but higher than in three cultivars of soft wheat (2.5% db). All the samples were cultivated in the same experimental field under the same agronomical conditions. The difference between the hulled and soft wheats could be mainly attributed to the larger amount of free lipid fraction, as also found by Ruibal-Mendieta et al 2002) in numerous accessions of spelt and soft wheat. Lower lipid values were found by Piergiovanni et al (1996) in 50 accessions of emmer (average 2.0% db; range 1.4–2.8% db), in 37 accessions of spelt (mean 2.1% db; range 1.7–2.5% db), and in three durum wheat varieties (1.5% db). This difference could be due to the different analytical methods used for lipid determination (Cubadda and Marconi, 2001).

Fatty Acids

The fatty acid composition of emmer compared with those of spelt and modern wheats (Table 7) shows that, as in the reference wheats, the primary fatty acid is linoleic (C18:2) (60% of total fatty acids), followed by oleic (C18:1) (19%), palmitic (C16:0) (16%), linolenic (C18:3) (4%), and stearic acid (C18:0) (1%). In addition, Marconi et al (2001) found a limited variability in the percentage of fatty acids between genotypes of the same species (CV $< 10\%$). With regard to the various species analyzed, on the one hand, oleic acid content (C18:1) was found to be higher in hulled wheats and durum wheats (17–19%) than in soft wheat (13%). On the other hand, soft wheat had higher linoleic acid (C18:2) and linolenic acid (C18:3) values. No differences were found in the total unsaturated/saturated fatty acid ratios (TUFA/SFA) and in the polyunsaturated/monounsaturated ratios (PUFA/MUFA) among emmer, spelt, and durum wheats.

TABLE 7
Fatty Acid Composition (% of total fatty acids) of Emmer and Reference Wheats[a]

Fatty Acid[b]	Emmer[c] Mean	Emmer[c] Range	Spelt[d]	Durum Wheat	Bread Wheat
Myristic C14:0	trace	trace	trace	trace	trace
Palmitic C16:0	16.3	15.5–18.0	16.3	16.5	16.3
Palmitoleic C16:1	trace	trace	trace	trace	trace
Stearic C18:0	0.9	0.7–1.0	0.8	1.2	0.8
Oleic C18:1	18.8	17.6–21.3	17.1	17.8	12.7
Linoleic C18:2	59.8	57.0–61.4	62.0	59.7	64.9
Linolenic C18:3	4.2	3.8–4.8	3.8	4.8	5.1
Eicosenoic C20:1	trace	trace	trace	trace	trace
SFA	17.2	16.2–19.0	17.1	17.7	17.1
MUFA	18.8	17.6–21.3	17.1	17.8	12.7
PUFA	64.0	60.8–66.2	65.8	64.5	70.0
TUFA:SFA ratio	4.8	4.6–4.8	4.8	4.6	4.8
PUFA:MUFA ratio	3.4	3.1–3.4	3.6	3.7	5.5

[a] Data from Marconi et al (2001).
[b] SFA = saturated fatty acids; MUFA = monounsaturated fatty acids; PUFA = polyunsaturated fatty acids; TUFA = total unsaturated fatty acids.
[c] Nine varieties.
[d] Twelve varieties.

Phytosterols

Phytosterols may have a role in preventing colon cancer and reducing total serum cholesterol (Piironen et al 2000). Cereals contain free sterols and stanols (saturated sterols) and conjugated sterols (steryl fatty acid esters and steryl glycosides). The total sterol and free sterol composition of emmer (whole meal) was characterized by Iafelice et al (2004a) and Pelillo et al (2003). The total and free sterol content of hulled (emmer and spelt) and hulless (soft and durum wheat) wheat species, summarized in Table 8, show that the main sterol was β-sitosterol, followed by campesterol and stigmasterol. A considerable amount of stanols (campestanol and β-sitostanol) were also found. Tetraploid species (*T. dicoccon* and *T. durum*) contain significantly larger amounts of sterols and stanols than hexaploid species (*T. spelta* and *T. aestivum*). The sterol:stanol ratio, higher in hexaploids (3.4–4.5) than in tetraploids (2.2–2.5), due to the high stanol content of emmer and durum, could be a good marker for discriminating tetraploid from hexaploid wheats. A high similarity in phytosterol composition between spelt and winter wheat fine bran was also found by Rozenberg et al (2003).

These findings underline the genetic affinity between free-threshing species and their respective hulled progenitors (*T. aestivum* with *T. spelta,* and *T. durum* with *T. dicoccon*).

The steryl fatty acid ester characterization was successfully used for distinguishing durum from soft wheat and for detecting semolina adulteration with soft wheat flour, since sitosteryl palmitate is found almost exclusively in soft wheat (Sarwar and McDonald 1993, Lindhauer 2001).

TABLE 8
Phytosterol Content (mg/100 g, db) of Hulled and Free-Threshing Wheat Species[a]

Species	Campesterol		Campestanol		Stigmasterol		β-Sitosterol		β-Sitostanol		Other Sterols		Sterol/Stanol		Σ Sterol + Stanol	
	Total[b]	Free[c]	Total[b]	Free[c]	Total[b]	Free[c]	Total[b]	Free[c]	Total[b]	Free[c]	Total[b]	Free[c]	Total[b]	Free[c]	Total[b]	Free[c]
Emmer	12.4	7.9	10.0	4.0	1.4	1.1	33.6	22.7	15.1	9.7	3.1	1.5	1.9	2.3	75.7	46.9
Spelt	10.4	4.5	6.2	1.6	1.2	1.0	38.9	14.2	10.9	3.9	2.7	1.5	2.9	2.6	70.1	26.7
Durum wheat	13.7	8.8	11.0	5.7	1.5	1.7	38.2	25.7	12.3	8.3	2.7	1.8	2.3	2.6	79.3	52.0
Soft wheat	11.4	5.7	3.9	1.3	0.8	0.9	37.5	17.8	7.0	3.6	2.7	1.5	4.6	5.0	63.4	30.8

[a] Data from Pelillo et al (2003) and Iafelice et al (2004a).
[b] Mean of five varieties.
[c] One variety.

TABLE 9
Steryl Fatty Acid Ester Composition (mg/100 g, db) of Hulled and Free-Threshing Wheat Species[a,b]

	Steryl Fatty Acid Esters				
	C16:0		C18:1		
Species	**Peak 1**	**Peak 2**	**Peak 3**	**Peak 4**	**Total**
Emmer	trace	trace	7.8	12.0	19.8
Spelt	4.9	18.2	6.4	14.0	43.5
Durum wheat	trace	trace	7.8	12.6	20.4
Soft wheat	4.0	14.0	5.5	14.4	37.9

[a] Data from Iafelice et al (2004b).
[b] The data are the average of five varieties per each species.

Caboni et al (2003) and Iafelice et al (2004b) found that emmer and spelt had similar steryl fatty acid ester compositions, as shown in Table 9. In fact, spelt and soft wheat had four major compounds (peaks) (two compounds esterified with oleic acid [C18:1] and two compounds esterified with palmitic acid [C16:0]), whereas emmer and durum wheat only had two compounds esterified with oleic acid (C18:1). In addition, the total steryl ester content of tetraploid wheats (*T. dicoccon* and *T. durum*) is significantly lower (≈20 mg/100 g db) than that of hexaploid wheats (*T. spelta*, and *T. aestivum*) (≈40 mg/100 g db).

This result further confirms the genetic affinity between hulled and free-threshing species and suggests a possible application of steryl fatty acid ester composition for detecting authenticity or adulteration in wheat products (soft or spelt flour in emmer products).

Minerals

The ash content in emmer and spelt was usually higher (>2.0% db) than in durum and soft wheats (1.7–1.8% db) (Piergiovanni et al 1996, Galterio et al 1999). This can be attributed to the lower starch accumulation capacity of the hulled species (as the low yields and low test weights imply) and to the fact that the minerals are located mainly in the outer layer of the kernel (aleurone layer). The low ash content of modern wheat species and cultivars is the result of selection, in order to increase the milling yield (Rasmusson et al 1971). Therefore, this parameter could be an indicator of the primitiveness of hulled wheats. Breeding for low mineral content might be possible for emmer since a broad range of ash contents was observed in hulled-wheat germ plasm; Piergiovanni et al (1996) found an ash content ranging from 1.75 to 2.33% db (mean value 2.00% db) in 50 emmer accessions.

The mineral composition of whole-meal emmer was thoroughly studied by Cubadda et al (2004) and Piergiovanni et al (1997); the latter study used appropriate sampling procedures (an agate laboratory mill and closed-vessel microwave digestion to avoid sample contamination) and advanced analytical technologies (inductively coupled plasma-mass spectrometry). The analysis (Table 10) shows that the Zn, Cu, Se, Li, Co, Mo, Fe, and Mn contents of

TABLE 10
Trace Element Content (mg/kg, db) in Whole Meal of Emmer and Reference Wheats According to Different Authors

	Grela (1996)		Piergiovanni et al (1997)				Cubadda et al (2004)		
Mineral	Spelt[a]	Soft Wheat	Emmer[b]	Durum Wheat	Spelt[b]	Soft Wheat	Emmer[c]	Durum Wheat	Spelt[d]
Zn	47.2	25.8	20.6	15.8	27.3	19.6	38.6	40.17	43.7
Cu	11.0	4.5	5.4	5.8	6.8	4.8	6.7	7.9	9.3
Se	0.37	0.43	0.03	0.02	0.04	0.01	0.49	0.40	0.53
Li	nd[e]	nd	5.8	6.0	8.7	8.4	nd	nd	nd
Co	1.2	1.6	nd	nd	nd	nd	0.06	0.07	0.11
Mo	0.54	0.29	nd	nd	nd	nd	1.1	1.8	1.4
Fe	0.07	0.14	nd	nd	nd	nd	42.4	38.3	57.7
Mn	51.2	35.6	nd	nd	nd	nd	30.9	26.4	35.7

[a] Mean of four varieties.
[b] Mean of ten accessions.
[c] Mean of eight accessions.
[d] Mean of twelve accessions.
[e] Not determined.

emmer and durum wheat do not substantially differ, whereas several studies (Grela 1996, Piergiovanni et al 1997, Moudry and Dvoracek 1999, Cubadda et al 2004) agree that spelt is higher in trace elements, particularly zinc, than soft wheat and tetraploid wheat. The absence of the D genome in tetraploid wheats may be related to their low Zn efficiency (Cakmak et al 1999).

With regard to the above, it should be noted that the content of single trace elements can be significantly influenced by the characteristics of the kernel (surface/volume ratio, test weight, etc.).

Vitamins

The riboflavin (vitamin B-2), thiamin (vitamin B-1), carotenoid (provitamin A), and tocochromanol (vitamin E) contents in whole-meal emmer, compared to those in the reference wheats, are reported in Table 11.

With regard to tocochromanols, the main vitamers found were, in decreasing order, β-tocotrienol, α-tocopherol, β-tocopherol, and α-tocotrienol (Panfili et al 2004). No appreciable levels of γ-tocopherol, γ-tocotrienol, δ-tocopherol, or δ-tocotrienol were found in any of the species analyzed. The tocotrienol/-tocopherol ratio was much higher in emmer and durum wheat (3.6 and 3.5, respectively) than in spelt and soft wheat (2.0). This ratio could be used as an index to make distinctions between spelt and emmer as well as between durum and soft wheats (Marconi et al 2001).

α-Tocopherol, considered the most biologically active form of tocochromanol, varied from a mean value of 7.10 mg/kg (db) in emmer to 10.01 and

TABLE 11
Vitamin Content (mg/kg, db) of Different Wheat Species[a]

Vitamins	Emmer	Spelt	Durum Wheat	Soft Wheat
Riboflavin	0.73	1.40	1.51	1.19
Thiamin	3.84	0.64	3.51	3.33
Carotenoids				
β-Carotene	0.05	0.04	0.14	0.05
Lutein	2.12	1.42	2.65	1.31
Zeaxanthin	0.17	0.12	0.26	0.13
Total carotenoids	2.34	1.58	3.05	1.49
Tocochromanols				
α-Tocopherol	7.10	10.01	8.40	15.90
β-Tocopherol	4.51	7.42	4.81	9.51
Total tocopherols	11.61	17.43	13.21	25.41
α-Tocotrienol	6.31	5.10	6.92	6.41
β-Tocotrienol	35.20	30.10	39.60	42.50
Total tocotrienols	41.51	35.20	46.52	48.91
Tocotrienol/tocopherol	3.6	2.0	3.5	2.0
Vitamin E activity (TE)[b]	13.2	16.9	15.1	24.9

[a] Data from Panfili et al (2004).
[b] Expressed as tocopherol equivalents, calculated as in Eldin and Appelqvist (1996): α-tocopherol = 1.00; β-tocopherol = 0.50; α-tocotrienol = 0.33; β-tocotrienols = 0.05; δ-tocopherol = 0.01.

15.90 mg/kg (db) in spelt and soft wheat, respectively. Thus, vitamin E activity in spelt was about 30% more than in emmer.

Carotenoids are a group of compounds that are both nutritionally and technologically important, since they influence the chromatic characteristics of the meals (yellow index). Lutein was the predominant compound found (making up about 90% of total carotenoids). Total carotenoids were lower in emmer (2.34 mg/kg db) and, as expected, in spelt (1.58 mg/kg db) and soft wheat (1.49 mg/kg db) than in durum wheat (3.05 mg/kg db) (Panfili et al 2004). *T. durum* was genetically improved for yellowness because it is intended for pasta-making. Similar findings were found by Fares et al (2003) (3.3 mg/kg for emmer vs. 5.4 mg/kg for durum wheat Simeto) and by Piergiovanni et al (1996) upon assessment of several accessions of emmer and spelt. The carotenoid values they found in emmer (mean 2.9 mg/kg, range 2.0–4.2 mg/kg) and in spelt (mean 3.4 mg/kg, range 2.2–5.0 mg/kg) were lower than in durum wheats (4.7 mg/kg). On the other hand, Somma et al (2004) did not find any significant differences between the carotenoid contents of emmer and durum wheats (6.17 vs. 6.34 mg/kg, respectively).

Emmer Processing

Storage

After harvesting and threshing, the spikelets are usually stored in traditional or industrial warehouses, generally without any particular control measures against pests and fungi. Most studies on insects and fungi regarding stored grain have focused on modern wheats, but relatively few have been made on hulled wheats. As in the case of the other cereals, the biotic infestation of stored emmer grain can have considerable economic repercussions because product quality and safety may be significantly reduced. Trematerra and Gentile (2002) found a greater number of pest species infesting emmer in traditional than in industrial warehouses since farmers are mostly unaware of safe storage practices. The insect species mainly found in emmer grain stored in silos and warehouses located in the Molise and Basilicata regions were *Ephestia elutella* (Hb.), *Plodia interpunctella* (Hb.), *Sitotroga cerealella* (Olivier), *Oryzaephilus surinamensis* (L.), *Sitophilus granarius* (L.), *Sitophilus oryzae* (L.), and *Tribolium castaneum* (Herbst) (Trematerra and Gentile 2002). Emmer stored in traditional conditions contained mycotoxigenic fungi belonging to the *Fusarium* species with related mycotoxins (fumonisins B1 and B2, ochratoxin A, and beauvericin) (R. Castoria, G. Lima, and A. Ritieni, *unpublished data*).

Thus, emmer storage is a crucial phase in the emmer market chain, and it would be advisable for the grain to be stored under controlled conditions, using mainly physical treatments such as refrigeration or controlled atmosphere.

Dehulling

Dehulling is the process used to remove husks (glumes, lemmas, and paleas) from the hulled kernel, since, after threshing, the emmer grain is still covered by the spikelet chaff. Clean, whole spikelets are the primary raw material that undergoes this typical process for hulled wheats. The dehulled grain yield varied from 65 to 75% (D'Antuono 1989, Castagna et al 1996, Laghetti et al 1999) and may depend on the genotypes and on the test weight of the dehulled kernel.

Although basically simple, the procedure still represents a major bottleneck for hulled wheat manipulation, production, and processing. In fact, virtually no farmers and very few factories have dehulling machinery. Dehulling should be done after the storage period because the chaff prevents direct contact between kernel and contaminants (mycotoxins, heavy metals, chemicals, etc.), and hulled grain is less susceptible to pests than dehulled grain (Trematerra et al 1999). The chaff decreases the release of volatile compounds and therefore is less attractive to *S. oryzae* (Trematerra et al 1999). The disposal of the dehulling by-products (chaff) is another concern when dealing with hulled wheats. Potential uses of chaff include animal feed, bedding, fuel, tempering mudbricks, plaster, and dung-cakes (Nesbitt et al 1996).

Parboiling

Parboiling, a process frequently used to protect rice from nutrient loss during polishing and to increase milling performance and shelf life, was applied to emmer grain to improve its milling performance, nutrient retention, and cooking quality (D'Onofrio 2001, Marconi et al 2002b, Messia et al 2003). Emmer was parboiled both in hulled and dehulled form, using a pilot parboiling system consisting of a thermostatic bath for steeping the cereal and an autoclave for cooking. Parboiled grains were then dehulled and polished, using a rice laboratory polisher to remove the same amount of product (15%) from each grain, in order to compare the nutritional, cooking, and sensory properties of processed and unprocessed grain. A flow diagram of the emmer parboiling process is shown in Figure 2, and the main physicochemical and sensory properties of the parboiled emmer samples are provided in Table 12.

The complete starch gelatinization and translucency of emmer kernel or endosperm were achieved under both parboiling conditions (parboiling of hulled and dehulled emmer grains). In addition, parboiling significantly increased the yield of dehulled grain and, at the same time, reduced kernel breakage as a result of the increased hardness of the kernel due to the hydrothermal treatment (hardness index, 110 vs. 79). Parboiled grains were darker (L^* and a^* values) than the reference sample due to the development of nonenzymatic browning (the Maillard reaction, assessed by the furosine index) and the diffusion of the coloring pigments contained in the husk and bran. Parboiled emmer produced a cooked product with excellent cooking quality (in terms of firmness, bulkiness, stickiness, water uptake, and solids loss in cooking water). The major advantages of hydrothermal treatment are actually reached with hulled grain, where the glumes help protect against hydrothermal stress.

In conclusion, it may be worthwhile to exploit this process to promote the marketing of parboiled emmer, an innovative product with particular sensory and nutritional properties, that may have wider appeal than natural emmer.

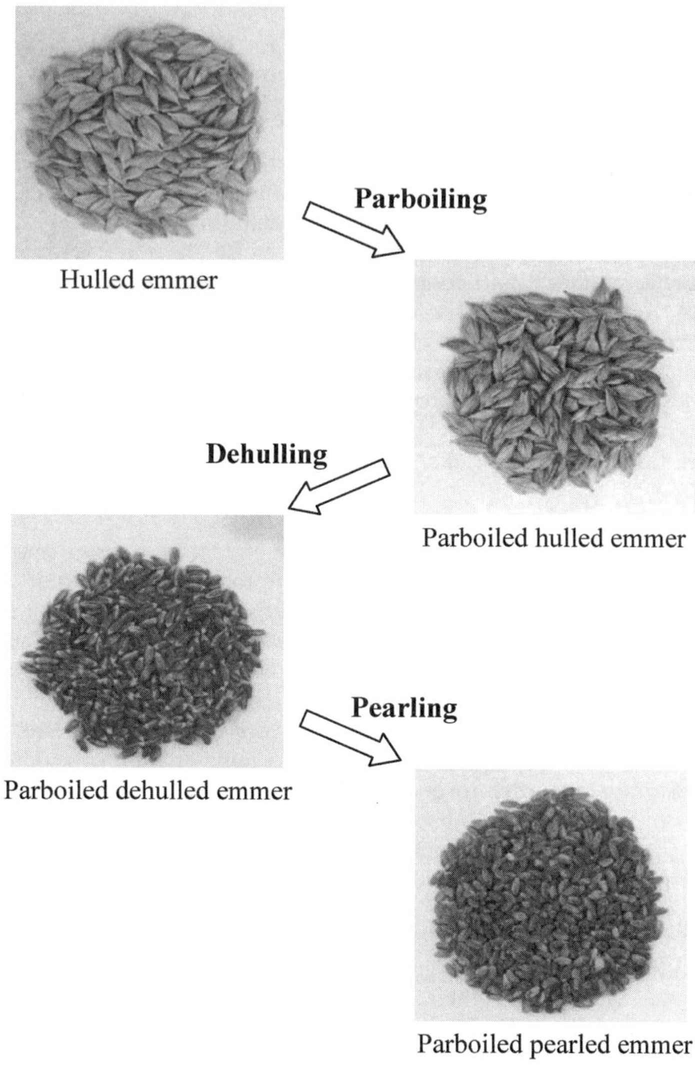
Hulled emmer
Parboiling
Parboiled hulled emmer
Dehulling
Parboiled dehulled emmer
Pearling
Parboiled pearled emmer

Fig. 2. Process for producing parboiled emmer.

Malting and Brewing

Emmer beer, which has particular sensory properties, has been successfully produced in Tuscany (Garfagnana), and Molise (Ortenzio 2002). Emmer spikelets are ideal for malting purposes: as with hulled barley, the husk holds the solid parts of the grain together during the malting process. Emmer was used in Ancient Egypt to produce malt and beer (Samuel 1993, Nesbitt and Samuel 1996) and, in the United Kingdom, some archeologists tried to repro-

TABLE 12
Physicochemical and Sensory Characteristics of Parboiled Emmer[a]

Parameter	Parboiled Emmer (hulled)[b]	Parboiled Emmer (dehulled)[c]	Reference Emmer (not parboiled)
Dehulled yield (%)	70	. . .	66
Translucency (%)	98	94	0
Hardness index (HI, by SKCS[d])	107	117	79
Ash (%, db)	1.18	1.17	0.32
Cooking time (min)	20	20	18
Cooking loss (%)	5.3	5.3	6.9
Water uptake (%)	132	119	143
Sensory judgment			
Firmness	Good	Good	Satisfactory
Stickiness	Almost absent	Almost absent	Very high
Bulkiness	Almost absent	Almost absent	High
Color			
L^*	79.0	78.4	85.8
a^*	1.2	0.7	0.6
b^*	15.0	16.0	12.2
Furosine (mg/100 g protein)	28.2	46.2	4.1

[a] Data from Messia et al (2003).
[b] Parboiling was carried out on hulled grain.
[c] Parboiling was carried out on hulless grain.
[d] SKCS = single-kernel characterization system.

duce the brewing process of the ancient Egyptians to obtain the so-called Pharaohs beer (Fairley 1992). The good malting potential of emmer (*T. dicoccon*) (high-amylase formation) was also reported by Singh et al (1983).

Pearling

Pearling is an abrasive scouring process that gradually removes the pericarp, seed coat, aleurone and subaleurone layers, and the embryo; thus, the content of total and insoluble dietary fiber, minerals, protein, lipids, and vitamins decreases as the pearling rate increases. For this reason, the use of low-pearled grain is advisable in order to maintain a higher nutritional value of the whole kernel. The degree of pearling best suited to producing emmer soups is 10–20%, which ensures satisfactory cooking and sensory characteristics (texture, firmness) and good nutritional properties. Pearled or whole kernels are used to make both homemade and commercial soups and salads. The pearled grain, whole grain, or broken grain ("*farricello*") is still used, as in ancient Rome, for making porridge (*puls*) and in soup and salad. Emmer grain intended for pearling should be uniform, plump, and of medium hardness and have a kernel weight of >40 mg.

Vacuum packaging is the standard form of packing found today in commerce for whole, pearled, and coarsely broken grains. Besides being sold separately, pearled whole grains are often marketed within an assortment of cereals and dried legumes, as basic ingredients for soups.

Debranning

Today, debranning (also referred to as preprocessing or premilling) is being increasingly used as a means of improving the milling performance of wheat. It involves preprocessing the wheat to remove the bran layers by

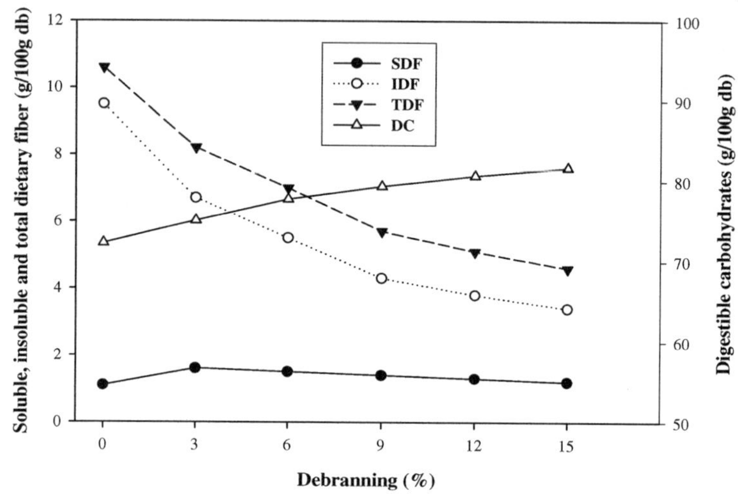

Fig. 3. Relationship between degree of emmer debranning and relative concentrations of insoluble dietary fiber (IDF), soluble dietary fiber (SDF), total dietary fiber (TDF), and digestible carbohydrates (DC). (E. Marconi and R. Cubbada, *unpublished data*)

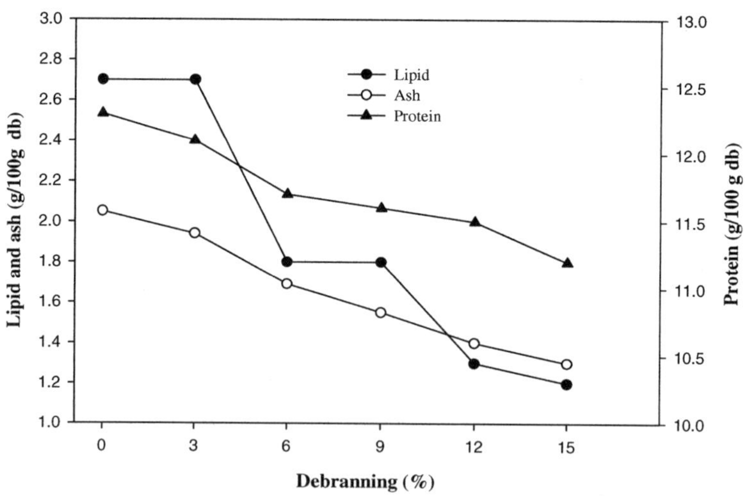

Fig. 4. Relationship between degree of emmer debranning and relative concentrations of lipid, ash, and protein. (E. Marconi and R. Cubbada, *unpublished data*)

sequential friction and abrasion passages through modified rice polishers. The preprocessed wheat is then milled by conventional roller milling equipment (Dexter et al 1994). In the case of durum wheat, the yield and degree of refinement of the semolina produced after debranning are significantly improved. Moreover, this process considerably simplifies the subsequent milling process and produces added-value by-products (Dexter and Wood 1996, Pagani et al 2003).

Variations in emmer grain composition, dependent on the degree of debranning, are shown in Figures 3 and 4, based on studies by the authors. A debranning degree between 6 and 9%, which means that the part removed was mostly insoluble fiber (lignin and cellulose), could be considered the perfect compromise between removing the peripheral parts of the grain and achieving good milling yields.

Hulled wheats could benefit from debranning since this helps maintain the nutritional properties and reduces manipulation of the kernel during milling. Manufacturers that process hulled wheats are mainly small enterprises that do not have all the machinery needed to process modern wheats, besides which consumers demand that hulled wheats undergo as little processing and manipulation as possible to maintain their natural characteristics.

Milling

Emmer can be milled using both conventional processes and the innovative premilling process, debranning. The authors performed milling tests on emmer using 6% debranned kernels and the corresponding whole kernels. A Buhler MLU 202 mill was used for the purpose; it was equipped with a laboratory semolina purifier with three breaking and regrinding passages. The milling performances of two emmer genotypes, characterized by different test weights, are reported in Table 13.

As for durum wheat, introducing an appropriate degree of debranning into emmer milling considerably improved both the apparent and the effective semolina yield. Similar values of emmer semolina yield were found by Fares et al (2003) (62–68%) and by Schlichting et al (2003) (69.3%), using classic milling processes.

The ash content of the semolina obtained from milling debranned kernels was similar to that obtained from milling the corresponding whole kernels. This indirectly shows that, at the same yield level, the semolina from debranned kernels contained less bran. The physical (particle size) and rheological (alveograph and farinograph parameters, gluten quality) characteristics of the semolina were not subject to any significant change when the debranning process was used (Table 14).

Alternatively, whole or pearled meals of emmer can be obtained by milling whole or pearled kernels in hammer or stone mills, in conjunction with a sifter. Oversized particles are fed back into the mill for further grinding. These types of meal are preferable for hulled wheats since more of the nutrients of the whole kernel are maintained.

TABLE 13
Kernel Characteristics and Milling Performances of Unprocessed (UP) and Debranned (DP) Emmer Grains[a]

Sample	Test Weight (kg/hl)	1,000 Kernel Weight (g)	Kernel Ash (%, db)	Semolina Yield[b] (%)	Flour Yield[b] (%)	Semolina Ash (%, db)	Flour Ash (%, db)	Semolina Particle Size (%)		
								>300 µm	>215–<300 µm	<215 µm
Molise Colli										
UP	73.2	50.8	2.05	57.5	8.1	0.87	1.11	86.0	13.4	0.6
DP	...	47.5	1.69	65.3	6.5	0.82	1.20	84.2	14.9	0.9
Lucanica										
UP	69.4	38.9	2.08	50.8	7.9	0.87	1.23	...	...	...
DP	...	36.4	1.66	57.5	7.6	0.88	1.25	...	...	...

[a] Source: E. Marconi and R. Cubadda, *unpublished data.*
[b] Real yield.

TABLE 14
Rheological Properties and Amylase Activity (Falling Number) of Unprocessed (UP) and Debranned (DP) Emmer Grains

	Alveograph Parameters		Farinograph Parameters[a]				
Sample	W (10^{-4} J)	P/L	WA (%)	DT (min)	Stability (min)	DS (FU)	Falling Number (sec)
Molise Colli							
UP	74	0.35	53	1.0	1.0	170	538
DP	75	0.37	55	1.0	1.0	180	525
Lucanica							
UP	81	0.17	56	1.5	3.5	110	515
DP	109	0.21	56	1.5	3.5	110	510

[a] WA = water absorption; DT = development time; DS = degree of softening after 12 min; FU = farinograph units.

Flour/Semolina Properties

Information on gluten quality and dough properties is useful in understanding the technological properties and in adopting adequate formulations and processing methods. Several physicochemical and rheological methods have been standardized to assess the technological aptitude of durum wheat meal (sodium dodecyl sulfate [SDS] sedimentation value, gluten index, and alveograph and farinograph tests) (Dexter and Matsuo 1980, Cubadda 1988, Dick and Youngs 1988, D'Egidio et al 1990, Kovacs et al 1997). The authors, studying the gluten quality and the rheological properties of the dough of three emmer varieties, found that emmer flour has poor technological potential because of its low values for the SDS sedimentation test, gluten index, alveograph and farinograph parameters, and yellow index (Table 15). Gluten was often so weak that it was impossible to extract or to work the dough with the alveograph. All studies concur on the poor technological potential of emmer when classic methods for assessing modern wheats are used.

Several studies and experiments have found low and exceedingly low SDS values, as reported in Table 4. The poor gluten quality of emmer is even more apparent when the specific sedimentation volume (the SDS sedimentation volume per unit of protein) is calculated. The high protein content of emmer can, in some cases, mask its real gluten strength, since the SDS sedimentation test is influenced by protein content (Halverson and Zeleny 1988, Cubadda and Marconi 2001).

Low values for the gluten index (GI) of emmer were also found by Cubadda and Marconi (1996) (GI = 37), Marconi and Schiavone (1997) (GI from unextractable to 45), Galterio et al (1999) (GI from 6 to 35, mean 17), Schlichting et al (2003) (GI = 16), and Fares et al (2003) (GI = 24).

Inadequate alveograph and farinograph values were also reported by Galterio et al (1994) ($W < 50 \times 10^{-4}$ J), Cubadda and Marconi (1996) ($W = 67 \times 10^{-4}$ J), Marconi and Schiavone (1997) (W from unworkable to 118×10^{-4} J; P/L from 0.95 to 1.97), and Schlichting et al (2003) ($W = 74 \times 10^{-4}$ J; P/L =

TABLE 15
Technological Properties of Three Italian Emmer Varieties[a,b]

	Whole Meal		Semolina											
	SDS[c] Sedimentation Test				Alveograph Parameters		Farinograph Parameters[e]					Color		
Emmer	Volume (ml)	Volume/ Protein[d]	Protein (%, db)	Gluten Index	W (10^{-4} J)	P/L	WA (%)	DT (min)	Stability (min)	DS (FU)	Falling Number (sec)	L^*	a^*	b^*
Farvento	17	1.27	14.5	0	UW	UW	49.5	1.7	1.0	166	660	82.5	1.3	14.9
Lucanica	28	1.39	12.4	5	98	0.20	52.8	2.6	2.3	68	719	84.8	−0.8	18.4
Molise Colli	19	1.86	11.1	UE	UW	UW	50.3	1.7	1.1	119	572	83.8	0.1	16.5

[a] Source: E. Marconi and R. Cubadda, *unpublished data.*
[b] UE = unextractable; UW = unworkable.
[c] Sodium dodecyl sulfate.
[d] Determined at 15% db.
[e] WA = water absorption; DT = development time; DS = degree of softening after 12 min; FU = farinograph units.

0.17 from alveogram, water absorption = 58%, development time = 2.5 min, and stability = 2.0 min from farinogram).

All the above-mentioned values are lower than those desirable for good-quality durum wheat: SDS sedimentation value > 35 mL; GI > 70; alveograph $W > 200 \times 10^{-4}$ J; farinograph stability > 5 min (Dexter and Matsuo 1980, Cubadda 1988, Dick and Youngs 1988, Kovacs et al 1997).

The yellow index (b^*) of emmer semolina/flour ($b^* = 14.9$–18.4) was also lower than for commercial durum wheat semolina ($b^* = 25$) due to the lower carotenoid content (see section on vitamins).

Given the poor technological quality of emmer flour, breeding programs have been undertaken by some researchers to genetically improve emmer gluten strength, crossing emmer with durum wheat. Some of the hybrid emmers (emmer-durum lines), as expected, have attained significantly higher SDS sedimentation, GI, and alveograph and farinograph values compared to true emmer (Galterio et al 1999, Fares et al 2003, Schlichting et al 2003).

There are two options for improving technological characteristics of emmer grain to obtain a high-quality emmer-based end-product: breeding programs to improve quality by crossing it with durum wheat, as some researchers have proposed (Galterio et al 2001, Fares et al 2003), or the use of appropriate technologies and formulations to enhance the technological characteristics of the raw material. The second option seems the more appropriate, given that the former would only be a rerun of the genetic improvements made for the selection of soft and durum wheats. In fact, it is essential that the specific and special characteristics of hulled wheats be preserved unaltered.

Transformation technology could, in fact, be the answer. For instance, certain adjustments could be made to various processes, such as combining high drying temperatures with flour exhibiting a high protein content for pasta-making, the addition of vital gluten, or the use of sourdough for bread-making.

Food Uses

Breadmaking

Very little information is available on the breadmaking potential of emmer. Marconi and Schiavone (1997) found that emmer breads (from two genotypes), baked according to the Italian straight-dough procedure (Cubadda and Pasqui 1984), had a lower baking quality (volume, break and shred, texture, crust and crumb color, and symmetry) than spelt and soft wheat breads but had a distinct flavor and taste.

Similar results were obtained by Schlichting et al (2003) on emmer bread (one emmer line) baked using the Canadian short-process baking test (Preston et al 1982) and the remix-to-peak baking test (straight-dough procedure) (Kilborn and Tipples 1981). In both cases, absorption, mixing time, loaf volume, and crumb structure were poorer than in the control durum wheat. In a study by the chapter authors, on bread-making potential of hulled wheats

TABLE 16
Qualitative Properties of Pasta and Bread Produced with Emmer and Spelt Wheats[a]

	Pasta Characteristics								Bread Characteristics[d]			
	Cooking Quality					Color						
	Sensory Judgment				TOM[c] (g starch/ 100 g dry pasta)				Volume (ml)	Moisture (%)	Firmness (N)	
	Firmness	Bulkiness	Stickiness	Total Score[b]		L^*	a^*	b^*			2 hr	24 hr
Emmer (Molise Colli)	80	80	80	80	1.26	59.3	2.1	40.1	708	30.0	9.3	19.7
Spelt (Forenza)	80	80	70	80	1.39	66.7	1.1	45.1	794	28.9	4.8	12.3
Durum wheat	100	100	100	100	1.00	66.7	0.5	50.2	...	...	...	...
Soft wheat	...	...	...	...	...	...	...	...	852	29.7	5.1	12.5

[a] Source: E. Marconi and R. Cubadda, *unpublished data*.
[b] ≤40 = poor or mediocre quality; >40–50 = not completely satisfactory, >50–70 = fair; >70–80 = good; >80 = excellent.
[c] TOM = total organic matter. >2.1 = low quality; ≥1.4 to ≤ 2.1 = good quality; and <1.4 = very good quality.
[d] Sourdough procedure.

using the sourdough procedure, interesting properties for emmer and spelt breads were found (Table 16). Spelt bread of good quality was also obtained using the remix straight-dough procedure (Abdel-Aal et al 1997). However, the sourdough procedure is preferable for emmer or hulled wheat breadmaking, since it meets the requirements of natural, organic products.

Pasta-Making

Durum wheat semolina is the best raw material for pasta-making because of the rheological properties of the protein and gluten and the high yellow pigment content. Other wheat species can be used, but adequate pasta processing and balanced formulations are needed to counteract their poor technological properties (Marconi and Carcea 2001).

To make pasta from emmer, which is characterized by rather weak gluten, and obtain a quality end product, emmer flours characterized by high protein content (>13.5% db) should be used (otherwise, vital wheat gluten should be added to reach the same protein level) and high-temperature drying (>80°C) should be adopted. In fact, the combined use of high protein content and high-temperature drying produces a coagulated and diffused protein network capable of preventing starch granules from exuding from pasta during cooking (Resmini and Pagani 1983, D'Egidio et al 1990, Novaro et al 1993, Cubadda 1996). By making these adjustments, Marconi et al (1999a, 2000b, 2002a) obtained spelt and barley pastas with excellent cooking properties.

Values that indicate the cooking quality of emmer and spelt pastas, obtained by the authors by adding 3% vital gluten to reach a semolina protein content of 14% and adopting the high-temperature drying diagram (>85°C) reported by Marconi et al (2002a), are given in Table 16. The cooking quality of emmer and spelt pastas was satisfactory, considering the poor quality of the raw materials; in fact, all the sensory (bulkiness, stickiness, firmness), chemical (total organic matter [TOM], i.e., the amount of surface material released from cooked pasta into the washing water), and instrumental (firmness, stickiness) parameters gave more than satisfactory values.

Emmer and spelt pastas were not as yellow (lower b^* index) as the durum wheat pasta, due to the lower carotenoid content of the emmer and spelt semolina/flour. This lack of yellowness, however, is not a problem because consumers of whole meal, health, or fashionable foods are prepared to accept the natural brownish color of these pastas (Marconi and Carcea 2001).

The above-mentioned findings concur with other test results. Galterio et al (1994) judged the cooking quality of pasta, obtained from a study of three emmer landraces with low protein content (<10.5%) and using low-temperature drying (50°C for 16 hr), as low and having poor sensory attributes. Cubadda and Marconi (1996) found that emmer pasta made at a high temperature, but with a low protein content of 12.3%, had poor cooking properties, whereas Marconi and Schiavone (1997) found very good pasta cooking-quality performances (TOM = 1.1–1.3 g of starch per 100 g of dry pasta; sensory total score of 75–80) for emmer and spelt pasta made with a high protein content of >18% db and using high-temperature drying (85°C). Schlichting et al (2003), testing an emmer pasta produced with 14.5% protein but using a drying cycle at 70°C, found that the firmness and yellowness values were significantly lower than for durum wheat spaghetti. Fares et al (2003) found low TOM values for two emmer pastas obtained from semolina with a high protein content (>14% db) but dried at a low temperature (50°C for 18 hr).

In Italy, several forms of emmer pasta-type products (in the Italian legislation, the term "pasta" is reserved exclusively for 100% durum wheat products) are available in different shapes (e.g., spaghetti, sedani, rigatoni).

Production of Cookies (Biscuits)

The production technologies for cookies (in British English, "biscuits") vary a great deal, ranging from conventional industrial procedures (use of hydrogenated fats and artificial flavoring, etc.) to specialized, small-scale activities, where only selected natural ingredients are used, resulting in rather unconventional and truly original or fashionable products. The latter processing, which was used at the Scientific and Technological Park, "Moliseinnovazione," in Campobasso, Molise, Italy, produced a wide range of emmer cookies (*frollini*, *cantucci*, biscuit fingers, almond biscuits, ring-shaped almond biscuits, *taralli*, and filled *panzerotti*) characterized by specific and often superior sensory properties (flavor, crunchiness, and friability) compared to cookies made with traditional raw materials (soft wheat). Emmer flours with low protein content, which were suitable for this type of product, were used. Such products could be another market opportunity for emmer if further developed and improved.

On the Indian subcontinent, emmer is widely used for producing traditional and savory sweet products—*rawa idli*, *upma*, *halwa*, etc. (Sidhu 1995). Reddy et al (1998) showed that *godi huggi* and *gulladiki laddu* had a relatively better taste and flavor when prepared with emmer semolina.

Other Products

Emmer meal is also suitable for use in many other food products, such as pizza, breakfast cereals (flakes, popped), extruded-cooked products, snacks, cakes, etc (D'Antuono 1995, D'Antuono and Bravi 1996, Abdel-Aal et al 1998, Cubadda and Marconi 2001, Schiavone et al 2001).

Thus, emmer flour can be used to advantage in the production of bread, pasta, breakfast cereals, snacks, and cookies, without having to resort to genetic improvement by crosses with durum wheat, simply by using appropriate formulations and transformation processes. The increasing popularity of hulled wheats as environmentally friendly cereal crops for the production of niche products is prompting research into new nutritious and attractive foods.

Old and new emmer recipes can be found in specialized books (Perrino et al 1994, Marconi and Colonna 2001, Padulosi et al 1996) and websites (Italian keywords: *farro*, *ricette*; English keywords: emmer, recipes).

Conclusion

The potential of emmer does not reside in its capacity to mimic attributes that are already present in modern wheats but in its own special characteristics (adaptability to marginal areas, resistance to biotic and abiotic stress, absence of dwarf genes, hulled kernel, chemical and physical properties, etc). Those characteristics that distinguish it from modern free-threshing wheats should be further developed by appropriate selection and breeding programs and not leveled out by crosses that merely aim to reproduce the same characteristics of modern wheats.

High production levels and agronomic characteristics approaching those of modern wheats will lead to overproduction and a supply above the market demand for niche products, resulting in loss of value and specialty characteristics.

Another problem inhibiting development of a market for emmer is the presence of products, at inflated prices, with inadequate quality characteristics (e.g., high contamination with other cereals such as soft wheat, durum, wheat barley, spelt) that don't satisfy consumers' expectations.

Enhancement of the qualities of emmer must be achieved through a proper understanding of the product, its correct characterization (certification, chain traceability, technological adjustment) and the introduction of protective measures for the cultivation of local types and certified varieties in the areas of origin. This will combine economic and commercial considerations with the advantages of protecting and safeguarding marginal growing areas and giving the consumer greater food quality and choice.

Acknowledgments

We wish to thank P. Perrino and G. Laghetti (Germplasm Institute of Bari), and G. Figliuolo (University of Basilicata, Potenza) for bibliographical material and genetic information and M. Colonna (Ersam, Campobasso) for information provided on the cultivation areas and the agronomic and storage methods.

References

AAVV. 1997. Farro: Scelta varietale. Risultati della sperimentazione 1996-97. Inf. Agrario 37:51-56.

AAVV. 1998. Farro: Scelta varietale. Risultati della sperimentazione 1997-98. Inf. Agrario 37:44-48.

AAVV. 1999. Confronto fra genotipi di farro. Risultati della sperimentazione nazionale 1998-99. Inf. Agrario 37:45-47.

Abdel-Aal, E-S. M., Hucl, P., Sosulski, F. W., and Bhirud, P. R. 1997. Kernel, milling and baking properties of spring-type spelt and einkorn wheats. J. Cereal Sci. 26:363-370.

Abdel-Aal, E-S. M., Hucl, P., and Sosulski, F. W. 1998. Food uses for ancient wheats. Cereal Foods World 43:763-766.

Barcaccia, G., Molinari, L., Porfiri, O., and Veronesi, F. 2002. Molecular characterization of emmer (*Triticum dicoccon* Schrank) Italian landraces. Genet. Resour. Crop Evol. 49:415-426.

Behall, K. M., and Hallfrish, J. 2002. Effects of grains on glucose and insulin responses. Pages 269-281 in: Whole-Grain Foods in Health and Disease. L. Marquart, J. L. Slavin, and R. G. Fulcher, Eds. Am. Assoc Cereal Chem., St. Paul, MN.

Bertin, P., Gregoire, D., Massart, S., and de Froidmont, D. 2001. Genetic diversity among European cultivated spelt revealed by microsatellites. Theor. Appl. Genet. 102:148-156.

Blanco, A., Giorgi, B., Perrino, P., and Simeone, R. 1990. Risorse genetiche e miglioramento della qualità del frumento duro. Agric. Ricerca 144:41-58.

Boggini, G., and Pogna, N. E. 1989. The breadmaking quality and storage protein composition of durum wheat. J. Cereal Sci. 9:131-138.

Bozzini, A., Francia, U., and Iannelli, P. 1994. Farro "Basian" *Triticum dicoccum*. Inf. Agrario 37:48.

Braun, T. 1995. Barley cakes and emmer bread. Pages 25-37 in: Food in Antiquity. J. Wilkins, D. Harvey and M. Dobson, Eds. University of Exeter Press, Exeter.

Caboni, M. F., Iafelice, G., Marconi, E., and Cubadda, R. 2003. Sterol esters in durum wheat compared to soft and hulled wheats (*T. dicoccon* Schrank, *T. spelta* L.): analysis and identification. Pages 185-188 in: Durum Wheat and Pasta Quality: Recent Achievements and New Trends. M. G. D'Egidio, Ed. Istituto Sperimentale per la Cerealicoltura, Rome, Italy.

Cakmak, I., Tolay, I., Ozdemir, A., Ozkan H., Ozturk L., and Kling, C. I. 1999. Differences in zinc efficiency among and within diploid, tetraploid and hexaploid wheats. Ann. Bot. 84:163-171.

Castagna, R., Minoia, C., Porfiri, O., and Rocchetti, G. 1996. Nitrogen level and seeding rate effects on the performance of hulled wheats (*Triticum monococcum* L., *T. dicoccum* Schubler and *T. spelta* L.) evaluated in contrasting agronomic environments. J. Agron. Crop Sci. 176:173-181.

Codianni, P., Troccoli, A., Galterio, G., Pogna, N. E., and Di Fonzo, N. 1998. Davide, prima varietà di farro migliorata geneticamente. Inf. Agrario 25:46-48.

Codianni, P., Galterio, G., Pogna, N. E., and Di Fonzo, N. 2000. Mosè e Padre Pio, due nuovi genotipi di farro. Inf. Agrario 24:37-38.

Colonna, P., Leloup, V., and Buleon, A. 1992. Limiting factors of starch hydrolysis. Eur. J. Clin. Nutr. 46(Suppl. 2):S17-S32.

Corazza, L., Pasquini, M., and Perrino, P. 1986. Resistance to rusts and powdery mildew in some strains of *Triticum monococcum* L. and *Triticum dicoccum* Schubler cultivated in Italy. Genet. Agraria 40:243-254.

Cubadda, F., Baldini, M., Raggi, A., Colonna, M., and Marconi, E. 2004. Microelementi nutrizionali in genotipi di frumenti vestiti esaploidi e tetraploidi (*Triticum spelta* L. e *T. dicoccon* Schrank). Pages 167-172 in: Atti del 5° Convegno AISTEC Cereali: Scienza e Benessere dal Campo alla Tavola. R. Cubadda and E. Marconi, Eds. University of Molise, Campobasso, Italy.

Cubadda, R. 1988. Evaluation of durum wheat, semolina and pasta in Europe. Pages 217-228. in: Durum Wheat: Chemistry and Technology. G. Fabriani and C. Lintas, Eds. Am. Assoc. Cereal Chem., St. Paul, MN.

Cubadda, R. 1996. Pasta quality: The relationship between raw material properties and production technologies. Pages 164-168 in: Proc. World Pasta Congress, 1st. G. Mondelli, Ed. Chiriotti Editori, Pinerolo, Italy.

Cubadda, R., and Marconi, E. 1996. Technological and nutritional aspects in emmer and spelt. Pages 203-212 in: Hulled Wheats. Promoting the Conservation and Use of Underutilized and Neglected Crops. S. Padulosi, K. Hammer, and J. Heller, Eds. International Plant Genetic Resources Institute, Rome, Italy.

Cubadda, R., and Marconi, E. 2001. Spelt wheat. Pages 153-175 in: Pseudocereals and Less Common Cereals. P. Belton and J. Taylor, Eds. Springer-Verlag, Berlin.

Cubadda, R., and Pasqui, A. 1984. Risultati di una Sperimentazione Quadriennale sulle Caratteristiche Tecnologico-Qualitative della Produzione Nazionale di Frumento Tenero. Istituto Nazionale della Nutrizione, Rome, Italy.

Damania, A. B., Hakim, S., and Moualla, M. Y. 1992. Evaluation of variation in *Triticum dicoccum* for wheat improvement in stress environments. Hereditas 116:163-166.

D'Antuono, L. F. 1989. Il farro: Areali di coltivazione, caratteristiche agronomiche, utilizzazione e prospettive colturali. Inf. Agrario 24:49-57.

D'Antuono, 1995. Evoluzione del mercato del farro e salvaguardia della tipicità. Inf. Agrario 38:47-52.

D'Antuono, L. F., and Bravi, R. 1996. The hulled wheat industry: Present developments and impact on genetic resources conservation. Pages 221-223 in: Hulled Wheats. Promoting the Conservation and Use of Underutilized and Neglected Crops. S. Padulosi, K. Hammer and J. Heller, Eds. International Plant Genetic Resources Institute, Rome, Italy.

D'Antuono, L. F., and Pavoni, A. 1993. Technology and grain growth of *Triticum dicoccum* and *T. monococcum* from Italy. Pages 273-286 in: Biodiversity and Wheat Improvement. A. B. Damania, Ed. International Center for Agricultural Research in the Dry Areas, Aleppo, Syria.

D'Antuono, L. F., Galletti, G. C., and Bocchini, P. 1998. Fiber quality of emmer (*Triticum dicoccum* Schubler) and einkorn wheat (*T. monococcum* L.) landraces as determined by analytical pyrolysis. J. Sci. Food Agric. 78:213-219.

D'Egidio, M. G., Mariani, B. M., Nardi, S., Novaro, P., and Cubadda, R. 1990. Chemical and technological variables and their relationships: A predictive equation for pasta cooking quality. Cereal Chem. 67:275-281.

Dexter, J. E., and Matsuo, R. R. 1980. Relationship between durum wheat protein properties and pasta dough rheology and spaghetti cooking quality. J. Agric. Food Chem. 28:899-902.

Dexter, J. E., and Wood, P. J. 1996. Recent applications of wheat before milling. Trends Food Sci. Technol. 7:35-41.

Dexter, J. E., Martin, D. G., Sadaranganey, G. T., Michaelides, J., Mathieson, N., Tkac, J. J., and Marchylo, B. A. 1994. Preprocessing: Effects on durum wheat milling and spaghetti-making quality. Cereal Chem. 71:10-16.

Dick, J. W., and Youngs, V. L. 1988. Evaluation of durum wheat, semolina and pasta in the United States. Pages 237-248 in: Durum Wheat: Chemistry and Technology. G. Fabriani and C. Lintas, Eds. Am. Assoc. Cereal Chem., St. Paul, MN.

D'Onofrio, M. 2001. Applicazione del trattamento di parboilizzazione al farro: Sviluppo di un prodotto innovativo tipo parboiled. M.S. thesis, University of Molise, Campobasso, Italy.

EC. 2003. Directive 2003/89/EC of 10 November. Off. J. Eur. Un. L. 308, 25.11.2003.

EEC. 1996. EEC Council Regulation 1236/96 of 10 July. Off. J. Eur. Commun. L. 163 2.07.1996.

Eldin, A. K., and Appelqvist, L. A. 1996. The chemistry and antioxidant properties of tocopherols and tocotrienols. Lipids 31:671-701.

Fairley, P. 1992. Probably the oldest lager in the world… New Sci. 133:6.

FAO/WHO, 1991. Protein quality evaluation (Report of joint FAO/WHO expert consultation. FAO Food and Nutrition Paper 51). FAO/WHO, Rome, Italy

Fares, C., Codianni, P., Schiavone, M. G., Di Fonzo, N., and Galterio, G. 2003. Qualitative traits and storage protein composition in selected strains and new genotypes of hulled wheat (*T. turgidum* spp. *dicoccum*) compared with durum wheat (*T. turgidum* spp. *durum*). Pages 193-196 in: Durum Wheat and Pasta Quality: Recent Achievements and New Trends, M. G. D'Egidio, Ed. Istituto Sperimentale per la Cerealicoltura, Rome, Italy.

Feillet, P. 1988. Protein and enzyme composition of durum wheat. Pages 93-119 in: Durum Wheat: Chemistry and Technology. G. Fabriani and C. Lintas, Eds. Am. Assoc. Cereal Chem., St. Paul, MN.

Feldman, M., Millet, E., and Avivi, Y. 1996. Wild emmer wheat, *Triticum turgidum* var. *dicoccoides*—A rich genetic resource for the improvement of durum and common wheat. Pages 39-45 in: Premio Barilla dal Grano alla Pasta. R. Ranieri and R. Romano, Eds. Barilla Alimentare, Parma, Italy.

Ferrante, M. P., De Lisio, L., Colonna, M., Falasca, L., Marconi, E., and Cubadda, R. 2000. Caratterizzazione qualitativa di varietà europee di farro spelta (*T. spelta* L.). Pages 163-167 in: Materie Prime Transgeniche, Sicurezza Alimentare e Controllo Qualità nell'Industria Cerealicola. R. Cubadda and E. Marconi, Eds. Arti Grafiche la Regione, Campobasso, Italy.

Figliuolo, G., and Spagnoletti-Zeuli, P. L. 2000. A nested analysis to detect relationships between genetic markers and germplasm classes of durum wheat. Plant Genet. Resour. Newsl. 124:44-51.

Figliuolo, G., and Perrino, P. 2004. Genetic diversity and intra-specific phylogeny of *Triticum turgidum* L. subsp. *dicoccon* (Schrank) Thell. revealed by RFLPs and SSRs. Genet. Resour. Crop Evol. 51:513-527.

Galletti, G. C., Bocchini, P., and D'Antuono, L. F. 1996. Fiber composition of a neglected wheat species (*Triticum dicoccum* Schubler) as determined by pyrolysis/gas chromatography/mass spectrometry. J. Agric. Food Chem. 44:3133-3135.

Galterio, G., Cappelloni, M., Desiderio, E., and Pogna, N. E. 1994. Genetic, technological and nutritional characteristics of three Italian populations of "farrum" (*Triticum turgidum* subsp. *dicoccum*). J. Genet. Breed. 48:391-398.

Galterio, G., Codianni, P., Novembre, G., Saponaro, C., Di Fonzo, N., and Pogna, N. E. 1998. Storage protein composition and technological characteristics of F6 lines from the cross *Triticum turgidum* spp *durum* x *Triticum turgidum* spp *dicoccum*. Proc. Int. Wheat Genetic Symp., 9th. University of Saskatchewan, Saskatoon, SK, Canada.

Galterio, G., Colonna, M., Mariani, G., and Novembre, G. 1999. Technological and nutritional characteristics of *Triticum turgidum* ssp *dicoccum* and *Triticum spelta* grown in the Molise region. Agric. Med. 129:227-234.

Galterio, G., Colonna, M., Mariani, G., and Saponaro, C. 2000. Qualità merceologica e caratterizzazione genotipica di *T. turgidum* ssp *dicoccum* Schrank coltivati nel Molise. Pages 174-178 in: Materie Prime Transgeniche, Sicurezza Alimentare e Controllo Qualità nell'Industria Cerealicola. R. Cubadda and E. Marconi, Eds. Arti Grafiche la Regione, Campobasso, Italy.

Galterio, G., Cardarilli, D., Codianni, P., and Acquistucci, R. 2001. Evaluation of chemical and technological characteristics of new lines of *Triticum turgidum* ssp *dicoccum*. Nahrung-Food 45:263-266.

Galterio, G., Codianni, P., Giusti, A. M., Pezzarossa, B., and Cannella, C. 2003. Assessment of the agronomic and technological characteristics of *Triticum turgidum* ssp. *dicoccum* Schrank and *T. spelta* L. Nahrung-Food 47:54-59.

Grela, E. R. 1996. Nutrient composition and content of antinutritional factors in spelt (*Triticum spelta* L.) cultivars. J. Food Sci. Agric. 71:399-404.

Gupta, R. B., Batey, I. L., and MacRitchie, F. 1992. Relationship between protein composition and functional properties of wheat flours. Cereal Chem. 69:125-131.

Hakim, S., Damania, A. B., Moualla, M. Y., and Altunji, H. 1993. Variation for storage proteins in *Triticum dicoccum*. Pages 325-328 in: Biodiversity and Wheat Improvement. A. B. Damania, Ed. International Center for Agricultural Research in the Dry Areas, Aleppo, Syria.

Halverson, J., and Zeleny, L. 1988. Criteria of wheat quality. Pages 15-45 in: Wheat: Chemistry and Technology, 3rd ed. Vol. I. Y. Pomeranz, ed. Am. Assoc. Cereal Chem., St Paul, MN.

Hsam, S. L. K., Kieffer, R., and Zeller, F. J. 2001. Significance of *Aegilops tauschii* glutenin genes on breadmaking properties of wheat. Cereal Chem. 78:521-525.

Iafelice, G., Caboni, M. F., Marconi, E., and Cubadda, R. 2004a. Analisi e identificazione dei fitosteroli in frumenti esaploidi e tetraploidi. Pages 335-338 in: Ricerche e Innovazioni nell'Industria Alimentare. S. Porretta, Ed. Chiriotti Editori, Pinerolo, Italy.

Iafelice, G., Pelillo, M., Marconi, E., Caboni, M. F., and Cubadda, R. 2004b. Analisi e identificazione degli esteri degli steroli in frumenti tetraploidi e esaploidi. Pages 9-12 in: Atti del 5° Convegno AISTEC Cereali: Scienza e Benessere dal Campo alla Tavola. R. Cubadda and E. Marconi, Eds. University of Molise, Campobasso, Italy.

Jaradat, A. A., Kanbertay, M., Pena-Chocarro, L., Hammer, K., Stavropoulos, N., and Perrino, P. 1996. *Ex situ* conservation of hulled wheats. Pages 121-128 in: Hulled Wheats. Promoting the Conservation and Use of Underutilized and Neglected Crops. S. Padulosi, K. Hammer, and J. Heller, Eds. International Plant Genetic Resources Institute, Rome, Italy.

Karagoz, A. 1996. Agronomic practices and socioeconomic aspects of emmer and einkorn cultivation in Turkey. Pages 172-177 in: Hulled Wheats. Promoting the Conservation and Use of Underutilized and Neglected Crops. S. Padulosi, K. Hammer, and J. Heller, Eds. International Plant Genetic Resources Institute, Rome, Italy.

Kasarda, D. D. 2001. Grain in relation to celiac disease. Cereal Foods World 46:209-210.

Kasarda, D. D., Autran, J. C., Lew, E. J. L., Nimmo, C. C., and Shewry, P. R. 1983. N-terminal aminoacid sequences of ω-gliadins and ω-secalins. Implications for the evolution of prolamin genes. Biochim. Biophys. Acta 747:138-150.

Kilborn, R. H., and Tipples, K. H. 1981. Canadian test baking procedures. I. GRL remix methods and variations. Cereal Foods World 26:624-627.

Kimber, G., and Sears, E. R. 1987. Evolution in the genus *Triticum* and the origin of cultivated wheat. Pages 154-164 in: Wheat and Wheat Improvement, 2nd ed. E. G. Heyne, Ed. American Society of Agronomy, Madison, WI.

Kovacs, M. I. P., Poste, L. M., Butler, G., Woods, S. M., Leisle, D., Noll, J. S., and Dahlke, G. 1997. Durum wheat quality: Comparison of chemical and rheological screening tests with sensory analysis. J. Cereal Sci. 25:65-75.

Laghetti, G., Piergiovanni, A. R., Volpe, N., Semeraro, N., Falivene, M., Basile, M., and Perrino, P. 1997. Il farro, un'alternativa per la cerealicoltura lucana. Inf. Agrario 40:105-109.

Laghetti, G., Piergiovanni, A. R., Volpe, N., and Perrino, P. 1999. Agronomic performance of *Triticum dicoccon* Schrank and *T. spelta* L. accessions under southern Italian conditions. Agric. Med. 129:199-211.

Laghetti, G., Volpe, N., Perrino, P., Marconi, E., and Desiderio, E. 2001. Attitudine alla semina primaverile di una collezione di farro. Tec. Molitoria 52:793-797.

Levy, A. A., and Feldman, M. 1987. Increase in grain protein percentage in high-yielding common wheat breeding lines by genes from wild tetraploid wheat. Euphytica 36:353-359.

Lindhauer, M. G. 2001. Analytical methods utilized in the durum wheat chain. Pages 181-195 in: Durum Wheat, Semolina and Pasta Quality. Recent Achievements and New Trends. J. Abecassis, J.-C. Autran, and P. Feillet, Eds. Institut National de la Recherche Agronomique, Paris, France.

Luo, M. C., Yang, Z. L., and Dvorak, J. 2000. The Q locus of Iranian and European spelt wheat. Theor. Appl. Genet. 100:602-606.

Marconi, E., and Carcea, M. 2001. Pasta from non traditional raw materials. Cereal Foods World 46:522-530.

Marconi, E., and Colonna, M. 2001. Farro e benessere: Dal campo alla tavola. Quaderno Divulgativo Ente Regionale Sviluppo Agricolo Molise 14:7-47.

Marconi, E., and Schiavone, M. 1997. Valutazione tecnologica e qualitativa di genotipi di farro selezionati in ambienti meridionali. Pages 103-108 in: Atti del Convegno I Cereali Minori Aspetti Genetici, Agronomici, Nutrizionali e Strategie per una Loro

Valorizzazione. O. Porfiri, R. Castagna, S. Padulosi, and D. Codoni, Eds. Cogecstre Edizioni, Pescara, Italy.

Marconi, E., Carcea, M., Graziano, M., and Cubadda, R. 1999a. Kernel properties and pasta-making quality of five European spelt wheat (*Triticum spelta* L.) cultivars. Cereal Chem. 76:25-29.

Marconi, E., Schiavone, M., Ferrante, M. P., and Cubadda, R. 1999b. Qualitative characterization of varieties and landraces of *Triticum dicoccon* Schrank and *T. spelta* L.). Tec. Molitoria 5:551-556.

Marconi, E., Carcea, M., Bassotti, G., Bartoli, L., and Cubadda, R. 2000a. Composizione amminoacidica di sfarinati integrali e raffinati di spelta (*T. spelta* L.). Pages 184-187 in: Materie Prime Transgeniche, Sicurezza Alimentare e Controllo Qualità nell'Industria Cerealicola. R. Cubadda and E. Marconi, Eds. Arti Grafiche la Regione, Campobasso, Italy.

Marconi, E., Graziano, M., and Cubadda, R. 2000b. Composition and utilization of barley pearling by-products for making functional pastas rich in dietary fiber and β-glucans. Cereal Chem. 77:133-139.

Marconi, E., Panfili, G., Iafelice, G., Fratianni, A., Caboni, M. F., Colonna, M., and Cubadda, R. 2001. Valutazione quali-quantitativa della frazione lipidica in *Triticum dicoccon* Schrank e *T. spelta* L. Tec. Molitoria 52:826-831.

Marconi, E., Carcea, M., Schiavone, M., and Cubadda, R. 2002a. Spelt (*Triticum spelta* L.) pasta quality: Combined effect of flour properties and drying conditions. Cereal Chem. 79:634-639.

Marconi, E., D'Onofrio, L., Panfili, G., and Cubadda, R. 2002b. Parboiled emmer (*Triticum dicoccon* Schrank): Development of an innovative pearled product. (Online: http://www.aaccnet.org/meetings/2002/abstracts/a02ma441.asp)

Mariani, G., Belocchi, A., Bravi, R., and Bernardi G. 1992. Risultati di prove su farro condotte in Garfagnana. Inf. Agrario 37:67-71.

Mariani, G., Galterio, G., Colonna, M., and Saponaro, C. 2000. Caratterizzazione di popolazioni italiane di farro mediante analisi elettroforetiche. Pages 188-192 in: Materie Prime Transgeniche, Sicurezza Alimentare e Controllo Qualità nell'Industria Cerealicola. R. Cubadda and E. Marconi, Eds. Arti Grafiche la Regione, Campobasso, Italy.

Mariani, G., Galterio, G., Colonna, M., and Saponaro, C. 2001. Costituzione di una subpopolazione di farro (*Triticum dicoccum* Schübler) caratterizzata per qualità di prodotto. Tec. Molitoria 52:760-761.

Merezhko, A. F., Filatenko, A. A., and Funtov, K. A. 1997. The diversity of *Triticum dicoccum* Schuebl. for use in cool, wet regions of Europe. Pages 38-51 in: Small Grain Cereals and Pseudo-Cereals, O. Stolen, K. Bruhn, K. Pithan, and J. Hill, Eds. European Commission, Luxembourg.

Messia, M. C., Panfili, G., and Marconi, E. 2003. Effect of hydrothermal processing on non-enzymatic browning of tetraploid wheats. Pages 325-328 in: Durum Wheat and Pasta Quality: Recent Achievements and New Trends. M. G. D'Egidio, Ed. Istituto Sperimentale per la Cerealicoltura, Rome, Italy.

Mohammadkani, A., Stoddart, F. L., and Marshall, D. R. 1998. Survey of amylose content in *Secale cereale*, *Triticum monococcum*, *T. turgidum* and *T. tauschii*. J. Cereal Sci. 28:273-280.

Mohammadkani, A., Stoddart, F. L., and Marshall, D. R. 1999. Amylose content in segregating populations of einkorn, emmer, and rye. Starch/Starke 51:66-73.

Morris, R., and Sears, E. R. 1967. The cytogenetics of wheat and its relatives. Pages 19-87 in: Wheat and Wheat Improvement. L. P. Reitz and K. S. Quisenberry, Eds. American Society of Agronomy, Madison, WI.

Moudry, J., and Dvoracek, V. 1999. Chemical composition of grain of different spelt (*Triticum spelta* L.) varieties. Rostl. Vyroba 45:533-538.

Nesbitt, M., and Samuel, D. 1996. From staple crop to extinction? The archaeology and history of the hulled wheats. Pages 41-100 in: Hulled Wheats. Promoting the Conservation and Use of Underutilized and Neglected Crops. S. Padulosi, K. Hammer, and J. Heller, Eds. International Plant Genetic Resources Institute, Rome, Italy.

Nesbitt, M., Hillman, G., Pena-Chocarro, L., Samuel, D., and Szabo, A. T. 1996. Checklist for recording the cultivation and uses of hulled wheats. Pages 234-245 in: Hulled Wheats. Promoting the Conservation and Use of Underutilized and Neglected Crops. S. Padulosi, K. Hammer, and J. Heller, Eds. International Plant Genetic Resources Institute, Rome, Italy.

Novaro, P., D'Egidio, M. G., Mariani B. M., and Nardi, S. 1993. Combined effect of protein content and high temperature drying systems on pasta cooking quality. Cereal Chem. 70:716-719.

Ortenzio, M. 2002. Selezione di lieviti per la produzione di birra da *Triticum dicoccum*. M.S. thesis, University of Molise, Campobasso, Italy.

Padulosi, S., Hammer K., and Heller, J. 1996. Pages 178-181 in: Hulled Wheats. Promoting the Conservation and Use of Underutilized and Neglected Crops. S. Padulosi, K. Hammer, and J. Heller, Eds. International Plant Genetic Resources Institute, Rome, Italy.

Pagani, M. A., De Noni, I., D'Egidio, M. G., and Cecchini, C. 2003. Effectiveness of debranning process of durum wheat for improving semolina quality. Pages 157-161 in: Durum Wheat and Pasta Quality: Recent Achievements and New Trends. M. G. D'Egidio, Ed. Istituto Sperimentale per la Cerealicoltura, Rome, Italy.

Panfili, G., Fratianni, A., and Irano, M. 2004. Vitamine come indici di prodotto e di processo nei cereali e derivati. Pages 247-256 in: Atti del 5° Convegno AISTEC Cereali: Scienza e Benessere dal Campo alla Tavola. R. Cubadda and E. Marconi, Eds. University of Molise, Campobasso, Italy.

Papa, C. 1996. The "farre de Montelione": landrace and representation. Pages 154-168 in: Hulled Wheats. Promoting the Conservation and Use of Underutilized and Neglected Crops. S. Padulosi, K. Hammer, and J. Heller, Eds. International Plant Genetic Resources Institute, Rome, Italy.

Payne, P. I., Jackson, E. A., and Holt, L. 1984. The association between gliadin 45 and gluten strength in durum wheat varieties: A direct casual effect on the result of genetic linkage. J. Cereal Sci. 2:73-81.

Pelillo, M., Iafelice, G., Marconi, E., and Caboni, M. F. 2003. Identification of plant sterols in tetraploid and hexaploid wheats using GC mass spectrometry. Rapid Commun. Mass Spectrom. 17:1-8.

Pena, R. J., Skovmand, B., and Amaya, A. 1993. Glutenin (HMW and LMW) subunit composition, quality characteristics and their relationship in *Triticum dicoccon* populations. Pages 781-786 in: Proc. Int. Wheat Genetic Symp., 8th. China Agric. Scientech Press, Beijing, China.

Pena-Chocarro, L. 1996. *In situ* conservation of hulled wheat species: The case of Spain. Pages 129-152 in: Hulled Wheats. Promoting the Conservation and Use of Underutilized and Neglected Crops. S. Padulosi, K. Hammer, and J. Heller, Eds. International Plant Genetic Resources Institute, Rome, Italy.

Perrino, P., and Hammer, K. 1982. *Triticum monococcum* L. and *T. dicoccum* Schubler (sin. di *T. dicoccon* Schrank) are still cultivated in Italy. Genet. Agric. 36:343-352.

Perrino, P., and Hammer, K. 1984. The farro: Further information on its cultivation in Italy, utilization and conservation. Genet. Agric. 38:303-311.

Perrino, P., Infantino, S., Laghetti, G., Volpe, N., and Di Marzio, A. 1991. Valutazione e selezione di farro in ambienti marginali dell'Appennino molisano. Inf. Agrario 43:41-44.

Perrino, P., Infantino, S., Basso, P., Di Marzio, A., Volpe, N., and Laghetti, G. 1993. Valutazione e selezione di farro in ambienti marginali dell'Appennino molisano (II nota). Inf. Agrario 42:57-62.

Perrino, P., Semeraro, D., and Laghetti, G. 1994. Pages 137-145 in: Atti del Convegno Il Farro un Cereale della Salute. P. Perrino, D. Semeraro, and G. Lagnetti, Eds. Istituto del Germoplasma, Bari, Italy.

Perrino, P., Laghetti, G., D'Antuono, A., Ajlouni, M., Kanbertay, M., Szabò, A. T., and Hammer, K. 1996a. Ecogeographical distribution of hulled wheat species. Pages 101-119 in: Hulled Wheats. Promoting the Conservation and Use of Underutilized and Neglected Crops. S. Padulosi, K. Hammer, and J. Heller, Eds. International Plant Genetic Resources Institute, Rome, Italy.

Perrino, P., Volpe, N., and Laghetti, G. 1996b. Lucanica e Forenza: Due nuove varietà di farro. Inf. Agrario 47:34-35.

Piergiovanni, A. R., Laghetti, G., and Perrino, P. 1996. Characteristics of meal from hulled wheats (*Triticum dicoccon* Schrank and *T. spelta* L.): An evaluation of selected accessions. Cereal Chem. 73:732-735.

Piergiovanni, A. R., Rizzi, R., Pannacciulli, E., and Della Gatta, C. 1997. Mineral composition in hulled wheat grains: A comparison between emmer (*Triticum dicoccon* Schrank) and spelt (*T. spelta* L.) accessions. Int. J. Food Sci. Nutr. 48:381-386.

Piergiovanni, A. R., and Volpe, N. 2003. Capillary electrophoresis of gliadins as a tool in the discrimination and characterization of hulled wheats (*Triticum dicoccon* Schrank and *T. spelta* L.). Cereal Chem. 80:269-273.

Piironen, V., Lindsay, D. G., Miettinen, T. A., Toivo, J., and Lampi, A.-M. 2000. Plant sterols: Biosynthesis, biological function and their importance to human nutrition. J. Sci. Food Agric. 80:939-966.

Piironen, V., Toivo, J., and Lampi, A.-M. 2002. Plant sterols in cereals and cereal products. Cereal Chem. 79:148-154.

Pisante, M., Basso, B., Carafa, A. C., and Stornaiuolo, S. 1996. Coltivazione di popolazioni di farro (*Triticum dicoccon* e *T. spelta*) in ambiente arido dell'Italia meridionale. Riv. Agron. 12:25-30.

Pogna, N. E., Autran, J. C., Mellini, D., Lafiandra, D., and Feillet, P. 1990. Chromosome 1B-encoded gliadin and glutenin subunits in durum wheat genetics and relationship to gluten strength. J. Cereal Sci. 11:15-34.

Pomeranz, Y. 1988. Chemical composition of kernel structures. Pages 97-158 in: Wheat Chemistry and Technology, 3rd ed. Vol. I. Y. Pomeranz, Ed. Am. Assoc. Cereal Chem., St Paul, MN.

Porceddu, E., and Lafiandra, D. 1986. Origin and evolution of wheats. Pages 143-178 in: The Origin and Domestication of Cultivated Plants. C. Barigozzi, Ed. Elsevier, Amsterdam, Netherlands.

Porfiri, O., Petrini, A., Fuselli, D., Minoia, C., Borghi, B., D'Antuono, L. F., Minelli, M., Codoni, D., and Mazzocchetti, A. 1996. Farro: Scelta varietale. Risultati della sperimentazione 1995-96. Inf. Agrario 36:58-62.

Preston, K. R., Kilborn, R. H., and Black, H. C. 1982. The GRL pilot mill II. Physical dough and baking properties of flour streams milled from Canadian red spring wheat. Can. Inst. Food Sci. Technol. J. 115:29-36.

Rasmusson, D. C., Hester, A. J., Fick, G. N., and Byrne, I. 1971. Breeding for mineral content in wheat and barley. Crop Sci. 11:623-627.

Reddy, M. M., Yenagi, N. B., Rao, M., Srinivasan, C. N., Hanchinal, R. R. 1998. Grain and gluten quality of some cultivars of wheat species and their suitability for preparation of traditional South Indian sweet products. J. Food Sci. Technol. 35:441-444.

Resmini, P., and Pagani, M. A. 1983. Ultrastructure studies of pasta. A review. Food Microstruct. 2:1-12.

Rozenberg, R., Ruibal-Mendieta, N. L., Petitjean, G., Cani, P., Delacroix, D. L., Delzenne, N. M., Meurens, M., Quetin-Leclercq, J., and Habib-Jiwan, J-L. 2003. Phytosterol analysis and characterization in spelt (*Triticum aestivum* ssp. *spelta* L.) and wheat (*T. aestivum* L.) lipids by LC/APCI-MS. J. Cereal Sci. 38:189-197.

Ruibal-Mendieta, N. L., Delacroix, D. L., and Meurens, M. 2002. A comparative analysis of free, bound and total lipid on spelt and winter wheat wholemeal. J. Cereal Sci. 35:337-342.

Samuel, D. J. 1993. Ancient Egyptian cereal processing: Beyond the artistic record. Camb. Archaeol. J. 3:276-283.

Sarwar, M., and McDonald, C. E. 1993. Detection of bread wheat farina adulterant in durum wheat semolina and pasta dried at low, high, and ultra-high temperatures. Cereal Chem. 70:405-411.

Schiavone, M., Marconi, E., Cubadda, R., Falasca, L., Perrino, P., Laghetti, G., and Colonna, M. 2000. Variabilità delle caratteristiche agronomiche e qualitative di differenti genotipi di farro (*T. dicoccon* Schrank e *T. spelta* L.) coltivati in ambienti meridionali. Pages 216-220 in: Materie Prime Transgeniche, Sicurezza Alimentare e Controllo Qualità nell'Industria Cerealicola. R. Cubadda and E. Marconi, Eds. Arti Grafiche la Regione, Campobasso, Italy.

Schiavone, M., Marconi, E., Cubadda, R., and Falasca, L. 2001. Utilizzazione di sfarinati di farro spelta per la produzione di cereali da colazione. Tec. Molitoria 52:793-797.

Schlichting, L. M., Dexter, J. E., Preston, K. R., Edwards, N. M., Marchylo, B. A., Hucl, P., and Perron, C. E. 2003. Quality characterization of lines from a cross between emmer (*T. dicoccum)* and durum (*T. durum*) wheat. Pages 71-76 in: Durum Wheat and Pasta Quality: Recent Achievements and New Trends. M. G. D'Egidio, Ed. Istituto Sperimentale per la Cerealicoltura, Rome, Italy.

Seilmeier, W., Valdez, I., Mendez, E., and Wieser, H. 2001. Comparative investigations of gluten proteins from different wheat species. II. Characterization of omega-gliadins. Eur. Food Res. Technol. 212:355-363.

Sidhu, J. S. 1995. Wheat usage in the Indian subcontinent. Pages 191-213 in: Wheat End Uses Around the World. H. Faridi, Ed. Am. Assoc. Cereal Chem., St. Paul. MN.

Siedler, H. M. M., Messmer, G. M., Schachermayr, H., Winzeler, H., Winzeler, M., and Keller, B. 1994. Genetic diversity in European wheat and spelt breeding material based on RFLP data. Theor. Appl. Genet. 88:994-1003.

Singh, T., Maninder, K., and Bains, G. S. 1983. Malting of *Triticum dicoccum* (Khapli) wheat: Response to gibberellic acid and use in baking. J. Food Sci. 48:1135-1144.

Sissons, M. J., and Hare, R. A. 2002. Tetraploid wheat—A resource for genetic improvement of durum wheat quality. Cereal Chem. 79:78-84.

Skerrit, J. H., and Hill, A. S. 1990. Monoclonal antibody sandwich enzyme immunoassays for determination of gluten in foods. J. Agric. Food Chem. 38:1771-1778.

Skovmand, B., Gilchrist, L. I., Pena, R. J., and Hede, A. R. 1997. Emmer wheat as a genetic resource in wheat improvement. Pages 66-69 in: Small Grain Cereals and Pseudo-Cereals. O. Stolen, K. Bruhn, K. Pithan, and J. Hill, Eds. European Commission, Luxembourg.

Slavin, J. L. 2002. Whole grains, dietary fiber, and resistant starch. Pages 283-299 in: Whole-Grain Foods in Health and Disease. L. Marquart, J. L. Slavin, and R. G. Fulcher, Eds. Am. Assoc Cereal Chem., St. Paul, MN.

Somma, S., Cenci, A., Simeone, R., and Blanco, A. 2004. I carotenoidi in una collezione di frumenti coltivati e selvatici. Pages 95-104 in: Atti del 5° Convegno AISTEC Cereali: Scienza e Benessere dal Campo alla Tavola. R. Cubadda and E. Marconi, Eds. University of Molise, Campobasso, Italy.

Stallknecht, G. F., Gilbertson, K. M., and Ranney, J. E. 1996. Alternative wheat cereals as food grains: Einkorn, emmer, spelt, kamut, and triticale. Pages 156-170 in: Progress in New Crops. J. Janick, Ed. ASHS Press, Alexandria, VA.

Szabò, A. T., and Hammer, K. 1996. Notes on the taxonomy of farro: *Triticum monococcum, T. dicoccon* and *T. spelta*. Pages 2-40 in: Hulled Wheats. Promoting the Conservation and Use of Underutilized and Neglected Crops. S. Padulosi, K. Hammer, and J. Heller, Eds. International Plant Genetic Resources Institute, Rome, Italy.

Trematerra, P., and Gentile, P. 2002. Stored insect pests in traditional cultivated hulled wheat crop areas of Central-Southern Italy with emphasis on *Sitotroga cerealella* (Oliver). Int. Org. Biol. Integr. Control/W. Paleartic Reg. Sect. Bull. 25:27-32.

Trematerra, P., Fontana, F., Mancini, M., and Sciarretta, A. 1999. Influence of intact and damaged cereal kernels on the behaviour of rice weevil, *Sitophilus oryzae* (L.) (*Coleoptera: Curculionidae*). J. Stored Prod. Res. 35:265-276.

Vallega, V., and Waines, P.I. 1987. High molecular weight glutenin subunit variation in *Triticum turgidum* var. *dicoccum*. Theor. Appl. Genet. 74:706-710.

Wasik, R. J., and Bushuk, W. 1975. Relationship between molecular weight distribution of endosperm proteins and spaghetti-making quality of wheats. Cereal Chem. 51:322-328.

Wieser, H. 2000. Comparative investigations of gluten proteins from different wheat species. I. Qualitative and quantitative composition of gluten protein types. Eur. Food Res. Technol. 211:262-268.

Wieser, H. 2001. Comparative investigations of gluten proteins from different wheat species. III. N-terminal amino acid sequences of alpha-gliadins potentially toxic for celiac patients. Eur. Food Res. Technol. 213:183-186.

Wrigley, C. W., and Bietz, J. A. 1988. Proteins and amino acids. Pages 159-275 in: Wheat Chemistry and Technology, 3rd ed. Vol. I. Y. Pomeranz, Ed. Am. Assoc. Cereal Chem., St Paul, MN.

Zohary, D., and Hopf, M. 1993. Domestication of plants in the Old World. Pages 32-38 in: The Origin and Spread of Cultivated Plants in West Asia, Europe, and the Nile Valley. Clarendon Press, Oxford, England.

CHAPTER 5

Spelt: A Specialty Wheat for Emerging Food Uses

E-S. M. Abdel-Aal[1] and P. Hucl[2]

[1]Agriculture and Agri-Food Canada, Food Research Program, Guelph, ON, Canada N1G 5C9; [2]Crop Development Centre, Department of Plant Sciences, University of Saskatchewan, Saskatoon, SK, Canada N7S 5A8

Classification of Spelt

Spelt is a hulled wheat with lax spikes that disarticulate when threshed. The glumes adhere to the grain; thus, the harvested sample consists of intact spikelets known as covered grains or florets. In contrast to wild wheat, the rachis is semibrittle. The spelt spike disarticulates when the crop is left standing for an extended period. The chaff comprises 21–32% of the harvested product (Percival 1921).

Spelt is a hexaploid with the genomic designation AABBDD. It was originally classified as a species (*Triticum spelta*) separate from common wheat (*Triticum aestivum* L.) (Percival 1921), based on its distinct morphology. Subsequently, spelt was classified as a subspecies of *T. aestivum* (MacKey 1966). More recently, spelt wheat has been classified as a morphological subgroup of common wheat (Barnes and Beard 1992). The latest taxonomic grouping is borne out by research demonstrating that common wheat and spelt wheat form hybrids with very high levels of chromosome pairing (Cao et al 2000). Similarly, Schmid and Winzeler (1990) detected hybrid vigor for grain yield per spike and kernel weight in spelt-wheat crosses. Heterosis would likely not have been evident if the hybrids suffered from poor reproductive fertility. The morphological traits that most differentiate common wheat from spelt (free-threshing, square spikes with nonbrittle rachis) are controlled by a series of loci. The Q locus (Muramatsu 1963) on the long arm of chromosome 5A was originally thought to account for most of the spelt spike morphology. However, more recent research indicates that loci not linked to the Q locus also influence spike threshability and rachis brittleness (Luo et al 2000). The interaction between the Q locus and these other loci remains to be elucidated in full.

[1] For the Department of Agriculture and Agri-Food Canada, Food Research Program, Government of Canada. Publication number S176.

Recently, numerous studies of genetic diversity based on DNA or protein variability (Siedler et al 1994, Harsch et al 1997, Radic et al 1997, Cao et al 1998, Bertin et al 2001) have demonstrated that there is a clear divergence between spelt and common wheat, indicating that these two wheat types evolved in separate gene pools despite being of the same species. Although spelt and common wheat are genetically divergent (Siedler et al 1994), the magnitude of that divergence (approximately 0.132 on a 0.00–1.00 scale) is not very large. Modern literature continues to assign separate species status to spelt wheat, more from an end use than from a genetic viewpoint.

Origin and Production

Spelt wheat features prominently in the southern German and Swiss Bronze Age (1800–1200 B.C.) archeological record (Nesbitt and Samuel 1996). Kuckuck and Schiemann (1957) reported on the cultivation of spelt in the Bakhtiari region of western Iran during the 1950s. Subsequently, it was assumed that spelt originated in the Middle East and migrated north of the Black Sea and along the Danube River from east to west, ending up in what is now Austria, southern Germany, and northern Switzerland (Andrews 1964). However, no clear archeological evidence links the Iranian spelt source with European spelts (Nesbitt and Samuel 1996).

Subsequently, spelt wheat displaced einkorn and emmer wheat in Europe during a period of climatic cooling. This change started during the Bronze Age and was completed by the Iron Age (750–15 B.C.). It is speculated that fall-sown spelt wheat would have outyielded emmer wheat, the latter being spring-sown (Nesbitt and Samuel 1996).

Free-threshing hexaploid wheat was detected in archeological sites dating to 7,000 B.C. in what is now Turkey (Nesbitt and Samuel 1996). Because free-threshing wheat is much easier to process, this begs the question why a hulled wheat such as spelt would have persisted in production when free-threshing types were available. The answer may reside in the resistance of spelt wheat to common bunt (*Tilletia caries*), a fungus that reduces the palatability of wheat grain and flour due to a fishy odor and off-flavor. Common bunt is a soil-borne fungal pathogen that tends to be a production problem when wheat is sown into cool soils. Research at the University of Saskatchewan revealed that a significant proportion of spring spelt wheat accessions under evaluation were highly resistant to the common bunt pathogen (*unpublished data*). Percival (1921) mentioned that spelt wheat was considered resistant to common bunt. Two of the spelt accessions were subsequently studied in detail (He and Hughes 2003) and found to carry a single major gene conferring resistance. In addition, the tight-glumed nature of the spelt spikelet likely acted as a deterrent to infection by ergot (*Claviceps purpurea*). The latter can infest einkorn and became a problem in rye when that species was domesticated.

The area of production of spelt spread from west-central Europe to Belgium, France, Spain, and England. Using random amplified polymorphic

DNA (RAPD) analysis, Cao et al (1998) clustered 69 spelt accessions into three groups. The first group comprised accessions primarily from Spain, the second group from Belgium, Germany, and Switzerland, and the third group mainly from Hungary, Romania, and Yugoslavia. The latter group also contained accessions identified as originating in the United Kingdom and the United States. The accessions in group one had a spring growth habit, while those in the other two groups were primarily winter wheats. Thus, European spelts appear to have three gene pools: Spanish, western European, and eastern European. Using pedigree and microsatellite analyses, Bertin et al (2001) were able to obtain somewhat separate clusters for modern Belgian and Swiss spelt cultivars. However, the Swiss cultivar Oberkulmer has been used as a parent in the development of modern Belgian spelt cultivars, resulting in reduced cluster separation.

In Spain, spelt was first detected in archeological sites dating to the Iron Age (1000 B.C.) (Oliveira, 2001). Spelt wheat is still grown in traditional small farm holdings in northern modern Spain in the mountain areas of Asturias at altitudes of 200 to 1,000 m above sea level (Oliveira 2001). The latitude and the milder climate in which Spanish spelt is grown, relative to the growing conditions of northern European spelts, likely explains the divergence in growth habit between the groups identified by Cao et al (1998). Spelt has traditionally been used as a source of flour for breadbaking in Spain. *Escanda* (spelt) bread is currently considered a delicacy and served on special occasions such as religious feasts or family occasions (Peña-Chocarro 1996). The production, however, appears to be very limited (15 ha).

In medieval France, in addition to free-threshing types of common wheat, a red-awned variety of winter spelt (*épeautre*) called *rousset* was grown. Bread made from spelt wheat was preferred to that made from rye or rye-barley blends (Grand 1935). Rye was considered higher yielding than wheat, producing seven bushels per bushel sown compared to five to one for wheat and was better suited for production on lower-fertility soils, while wheat is reported to have been grown on heavier-textured soils. In some areas, wheat flour was used solely for making pastry. Spelt had largely disappeared as a cultivated crop by the twentieth century in France.

In Switzerland, spelt wheat was grown on 39,000 ha at the turn of the last century (Percival 1921) and was the dominant wheat until 1910 or so, after which it was rapidly replaced by common wheat, dropping to 3,000 ha by the late 1980s (Winzeler and Ruegger 1990) and 2,000 ha in the 1990s (Messmer et al 1996). In Germany, spelt was grown on 314,000 ha at the turn of the twentieth century (Percival 1921), declining to 231,000 ha in 1913 (Campbell 1997) and nearly ceasing by the end of World War II before recovering to approximately 5,000 ha in the early 1980s (Winzeler and Ruegger 1990). The states of Bavaria, Wurtemberg, and Baden are the primary growing regions (Percival 1921). In Belgium, the area sown to spelt was in the 8,000–10,000 ha range during the 1980s (Winzeler and Ruegger 1990). Current spelt production in Europe is estimated to occupy 25,000–30,000 ha (Dekeyser and Goenaga 2001).

While spelt was used primarily for human consumption in most countries, it was used as animal feed in Belgium and in Ohio. Winter spelt was introduced to Ohio by immigrants from Switzerland (Campbell 1997). Winter spelt produced grain yields and hulled test weights that were competitive with those of winter oat cultivars of the early twentieth century (Campbell 1997). This, combined with the greater degree of winter hardiness in wheat, would have made winter spelt an economically viable feed crop. Production in Ohio reached 100,000 ha in the mid-1980s, with minor production in Indiana, Michigan, Minnesota, Montana, and Pennsylvania (Campbell 1997). By 1995, the area sown to spelt in Ohio had dropped to 8,000 ha (Campbell 1997). The decline of winter spelt as a feed crop in the eastern United States was a result of displacement by higher-value crops as land costs increased. The production that remains is likely aimed largely at the organic food market (Perrino et al 1996). According to Stallknecht et al (1996), spelt production for human consumption in the United States increased from 40 to 3,200 ha between 1987 and the mid-1990s.

Information on the feed value of the hulled mature spelt grain appears to be limited in scope. Campbell (1997) presented data from the National Academy of Science indicating that the spelt is similar in feed value to oat. Spelt has been used as a green fodder in Spain (Peña-Chocarro 1996). The smaller spikelets were put to use as seed source for planting the green feed crop. In some cases, the green crop arose from shattered spikelets supplemented by sown small spikelets. No published data on the green feed quality of spelt exists. However, unpublished data from the University of Saskatchewan indicates that the feed value of spring spelt harvested at the early grain-filling stage is inferior to that of barley, oat, and common wheat.

In Canada, spelt production reached 2,000 ha in 2001, twice the area sown in 1996. The majority of this production, if not all, would likely have been for the organic market.

Cultivars

The vast majority of registered spelt cultivars have a winter growth habit. In Europe, 24 winter spelt cultivars are currently eligible for seed certification (OECD 2002). Of the 24 cultivars, seven are registered in Luxembourg or Belgium, seven in Switzerland, seven in Germany, two in Hungary, and one each in Austria and the Netherlands. The Swiss cultivar Ostro is listed in both Switzerland and Austria.

In the United States, two winter spelt cultivars are listed by the U.S. Department of Agriculture (USDA) as being under "Plant Variety Protection." One is GR900, an Ohio State University cultivar, and the other is Franckenkorn, a Belgian cultivar marketed by a German company. The spelt-common wheat-derived cultivar Champ was released in the mid-1980s by Ohio State University (Lafever 1988). Subsequently, Lafever has been developing winter spelt cultivars for the Sunbeam Extract Company (Stallknecht et al 1996). A number of cultivars (Comet, Maverick, Sammy,

Sava, and Sungold) have been developed (Sunbeam Extract Co. 2002) and released for seed multiplication in Ohio (OSIA 2002). It is not clear whether these five cultivars are derived from spelt-common wheat crosses. In addition to these recently developed cultivars, Champ and Oberkulmer (a Swiss landrace reselection dating from 1948) are eligible for seed production in Ohio (OSIA 2002).

In Canada, there are two registered cultivars: Heritage (winter type) and CDC Nexon (spring type). Heritage is the U.S. cultivar Sava (CFIA 2001). CDC Nexon was previously interim-registered as CDC Bavaria. Franckenkorn has been submitted for Canadian Plant Breeders Rights Protection (CFIA 2002) but is not registered.

Agronomic Properties

The majority of winter spelts are awnless (Campbell 1997), while spring spelts are largely awned (*unpublished data*). Spelt tends to be 30–40 cm taller than modern common wheat cultivars. This relationship has been observed with both winter (Campbell 1997) and spring spelt cultivars (Hucl et al 1995). Spelt cultivars tend to have a higher tillering rate and higher tiller mortality rate than common wheat cultivars (Ruegger et al 1990, Ruegger and Winzeler 1993). Thus, spelt cultivars may or may not produce more spikes per unit area than common wheat cultivars. Winter spelt grown in Ohio tended to be later maturing than common wheat (Lafever and Campbell 1977, Rimle 1995). A similar trend was observed with spring spelt (Hucl et al 1995). Because of its long, weaker straw, spelt wheat is prone to lodging (Ruegger et al 1993). This has led to fertilizer recommendations that involve lower nitrogen levels (Oplinger et al 1990) than would be recommended for common wheat. Spelt has a lower harvest index (–8 to 12% units) than modern common wheat cultivars (Ruegger et al 1993, Rimle 1995, Ehsanzadeh 1999) but larger kernels (Ruegger et al 1993).

The hulled grain yield of winter spelt is higher than that of common wheat under low-input conditions (Ruegger and Winzeler 1993). A similar trend was observed for spring spelt (Hucl et al 1995, Ehsanzadeh et al 1998). In the study by Ruegger and Winzeler (1993), the spelt cultivar Oberkulmer had a hulled grain yield equal to that of the common wheat Arina in a low-yield environment but was approximately 9% lower yielding in a higher-yield environment. In spring spelt, two cultivars (CDC Nexon, PGR8801) yielded, on average, 20% higher than the common wheat cultivar Katepwa (Ehsanzadeh et al 1998). Assuming that the hull accounts for roughly 25% of the harvested spelt yield, the net yields of spring spelt and common wheat were similar, while the net yield of winter spelt was 25–35% lower than that of common wheat. In spelt cultivars derived from spelt-common wheat crosses, the net grain yields have been superior to those of straight-spelt cultivars. This is evident from yield potential of the spelt-common wheat-derived cultivar Hercule (Ruegger and Winzeler 1993) and the cultivar Champ (Lafever 1988, Oplinger et al 1990).

Seeding

Seeding rates for winter spelt (90–120 kg/ha) (Campbell 1997) are generally similar to those used for common wheat. Ruegger and Winzeler (1993) compared two cultivars each of fall-sown spelt and common wheat at two seeding rates and found no differential response to seeding rate. In a study comparing two spring spelts and one common wheat cultivar, Ehsanzadeh et al (1998) determined that the optimal seeding rate for spelt wheat was no different than that of common wheat.

Unlike common wheat, in which the naked grain is planted, the planting propagule for spelt is a polished spikelet. The spikelet is polished via moderate abrasion to remove excess chaff that would interfere with seed-dispensing mechanisms in drills (Bleiker and Winzeler 1991). The spelt hull may result in better seedling establishment under cold-wet seed bed conditions due to seed protection from fungal colonization. Riesen et al (1986) conducted a controlled environment study that demonstrated a significantly higher percentage of seedling establishment for hulled spelt relative to naked spelt or common wheat grain. In a subsequent field study in waterlogged soil (Ruegger et al 1990), hulled spelt grain had a significant seedling establishment advantage. Subsequently, Beglinger (1995) demonstrated under controlled laboratory conditions that spelt seedlings had a higher tolerance to hypoxia (reduced oxygen supply) than common wheat. Furthermore, the coleoptile growth rate of spelt wheat appears to be higher than that of common wheat under controlled conditions (Beglinger 1995).

There do not appear to be any published studies on the effect of sowing date on winter spelt performance. Ehsanzadeh (1999) determined that spring spelt wheat had an optimal sowing date that is earlier than that of common wheat in trials conducted at Saskatoon, Saskatchewan. The spring spelt cultivar CDC Nexon had a slower development rate (longer phyllocron interval) than the common wheat cultivar Katepwa. Although both CDC Nexon and Katepwa reached the double-ridge stage of plant development at the same time, the spelt cultivar required three extra days for spike differentiation. On average, the spelt cultivar was 14 days later maturing than the common wheat cultivar (Ehsanzadeh 1999). In addition to being later maturing, the spelt cultivar CDC Nexon was significantly more prone to lodging than the common wheat cultivar. However, an accession of spring spelt wheat, PGR8801, had significantly better straw strength than CDC Nexon (Ehsanzadeh 1999).

In a growth analysis of the cultivars CDC Nexon and PGR8801, along with the wheat cultivar Katepwa, Ehsanzadeh et al (1998) found that the two spelt wheat cultivars had significantly higher leaf area indices, leaf area duration, crop-growth rate, and crop biomass at maturity than the common wheat cultivar. The two spelt wheat lines had a more horizontal leaf attitude than the common wheat cultivar (Ehsanzadeh 1999). In a study of spring wheat cultivar differences in competitive ability, Hucl et al (1997) determined that the spelt cultivar CDC Nexon was more competitive than common or durum wheats, approaching spring barley in ability to compete against tame oat and mustard. The competitive ability of spelt wheat appears related to its greater leaf production capacity and leaf orientation, which has a greater shading effect. This morphological trait would make spelt wheat well suited to organic crop-production systems.

In an attempt to overcome the lodging problems and lower grain yields typical of winter spelt landraces, European breeders have made use of spelt-common wheat crosses (Bertin et al 2001). The introduction of dwarfing genes has reduced the degree of lodging. The majority of European winter spelt wheat cultivars currently have a common wheat parent in their pedigree. However, current market demand is for spelt-spelt derivatives.

Harvesting

Spelt can be threshed using conventional combines. The spike disarticulates into spikelets with 10–20% of the grain threshing out, depending on the cultivar and harvest conditions. Once the hulled seed is dried to 13–15% moisture, it can be stored safely. If the spelt crop is left standing for an extended period, the spikes will shatter near the base, resulting in severe yield losses and excessive volunteering in the subsequent growing season. It is recommended that the crop be swathed as it reaches physiological maturity.

Disease Resistance

Primitive wheats are often assumed to be more disease resistant than modern cultivars, but this is generally a misconception. Spelt was shown to have an intermediate response to leaf and glume blotch caused by the fungal pathogen *Septoria nodorum* (Arseniuk et al 1991). Similarly, spelt cultivars were comparable in reaction range to strip rust (Schmid et al 1994) caused by *Puccinia striiformis*. However, individual spelt accessions can provide new genes for resistance to the stripe rust pathogen (Kema 1992). McVey (1990) screened the USDA spelt collection for reaction to stem rust (*Puccinia graminis*) and found a number of accessions that were resistant to a wide array of isolates. Spelt produced in Ohio is reported as being very susceptible to loose smut (Lipps 1996). Conversely, spelt tends to be resistant to common bunt (stinking smut) (Percival 1921).

Milling Performance

Spelt is a covered or hulled wheat and needs to be dehulled before milling or processing. Removal of hulls is usually done by passing the hulled grains through pairs of rubber-coated rolls, pearling stones, or abrasive mills, followed by air aspiration. Nowadays more efficient and specifically constructed dehullers are being developed to remove hulls from spelt and other hulled grains (Kaiser 1992). The hulls make up 24–28% of the grains, averaging approximately 26% (Hucl et al 1995).

The wheat hulls may be of some economic value in feed and industrial applications. The hulls may also provide physical protection to the grains during planting and storage. On the other hand, the hulled grains are bulky and require more storage space during transportation and handling, which results in increased processing costs. The premium obtained for spelt products compared to common wheat products currently still generates higher profits for spelt products, especially in the organic and health-food markets. In the marketplace, spelt flours are almost twice as expensive as common wheat flours. In Germany, spelt flour is about 80% more expensive than wheat flour (Federmann et al 1992).

Spelt is a wheat that can be milled into flour at several extraction rates for various end uses (e.g., white flour, 65%, 72%) and whole-meal flour (100%). The same basic types of equipment used for milling common wheat can also be used in milling of spelt and other ancient wheats. As in common wheat, the kernel properties of spelt determine its milling performance (i.e., flour yield). Some spelt and other ancient wheats may possess desirable flavors that could require special care in milling to reduce the loss of flavor caused by heat damage. In this respect, stone mills are being used to reduce the greater heat damage generated by metal mills and to maintain flavor.

An early study (LeClerc et al 1918) showed that a variety of ancient wheats including spelt, emmer, einkorn, and polish wheat were comparable to a hard red spring wheat when milled on an Allis-Chalmers experimental flour mill to 65% flour yield, but the ancient wheat flours were slightly darker than that of spring wheat. The spelt cv. Alstroum produced an acceptable flour for baking purposes. More recently, five accessions of hard and soft spring spelt, adapted for growing under Western Canadian conditions, gave flour yields of approximately 70%, comparable to those of hard red spring wheat using standard experimental milling procedures (Abdel-Aal et al 1997). The spelt flours were similar in whiteness (Hunter L values = 90) to those of common wheat and exhibited similar or finer particle-size distributions. One of the soft wheat accessions with reasonable baking quality was registered in Canada under the name CDC Nexon in 2002. Ranhotra et al (1995) obtained lower flour yields for a sample of spelt compared to a hard red winter wheat check over a range of tempering moisture levels. The investigators associated differences in flour yield to variation in test weight, particularly at lower weights (i.e., less than 57 lb/bu). However, the maximum flour yields of spelt were still comparable to those obtained with commercial milling. In other words, the maximum flour yields obtained at 100 g/kg grain moisture content were approximately 78% for spelt versus 82% for common winter wheat. These studies suggest that milling performance of spelt is somewhat similar to common wheat when standard milling procedures are used.

Nutrient Composition

Starch

Starch is the principal storage carbohydrate in wheat kernels, including spelt, and its content and characteristics are known to substantially affect the quality of wheat grains and their end products. A study of five accessions of

TABLE 1
Average Nutrient Composition of Whole Spelt, Durum, and Common Wheat (%, db)

Wheat	Starch	Protein[a]	TDF[b]	Ash	Fat	Reference
Soft spelt (*n* = 3)[c]	65.3	14.9	9.8	1.7	2.5	Abdel-Aal et al (1995)
Hard spelt (*n* = 2)	61.6	16.0	10.3	1.8	2.3	Abdel-Aal et al (1995)
Spelt (*n* = 4)	66.7	12.2	…	2.1	3.8	Grela (1996)
Spelt (*n* = 37)	…	17.1	…	2.1	2.1	Piergiovanni et al (1996)
Spelt (*n* = 9)	62.1[d]	12.8	11.4	1.8	2.0	Ranhotra et al (1996a)
Spelt (*n* = 5)	65.2[d]	15.7	12.7	1.9	4.4	Marconi et al (1999)
Spelt[e] (*n* = 10)	…	12.1	…	2.4	1.7	Moudry and Dvoracek (1999)
Spelt (*n* = 3)	…	16.4	13.2	1.8	…	Bonafaccia et al (2000)
Spelt (*n* = 1)	63.2	14.0	…	…	…	Skrabanja et al (2001)
Durum	64.9	15.1	11.1	1.6	2.1	Abdel-Aal et al (1995)
Common HRS	62.4	15.3	12.5	1.7	2.1	Abdel-Aal et al (1995)

[a] N × 5.7, except N × 6.25 for data from Grela (1996).
[b] Total dietary fiber.
[c] Number of accessions/cultivars in the test.
[d] Digestible carbohydrates (starch plus sugars).
[e] Grown in low-input system.

spring spelt found that starch content varied from 61 to 66%, compared to 62% in common wheat grown side by side with the spelt lines in western Canada (Abdel-Aal et al 1995). The digestible carbohydrate content (calculated by difference) in five European winter spelt cultivars grown in different European countries (Austria, Belgium, Italy, and Switzerland) ranged from 60 to 69%, with an average of 65% (Marconi et al 1999). Ranhotra et al (1995) reported slightly higher contents of carbohydrate and energy contents for a spelt wheat sample compared to those of hard red winter wheats. In a subsequent study of eight spelt samples, carbohydrate content ranged from 60 to 64%, with an average of 62%, and energy content ranged from 312 to 319 kcal/100 g, with an average of 316 kcal/100 g (Ranhotra et al 1996a). In general, the starch content of spelt has been found to vary among accessions and cultivars, ranging from 62 to 67% (Table 1). The variation in starch content among spelt wheats is most likely similar to those differences found between soft and hard common wheat cultivars.

Protein and Amino Acids

Analyses of spring-sown soft and hard spelt revealed significant differences in protein content (Abdel-Aal et al 1995). The hard spelt accessions contained significantly higher levels of protein than soft spelt cultivars, exhibiting a similar trend as in common wheat. However, the breadmaking quality of soft spelt exceeded that of hard spelt, contrary to the pattern found with common wheat (Abdel-Aal et al 1997). Likewise, winter-type spelt wheats show considerable variability in protein contents, reflecting both varietal and environmental effects. Cubadda and Marconi (1996) cited nine investigations in which protein contents of emmer landraces ranged from

9.3 to 21.3% and four studies in which the protein levels in winter spelts ranged from 13.4 to 16.1%. Analyses of four commercial winter spelt cultivars indicated that protein content varied from 11.0 to 14.4%, compared with 13.4% in common wheat (Grela 1996). Piergiovanni et al (1996) reported that the average protein contents of 50 emmer and 37 spelt accessions were similar, averaging 16.7 and 17.1%, respectively, both exceeding the mean for three durum cultivars (15.3%). Several studies have shown substantial variation among spelt cultivars in protein content (Table 1). This indicates potential genetic diversity among spelt wheats for breeding high- or low-protein spelt cultivars.

Clamot (1984) found considerable genetic differences in protein and lysine contents among 164 spelts, including 77 selections from old Belgian landraces, 72 introductions from various countries, and 15 induced mutants. Protein content in spelt was also influenced by year-to-year environmental variation. The genetic and environmental factors influence the protein content and composition of spelt wheats and should be considered when comparisons are made between spelt and durum or common wheat.

In general, wheat proteins are known to be low in some amino acids that are considered essential in the human diet, especially lysine (the first most deficient amino acid) and threonine (the second most deficient amino acid) (Kies and Fox 1970), but they are rich in glutamic acid and proline, the major

TABLE 2
Average Amino Acid Composition of Whole Spelt and Common Wheat (g/100 g of protein)

Amino Acid	Spelt[a]	Wheat[a]	Spelt[b]	Wheat[b]	Soft Spelt[c]	Hard Spelt[c]	Wheat[c]
Alanine	3.8	3.5	3.4	3.6	3.1	2.9	3.2
Arginine	5.1	4.6	4.5	4.6	4.2	4.1	4.4
Aspartic acid	6.0	5.3	5.2	4.9	4.3	4.6	4.3
Cystine	2.1	2.2	2.1	2.5	2.2	2.3	1.9
Glutamic acid	26.8	28.5	36.0	29.9	35.2	34.9	34.9
Glycine	3.9	4.0	3.8	3.9	3.9	3.7	3.8
Histidine	2.3	2.8	2.4	2.3	2.4	2.3	2.4
Isoleucine	4.2	3.9	3.8	3.3	2.5	2.6	2.7
Leucine	7.1	7.3	7.1	6.7	6.8	6.8	6.9
Lysine	3.2	2.9	2.7	2.9	2.2	2.2	2.4
Methionine	1.7	2.3	1.7	1.5	1.6	1.8	1.5
Phenylalanine	4.5	5.2	5.1	4.5	4.9	5.1	4.8
Proline	7.6	8.4	11.9	9.9	8.6	8.9	8.8
Serine	4.6	5.0	4.7	4.9	4.5	4.4	4.4
Threonine	3.7	3.6	2.7	2.9	2.9	2.9	3.0
Tryptophan	1.5	1.5	...	...	1.5	1.3	1.4
Tyrosine	3.5	3.4	2.7	3.0	2.8	2.6	2.6
Valine	5.0	4.5	4.7	4.4	4.0	3.9	3.9

[a] Data from Grela (1996).
[b] Data from Bonafaccia et al (2000).
[c] Data from Abdel-Aal and Hucl (2002).

functional amino acids in the formation of dough. The amino acid composition of the proteins from spelt differs slightly from that of modern bread wheat (Table 2) and pasta wheat (Cubadda and Marconi 1996). Milling and processing of spelt and common wheat were found to adversely influence lysine content of the end products (Abdel-Aal and Hucl 2002). The reduction in lysine content varied with the type of processing and the wheat species. Lysine content was also found to significantly negatively correlate with glutamic acid, the major amino acid in wheat proteins, indicating the importance of glutamic acid in wheat quality and in processing as an indication for lysine loss. The *in vitro* protein digestibility of spelt was similar to that of other ancient and modern wheat samples, averaging 86.7% compared to 97.6% for casein (Abdel-Aal and Hucl 2002).

Dietary Fiber

Several reports have shown that spelt wheats contain lower or similar levels of insoluble dietary fiber compared to durum and common wheats (Abdel-Aal et al 1995, Ranhotra et al 1996a,b, Bonafaccia et al 2000), which would not support claims that spelt has superior benefits in weight control or elimination of obesity (D'Antuono and Bravi 1996). The insoluble dietary fiber fraction acts as a bulking agent in the gastrointestinal tract and improves colonic health, whereas soluble dietary fiber may have a cholesterol-lowering effect. The levels of soluble dietary fiber in spring- and winter-type spelt were similar or slightly higher than those of modern wheats (Abdel-Aal et al 1995, Bonafaccia et al 2000), but as a percentage of total dietary fiber, soluble dietary fiber is slightly higher in spelt than in common wheat. Consumption of whole-grain or bran products of spelt and other wheat species would reduce caloric density and possibly intake, and the incidence of diseases of the lower digestive tract, but other components of the diet would be needed to supply soluble dietary fiber to reduce blood lipids. More generally, in the United States, a health claim associating consumption of whole-grain products with a lower risk of heart disease and certain cancers is allowed. Some of these benefits may be related to dietary fiber. The total dietary fiber content in different spelt cultivars varies from 9.8 to 13.2% (Table 1).

Lipids and Fatty Acids

Lipids are minor constituents in wheat grains (about 2%) and are more concentrated in the germ and aleurone than in the endosperm. The nonpolar lipids constitute about 70% of whole-wheat lipids. The other lipids are glycolipids (20%) and phospholipids (10%), in addition to small percentages of sterols, tocopherols, and other fat-soluble vitamins. The whole-meal flours of 50 emmer and 37 spelt wheats were higher than the control durum wheats in fat content, averaging 2.0, 2.1, and 1.5%, respectively (Piergiovanni et al 1996). A recent study of 91 samples of true and hybrid spelt and 78 samples of winter wheat showed that spelt contains significantly higher levels of free (crude) and total lipid than common winter wheat (Ruibal-Mendieta et al 2002), and that true spelt may contain more lipid than hybrid spelt, although

TABLE 3
Average Fatty Acid Composition of Whole Spelt and Common Wheat (% of total fatty acids)[a]

Fatty Acid (FA)	Spelt (n = 4)	Wheat (n = 1)
Palmitic, C16:0	18.5	16.7
Oleic, C18:1 n-9[b]	20.4	11.3
Linoleic, C18:2 n-6	55.1	62.8
Linolenic, C18:3 n-3	3.0	7.1
Saturated FA	20.5	18.0
Monounsaturated FA	21.5	12.1
Polyunsaturated FA	58.1	69.9

[a] Source: Grela (1996); used by permission.
[b] Chain length and number and location of the double bond(s).

that difference was significant in only two out of three harvest years. It was also suggested that free lipid could be used to differentiate between spelt and common winter wheat.

The predominant fatty acids in wheat are linoleic, palmitic, oleic, and linolenic (Table 3). The whole-meal flours of four winter-type spelt cultivars appeared to contain more monounsaturated and less polyunsaturated fat than that of common wheat (Grela 1996). In other words, spelt whole-meal flours contained more oleic acid (on average 20 vs 11% of total fatty acids) and less linoleic and linolenic acids (on average, 55 and 3% vs 63 and 7% of total fatty acids) than common wheat.

Vitamins and Minerals

The contents of total tocopherol and tocotrienols, which are responsible for vitamin E activity, in eight market classes of wheat ranged from 2.8 to 9.9 mg/100 g (Chung 1991). The mean concentration of total tocopherols in four winter spelt cultivars was 4.2 mg/100 g, compared to 2.3 mg/100 g in common winter wheat (Grela 1996). Because one-third of the tocopherols in the spelts was α-tocopherol while α-tocopherol constituted one-half of the tocopherols in common wheat, the vitamin E activities were 3.3 IU/100 g and 2.3 IU/100 g in spelts and common wheat, respectively. These levels are quite significant relative to the human requirements of 9 mg/day (Guthrie 1993). Because most of the tocopherol derivatives are concentrated in the germ, and wheat flours contain about 40% of the level in the grain (Chung 1991), more data are needed on the tocopherol composition in spelt as well as in other ancient grains.

Wheat grains are recognized as important dietary sources of B vitamins. For example, Hoppner et al (1968) demonstrated that two common spring wheat cultivars grown at 16 locations in two years contained 0.5, 0.2, and 6.8 mg/100 g of thiamin, riboflavin, and niacin, respectively. These thiamin and niacin levels would provide a substantial proportion of the human requirements in balanced diets, but the riboflavin level would not supplement defi-

TABLE 4
Average Vitamin Contents of Whole Spelt and Common Wheat (mg/100 g, db)

Vitamin	Soft Spelt[a]	Hard Spelt[a]	Wheat[a]	Spelt[b]	Wheat[b]
Thiamin	0.54	0.61	0.57	0.41	0.38
Riboflavin	0.16	0.15	0.55	0.21	0.17
Niacin	3.70	5.70	2.30	6.90	7.20
Pyridoxine	0.35	0.42	0.36	...	...

[a] Data from Abdel-Aal et al (1995).
[b] Data from Ranhotra et al (1995).

TABLE 5
Mineral Content Ranges in Whole Spelt, Emmer, Durum, and Common Wheat (mg/100 g, db)[a]

Mineral	Spelt (n = 10)[b]	Emmer (n = 10)	Durum (n = 3)	Wheat (n = 2)
Macro elements				
Potassium	394–450	337–450	335–449	280–393
Phosphorus	363–571	293–358	335–361	350–377
Sulfur	151–196	138–175	129–134	95–103
Magnesium	140–190	130–171	107–144	117–134
Calcium	26–52	25–42	39–44	35–50
Trace elements				
Zinc	2.25–3.94	1.38–2.53	0.84–2.24	1.68–2.24
Copper	0.56–0.79	0.39–0.67	0.56–0.62	0.45–0.50
Lithium	0.22–1.36	0.11–0.96	0.56–0.67	0.56–1.12
Selenium ($\times 10^{-2}$)	0.19–0.58	0.18–0.35	0.14–0.23	0.06–0.18

[a] Source: Piergiovanni et al (1997); used by permission.
[b] Number of accessions/cultivars in the test.

ciencies in other components of the diet. An early study on spelt or *dinkel* (the German name for spelt) showed that spelt is richer in thiamin and niacin than common wheat, but the riboflavin content of both is similar (Jacquot et al 1960). Bognár and Kellermann (1991) also found high levels of thiamin, riboflavin, and pyridoxine in winter spelt. On the other hand, Ranhotra et al (1995, 1996a) found similar concentrations of thiamin, riboflavin, and niacin in spelt and common wheat (Table 4). Abdel-Aal et al (1995) reported similar contents of thiamin and pyridoxine in spelt and common wheat, significantly higher levels of riboflavin in common wheat, and significantly higher concentrations of niacin in spelt (Table 4). The limited data in the literature on B-complex vitamins in spelt and other ancient wheats does not support claims of superior nutritional value, at least on the basis of these vitamin contents. A larger number of studies on vitamins and minerals in spelt cultivars is required to better assess the nutritional quality and possible advantages of this primitive grain.

Several investigators have found that spring and winter spelt wheats were generally comparable to the common wheat control in calcium, zinc, copper, potassium, manganese, and sodium composition (Abdel-Aal et al 1995, Grela 1996, Ranhotra et al 1996b). The mineral composition of 10 emmer and 10 spelt accessions was evaluated and compared to that of two common wheat cultivars and three durum cultivars grown in the same experimental field in Southern Italy (Table 5). Emmer and spelt wheats differed from common and durum wheat cultivars in having higher levels of lithium, magnesium, phosphorus, selenium, and zinc. The highest levels for all minerals tested were found in spelt accessions, suggesting a higher uptake in spelt. In another study of 10 cultivars of spelt and one cultivar of common wheat cultivated in a low-input system, spelt was significantly higher than common wheat in total ash, zinc, and phosphorus of the eight analyzed elements (sodium, potassium, calcium, magnesium, phosphorus, copper, zinc, and iron) (Moudry and Dvoracek 1999). The other minerals were higher in spelt by 5–25%, except for calcium, which was lower by approximately 3%.

Bioactive Constituents

Besides providing basic nutrients, wheat is also known as a source of potentially health-enhancing and physiologically active components such as dietary fiber, phenolics, phytates, enzyme inhibitors, tocopherols, and carotenoids. These may have both adverse and beneficial health effects, but in general, the effects of these components in promoting good health and reducing the risk of degenerative chronic diseases are becoming scientifically documented. For example, phytates were found to lower blood glucose response to starchy foods (Yoon et al 1983), and to reduce plasma cholesterol and triacylglycerol levels in rats (Jariwalla et al 1990) and cancer risk in rats (Shamsuddin et al 1988, 1989). Several reports also indicated that flavonoids and phenolics may be inversely associated with the risk of coronary heart disease (Hollman et al 1996), possibly by protection against oxidation of low-density lipoprotein and liposome (Heinonen et al 1998, Chang et al 2000). Antioxidant activity of these compounds may also reduce the risk of cancer (Block 1992). Phenolic components are also recognized to play a protective role for plants against diseases and pests. For instance, resistance to mold damage in sorghum (Hahn et al 1983), insect consumption of corn (Arnason et al 1992), aphid infestation of barley (Cabrera et al 1995), and midge damage in wheat (Abdel-Aal et al 2001) have been linked to a high level of phenolic acids in those grains. Little information is available with regard to bioactive components in spelt or other primitive grains. Cubadda and Marconi (1996) found that emmer and spelt flours contained higher levels of phytate (236 and 313 mg/100 g, respectively) than soft wheat flours (142 mg/100 g), and suggested that these higher levels could be attributed to aleurone and bran contamination in the flours. In the same study, trypsin inhibitor activities in the hulled wheats were similar to those of durum but lower than those of soft wheat. Grela (1996) evaluated four spelt cultivars for their alkylresorcinol, tannin, and trypsin inhibitor content. The trypsin inhibitor activities were similar among spelt cultivars, at a level of 1.0 trypsin inhibitor units (TIU)/mg compared to 1.3 TIU/mg in common wheat. The alkylresorcinol content ranged from 34 to 49 mg/100 g in spelt, averaging 40 mg/100 g, which was mostly less than that in common wheat (47 mg/100 g), while tannin concentration varied from 1.4 to 2.4 g/kg, with an average of 2.0 g/kg, which was similar to that of common wheat. The small concentrations of these bioactive components in spelt as in common wheat would not reduce palatability or nutrient digestibility. Long-term health effects are not known, but it seems unlikely that there would be a difference between spelt and common wheat based on these components.

Storage Proteins

The prolamin storage proteins in the wheat kernel are a key factor that determines the quality of products and end uses. They represent a diverse group of polymers with different molecular structures and functions. The quantity, amino acid composition, and molecular structure of wheat-storage proteins have been investigated extensively in an attempt to understand their functionality and to establish roles in cultivar identification, quality, and processing of grains and in human nutrition. Traditionally, wheat-storage proteins have been classified primarily into two major groups, gliadins and glutenins, based on solubility. Gliadins are alcohol-soluble proteins and glutenins are soluble in dilute acids or bases. Gliadin and glutenin proteins constitute about 80–85% of the total grain proteins, with a ratio of approximately 1:1 in common wheat. Gliadins are monomer components of peptides that are further categorized into α-, β-, γ-, and ω-gliadin on the basis of their mobility in acid-polyacrylamide gel electrophoresis (A-PAGE) (Wall 1979), while glutenins are polymers of peptide chains that are subdivided into high-molecular-weight (HMW) (100–140 kDa) and low-molecular-weight (LMW) (30–50 kDa) protein subunits by sodium dodecyl sulfate-polyacrylamide gel electrophoresis (SDS-PAGE) (Bietz and Simpson 1992). The α-, β-, and γ-gliadins and LMW glutenins are sulfur-rich proteins, while ω-gliadin and HMW glutenins are sulfur-poor proteins. The molecular weight range of ω-gliadins has been estimated at 44–78 kDa by SDS-PAGE (Tatham et al 1990). Several reports have shown that spelt contains gliadins and glutenins with structures distinct from those of common wheat (Abdel-Aal et al 1996a, Harsch et al 1997, Radic et al 1997, von Buren et al 2000). In addition, spelt storage proteins are found to form gluten, the well-known cohesive viscoelastic dough of wheat, but with different properties and quality (Abdel-Aal et al 1995, Schober et al 2002).

The prolamins are encoded by genes at three major locations in all three chromosome sets: HMW glutenins on the long arms of chromosomes of homologous group 1 (Glu-1 loci); LMW glutenins, γ- and ω-gliadins on the short arms of group 1 (Glu-3 and Gli-1, respectively); and α- and β-gliadins on the short arms of group 6 (Gli-2 loci) (Payne 1987). HMW and LMW glutenins have been associated with bread- and pasta-making quality in common and durum wheat, respectively (Pogna et al 1990, Shewry et al 1995), while the triggering agents in celiac disease are found in the gliadin fraction (Skerritt et al 1990, Sturgess et al 1991). Moreover, Maruyama et al (1998) found that different prolamin fractions exhibited allergenic activity. The prolamin protein subunits determined by A-PAGE, SDS-PAGE, capillary electrophoresis, reversed-phase high performance liquid chromatography (RP-HPLC), or enzyme-linked immunosorbent assay (ELISA) have been employed for cultivar identification (Payne and Lawrence 1983), detection of adulteration of spelt flour with common wheat flour (Federmann et al 1992), and detection of ω-gliadin or gluten contamination in gluten-free products made for celiac patients or individuals with gluten intolerance (Skerritt and Hill 1990, 1991). The polymerase chain reaction (PCR) analytical approach was applied to 35 hexaploid cultivars, including 11 spelts, seven spelt-wheat crosses, and 17 wheats to study differences in gliadin gene patterns between spelt and wheat (von Buren et al 2000). The 18 spelts tested and the wheat cv. Chinese Spring were found to carry an unknown γ-gliadin gene, while the 16 wheat cultivars possessed a previously documented allele.

Analysis of the gliadin composition of 95 spring spelts and five winter spelts in comparison with the hard red spring (HRS) wheat cv. Neepawa by A-PAGE and SDS-PAGE techniques showed that both spelt types diverged widely from HRS wheat based on scoring and analysis of 13 gliadin bands by similarity for qualitative data (SIMQUAD) to generate Jaccard similarity coefficients (Abdel-Aal et al 1996a). None of the spelts evaluated had a gliadin profile similar to that of the common wheat. Spelt gliadins are characterized by the absence of a slow-moving ω-gliadin and a strong-staining fast-moving ω-gliadin. These two ω-gliadins are present in common wheat. The same observations were made by Federmann et al (1992), who reported that slow-moving ω-gliadins are the most suited for discrimination between spelt and common wheat. Abdel-Aal et al (1996a) identified two types of spring spelt based on gliadin composition. One was characterized by the presence of γ-gliadin band and having soft endosperm kernels; the other type (hard-grained spelt) did not contain the γ-gliadin band. The latter study showed that the molecular weights of the spelt gliadins ranged from 34 to 75 kDa using SDS-PAGE. A study on 16 spelt cultivars, 12 spelt-wheat crosses, four German wheat cultivars, and four English wheat cultivars showed specific differences in the gliadin band patterns, providing a clear distinction between spelt and wheat (Harsch et al 1997). The investigators have developed a special nomenclature to show the gliadin differences between the two wheats. The new nomenclature is based on the one developed by Woychick et al (1961), which classifies the gliadins bands into A, B, C, and Z rather than α, β, γ, and ω, with the addition of another band group, between group C and Z, called D. The study indicated that the appearance of protein bands A1 and Z1 as well as the absence of the D-section can be taken as evidence for a strong wheat character. The spelt crosses showed differences in the intensity, mobility, occurrence, and splitting of single bands when compared to their corresponding parents. A majority of the spelt-common wheat derivatives showed more similarities with the maternal parent than with

TABLE 6
Wheat- and Spelt-Typical Protein Bands of All Sodium Dodecyl Sulfate-Soluble Proteins With and Without Preextraction in Chlorine Ethanol[a]

Band type	Area I	Area II
With the preextraction method		
Wheat-typical bands	43.9 and 45 kDa	59.5 kDa
Spelt-typical bands	45.7 and 47.5 kDa	60.5 kDa
Without the preextraction method		
Wheat-typical bands	40.7 and 43.1 kDa	56.0 kDa
Spelt-typical bands	41.4 and 44.6 kDa	60.4 kDa

[a] Source: Radic-Miehle et al (1998); used by permission.

the paternal one. Nevertheless, using either nomenclature, the latter observations agree with the above-mentioned differences in which the slow-moving ω-gliadins are the most suited for discriminating between spelt and common wheat.

Analysis of glutenin proteins of 28 spelts, 16 spelt-wheat crosses, and 10 winter wheat cultivars using SDS-PAGE showed differences between spelt and wheat (Radic et al 1997). The major differences are found in three distinct areas of the electropherograms, in which the molecular weight ranges from 40 to 49, 53 to 62, and 74 to 115 kDa. The wheat standard had protein bands of molecular weight 53, 56, 57, 59, 73, 84, 97, and 104 kDa but lacked the 30- and 40-kDa bands that appear in spelt. Spelt had protein bands of molecular weight 40, 45, 49, 60, 62, 82, 88, 95, 101, 108, and 109 kDa. Bands of 31, 32, 41, 44, and 79 kDa appear in both spelt and wheat standards but are of different intensities. In addition, the study indicated that the HMW bands of wheat and spelt-wheat crosses had weak intensities. In a following study (Radic-Miehle et al 1998), a large number of spelt and Central European winter wheats were analyzed, and glutenin and gliadin protein subunit compositions were compared. The differences in SDS soluble protein bands between spelt and common wheat are presented in Table 6. These investigators also classified spelt cultivars based on their strong or weak spelt or wheat character into spelt cultivars with typical spelt character, spelt cultivars with weak wheat character, and spelt cultivars with strong wheat character. Such classification is useful in cultivar identification and quality evaluation, and in selecting spelt for specific end uses. This might also help promote spelt on the basis of cultivar ancestry.

Gluten Quality

The wet gluten quality of 27 European spelt cultivars was evaluated using a diverse range of techniques, including fundamental rheological methods (oscillatory and creep tests), the SDS sedimentation test, moisture content of gluten (as an indication of swelling capacity), and a special baking test developed for evaluating spelt in the production of the traditional German spelt specialty bread called *Seelen* (Schober et al 2002). *Seelen* breads are prepared from a very soft yeast dough by using a higher amount of water (67% flour basis), and the dough is subjected to a long bulk fermentation time of 2.5 hr at low temperature (14°C) with reshaping after 1 and 2 hr. After fermentation, a dough portion of 65 g was weighed and machine-rounded into rolls that were final proofed for 35 min at 30°C and 90% rh and then baked for 20 min at 220°C. As for common wheat, significant correlations were found between the gluten properties and the baking quality of spelt bread. A high volume and round shape of the rolls are obtained if the gluten is firm at the larger deformations of the creep test, has more elastic components contributing to the rheological behavior, and has higher SDS sedimentation volumes and swelling capacity. The spelt cultivars evaluated varied significantly with regard to gluten properties. When 10 accessions of emmer and spelt were tested for quality based on γ-gliadins and HMW glutenin subunits, the gliadin γ-45, which is related to good gluten quality in durum, was found in all emmer accessions and in only seven accessions of spelt (Piergiovanni and Blanco 1999). With regard to the HMW glutenins, emmer was found to be more polymorphic than spelt. Some of the spelt accessions exhibited the highest SDS sedimentation volumes and the highest-quality index values, which are associated with the presence of the subunit pair 13 + 16 in the HMW glutenin fraction. In general, spelt and spelt-wheat crosses are widely different in gluten properties and quality, exhibiting genetic diversity for selection for specific characteristics and end uses.

Food Use

The world collections contain numerous landraces and biotypes of spelt, but a limited number of studies have characterized the range of quality properties among spelt accessions. Spelt has shown potential in a variety of end uses, including bread, pasta, and breakfast cereals (Abdel-Aal et al 1998a, 1998b, 1999, Marconi et al 1999, Bonafaccia et al 2000). As an ancient crop, niche marketing of spelt is well underway in North America and Europe, particularly in natural, organic, health, and specialty-food markets. Expansion in these markets will depend on the ability of spelt to compete directly with other wheats in productivity, functionality and applications, and nutritional and distinct characteristics.

Several spelt cultivars are commercially available for the production of spelt wheat for food uses. Segregation of these cultivars into market classes on the basis of kernel hardness, seed coat color, and growth habit, as is done for modern wheat, would help producers and processors select the best spelt samples for particular end uses. Additionally, segregation of commercial spelt on the basis of protein content may help determine quality and end uses of spelt. Hucl et al (1995) identified soft and hard endosperm spring-type spelt wheats and found that the soft spelts were intermediate in gluten strength and showed several desirable breadmaking properties (Abdel-Aal et al 1997), while the hard spelt biotypes were inferior in gluten strength but developed a unique taste and texture when drum-dried and broken into flakes for consumption as a breakfast cereal (Abdel-Aal et al 1998b).

A large-seeded spring-type soft spelt cv. CDC Nexon (formerly CDC Bavaria) with high protein content and flour yield was evaluated in breadmaking (Abdel-Aal et al 1999). The gluten strength of the spelt flour was intermediate, as indicated by sedimentation and mixograph tests, while loaf volumes were inferior to those of high-quality bread wheat (Abdel-Aal et al 1997). When a combination of 100 ppm ascorbic acid, 1% whey protein, and 0.3% blend of mono- and diglycerides was incorporated into a lean baking formula, the resultant spelt bread had loaf volume comparable to that of a high-quality bread wheat, softer crust and crumb textures, and improved sensory scores. In this study, the soft spelt flour showed a high baking response to ascorbic acid, resulting in improved bread properties. Abdel-Aal et al (1998b) used the same soft spelt cultivar in making pita bread that was comparable to that produced with a strong gluten HRS wheat flour without modifications in the baking formulations. In those studies, a short dough mixing time and a long fermentation process resulted in improved dough-handling properties and enhanced bread quality. A study in Italy reported that spelt and emmer flours produced breads with large loaf volume and better flavor, taste, and crust color than the bread wheat control (Cubadda and Marconi 1996). Spelt bread loaves possessed a relatively fine and uniform texture and a distinctive slight dark color of the crumb.

The nutritional quality of spelt bread baked from spelt flour, whole-meal flour, and scalded kernels was evaluated and compared with that made from a commercial white wheat flour (Skrabanja et al 2001). The spelt was organically grown without applying fertilizers or chemicals, and the breads were made using lean baking formulations (flour, whole meal, or flour plus scalded kernels; salt; yeast, and water). The spelt wheat flours and breads contained more protein than the white wheat flour and bread. The spelt white flour bread was shown to have a significantly more rapidly digestible starch than the whole-meal spelt bread, and more digestible starch than in white wheat bread and scalded grain-derived spelt bread. In general, and as for normal wheat, the most refined spelt flour resulted in a bread product that was significantly higher in starch hydrolysis index. Additionally, Bonafaccia et al (2000) found that spelt breads contain more rapidly digestible starch and a higher starch digestion index in comparison to common wheat bread. Compared to common wheat and spelt flour breads, whole-meal spelt bread had less total starch, as would be expected from the starting material, and proportionately more resistant starch and less-digestible protein. The quality of spelt breads was slightly lower than that of common wheat breads, based on loaf volume measurements (i.e., spelt flour bread loaf volume was 454 cm^3 and spelt whole-meal bread 446 cm^3 compared with 459 cm^3 for common wheat flour bread).

Five spelt cultivars were evaluated in relation to their potential in pasta production (Marconi et al 1999). Despite the low gluten strength in spelt as measured by SDS sedimentation, gluten index, and alveograph tests, spelt was found to produce high-quality pasta as evaluated by sensory and chemical measurements. That study indicated that the combination of high protein content and high drying temperature used in pasta processing could be responsible for the high quality of pasta products. Subsequently, Marconi et al (2002) verified that the combination of high protein in spelt (13.5%) with a high drying temperature is responsible for the production of reasonable-quality spelt pasta. Abdel-Aal et al (1998b) also found that a high-protein hard spelt produced pasta with cooking properties (cooking loss, stickiness, and firmness) comparable to those of a superior durum pasta, but in this study spelt pasta was scored significantly lower than durum pasta in sensory properties (i.e., appearance, color, and flavor).

A high-protein hard spelt was found to produce breakfast cereal flakes with appealing flavor and a unique, crispy, easy-to-break texture, and maintained firmness when served with cold milk (Abdel-Aal et al 1998b). The flaked breakfast cereal product was prepared by cooking and texturization of 15% homogenized slurries of spelt flours on a double-drum dryer under conditions of 2.8 kg cm^{-2} steam pressure, 1.0–1.5 rpm drum speed, and 1.2–1.4 mm spacing between drums, depending on the viscosities of the slurries as described by Abdel-Aal et al (1996b).

Celiac Disease

Spelt was the predominant bread wheat from the fifth century until the beginning of the twentieth century and was subsequently replaced by higher-yield free-threshing modern wheat. Spelt, emmer, and einkorn are among the earliest cultivated wheats and are commonly referred to as ancient wheats. Several nutritional and health claims have been made about these ancient wheats. A few studies have suggested that ancient wheats, particularly diploid (einkorn) and tetraploid (emmer) species, are nontoxic or inactive with regard to damage to small intestinal mucosa in celiac patients (Auricchio et al 1982, Favret et al 1984, 1987). Several health food companies and distributors labeled spelt food products as a wheat alternative for those with wheat sensitivity, or as "nonhybridized wheat" (Friedman et al 1994, Yunginger 1994). Nevertheless, spelt is a wheat that contains gluten proteins (Ranhotra et al 1995, 1996a) and is capable of provoking wheat allergy and gluten enteropathy (Friedman et al 1994, Yunginger 1994, Forssell and Wieser 1995, Kasarda and D'Ovidio 1999). Therefore, spelt is not safe for consumption by wheat-allergic individuals or by celiac disease patients, and it should be eliminated from their diets as recommended for common wheats and related cereals (e.g., barley, rye, triticale). The differences in protein structure between spelt and common wheat influence the quality of grains but not the ability to cause celiac disease.

Celiac disease, also known as celiac sprue, nontropical sprue, or gluten-sensitive enteropathy, is a dietary intolerance disease of the small intestine characterized by damage to the small intestinal mucosa, resulting in malabsorption of most nutrients. The disease was first reported by Samuel Gee in

1888 (Gee 1888), who described the features of the disease with remarkable accuracy and even suggested that the cure might be found in the diet. Later, in 1918, Still (1918) described the symptoms, pathogenesis, and treatment of celiac disease, focusing on avoiding some nutrients in the diet such as fats, cow's milk, and starch, particularly in bread form. Subsequently, Dicke et al (1953) demonstrated that a component of a normal diet, wheat, is toxic to celiac patients. Wheat proteins, particularly gliadin and its peptide digests, are known to cause the mucosal damage associated with celiac disease, which is characterized by flattened jejunal mucosa and intestinal malabsorption (DeRitis et al 1979). Other similar prolamins (alcohol-soluble proteins) from rye, barley, and triticale are also found to cause damaging effects in the celiac small intestine (Auricchio et al 1984, Kagnoff 1988). The reaction to prolamins in celiac disease is thought to be a humoral and cell-mediated immune response in the jejunal mucosa and in the peritoneal blood of celiac patients (Kagnoff 1988).

Most recent work has focused on gliadin proteins and their enzymatic peptide digests as being primarily responsible for triggering immunological changes in the epithelium leading to intestinal damage. In a clinical study on celiac patients, different doses of unfractionated gliadin and its fractions of α-, β-, γ-, and ω-gliadin were assessed for their toxicity based on the histological appearance of jejunal mucosal biopsies taken from the celiac patients before and after intraduodenal infusions (Ciclitira et al 1984). The study has shown that the unfractionated gliadin and its fractions of α-, β-, γ-, and ω-gliadin are toxic to celiac patients. The purity of each gliadin fraction was confirmed by PAGE and radioimmunoassay techniques. Characterization of wheat endosperm gliadins by using a combination of RP-HPLC and SDS-PAGE followed by immunoblotting with celiac serum has allowed the identification of five α-type, one γ_2-type, two γ_3-type and two γ-type gliadins, as well as a few unidentified LMW components as celiac immunoreactive proteins exhibiting similar antigenicity (Rocher et al 1995). Additionally, two major celiac disease-associated B-cell epitopes—peptide 9 (41QPYPQPQPFP50) in α- and α/β-gliadins and peptide 42 (206LGQGSFRPSQ215) only in α-gliadin—were identified (Lahdeaho et al 1995). The study suggested that specific regions of gliadin molecules may be involved in triggering the production of gliadin antibodies in celiac patients.

Forssell and Wieser (1995) separated α-gliadin fractions by RP-HPLC for N-terminal sequence analysis and found no significant differences between spelt and common wheat within the first 25 amino acid positions. The sequences of amino acids in gliadin peptides of spelt were also identical to those isolated from common wheat from positions 3 to 56. For these reasons, the authors concluded that spelt wheat contained immunoreactive gliadins that must be avoided by celiac patients. In a subsequent study by Kasarda and D'Ovidio (1999), comparison of the amino acid sequence of α-type gliadin from spelt and bread wheats, deduced from the cloned DNA sequence, have shown only very minor differences, with an identity of 98.5%. Both studies have indicated that spelt α-gliadin contains the toxic amino acid sequence that was previously identified using synthetic peptides in human trials (Sturgess et al 1994, Marsh et al 1995). In the latter studies, a 19-residue synthetic peptide corresponding to residues 31–49 of an α-type gliadin (Sturgess et al 1994) or a 13-residue synthetic peptide with sequence corresponding to residues 31–43 of α-gliadin (Marsh et al 1995) was instilled into the intestines of several patients who had been on a wheat-free diet, and the effects of the instillation were followed by taking intestinal biopsies and demonstrated changes in the mucosal tissues indicative of toxicity for the peptide. The toxic amino acid sequences tested by Sturgess et al (1994) and Marsh et al (1995) and those isolated from spelt and common wheat (Kasarda and D'Ovidio 1999) were identical, having sequences of LGQQQPFPPQQPYPQPQPF and LGQQQPFPPQQPY for the 19 and 13 amino acid residues (F, phenylalanine; G, glycine; L, leucine; P, proline; Q, glutamine; Y, tyrosine).

Celiac disease is activated when a susceptible person ingests food products that contain wheat, barley, and rye. Therefore, elimination of these grains from the diets of celiac patients is recommended as a remedy. A lifelong gluten-free diet is the recommended treatment for celiac patients regardless of symptoms. According to the level of gluten sensitivity of the patient, an absolute or tailored gluten restriction will be applied to the diet. It may be worth mentioning that the term *gluten* given by physicians and paramedics means prolamins from grains that are capable of activating celiac disease, and not the dough-forming proteins as defined by cereal scientists and bakers. The presence of gluten or more specific gliadins in food will determine celiac toxicity, and accordingly, detection of gluten in foods is of importance especially to patients with severe conditions of gluten sensitivity. Skerritt and Hill (1990, 1991) developed two simple monoclonal antibody-based test kits using enzyme-labeled antibodies for detecting and quantifying gluten in diets. The first test is the Gluten Lab-Test, which is able to quantify gluten in uncooked, cooked, and processed foods and is intended for laboratory use by professionals. The second Gluten Test Kit provides rapid qualitative or semiquantitative results and is appropriate for use either at home or in process quality by food and wheat starch manufacturers. The antibodies in these tests were selected to bind certain prolamins from wheat, durum, triticale, rye, and barley and to react with heat-stable ω-gliadin in spite of its lower toxicity compared with α-, β-, and γ-gliadins. The α-, β-, and γ-gliadins lose much of their antigenicity after heating, especially baking, yet retain their toxicity. Testing for those gliadins in cooked foods is not practical. The advantage of ω-gliadin antibodies is that they bind with raw and heat-treated or processed proteins.

A few investigations have shown that einkorn (diploid wheat) and durum (tetraploid wheat) exhibit lower celiac toxicity (Auricchio et al 1982, Frisoni et al 1995). If these observations are valid, the gluten in these wheat species may be deficient in the wheat allergen or the IgE-binding epitope in their gliadins, the causative factors in celiac disease. It was also reported that mannan or sugar derivatives like N-acetylglucosamine oligomers might protect the villi in walls of the small intestine from the damaging effects of gliadin peptides (Auricchio et al 1987). An investigation of 30 grain samples, including einkorn, durum, spelt, common wheat, barley, naked barley, rye, triticale, oat, naked oat, millet, and corn have shown intense reactivities against rabbit antigliadin antibodies for all wheat species, barley, rye, triticale, and oat, but not for corn and millet samples (Matuz et al 2000). Other reports found that pure oats are safe to celiac patients, and more details on using pure oats to serve celiac patients are given in Chapter 9. In general, more studies are required to quantitatively assess the levels of celiac toxicity in wheat species and to confirm the hypothesis that some sugars may exert a protective effect on the toxic activity of cereal prolamin peptides on the human celiac intestine. The development of a reliable *in vitro* method for the quantification of the degree of celiac toxic peptides in wheat and related cereals would help resolve some of the controversy and would aid in identifying low-allergen wheat species or genotypes if they do indeed exist.

Recent attempts to use sourdough lactic acid bacteria as a means to break down the A-gliadin, the most toxic α-gliadin fraction in celiac disease, were investigated (Di Cagno et al 2002). The preliminary experiments appear to be very promising. A toxic peptic-tryptic (PT) gliadin digest was used for *in vitro* agglutination test on K 562 (S) cells of human myelogenous leukemia origin, and the lowest concentration of PT digest that agglutinated 100% of the cells was 0.218 g/L. Digestion of the PT digest with proteolytic enzymes of *Lactobacillus alimentarius* 15M and *L. brevis* 14G completely prevented agglutination of the K 562 (S) cells at a concentration of 0.875 g/L. Other *Lactobacillus* strains produced considerable inhibitory effects at higher concentrations of the PT gliadin digest. Shan et al (2002) identified a 33-amino acid peptide in gluten containing the major immunogenic epitopes that trigger celiac disease in susceptible individuals. The peptide was resistant to breakdown by all gastric, pancreatic, and intestinal brush border membrane proteases in *in vitro* and *in vivo* rat and human studies. The investigators hypothesized that the peptide could be detoxified by exposure to a bacterial prolyl endopeptidase, suggesting a strategy for oral peptidase supplement therapy for treating celiac disease. Addition of a bacterial prolyl endopeptidase caused degradation and loss of the antigenicity of the peptide, which would open the possibility to use these enzymes for detoxification of the toxic peptides and developing therapeutic dietary strategies to treat celiac disease (Schuppan and Hahn 2002).

Wheat Allergy

Large numbers of proteins are found in foods, but only a very small percentage are capable of evoking allergic reactions or cannot be tolerated by certain individuals. Virtually all food allergens are proteins, but most proteins are not allergenic to sensitive individuals. The structural properties of allergenic food components have not been thoroughly characterized, but most food allergens generally have molecular weights between 10 and 70 kDa, stimulate the immune response or induce the production of allergen-specific

IgE, and are resistant to the effects of processing, cooking, and digestive processes (Lehrer et al 1996). Food allergy involves abnormal immunological responses within certain individuals to specific foods or, more specifically, to certain food protein(s) that may be of plant or animal origin. Taylor (1992) summarized the most common allergenic foods and their allergenic substances or allergens. Cow's milk, eggs, peanuts, and soybeans are among the most common allergenic foods. Cereal grains are not particularly common causes of allergic reactions; however, wheat, barley, rye, and rice are found to be allergenic to sensitive individuals, causing adverse reactions. Wheat allergy is different from celiac disease, and the causing factors and pathogenesis are not the same.

Several studies have demonstrated IgE binding by the water-soluble albumins and salt-soluble globulins of wheat (Hoffman 1975, Sutten et al 1982, Donovan and Baldo 1990). In addition, binding of wheat proteins to IgE may occur in many individuals with allergies to grass pollens (Donovan and Baldo 1990). Maruyama et al (1998) fractionated and purified wheat proteins into salt-soluble, gluten-rich, and gliadin-rich fractions to examine their allergenic reactions with sera of persons having wheat allergies. The relative reactivity of the fractions was variable among patients and reaction conditions but, in general, gluten-rich proteins were higher than gliadin-rich proteins, which were both higher than salt-soluble proteins.

The role of trypsin and α-amylase inhibitors as wheat allergens in baker's asthma has been demonstrated (Walsh et al 1987). These inhibitors along with many other physiological proteins belong to water- and salt-soluble or non-storage proteins in the wheat kernel. In general, little information is available on albumin and globulin proteins in common wheat or spelt and their role in wheat allergy. The albumins and globulins in wheat, particularly those that appeared to be specific to particular chromosomes, were characterized using several techniques of separation, purification, and identification, such as SDS-PAGE, isoelectric focusing, RH-HPLC, immunoaffinity chromatography, library of monoclonal antibodies, and protein sequencing (Singh et al 2001, Singh and Skerritt 2001). These studies indicate that most of the water-soluble proteins belong to a family of α-amylase inhibitors. One protein that is assigned to chromosome 4BS was homologous to serine carboxypeptidase III. Some salt-soluble proteins had N-terminal sequences similar to that of barley embryo globulin, and other proteins were identified as lipid transfer protein, peroxidase BP-1 precursor, and histone H4 proteins. It was suggested that chromosome-specific proteins can be used to develop chromosome-specific markers, and protein sequences could be used for making antibody or DNA probes for use in breeding program selection.

Spelt as an Organic Grain

The term *organic* refers to the way agricultural commodities are produced and processed in which synthetic fertilizers, pesticides, growth regulators, genetically modified materials, sewage sludge, and feed and food additives are not used. The organic farming system relies on crop rotation, manures, manual weeding, and biological pest control. Additionally, the organic integrity should be maintained during handling and processing by avoiding the use of artificial ingredients, preservatives, and irradiation. In theory, such a production system should assist in maintaining a healthier environment and in providing a food supply with fewer pesticide and chemical residues. This may rationalize the increasing demand for organic food.

The organic food market is growing rapidly worldwide, particularly in North America and Europe. In Canada, the organic food market is expected to rise from a $0.7 billion retail value in 1997 to $3.1 billion in 2005, with an average growth of about 20% annually (AAFC 2001). In 2001, natural and organic food sales in the United States were estimated at $12.9 billion (up 9.3% since 2000), organic foods at $6.95 billion (up 19.9%), and natural foods at $5.95 billion (down 0.9%) (Sloan 2002). The natural and organic food markets are expected to reach $25.8 billion by 2010, with organic foods at $21.9 billion (3.7% of all food industry sales), while natural foods will drop to $3.9 billion. The terms *natural* and *organic* appear to have been used interchangeably in earlier literature. Currently, the term *organic* describes a process covered by a formal certification, while the term *natural* does not. The overall annual growth rate of U.S. organic food is estimated at 20% for 2001–2004, with breads and grains at 21.9% (Sloan 2002). Austria, Sweden, and Switzerland have well-established organic production sectors, with approximately 10.2, 7.5 and 6.6%, respectively, of total agricultural land in organic production (Emerald 2001). The organic grains and products produced in Europe and North America are discussed in detail in Chapter 2.

With so much interest in the sector, organically grown spelt could be a major source for making organic baked goods. In Canada, organic spelt is being used for the production of a diverse array of bread and pastry products. The agronomic properties of spelt are a determining factor in the organic production of spelt. Spelt was found to perform well under suboptimal growing conditions (Ruegger et al 1990) and to better utilize nutrients when grown in a low-input system (Moudry and Dvoracek 1999) compared to common wheat. As previously mentioned, spelt is also resistant to some diseases and pathogens such as common bunt and ergot.

Organic spelt is being produced and processed in different food forms. The organic spelt food market is driven by a consumer demand for organically produced wheat-based food products. Spelt products are perceived to be better tolerated than their counterpart wheat products. Additionally, consumers believe that organic products contribute to their overall health rather than ascribe any specific health effect to them. Some spelt cultivars were found to produce a unique flavor that contributes to the overall differentiation of organic food products.

Conclusions

Spelt appears to be comparable but not unique relative to common wheat in most of its nutrient composition. In general, spelt may contain higher levels of protein, soluble dietary fiber, and minerals (zinc, selenium, lithium, phosphorus, magnesium), depending on genotype. No evidence suggests that spelt is superior to common wheat in health benefits and disease prevention. Recent studies show that spelt gliadins contain the toxic amino acid sequence in celiac disease, similar to common wheat, and must be avoided by celiac patients. To some extent, spelt has unique agronomic characteristics that make it a good potential choice for organic crop production. Research is needed to evaluate organic spelt products in nutritional quality, phenolic composition and antioxidant properties, absence of hazardous substances, and shelf stability. Additionally, segregation of commercial spelt on the basis of grain hardness, growth habit, seed coat color, and protein content, as is done for common wheat, would help promote the spelt market and would aid producers and processors in selecting the best grains for specific end uses.

References

Agriculture and Agri-Food Canada (AAFC). 2001. Canada's organic industry. Online: http://ats-sea.agr.gc.ca/supply/3313_e.pdf

Abdel-Aal, E.-S. M., Hucl, P., and Sosulski, F. W. 1995. Compositional and nutritional characteristics of spring einkorn and spelt wheats. Cereal Chem. 72:621-624.

Abdel-Aal, E.-S. M., Salama, D. A., Hucl, P., Sosulski, F. W., and Cao, W. 1996a. Electrophoretic characterization of spring spelt wheat gliadins. J. Agric. Food Chem. 44:2117-2123.

Abdel-Aal, E.-S. M., Sosulski, F. W., Shehata, A. Y., and Youssef, M. M. 1996b. Nutritional, functional and sensory properties of wheat, rice and faba bean blends texturized by drum drying. Int. J. Food Sci. Technol. 31:257-266.

Abdel-Aal, E-S. M., Hucl, P., Sosulski, F. W., and Bhirud, P. R. 1997. Kernel, milling and baking properties of spring-type spelt and einkorn wheats. J. Cereal Sci. 26:363-370.

Abdel-Aal, E.-S. M., Sosulski, F. W., and Hucl, P. 1998a. Origins, characteristics and potentials of ancient wheats. Cereal Foods World 43:708-715.

Abdel-Aal, E-S. M., Hucl, P., and Sosulski, F.W. 1998b. Food uses for ancient wheats. Cereal Foods World 43:763-767.

Abdel-Aal, E.-S. M., Hucl, P., and Sosulski, F. W. 1999. Optimizing the bread formulation for soft spelt wheat. Cereal Foods World 44:480-483.

Abdel-Aal, E.-S. M., Hucl, P., Sosulski, F. W., Graf, R., Gillott, C., and Pietrzak, L. 2001. Screening spring wheat for midge resistance in relation to ferulic acid content. J. Agric. Food Chem. 49:3559-3566.

Abdel-Aal, E.-S. M., and Hucl, P. 2002. Amino acid composition and in vitro protein digestibility of selected ancient wheats and their end products. J. Food Comp. Anal. 15:737-747.

Andrews, A. C. 1964. The genetic origin of spelt and related wheats. Züchter 34:17-22.

Arnason, J. T., Gale, J., Conilh de Beyssac, B., Sen, A., Miller, S. S., Philogene, B. J. R., Lambert, J. D. H., Fulcher, R. G., Serratos, A., and Mihm, J. 1992. Role of phenolics in resistance of maize grain to stored grain to the stored grain insects, *Prostephanus truncatus* (Horn) and *Sitophilus zeamais* (Motsch). J. Stored Prod. 28:119-126.

Arseniuk, E., Fried, P. M., Winzeler, H., and Czembor, H. J. 1991. Comparison of resistance of triticale, wheat and spelt to Septoria nodorum blotch at the seedling and plant stage. Euphytica 55:43-48.

Auricchio, S., Cardelli, M., De Ritis, G., De Vincenzi, M., Latte, F., and Silano, V. 1984. An *in vitro* animal model for the study of cereal components toxic in celiac disease. Pediatric Res. 18:1372-1378.

Auricchio, S., De Ritis, G., De Vincenzi, M., Latte, F., Maiuri, L., Pino, A., Raia, V., and Silano, V. 1987. Prevention by mannan and other sugars of *in vitro* damage of rat fetal small intestine induced by cereal prolamin peptides toxic for human celiac intestine. Pediatric Res. 22:703-707.

Auricchio, S., De Ritis, G., De Vincenzi, M., Occorsio, P., and Silano, V. 1982. Effects of gliadin-derived peptides from bread and durum wheat on small intestine cultures from rat fetus and coeliac children. Pediatric Res. 16:1004-1010.

Barnes, R. F., and Beard, J. B. 1992. A Glossary of Crop Science Terms. Crop Science Society of America, Inc., Madison, WI.

Beglinger, C. 1995. Physiological and genetic studies on early vigour of *Triticum aestivum* L. and *Triticum spelta* L. Dissertation Eidgenössische Technische Hochschule No. 11286. Eidgenössische Technische Hochschule, Zürich.

Bertin, P., Gregoire, D., Massart, S., and de Froidmont, D. 2001. Genetic diversity among European cultivated spelt revealed by microsatellites. Theor. Appl. Genet. 102:148-156.

Bietz, J. A., and Simpson, D. G. 1992. Electrophoresis and chromatography of wheat proteins: Available methods and procedures for statistical evaluation of the data. J. Chromatogr. 624:53-80.

Bleiker, U., and Winzeler, H. 1991. A simple device to prepare single ears of spelt (*Triticum spelta* L.) for seeding with the "seedmatic-system." Plant Breeding 106:258-260.

Block, G. 1992. The data support role for antioxidants in reducing cancer risk. Nutr. Rev. 50:207-213.

Bognár, A., and Kellermann, C. 1991. Vergleichende untersuchung uber den gehalt an vitaminen in vier verschiedenen Dinkelsorten, in Weizen und Roggen. 2. Hohenheimer Dinkelkolloquium an der Universitat Hohenbeim, Germany, Dinkellacker Stifung, Stuttgart.

Bonafaccia, G., Galli, V., Francisci, R., Mair, V., Skranbanja, V., and Kreft, I. 2000. Characteristics of spelt wheat products and nutritional value of spelt wheat-based bread. Food Chem. 68:437-441.

Cabrera, H. M., Munoz, O., Zuniga, G. E., Corcuera, L. J., and Argandona, V. H. 1995. Changes in ferulic acid and lipid content in aphid-infested barley. J. Phytochem. 39:1023-1026.

Campbell, K. G. 1997. Spelt: Agronomy, genetics and breeding. Plant Breed. Rev. 15:187-213.

Canada Food Inspection Agency (CFIA). 2001. Variety Registration Office. Notifications of Variety Registration, April 1, 2001 to June 30, 2001. Online: http://www.inspection.gc.ca

Canada Food Inspection Agency (CFIA). 2002. Plant Breeders Rights Office. Online: http://www.inspection.gc.ca

Cao, W., Hucl, P., Scoles, G., and Chibbar, R. N. 1998. Genetic diversity within spelta and macha wheats based on RAPD analysis. Euphytica 104:181-189.

Cao, W., Scoles, G., and Hucl, P. 2000. Phylogenetic study of five morphological groups of wheat (*Triticum aestivum* L. em Thell.) based on cytological analysis. Wheat Inf. Ser. 90:37-41.

Chang, S., Tan, C., Frankel, E. N., and Barrett, D. M. 2000. Low-density lipoprotein antioxidant activity of phenolic compounds and polyphenol oxidase activity in selected clingstone peach cultivars. J. Agric. Food Chem. 48:147-151.

Chung, O. K. 1991. Cereal lipids. Pages 497-553 in: Handbook of Cereal Science and Technology. K. J. Lorenz and K. Kulp, Eds. Marcel Dekker, New York.

Ciclitira, P. J., Evans, D. J., Fagg, N. L. K., Lennox, E. S., and Dowling, R. H. 1984. Clinical testing of gliadin fractions in coeliac patients. Clin. Sci. 66:357-364.

Clamot, G. 1984. Genetic variability of the protein and lysine content of spelt (*Triticum spelta*). Z. Pflanzenzuchtg. 93:106-114.

Cubadda, R., and Marconi, E. 1996. Technological and nutritional aspects in emmer and spelt. Pages 203-211 in: Hulled Wheats: Proc. First Int. Workshop on Hulled Wheats. S. Padulosi, K. Hammer, and J. Heller, Eds. International Plant Genetic Resources Institute, Rome.

D'Antuono, L. F., and Bravi, R. 1996. The hulled wheat industry: Present developments and impact on genetic resources conservation. Pages 221-233 in: Hulled Wheats: Proc. First Int. Workshop on Hulled Wheats. S. Padulosi, K. Hammer, and J. Heller, Eds. International Plant Genetic Resources Institute, Rome.

Dekeyser, A., and Goenaga, X. 2001. Spelt: A protein-rich cereal for animal feed and health foods.Online: http:europa.eu.int/comm./research/press/2001/pr1110-spelt.en

De Ritis, G., Occorsio, P., Auricchio, S., Gramenzi, F., Morisi, G., and Silano, V. 1979. Toxicity of wheat flour proteins and protein-derived peptides for *in vitro* developing intestine from rat fetus. Pediatr. Res. 13:1255-1261.

Di Cagno, R., De Angelis, M., Lavermicocca, P., De Vincenzi, M., Giovanni, C., Faccia, M., and Gobbetti, M. 2002. Proteolysis of sourdough lactic acid bacteria: Effects on wheat flour protein fractions and gliadin peptides involved in human cereal intolerance. Appl. Env. Micro. 68:623-633.

Dicke, W. K., Weijers, H. A., and Van de Kamer, J. H. 1953. Coeliac disease: Presence in wheat of factor having deleterious effect in cases of coeliac disease. Acta Pediatr. 42:34-43.

Donovan, G. R., and Baldo, B. A. 1990. Cross-reactivity of IgE antibodies from sera of subjects allergic to both ryegrass pollen and wheat endosperm proteins: Evidence for common allergenic determinants. Clin. Exp. Allergy 20:501-509.

Ehsanzadeh, P. 1999. Agronomic and growth characteristics of spring spelt compared to common wheat. Ph.D. dissertation, University of Saskatchewan, Saskatoon.

Ehsanzadeh, P., Hucl, P., and Simpson, G. M. 1998. Agronomic characteristics of spelt wheat: Seeding rate effects. Pages in 147-153: Proc. Soils and Crops Workshop. University of Saskatchewan, Saskatoon.

Emerald. 2001. Food facts. Online: Emeraldinsight.com/ft

Favret, E. A., Cervetto, J. L., Solari, R. M., Bolondi, A., Nunez, H. Manghers, L. E., Boffi, A., and Ortiz, J. P. 1984. Influence of wheat ploidy on the induction of coeliac disease. Page 116 in: Proc. Meeting Latin-American Society of Pediatric and Gastroenterological Nutrition, 7th. The Society, Sao Paolo, Brazil.

Favret, E. A., Cervetto, J. L., Solari, R. M., Bolondi, A., Manghers, L. E., Boffi, A., and Ortiz, J. P. 1987. Comparative effect of diploid, tetraploid and hexaploid wheat on the small intestine of coeliac patients. Page 13 in Proc. Meeting Latin-American Society of Pediatric and Gastroenterological Nutrition, 8th. The Society, Sao Paolo, Brazil.

Federmann, G. R., Goecke, E. U., and Steiner, A. M. 1992. Research note: Detection of adulteration of flour of spelt (*Triticum spelta* L.) with flour of wheat (*Triticum aestivum* L. emend. Fiori et Paol.) by electrophoresis. Plant Var. Seeds 5:123-125.

Friedman, H. M., Tortolani, R. E., Glick, J., and Burtis, R. 1994. Spelt is wheat. Allergy Proc. 15:217-218.

Frisoni, M., Vallega, V., D'Egidio, M. G., Corazza, G. R., and Gasbarrini, G. 1995. *In vitro* toxicity of gluten of three wheat species on the intestinal mucosa of coeliac patients. Page 8 in: ICC Jubilee Conference Proceedings. International Association for Cereal Science and Technology (ICC), Vienna, Austria.

Forssell, F., and Wieser, H. 1995. Spelt wheat and coeliac disease. Z. Lebensm. Unters Forsch. 201:35-39.

Gee, S. 1888. On the coeliac affliction. St. Bartholomew's Hospital Rep. 24:17.

Grand, R. 1935. L'Agriculture à travers les âges, histoire des faits, des institutions, de la pensée et des doctrines economique et socials, vol 3: L'Agriculture au moyen age de la fin de l'empire romain au XVIe siecle. E. De Boccard, Paris.

Grela, E. R. 1996. Nutritional composition and content of antinutritional factors in spelt (*Triticum spelta* L) cultivars. J. Sci. Food Agric. 47:399-404.
Guthrie, H. A. 1993. Dietary requirements of adults. Pages 1393-1396 in: Encyclopaedia of Food Science, Food Technology and Nutrition. Vol 2. R. Macrae, R. K. Robinson, and M. J. Sadler, Eds. Academic Press, London.
Hahn, D. H., Faubion, J. M., and Rooney, L. W. 1983. Sorghum phenolic acids, their high performance liquid chromatography separation and their relation to fungal resistance. Cereal Chem. 60:255-259.
Harsch, S., Günther, T., Kling, Ch. I., Rozynek, B., and Hesemann, C. U. 1997. Characterization of spelt (*Triticum spelta* L.) Forms by gel electrophoretic analyses of seed storage proteins. I. The gliadins. Theor. Appl. Genet. 94:52-60.
He, C., and Hughes, G. R. 2003. Inheritance of resistance to common bunt in spelt and common wheat. Can. J. Plant Sci. 83:47-56.
Heinonen, I. M., Meyer, A. S., and Frankel, E. N. 1998. Antioxidant activity of berry phenolics on human low-density lipoprotein and liposome oxidation. J. Agric. Food Chem. 46:4107-4112.
Hoffman, D. R. 1975. The specifics of human IgE antibodies combining with cereal grains. Immunochemistry 12:535-538.
Hollman, P. C. H., Hertog, M. G. L., and Katan, M. B. 1996. Analysis and health effects of flavonoids. Food Chem. 57:43-46.
Hoppner, K. H., Owen, B. D., and Sosulski, F. W. 1968. Proximate principles and B-vitamins in Saskatchewan feed grains. Can. J. Anim. Sci. 48:135.
Hucl, P., Abdel-Aal, E.-S. M., and Sosulski, F. W. 1995. Specialty wheats. Page 40-47 in: Proc. Croppotunities III Conference. University of Saskatchewan, SK, Canada.
Hucl, P., Holm, F. A., Kirkland, K., and Johnson, E. 1997. Spring wheat cultivars that differ in competitive ability. Pages 62-68 in: Proc. Soils and Crops Workshop, University of Saskatchewan, Saskatoon.
Jacquot, R., Adrian, J., and Rerat, A. 1960. A forgotten cereal species: Spelt or Dinkel. Z. Acker. Pflanzenb 3:279.
Jariwalla, R. J., Sabin, R., Lawson, S., and Herman, Z. S. 1990. Lowering of serum cholesterol and triglycerides and modulation of divalent cations by dietary phytate. J. Appl. Nutr. 42:18-28.
Kagnoff, M. F. 1988. Celiac disease: A model of an immunologically mediated intestinal disease. Gut Intest. Immunol. 8:505-520.
Kaiser, H. G. 1992. Use of emery and frictional grinding machines for husking spelt. Getreide Mehl Brot 46:296-298.
Kasarda, D. D., and D'Ovidio, R. 1999. Deduced amino acid sequence of an α-gliadin gene from spelt wheat (spelta) includes sequences active in celiac disease. Cereal Chem. 76:548-551.
Kema, G. H. J. 1992. Resistance in spelt wheat to yellow rust. I. Euphytica 63:207-217.
Kies, C., and Fox, H. M. 1970. Determination of the first-limiting amino acid of wheat and triticale grain for humans. Cereal Chem. 47:615-622.
Kuckuck, H., and Schiemann, E. 1957. Ubder das Vorkommen von Speltz und Emmer (*Triticum spelta* L. und *Tr. dicoccum* Schubl.) Iran. Z. Pflanzenzuchtg. 38:383-396.
Lafever, H. N., and Campbell, L. G. 1977. Spelt: A new look at old crop. Crops Soils 29:15-16.
Lafever, H. N. 1988. Registration of 'Champ' spelt. Crop Sci. 28:377-378.
Lahdeaho, M-L., Vainio, E., Lehtinen, M., Parkkonen, P., Partanen, J., Koskimies, S., and Maki, M. 1995. Activation of celiac disease immune system by specific α-gliadin peptides. Cereal Chem. 72:475: 479.
LeClerc, J. A., Bailey, L. H., and Wessling, H. L. 1918. Milling and baking tests of einkorn, emmer, spelt, and polish wheat. J. Am. Soc. Agron. 10:215-217.

Lehrer, S. B., Horner, W. E., and Reese, G. 1996. Why are some proteins allergenic? Implications for biotechnology. Crit. Rev. Food Sci. Nutr. 36:553-564.

Lipps, P. E. 1996. Loose smut of wheat, spelt and barley. Ohio State University. Extension Factsheet AC-12-96.

Luo, M. C., Yang, Z. L., and Dvoøák, J. 2000. The *Q* locus of Iranian and European spelt wheat. Theor. Appl. Genet. 100:602-606.

MacKey, J. 1966. Species relationships in *Triticum*. Proc. Int. Wheat Genet. Symp., 2nd. (Hereditas Suppl.) 2:237-276.

Marconi, E., Carcea, M., Schiavone, M., and Cubadda, R. 2002. Spelt (*Triticum spelta* L.) Pasta quality: Combined effect of flour properties and drying conditions. Cereal Chem. 79:634-639.

Marconi, E., Carcea, M., Graziano, M., and Cubadda, R. 1999. Kernel properties and pasta-making quality of five European spelt wheat (*Triticum spelta* L.) cultivars. Cereal Chem. 76:25-29.

Marsh, M. N., Morgan, S., Ensari, A., Wardle, T., Lobley, R., Mills, C. and Auricchio, S. 1995. In vivo activity of peptides 31-43, 44-55, 56-68 of α-gliadin in gluten sensitive enteropathy (GSE). Gastroenterology 108:A871.

Maruyama, N., Ichise, K., Katsube, T., Kishimoto, T., Kawase, S. I., Matsumura, Y., Takeuchi, Y., Sawada, T., and Utsumi, S. 1998. Identification of major wheat allergens by means of the *Escherichia coli* expression system. Eur. J. Biochem. 255:739-745.

Matuz, J., Poka, R., Boldizsar, I., Szerdahelyi, E., and Hajos, G. 2000. Structure and potential allergenic character of cereal proteins. II. Potential allergens in cereal samples. Cereal. Res. Comm. 28:433-442.

McVey, D. V. 1990. Reaction of 578 spring spelt wheat accessions to 35 races of wheat stem rust. Crop Sci. 30:1001-1005.

Messmer, M. M., Boller, S., Winzeler, M., Schmid, J. E., and Winzeler, H. 1996. Breeding and research activities with spelt at the Swiss Federal Research Station for Agroecology (FAL). Pages 9-18 in: Small Grain Cereals and Pseudo-Cereals Workshop, Copenhagen, Denmark.

Moudry, J., and Dvoracek, V. 1999. Chemical composition of grain of different spelt (*Triticum spelta* L.) varieties. Rostlinna Vyroba 45:533-538.

Muramatsu, M. 1963. Dosage effect of the spelta gene *q* of hexaploid wheat. Genetics 18:469-482.

Nesbitt, M., and Samuel, D. 1996. From staple crop to extinction? The archaeology and history of hulled wheats. Pages 41-100 in: Hulled Wheats: Proc. First Int. Workshop on Hulled Wheats. S. Padulosi, K. Hammer, and J. Heller, Eds. International Plant Genetic Resources Institute, Rome.

OECD. 2002. OECD List of varieties eligible for Certification – 2002/2003. Online: http://www.oecd.org /pdf/M00037000/M00037693.pdf

OSIA. 2002. Seed certification regulations. Online: http://www.ohseed.org/downloads/summer2002.pdf

Oliveira, J. A. 2001. North Spanish emmer and spelt wheat land races: Agronomical and grain quality characteristic evaluation. Plant Genet. Res. Newsl. 125:16-20.

Oplinger, E. S., Oelke, E. A., Kaminski, A. R., Kelling, K. A., Doll, J. D., Durgan, B. R., and Shuler, R. T. 1990. Spelt. In: Alternative Field Crops Manual. Univ. of Minnesota Center Alt. Plant Animal Prod., Coop Ext. Serv., St. Paul, MN.

Payne, P. I. 1987. Genetics of wheat storage proteins and the effect of allelic variation on bread-making quality. Annu. Rev. Plant Physiol. 38:141-153.

Payne, P. I., and Lawrence, G. J. 1983. Catalogue of alleles for the complex gene loci, Glu-A1, Glu-B1 and Glu-D1 which code for high-molecular-weight subunits of glutenin in hexaploid wheat. Cereal Res. Commun. 11:29-35.

Peña-Chocarro, L. 1996. In situ conservation of hulled wheats: The case of Spain. Pages 129-146 in: Hulled Wheats: Proc. First Int. Workshop on Hulled Wheats. S. Padulosi,

K. Hammer, and J. Heller, Eds. International Plant Genetic Resources Institute, Rome.

Percival, J. 1921. The wheat plant: A monograph. Duckworth and Co., London.

Perrino, P., Laghetti, G., D'Antuono, L. F., Al Ajlouni, M., Kanbertay, M., Szabo, A. T., and Hammer, K. 1996. Ecogeographical distribution of hulled wheat species. Pages 101-119 in: Hulled Wheats: Proc. First Int. Workshop on Hulled Wheats. S. Padulosi, K. Hammer, and J. Heller, Eds. International Plant Genetic Resources Institute, Rome.

Piergiovanni, A. R., and Blanco, A. 1999. Variation of HMW glutenin and γ-gliadin subunits in selected accessions of *Triticum dicoccon* (Shrank) and *T. spelta* (L.). Cereal Res. Comm. 27: 205-211.

Piergiovanni, A. R., Laghetti, G., and Perrino, P. 1996. Characteristics of meal from hulled wheats (*Triticum dicoccon* Shrank and *T. spelta* L.): An evaluation of selected accessions. Cereal Chem. 73:732-735.

Piergiovanni, A. R., Rizzi, R., Pannacciulli, E., and Della Gatta, C. 1997. Mineral composition in hulled wheat grains: A comparison between emmer (*Triticum dicoccon* Shrank) and spelt (*T. spelta* L.) accessions. Int. J. Food Sc. Nutr. 48:381-386.

Pogna, N. F., Autran, J. C., Mellini, F., Lafiandra, D., and Feillet, P. 1990. Chromosome 1B-encoded gliadins and glutenin subunits in durum wheat: Genetics and relationship to gluten strength. J. Cereal Sci. 11:15-34.

Radic, H., Gunther, T., Kling, Ch. I., and Hesemann, C. U. 1997 Characterization of spelt (*Triticum spelta* L.) forms by gel-electrophoretic analyses of seed storage proteins. II. The glutenins. Theor. Appl. Genet. 94:882-886.

Radic-Miehle, H., Saam, C., Huls, R., Kling, Ch. I., and Hesemann, C. U. 1998. Characterization of spelt (*Triticum spelta* L.) forms by gel-electrophoretic analyses of seed storage proteins. III. Comparative analyses of spelt and Central European winter wheat (*Triticum aestivum* L.) cultivars by SDS-PAGE and acid-PAGE. Theor. Appl. Genet. 97:1340-1346.

Ranhotra, G. S., Gelroth, J. A., Glaser, B. K., and Lorenz, K. J. 1995. Baking and nutritional qualities of a spelt wheat sample. Lebensm. Wiss. Technol. 28:118-122.

Ranhotra, G. S., Gelroth, J. A., Glaser, B. K., and Lorenz, K. J. 1996a. Nutrient composition of spelt wheat. J. Food Comp. Anal. 9:81-84.

Ranhotra, G. S., Gelroth, J. A., Glaser, B. K., and Stallknecht, G. F. 1996b. Nutritional profile of three spelt wheat cultivars grown at five different locations. Cereal Chem. 73:533-535.

Riesen, T. H., Winzeler, H., Ruegger, A., and Fried, P.M. 1986. The effect of hulls on fungal infection of germinating seed of spelt (*Triticum spelta* L.) in comparison to wheat (*Triticum aestivum* L.). J. Phytopathol. (Berl.) 115:318-324.

Rimle, R. 1995. Agronomische und morphologische Characterisierung von Weizen (*Triticum aestivum* L.) und Dinkel (*Triticum spelta* L.) sowie von spezifischen Weizen/Dinkel-F_1-Hybriden und deren Folgengenerationen von der F_2 bis zur F_5. Dissertation, Dissertation Eidgenössische Technische Hochschule No. 11242. Eidgenössische Technische Hochschule, Zürich.

Rocher, A., Soriano, F., Molina, E., Gonzalez-Limas, G., and Mendez, E. 1995. Characterization of distinct α- and γ-type gliadins and low molecular weight components from wheat endosperm as coeliac immunoreactive proteins. Biochem. Biophys. Acta 1247:143-148.

Ruegger, A., Winzeler, H., and Nosberger, J. 1990. Studies on the germination behaviour of spelt (*Triticum spelta* L.) and wheat (*Triticum aestivum* L.) under stress conditions. Seed Sci. Technol. 18:311-320.

Ruegger, A., Winzeler, H., and Nosberger, J. 1993. Dry matter production and distribution of C^{14} assimilates of spelt (*Triticum spelta* L.) and wheat (*Triticum aestivum* L.) as influenced by different temperatures before and during grain filling. J. Agron. Crop Sci. 165:110-120.

Ruegger, A., and Winzeler, H. 1993. Performance of spelt (*Triticum spelta* L.) and wheat (*Triticum aestivum* L.) at two different seeding rates and nitrogen levels under contrasting environment conditions. J. Agron. Crop Sci. 170:289-295.

Ruibal-Mendieta, N. L., Delacroix, D. L., and Meurens, M. 2002. A comparative analysis of free, bound and total lipid content on spelt and winter wheat wholemeal. J. Cereal Sci. 35:337-342.

Schober, T. J., Clarke, C. I., and Kuhn, M. 2002. Characterization of functional properties of gluten proteins in spelt cultivars using rheological and quality factor measurements. Cereal Chem. 79:408-417.

Schmid, J. E., and Winzeler, H. 1990. Genetic studies of crosses between common wheat (*Triticum aestivum* L.) and spelt (*Triticum spelta* L.) J. Genet. Breed. 44:75-80.

Schmid, J. E., Winzeler, M., and Winzeler, H. 1994. Analysis of disease resistance and quality characters of F_1 hybrids of crosses between wheat (*Triticum aestivum* L.) and spelt (*Triticum spelta* L.). Euphytica 75:105-110.

Schuppan, D., and Hahn, E. G. 2002. Gluten and the gut—Lessons for immune regulation. Science 297:2218-2220.

Shamsuddin, A. M., Elsayed, A. M., and Ullah, A. 1988. Suppression of large intestinal cancer in F344 rats by inositol hexaphosphate. Carcinogenesis 9:577-580.

Shamsuddin, A. M., Ullah, A., and Elsayed, A. M. 1989. Inositol and inositol hexaphosphate. Suppress cell proliferation and tumor formation in CD-1 mice. Carcinogenesis 10:1461-1464.

Shan, L., Molberg, O., Parrot, I., Hausch, F., Filiz, F., Gray, G. M., and Solid, L. M. 2002. Structural basis for gluten intolerance in celiac sprue. Science 297:2275-2281.

Shewry, P. R., Tatham, A. S., Barro, F., Barcelo, P., and Lazzeri, P. 1995. Biotechnology of breadmaking: Unraveling and manipulating the multi-protein gluten complex. Bio/Technology 13:1185-1190.

Siedler, H., Messmer, M. M., Schachermayr, G. M., Winzeler, H., Winzeler, M., and Keller, B. 1994. Genetic diversity in European spelt and spelt breeding material based on RFLP data. Theor. Appl. Genet. 88:894-1003.

Singh, J., Blundell, M., Tanner, G., and Skerritt, J. H. 2001. Albumin and globulin proteins of wheat flour: Immunological and N-terminal sequence characterization. J. Cereal Sci. 34:85-103.

Singh, J., and Skerritt, J. H. 2001. Chromosomal control of albumins and globulins in wheat grain assessed using different fractionation procedures. J. Cereal Sci. 33:163-181.

Skerritt, J. H., Devery, J. M., and Hill, A. S. 1990. Gluten intolerance: Chemistry, celiac-toxicity, and detection of prolamins in foods. Cereal Foods World 35:638-644.

Skerritt, J. H., and Hill, A. S. 1990. Monoclonal antibody sandwich enzyme immunoassays for determination of gluten in foods. J. Agric. Food Chem. 38:1771-1778.

Skerrit, J. H., and Hill, A. S. 1991. Enzyme immunoassay for determination of gluten in foods: Collaborative study. J. Assoc. Off. Anal. Chem. 74:257-264.

Skrabanja, V., Kovac, B., Golob, T., Liljeberg Elmstahl, H. G. M., Bjorck, I. M. E., and Kreft, I. 2001. Effect of spelt wheat flour and kernel on bread composition and nutritional characteristics. J. Agric. Food Chem. 49:497-500.

Sloan, A. E. 2002. The natural and organic foods marketplace. Food Technol. 56:27-37.

Stallknecht, G. F., Gilbertson, K. M., and Ranney, J. E. 1996. Alternative wheat cereals as food grains: Einkorn, emmer, spelt, kamut and triticale. Pages 156-170 in: Progresss in New Crops. J. Janick, Ed. American Society for Horticultural Science Press, Alexandria, VA.

Still, G. F. 1918. Coeliac disease. Lancet 2:162

Sturgess, R. P., Ellis, H. J., and Ciclitira, P. J. 1991. Cereal chemistry, molecular biology and toxicity in coeliac disease. Gut 32:1055-1060.

Sturgess, R. P., Day, P., Ellis, H. J., Lundin, K. E. A., Gjertsen, H. A., Kontakou, M., and Ciclitira, P. J. 1994. Wheat peptide challenge in coeliac disease. Lancet 343:758-761.

Sunbeam Extract Company. 2002. Spelt varieties released by Sunbeam Extract Co. Online: http://www.sunbeamextract.com /spelt

Sutton, R., Hill, D. J., and Baldo, B. A. 1982. Immunoglobulin E antibodies to ingested wheat flour components: Studies with sera from subjects with asthema and eczema. Clin. Allergy 12:63-74.

Tatham, A. S., Shewry, P. R., and Field, J. M. 1990. Conformational studies of the repetitive domains of cereal prolamins. Pages 376-388 in: Gluten Proteins 1990. (Proc. Int. Workshop on Gluten Proteins, 4th.) W. Bushuk and R. Tkachuk, Eds. Am. Assoc. Cereal Chem., St. Paul, MN.

Taylor, S. L. 1992. Chemistry and detection of food allergens. Food Technol. 36:146-152.

von Buren, M., Luthy, J., and Hubner, P. 2000. A spelt-specific γ-gliadin gene: Discovery and detection. Theor. Appl. Genet. 100:271-279.

Wall, J. S. 1979. The role of wheat proteins in determining baking quality. Pages 275-311 in: Recent Advances in the Biochemistry of Cereals. D. L. Laidman and R. G. Wyn Jones, Eds. Academic Press, London.

Walsh, B. J., Baldo, B. A., Bass, D. J., Clancy, R., Musk, A. W., and Wrigley, C. W. 1987. Insoluble and soluble allergens from wheat and wheat dust: Detection of IgE binding in inhalant and ingestion allergy. New Engl. Regional Allergy Proc. 8:27-33.

Winzeler, H., and Ruegger, A. 1990. Dinkel: Renaissance einer altern Getreideart. Landwirtsch. Schweiz Band 3:503-511.

Woychick, J. H., Boundy, J. A., and Dimler, R. J. 1961. Starch gel electrophoresis of wheat gluten proteins with concentrated urea. Arch. Biochem. Biophys. 94:477-482.

Yoon, J. H., Thompson, L. U., and Jenkins, D. J. A. 1983. The effect of phytic acid on in vitro rate of starch digestibility and blood glucose response. Am. J. Clin. Nutr. 38:835-842.

Yunginger, J. W. 1994. Food ingredient labeling: How many ways can wheat be spelt? Allergy Proc. 15:219-220.

CHAPTER 6

Waxy Wheat

Ravindra N. Chibbar[1] and Monisha Chakraborty[2]

[1]Department of Plant Sciences, College of Agriculture, University of Saskatchewan, Saskatoon, SK, Canada S7N 5A8; [2]Department of Plant Sciences, College of Agriculture, North Dakota State University, Fargo, ND 58105

Starch is the major component of a wheat grain, composing two-thirds to three-quarters of the dry grain weight (Hucl and Chibbar 1996). The endosperm of the wheat grain is the storage site for the starch, which is used by the germinating embryo as an energy source until it can begin photosynthesis and produce its own carbohydrates. In harvested grain consumed by humans as food or by livestock as feed, starch is the major source of energy. Extracted starch is one of the most widely used ingredients in the food industry. It has multiple uses, such as a thickener in soups and gravy and as a binder in coatings to maintain the texture and stability of the processed food product. Its hydrolysis products are used as sweeteners in beverages and confectionery products. In addition, starch is a leading industrial chemical, used in papermaking, the production of biodegradable plastics, corrugated board and cardboard paper, in the textile industry, in seed coatings for agrochemicals, and as a filler and dusting powder for pharmaceutical products.

The multitude of food and industrial uses for starch can be partly ascribed to the diversity introduced by the botanical origin and the amenability of the starch molecule to physical, chemical, and enzymatic modifications, which alter its physical and chemical properties to meet the demands of changing markets and consumers. The market demand for starch has risen steadily, as has a need for producing modified starches *in planta*, so that expensive and environmentally unfriendly postharvest enzymatic and chemical treatments can be reduced (Davis et al 2003). Plant-breeding techniques have been used to alter starch structure in corn, which has resulted in the production of several types of starches with altered structure and functionalities. These modified starches have been used to produce several new types of food products and have diversified the markets for corn producers around the world (Johnson et al 2001a,b). Genetic techniques have also been used to alter starch structure in other cereal crops such as rice and barley, but until recently, the production of altered starch structure in wheat endosperm had not been achieved. Wheat is hexaploid (AABBDD; $2n = 6x = 42$), which precluded the development of an aberrant phenotype due to a spontaneous mutation in one genome, because of the compensatory effect of the genes present in the other two genomes. However, biochemical and molecular techniques have been used to detect null alleles in each of the three genomes. Subsequently, lines with null alleles have been crossed to develop a genotype with three null alleles. Waxy (amylose-free) wheat has been produced by combining three null GBSS1 alleles. In this chapter, we will summarize the development of waxy wheat, with emphasis on the genetics and genes and the utilization of waxy wheat and extracted waxy starch.

Starch Structure and Biosynthesis

Starch is the most common storage carbohydrate in plants (Kossmann and Lloyd 2000, Chibbar and Båga 2003). It is synthesized in the chloroplasts during the day and mobilized to the storage organs at night. In plants, amyloplasts in the storage organs such as seeds, tubers, fruits, and storage roots are the major sites of reserve starch synthesis. Plants store starch in highly organized water-insoluble granules, which contain glucan chains packed in clusters by an asymmetric distribution of α-(1→6) branches within the molecules. The tightly spaced glucan branches form a double helix at the bottom of each unit cluster, which imparts crystallinity to the starch molecule. Starch is a complex macromolecule composed of two glucan polymers, an essentially linear chain amylose, and a highly branched amylopectin. Amylose (molecular weight 10^5–10^6 Da) is composed of linear chains of 840–22,000 α-(1→4)-D-glucopyranosyl residues. However, a small amount of the glucose residues (approximately up to 0.5%) are branched by the α-(1→6)-glucosidic linkages in amylose chains. Amylopectin (molecular weight 10^7–10^9 Da) is more highly branched with 4–5% of the α-(1→6)-glucosidic linkages. Starch is normally made up of about one-quarter amylose and three-quarters amylopectin. Both the proportion of amylose to amylopectin and structure of amylose and amylopectin molecules vary with the plant species and its developmental stage, thus giving a natural diversity of starch molecules. Starch occurs in plants with amylose and amylopectin arranged in a three-dimensional semicrystalline structure—the starch granule. The granules contain, in addition to the glucan polymers, small amounts of lipids (0.1–1.0%), proteins (0.05–0.5%), and trace amounts of phosphates (Thomas and Atwell 1998).

Biosynthesis of starch in plants has been studied over the years (Preiss and Sivak 1996), but the biochemistry of amylopectin synthesis and the precise mechanism for starch granule initiation are not clearly understood. Studies of starch mutants have so far produced a general consensus that ADP-glucose pyrophosphorylase (AGPase), starch synthases (SS), starch branching enzymes (SBE), starch debranching enzymes (DBE; pullulanase; isoamylase), and possibly also disproportionating enzyme (D-enzyme) catalyze the final steps leading to amylopectin synthesis. Granule bound starch synthase 1 (GBSS1) is the only enzyme committed to amylose synthesis. Several of the enzymes exist in different isoforms, some of which vary in their subcellular distribution, enzyme specificity, temporal activity, and interaction with other enzymes, which increases pathway complexity. The priming mechanism for starch glucan polymerization in plants is unclear, but it likely involves short-chain maltodextrins that are extended and branched by the action of GBSS1, SBE1, and SS1 to form a molecule with an amylopectin-like backbone. The primary glucan polymer is further polymerized through cycles of chain extensions and branching catalyzed mainly by SS1 and SBE2. Two models have recently been proposed to explain the involvement of starch debranching enzymes in starch synthesis. In the glucan-trimming model (Myers et al 2000), debranching enzymes are required to debranch the ends of water-soluble, preamylopectin molecules to produce amylopectin that can be crystallized and packaged into granules. The glucan-recycling model (Smith 1999) suggests that the role of debranching enzymes is to degrade water-soluble glucans synthesized by starch synthases and starch branching enzymes to prevent accumulation of phytoglycogen. Observations made in *Chlamydomonas* suggest that the D-enzyme is involved in starch synthesis and granule formation in addition to starch degradation. Polymerization of amylose is initiated from soluble malto-oligosaccharides that serve as primers for GBSS1 (Ball et al 1998).

Genetics and Breeding of Waxy Wheat

Waxy Locus

The corn and rice *waxy* mutants lack amylose and were also found to be deficient in GBSS1, also known as the waxy protein (Nelson and Rines 1962, Murata et al 1965, Tsai 1974, Echt and Schwartz 1981). The chromosomal regions containing the gene encoding GBSS1 are the *waxy* (*wx*) loci, which were first mapped in corn (Nelson 1968). Genetic analyses have shown that the allohexaploid common bread wheat has three *waxy* loci, *Wx-A1*, *Wx-B1*, and *Wx-D1*, located on the chromosome arms 7AS, 4AL, and 7DS, respectively (Chao et al 1989, Ainsworth et al 1993, Yamamori et al 1994a). The 4A *waxy* locus was originally present on chromosome 7B, but during the evolution of present-day wheat, it got translocated to 4AL (Chao et al 1989); therefore, although it is present on chromosome 4A, it is still designated as *Wx-B1*. Molecular characterization of the *Wx* locus by DNA sequencing from several plant species such as corn (Shure et al 1983, Klösgen et al 1986), barley (Rohde et al 1988), rice (Wang et al 1990), pea (Dry et al 1992), potato (Hovenkamp-Hermelink et al 1987), and wheat (Ainsworth et al 1993, Murai et al 1999) has predicted that it codes for GBSS1. The *Wx* locus, at all the three homeologous loci in the common wheat and its diploid progenitors, codes the GBSS1 structural gene comprised of 11 exons interspersed by 10 introns (Murai et al 1999, Yan et al 2000). In wheat, the arrangement and the number of exons and introns are very similar to those reported in barley (Rohde et al 1988) and rice, but they differ from corn, which has 14 exons and 13 introns, for a total length of 3,718 bp (Klösgen et al 1986). The three homeologous waxy genes from common bread wheat and its three diploid progenitors exons have a very similar nucleotide sequence, but there is some degree of sequence variation in the introns (Murai et al 1999, Yan et al 2000, Yan and Bhave 2001). The nucleotide sequence of the introns 4 and 5 in the diploid wheat progenitors varies significantly, and these can be used to distinguish the three homeologous waxy genes in the hexaploid wheat (Yan et al 2000, Yan and Bhave 2000). The DNA sequence information is being used to develop molecular markers to help in marker-assisted breeding for introgressing waxy starch traits into well-adapted cultivars in various regions of the world.

The three waxy genes are transcribed as 1815 bp (*Wx-7A*), 1818 bp (*Wx-4A*), and 1815 (*Wx-7D*) transcripts, with the first 210 (*A* and *D*) and 213 (*B*) bp encoding a transit peptide, and the remaining 1605 bp encoding the mature peptide (Murai et al 1999). The predicted molecular masses for the transit peptide and the mature peptide are 7.62 and 58.95 kDa, 7.57 and 58.5 kDa, and 7.38 and 58.90 kDa for the *Wx-7A*, *Wx-7D,* and *Wx-4A* encoded GBSS1, respectively (Murai et al 1999). The three homoeoalleles show close to 96 and 90% sequence similarity in the coding and transit peptide sequences, respectively (Murai et al 1999).

Granule Bound Starch Synthase 1 (GBSS1)

Most of the enzymes participating in starch biosynthesis are associated with starch granules (Båga et al 1999). In wheat, SDS-PAGE analysis of starch granule proteins showed that GBSS1, with an apparent molecular mass of 59 kDa, was the most prominent polypeptide associated with starch granules (Schofield and Greenwell 1987). Modification of the SDS-PAGE (acrylamide:biacrylamide ratio of 30:0.135) resulted in the resolution of the GBSS1 polypeptide into two components with slightly different mobilities (Nakamura et al 1993b). Two-dimensional gel electrophoresis separates polypeptides based on net charge in the first dimension, and then the molecular mass of the separated polypeptides is determined by denaturing gel electrophoresis (SDS-PAGE) in the second dimension (O'Farrell 1975). Two-dimensional gel electrophoresis was used to separate the wheat GBSS1 into three defined subunit groups—SGA, SGB, and SGD—which corresponded to the *Wx-A1*, *Wx-B1,* and *Wx-D1* loci, encoded by the three wheat genomes (Nakamura et al 1993b). Wheat cv. Chinese Spring nullisomic-tetrasomic lines (Sears 1966) compensated for chromosomes 7A, 4A, and 7D were used to assign the GBSS1 polypeptides to the respective genomes. The *Wx-A1* had a higher molecular mass (61 kD) and a more basic isoelectric point (pI), while the *Wx-B1* and *Wx-D1* had very similar molecular masses (59 kD), but *Wx-D1* had a slightly basic pI as compared to *Wx-B1* (Nakamura et al 1993b). Zhao and Sharp (1996), by modifying the SDS-PAGE (acrylamide/biacrylamide ratio of 30:0.1) method, could resolve the wheat cv. Chinese Spring GBSS1 isotypes with apparent molecular masses of 62.8, 58.7, and 56.7 kDa. By using the appropriate nullisomic-tetrasomic wheat lines, the slowest-mobility isotype corresponded to *Wx-A1*, followed by *Wx-D1*, and the most mobile was

Wx-B1 (Zhao and Sharp 1996), concurring with the results reported by Nakamura et al (1993b). However, the apparent molecular mass estimated by SDS-PAGE is higher than that predicted by the cDNA clones, as described above (Murai et al 1999). Nevertheless, the SDS-PAGE (Zhao and Sharp 1996) has been used to screen wheat germ plasm to identify lines with null GBSS1 alleles.

Immunochemical Detection of Waxy Proteins

Rahman et al (1995) reported the characterization of two monoclonal antibodies that specifically reacted with GBSS1. These monoclonal antibodies against GBSS1 were used in a sandwich enzyme-linked immunoassay (ELISA) to quantitatively determine the amounts of water-extractable GBSS1 and its correlation with amylose concentration in wheat grains (Graybosch et al 1998, 1999). The ELISA-based assays could distinguish wheat lines with double GBSS1 null alleles and showed some degree of correlation between the amount of GBSS1 protein and the amylose concentration, but it could not distinguish wheat lines with single GBSS1 null alleles. In another approach to distinguish GBSS1 *Wx-B1b* allele, which has been correlated with superior noodle-making qualities of wheat, polyclonal antibody (R12) was raised against a GBSS1 synthetic peptide incorporating amino acid sequences unique to GBSS1-*Wx-B1b* protein (Gale et al 2001). The specific antibodies were used in a 96-well microtitre plate format sandwich ELISA to assess the GBSS1-*Wx-B1b* protein in a doubled haploid mapping population characterized for *Wx-B1* locus on chromosome 4A. The assay unambiguously identified 153 of the 161 lines analyzed, thus validating its utility for use in wheat-improvement programs for development of noodle-quality wheat. This assay was also applicable to GBSS1 extracted from crude flour extracts. The ELISA results were also in conformity with flour swelling volume, another important determinant of grain quality for noodle-making properties (Gale et al 2001).

DNA-Based Markers for Waxy Loci

Recently, several attempts have been made to develop polymerase chain reaction (PCR)-based DNA markers to distinguish each homoeoallele of GBSS1. DNA-based markers have a distinct advantage in detecting the presence of each homoeoallele at an early stage, thus reducing the number of plants to be carried to maturity. As mentioned above, the three GBSS1 homoeoalleles (Mason-Gamer et al 1998, Yan et al 2000) show a very high degree of nucleotide sequence similarity in their coding sequences; thus, these are of limited use in developing molecular markers. A close examination of the cDNA sequence of wheat GBSS1 (Accession X07931) (Clark et al 1991), by Shariflou and Sharp (1999), detected the presence of an imperfect $(AT)_n$ repeat $[(AT)_6A(AT)_2]$ near the 3′ end of the gene (Accession X57233, bases 2010–2027) that was partly aligned with an $(AT)_4$ in the barley waxy gene (Accession X07931) (Rohde et al 1988) in a similar position. This polymorphic microsatellite marker is codominant for the *Wx-A1* locus, but dominant for the *Wx-D1* locus, where it is absent in the lines that have the *Wx-*

D1 null allele (Shariflou and Sharp 1999). The utility of this microsatellite as a dominant marker for the *Wx-D1* locus was further confirmed in a subsequent study (McLauchlan et al 2001). The nucleotide sequence divergence in the exons has been used to develop DNA markers for use in a PCR-based assay (Briney et al 1998, McLauchlan et al 2001). An oligonucleotide primer based on the intron 4 sequence of the *Wx-4b* locus (chromosome 4A), when used in a PCR-based assay, correctly identified 267 out of 268 genotypes tested for the presence or absence of GBSS1-*WxB* (Briney et al 1998). A primer pair targeting the amplification of DNA fragments from GBSS1 intron 1 has resulted in the identification of a dominant marker linked to the *Wx-B1* locus in most of the Australian wheats studied (McLauchlan et al 2001). The development of DNA-based markers and their validation using diverse germ plasm and in early stages of wheat improvement programs will help in the development of wheat lines with modified starch properties (McLauchlan et al 2001).

Genetic Variation for GBSS1 in Wheat

The identification of wheat germ plasm with GBSS1 null alleles is the first step in the development of waxy wheat cultivars. SDS-PAGE has been used to determine the distribution of wheat lines deficient in GBSS1 proteins (Table 1). In the first published study (Yamamori et al 1994a), SDS-PAGE

TABLE 1
Geographical Distribution of Wheat Germ Plasm Carrying GBSS1 Null Alleles

Region or Country	Number of Lines Characterized	Null A	Null B	Null D	Null A and B	Reference
Afghanistan	59	0	13			Yamamori et al (1994a)
Australia	127	1	51			Yamamori et al (1994a),
	126		18			Demeke et al (1997)
China	308	3	12	1		Yamamori et al (1994a)
India	50	3	25			Yamamori et al (1994a)
Japan	462	75	16			Yamamori et al (1994a),
	112	10	1		1	Demeke et al (1997)
North America						
United States	315	3	19			Yamamori et al (1994a)
	63	0	2			Demeke et al (1997)
	196	7	13		1	Graybosch et al (1998)
Canada	86		40			Demeke et al (2000)
Pakistan	85	0	13			Yamamori et al (1994a)
Russia	133	0	5			Yamamori et al (1994a)
South and North Korea	93	10	1			Yamamori et al (1994a)
Turkey	156	81				Yamamori et al (1994a)
Western Europe	172	1	4			Yamamori et al (1994a)
Spain (Iberian wheats)	606	24	96		4	Rodriguez-Quijano et al (1998)
Italy	288	1	63	1		Boggini et al (2001)

and two-dimensional electrophoresis were used to screen 1960 wheat cultivars originating from different geographic regions of the world. Among the cultivars screened, 9% lacked the *Wx-A1*, while 8% lacked the *Wx-B1* protein. Only one wheat cultivar, BaiHuo, from China, lacked the *Wx-D1* protein. Subsequent studies have detected *Wx-B1* null alleles at a higher frequency than *Wx-A1* (Table 1). However, *Wx-D1* null allele has been found in only one Italian wheat land race—Cologna Lunga (Boggini et al 2001), in addition to BaiHuo, reported before. The reason for the rare occurrence of null *Wx-D1* is not yet known. In addition to the spontaneous occurrence of single null GBSS1 alleles, the double null alleles for *Wx-A1* and *Wx-B1* have also been reported at a very low frequency (Table 1).

Production of Waxy and Partially Waxy Wheat

A historical perspective of waxy wheat development was recently published (Seib 2000) (Table 2). The world's first waxy wheat was produced by combining a double *Wx-A1/Wx-B1* null allele line, Kanto 107, with a *Wx-D1* null allele carrying line, BaiHuo, using standard plant-breeding techniques (Nakamura et al 1995). The completely waxy wheat line produced lacked the three GBSS1 isoforms, and the grain starch contained no detectable amylose. Subsequent to the first demonstration, using Bai Huo as the *Wx-D1* null allele donor, the process of genetic elimination of GBSS1 alleles by plant-breeding techniques has been used to produce waxy wheat lines in several other laboratories (Demeke et al 1999, Morris and Konzak 2001). Chemical mutagenesis has also been used to develop fully waxy wheat lines. Treatment of wheat cv. Kanto 107 (null *Wx-A1/Wx-B1*) seeds with a chemical mutagen ethyl methane sulfonate (EMS), resulted in few completely waxy seeds (Yasui et al 1997). In another approach, a low-amylose wheat line Tanikei A6099, obtained by EMS treatment of Kanto 107 (Oda et al 1992), was crossed with an elite Japanese wheat cultivar, Saikai 168, and subjected to a doubled-haploid program to speed up the introgression of waxy null alleles, which resulted in five waxy wheat lines with negligible amounts of amylose in the grain starch (Kiribuchi-Otobe et al 1997). The possible molecular mechanism for the inactivation of GBSS1 *Wx-D1* in these wheat lines is difficult to explain, but it could be due to the somaclonal variation introduced during the in vitro regeneration step of the doubled haploid production protocols.

Partial waxy wheat has one or two null alleles, which result in starch with reduced amylose concentration (Nakamura et al 1995). The reported ranges in amylose content of single null and wild-type wheats overlap, suggesting a differential effect of the individual GBSS isoforms (Graybosch 1998). Chinese Spring and its aneuploid lines in which the dosage of GBSS1 derived from different genomes was selectively reduced, revealed that GBSS1 B deficiency decreased the amylose concentration by 3% (Miura and Sugawara 1996). Deficiency in GBSS1 *A* and *D* did not significantly reduce the amylose concentration. The presence of two null alleles reduces the amylose content by about 5% relative to the wild type (Yamamori et al 1994b, Miura and Sugawara 1996). However, in another study, the deficiency in GBSS1 A and B reduced

TABLE 2
Significant Events Leading to the Development of Waxy and Partially Waxy Wheats

Year	Location	Event	References
1975	Christchurch, New Zealand	Starches from selected Australian wheats with 2–3% less amylose than New Zealand wheats had a high pasting peak.	Loney et al (1975)
1977	Tokyo, Japan	Flour of acceptable quality for salt noodles milled from Western Australian wheat produced an amylogram with low pasting temperature and high pasting peak.	Nagao et al (1977)
1980	North Ryde, Australia; Atsugi, Japan	High amylograph pasting peak or rapid time to reach pasting peak for starch from salt noodle flour was associated positively with eating quality of salt noodles and negatively with apparent amylose levels between 19 and 32%.	Moss (1980); Oda et al (1980)
1984	North Ryde, Australia	Wheat starch with high amylose level had a low pasting peak and no breakdown.	Moss and Miskelly (1984)
1987	Charleywood, United Kingdom	Granule-bound starch synthase (waxy protein) was confirmed in wheat starch.	Schofield and Greenwell (1987)
1989	Morioka, Japan	Japanese wheats Kanto 79 and Kanto 107 had 22% amylose in flour compared with ≥27% in 116 other Japanese wheats.	Kuroda et al (1989)
1989	South Perth, Australia	Flour swelling power and swelling volume tests were developed for breeders to identify noodle wheats.	Crosbie (1989, 1991)
1990s	Australia, Japan, Korea, and Hong Kong	Investigators verified that the quality of salt noodle flour was associated with enhanced swelling of wheat starch and reduced amylose level.	Moss and Miskelly (1984); Morris et al (1997a,b)
1993	Morioka, Okinawa, and Tsukuba, Japan	Waxy proteins in wheat starch produced by *Wx-A1*, *Wx-B1*, and *Wx-D1* loci in hexaploid wheats were separated; the term "partially waxy" wheat was coined; and waxy wheat was predicted.	Nakamura et al (1993a,b)
1994	Morioka, Okinawa, and Nara, Japan	Wheat cultivars (2,000) were screened for waxy proteins; 17% of wheats with a single null allele at *Wx* locus were identified (only one wheat had a null for *Wx-D1* locus); 0.05% double nulls at *Wx-A1* and *Wx-B1* were found, but no double nulls involving *Wx-D1* locus; no triple null was found; and distributions of waxy proteins in a total of eight types of wheat starches were assigned.	Yamamori et al (1994a)

Year	Location	Event	References
1994	Okinawa and Morioka, Japan	A durum (tetraploid) wheat Aldura was crossed with Kanto 107 (hexaploid with double null for *Wx-A1* and *Wx-B1* proteins) to produce the first waxy tetraploid wheat; Chinese Bai Huo wheat (null for *Wx-D1* protein) was crossed with Japanese Kanto 107 and Saikai 173 (null for *Wx-A1* and *Wx-B1* proteins) to obtain waxy hrexaploid wheat.	Yamamori et al (1994b); Nakamura et al (1995)
1996	Camden, Australia	An improved one-dimensional gel electrophoresis method was used to separate three waxy proteins in wheat starch.	Zhao and Sharp (1996)
1998	Western Australia and New South Wales, Australia, Nebraska, USA	Quality of wheat for salt noodle predicted by 1) separation of waxy proteins isolated from starch; 2) polymerase chain reaction-based assay for null *Wx-B1* locus in leaf DNA; 3) immunoassay (enzyme-linked immunosorbent assay) for total waxy proteins dissolved from starch.	Zhao et al (1998); Briney et al (1998); Graybosch et al (1999)
1999	Saskatoon, Canada	Wheat was produced with a double null for *Wx-B1* and *Wx-D1* proteins; starch contained 12.4% amylose.	Demeke et al (1999)
1999	Osaka, Japan	Complete genomic sequences of the waxy structural genes located on chromosomes 7A, 4A, and 7D	Murai et al (1999)
2000	Tsukuba, Japan	Isogenic lines of hexaploid wheats were produced with all combinations of waxy proteins; double nulls contained 7–10% less amylose compared with the wild-type.	Yamamori and Quynh (2000)
2001	Italy	A wheat line Cologna Lunga was found to be deficient in *Wx-D1* protein.	Boggini et al (2001)
2001	Pullman, WA, USA	Registration of hard and soft homozygous waxy wheat germplasm	Morris and Konzak (2001)

[a] Modified, with permission, from Seib (2000).

the amylose concentration by 2%, but the GBSS1 B and D deficiency reduced the amylose concentration to 12.5% as compared to 25% in the wild type (Demeke et al 1999). Wheat near-isogenic lines with the eight possible combinations of *wx* alleles have been produced (Zhao and Sharp 1998, Miura et al 2002). While the triple null *Wx* allele (waxy) line had less than 3% amylose, in the lines with null B and D *wx* alleles, the amylose concentration was reduced to 16%, as compared to 24% in the wild type (Miura et al 2002). This report also concurred with the earlier observations that deficiency in GBSS1 B and D caused the most reduction in amylose concentrations as compared to the combination of the other two alleles. These lines will be very useful for studying the biosynthetic mechanism underlying amylose biosynthesis, as well as for providing an opportunity to develop wheat lines with a wide spectrum of amylose/amylopectin concentrations. The waxy and partial waxy wheat offer unique starch functional properties that might extend the use of wheat in many food and nonfood applications as described below.

Characteristics of Waxy Wheat Starches

Starch-related functional attributes of waxy lines have been found to be extremely stable across environments, unlike protein-related quality traits that showed significant environmental and genotypic variances, similar to those typical of nonwaxy wheats (Graybosch et al 2003). The ratio of amylose to amylopectin determines the physicochemical properties of starch, and thereby, the end use of the grain. Amylose has a higher tendency to retrograde and consequently produces a firm gel after the starch has been cooked and cooled. Conversely, the branched, crystalline, "tumbleweedlike" structure of amylopectin impedes retrogradation and slows starch gel formation after cooking and cooling, and the resultant paste is cohesive with a gummy texture (Thomas and Atwell 1998). Cereal grain genotypes exhibiting altered amylose-to-amylopectin ratios may therefore affect end products, which depend on the unique performance properties of amylopectin. There has been much speculation about the use of full waxy wheat flour in various food end products. However, these applications are still under investigation due a limited understanding of the fundamental relationship between waxy starch structure and functional properties (Mua and Jackson 1997).

Structural Characteristics

The weight-average molecular weight (MW) and chain-length distribution of starch fractions influence starch crystallinity and affect the gelatinization, pasting, and retrogradation properties of starch (Shibanuma et al 1996, Jane et al 1999, Yoo and Jane 2002a). Yasui et al (1996) reported that the waxy trait had little effect on the chain-length distribution of amylopectin molecules, whereas Yoo and Jane (2002b) observed that waxy amylopectins had substantially higher MW and more branch-chains than their normal starch counterparts, which resulted in more densely packed molecules. They hypothesized that the presence of about 25% (by mass) amylose in normal starch granules probably limited space and resulted in lower MW of normal amylopectin.

X-ray diffraction patterns are related to differences in chain length and the arrangement of branch points in the amylopectin fraction (Rahman et al 2000). The typical A-type patterns of X-ray diffractograms were observed for waxy and nonwaxy wheats, although the relative crystallinity was significantly higher in waxy wheats (Hayakawa et al 1997, Demeke et al 1999, Kim et al 2003). Thermal analysis showed comparatively higher enthalpy values (ΔH) in waxy wheat, consistent with their degrees of crystallinity. DSC thermal properties were more significantly affected by the degree of crystallization than the granule size of waxy and normal wheat (Yasui et al 1996, Fujita et al 1998). Yoo and Jane (2002a) reported similar results and also noted the absence of amylose-lipid complex in waxy wheat endotherms. Compared to nonwaxy wheat starch, waxy wheat starch exhibits lower lipid content. X-ray diffraction studies confirmed the absence of amylose lipid complexes in waxy wheat starch (Abdel-Aal et al 2002). The surface lipids, if present on starch granules, have little influence on the fatty acid composition of starch lipid (Yasui et al 1996, Fujita et al 1998). The small amount of lipids detected in waxy wheat lines presumably represents lipids trapped in the interstices of the starch granule (Yasui et al 1996).

Functional Properties

The functional properties of waxy wheat starch are typically analyzed using the Rapid ViscoAnalyser (RVA), which measures the resistance of starch granules to shearing forces under defined hydration and temperature regimes. The overall process of gelatinization is similar in both nonwaxy and waxy starch granules, although the presence of amylose in nonwaxy starch restricts water movement and starch granule swelling, mediated through reduced mobility of amylose-lipid complexes in the granule (Rahman et al 2000). The pasting profile of waxy wheat is typically characterized by a high peak viscosity, low initial pasting temperature, and low setback (Kiribuchi-Otobe et al 1997, Yasui et al 1999, Grant et al 2001, Abdel-Aal et al 2002, Bhattacharya et al 2002, Kim et al 2003), although contrasting results for peak viscosity have been reported by Hayakawa et al (1997). The high amount of amylopectin, as well as the low amylose and lipid contents in waxy starch, facilitates rapid water uptake and higher granule swelling in a relatively shorter time and at a lower temperature (Tester and Morrison 1990). Waxy starches swell unrestrictedly and exhibit higher swelling power and solubility than the nonwaxy starches, indicating a loosely bound micellar network due to the absence of amylose (Grant et al 2001). Following complete gelatinization and subsequent cooling to ambient temperatures, waxy starches form viscous solutions rather than gels, which are typically translucent, and exhibit lower syneresis and higher resistance to retrogradation than nonwaxy starches (Hayakawa et al 1997, Kiribuchi-Otobe et al 1998, Rahman et al 2000).

Characteristics of Waxy Wheat Grains and Flours

End-use applications of waxy wheat are highly dependent on the wheat grain and endosperm characteristics. Therefore, the use of waxy wheat in various wheat-based products may be feasible only when the waxy trait is combined with other desirable grain and flour-quality characteristics (Graybosch 1998). Sayaslan et al (2001) reported that waxy wheats had lower protein content and weaker gluten strength than nonwaxy flours, but gave similar or higher loaf volumes than the controls. In contrast, Park et al (2001) observed that Korean waxy flours produced inferior-quality cereal products (bread, noodles, and cookies), despite high protein content and large sedimentation volumes. Abdel-Aal et al (2002) compared the properties of waxy wheat flour with those obtained from hard and soft wheat grown in the same environment. The waxy wheat flours absorbed significantly more water than hard or soft wheat flours and required less time to develop into optimum dough compared to bread flour. However, the dough exhibited medium gluten strength and lower stability to mechanical mixing than hard wheat, as also indicated by intermediate sedimentation volume. Weaker gluten strength was also observed in a set of waxy spring wheats of diverse parentage, grown at various North American environments (Graybosch et al 2003). The growing environment was the largest source of variance for seed weight, SDS sedimentation volume, flour ash, and mixograph peak time and tolerance.

Yasui et al (1999) compared the milling quality and flour properties of two Japanese waxy mutant lines with their parent bread wheat cultivar. The protein content and grain hardness did not differ markedly between them, yet the waxy lines had reduced flour flowability and about 20% lower flour yield than the nonwaxy parent, which was attributed to the elevated grain fat (20% higher than the nonwaxy parent) and β-glucan content seen in the waxy mutants. Lower flour yield has also been reported in waxy soft wheat (Kim et al 2003) and waxy spring wheat Graybosch et al (2003) compared to that in wild types, clearly indicating that flour yield is not related to gluten strength. Perhaps the lack of amylose confers higher endosperm crystallinity, which subsequently influences the milling properties of waxy wheat (Graybosch et al 2003). Higher starch damage has been reported in waxy wheat in comparison to nonwaxy wheat (Grant et al 2001, Abdel-Aal et al 2002, Guo et al 2003a,b). Waxy starch granules are less resistant to mechanical damage than normal starch granules and are consequently more susceptible to increased starch damage. The lack of amylose-related hydrogen bonding in waxy starch may cause a decreased resistance to crushing, with a concomitant increase in starch damage during milling (Bettge et al 2000). Starch damage and subsequent milling yield is mainly dependent on the endosperm texture of the wheat grain. Grain hardness is independent of starch amylose concentrations, and waxy wheat may be developed with desired endosperm texture (Morris and Konzak 2001). Higher kernel hardness has been reported in soft waxy wheats as compared to wild- type or single null genotypes (Kim et al 2003). However, waxy spring wheats with both hard- and soft-textured lines have been developed (Morris and Konzak 2001, Graybosch et al 2003). Developing waxy wheat with lower kernel hardness may help reduce the damaged starch content of milled waxy grain (Graybosch et al 2003).

The falling number (FN) test, which is a means for assessing preharvest sprouting and α-amylase activity in wheat grain and flour samples, is not applicable to waxy wheat (Graybosch et al 2000). Waxy wheat flours exhibit markedly and uniformly reduced FN, even when their α-amylase levels are identical to those of sound wheats. The aberrant FN number has been attributed to the unique starch-pasting properties of waxy wheat. The absence of amylose, which confers granular rigidity and increased sensitivity of amylopectin to mechanical shear and high temperature (95°C), in addition to low gelatinization temperature, facilitates rapid breakdown of waxy starch granules and contributes to the low-consistency flour slurry in the FN test (Abdel-Aal et al 2002). Consequently, the FN assay is not effective as a means of assessing sprout damage in waxy wheats but may still be a valuable tool in marketing channels as a means of segregating waxy grain. When screening waxy wheat for sprout damage, the use of RVA peak viscosity provides a more accurate assessment of α-amylase levels (Graybosch et al 2000). In contrast, when screening waxy wheat flour for its starch pasting properties, the use of an amylase inhibitor like silver nitrate instead of water may alleviate erroneous results associated with amylase activity, and significantly improve the viscosity of waxy wheat, with no change in temperature parameters (Yasui et al 1999, Abdel-Aal et al 2002, Bhattacharya et al 2002).

Uses of Waxy and Partial-Waxy Wheat

Asian Noodles

Starch is the key contributor to the textural quality of Japanese white salted noodles (WSN). WSN are typically produced from flour exhibiting high starch swelling volume and high peak viscosity (Zhao et al 1998), which confers a soft and elastic texture to the noodles. Miura and Tanii (1994) established a link between the presence of GBSS1 null alleles and superior eating quality of WSN. Reduced amylose content, increased flour swelling ability, decreased paste gel rigidity, and enhanced deformation of gelatinized starch granules contribute to soft texture in WSN (Oda et al 1980, Yamamori et al 1992, Miura and Tanii 1994, Wang and Seib 1996, Seib 2000, Guo et al 2003a). Conversely, partial waxy wheats are unsuitable for making Chinese yellow alkaline noodles (YAN), which require a firm, smooth, and springy texture (Akashi et al 1999). Thus, noodle texture preference varies markedly among noodle types.

Developing partial waxy wheats with varying amylose content will categorically provide a means for producing diverse noodle types with desired eating texture. Improved noodle textural properties, as determined by sensory tests, have been observed when amylose content was reduced by adding waxy wheat flour to regular wheat flour (Hoshino et al 2000, Yamaguchi et al 2000). An optimum amylose content range between 21 and 24% has been suggested for WSN (Batey et al 1997, Guo et al 2003a), although Batey et al (1997) found a nonlinear relationship between amylose content and noodle quality. Detailed analyses of partial waxy lines revealed that a single null allele at *Wx-B1* locus demonstrated lower amylose contents and elevated flour swelling volumes than nulls at *Wx-D1* and *Wx-A1* (Zhao et al 1998, Kim et al 2003), suggesting a higher potential of *Wx-B1* null for producing optimum WSN quality flour (Miura et al 1999). Epstein et al (2002) studied the relationship between GBSS1 genotype and WSN texture parameters among a set of genetically defined, advanced-generation recombinant inbred lines (RIL). Results indicated that W*x-B1b* null produced noodle firmness similar to that of the double nulls, whereas, W*x-D1b* null gave noodle texture similar to that of the nonwaxy starch samples. Addition of waxy flour to wild-type flours gave reduced cooked noodle firmness, gumminess, and chewiness values, whereas noodle cohesiveness, springiness, and resilience increased (Guo et al 2003a). Firmness of noodles made from reconstituted flours with waxy starch correlated positively with amylose content and setback and negatively with RVA peak viscosity and breakdown (Baik and Lee 2003). Furthermore, the positive effect of high protein content on noodle firmness was significantly diminished by changes in starch amylose content, indicating that high-protein flours can still produce soft-textured WSN of optimum quality when the amylose content of the base flour is reduced (Baik and Lee 2003).

Baking Industry

Starch contributes to the textural characteristics of bread through gelatinization and formation of three-dimensional networks with the gluten proteins (Zobel and Kulp 1996). On cooling and aging of bread, rearrangements in the starch fractions lead to a series of changes, including gelation and crystallization. This starch retrogradation is thought to be the major cause of bread crumb firming, commonly referred to as bread staling (Hug-Iten et al 1999). Conflicting results attribute the staling mechanism to retrogradation of either amylose or amylopectin. Hug-Iten et al (1999) related bread staling to reorganization of the intragranular amylose fraction, whereas Krog et al (1989) attributed it to reassociation of the amylopectin chains. However, bread aging is not directly correlated with the overall crystallinity of starch. Biliaderis (1992) stated that starch retrogradation was a biphasic phenomenon, consisting of early complexing of amylose, followed by a slow and gradual recystallization of amylopectin, and therefore reducing the amylose content would eliminate the rapid early component of staling. To understand the functionality of amylose and amylopectin in baked products, one approach would be to reduce or eliminate a starch fraction (mainly amylose) from the base flour and study its impact on the texture and keeping quality of bread. The availability of waxy wheat provides a unique opportunity to study bread staling in an amylose-free environment, without introducing the undesirable flavor and color factors associated with nonwheat cereals (Toufeilli et al 1999). A number of patents already exist on the use of flours with high amylopectin to improve the shelf life of baked goods (Zallie et al 1986, Hoshino et al 2000, Messager and Despre 2002).

Incorporation of waxy wheat starch could be helpful in retaining higher moisture in bread crumbs and has the potential to retard staling and extend the shelf life of baked goods (Graybosch 1998, Yasui et al 1999, Lee et al 2001, Bhattacharya et al 2002). Moreover, because of their slow retrogradation rates, waxy starches may function as fat replacers in baked products (Graybosch 1998, Bhattacharya et al 2002). However, the presence of some amylose appears to be essential to the production of acceptable-quality baked goods (Graybosch 1998). Lorenz (1995) observed that doughs made from 100% waxy barley resulted in breads with markedly reduced volume, poor appearance, and less desirable texture. Waxy wheat flour exhibited increased water absorption, reduced dough development time, and higher susceptibility to overmixing, and produced sticky and less stable dough (Abdel-Aal et al 2002, Morita et al 2002). Waxy wheat flour displayed higher gas production and lower gas retention, reflecting a weakened dough structure (Lee et al 2001). Fermentation proceeded faster with waxy wheat flours, possibly reflecting greater susceptibility of the branched starch molecules to α-amylase activity (Lee et al 2001, Abdel-Aal et al 2002). Breads made with waxy wheat flour resulted in an open-crumb structure with excessive shrinkage of the loaf upon cooling (Lee et al 2001), which was attributed to the lack of amylose concentration and excessive damaged starch, rather than to protein concentration or protein quality (Kim et al 2003).

There is a need to identify optimum amylose-to-amylopectin proportions, in which the benefits of lowered amylose levels outweigh its negative effects for specific bakery product applications. Bread prepared from 10–15% waxy wheat exhibited crumb structure similar to that of bread from regular wheat but retained higher crumb moisture and lower crumb hardness after seven days of storage. However, when the blending ratio was increased to 25–50% waxy wheat, the loaves exhibited greater volume, softer crumb, more porous crumb structure, and a higher level of starch retrogradation than regular wheat (Lee et al 2001). Similarly, Morita et al (2002) reported higher loaf volume in bread made from waxy wheat flour compared to nonwaxy wheat flour, although the crumbs had an open structure and the top of the loaf was wider than the bottom. SEM analyses revealed that bread made from waxy wheat flour had a rough and irregular appearance, whereas the control bread had an even and uniform pore structure. Despite inferior crumb texture, bread made from waxy wheat remained softer after seven days of storage, and the crumbs retained their softness after reheating. In contrast, the firmness of bread made from nonwaxy control flour and high-amylose wheat flour increased distinctly when refreshed by reheating. Waxy wheat flour appeared to suppress the formation of an insoluble network structure of starch during cooling, which improved the tolerance of gelatinized starch to the retrogradation process (Morita et al 2002). Addition of waxy durum flour to strong bread flour, in the ratio of 10, 20, and 30%, resulted in a significant decrease in the firming of bread (Bhattacharya et al 2002). Loaves produced from a 20% waxy flour blend displayed good external and internal texture comparable with the control flour. Waxy blends of 20 and 30% were most effective at reducing the rate of staling over a five-day storage period, as shown by lower firmness and enthalpy values of the loaves. The enhanced softness of loaves made with waxy blends was more pronounced than that obtained with 3% shortening, suggesting the possible use of waxy flour as an economical replacement for shortening in the baking industry (Bhattacharya et al 2002). Morita et al (2002) reported that Japanese consumers prefer bread with a sticky and glutinous texture, which can be achieved with a 40% waxy wheat flour blend. In contrast, high-amylose wheat flour could be used to replace durum wheat flour in pasta making or as an added ingredient in steamed Chinese processed foods, where a nonglutinous texture is desired.

Limited literature exists on the application of waxy wheat in cakes and cookies. Several characteristics of waxy flour, including higher ash, starch damage, and β-glucan, in addition to increased amylopectin levels, affect cookie quality. Park et al (2001) found that waxy wheat flour yielded cookies with smaller diameters than nonwaxy flours, which required a greater force to snap the cookie. Cookies formulated with the addition of waxy barley flour were also found to have smaller diameters than those from nonwaxy barley (Klamczynski and Czuchajowska 1999). For broader applications in the baking industry, it would be necessary to ascertain that the flavor and taste of waxy flour are not discernible in the final baked product (Toufeilli et al 1999).

Tortillas

Tortilla processing and product quality is also affected by waxy wheat flour. Blends with low proportions of waxy wheat flour (10–20%) improve product quality, whereas excessive levels (>40%) are detrimental, due in part to early puffing in the oven. The early puffing contributes to rolling and folding problems during tortilla baking and conveying (Guo et al 2003b). The increased water absorption and lower gelatinization temperature of waxy flour, in comparison to wild-type flour (Hayakawa et al 1997, Otobe et al 1997, Graybosch et al 2000), affect early puffing because of their effects on polymer mobility and steam generation (Guo et al 2003b). Machinability, described as baked tortilla shape and production yield, also degrades with waxy flour levels exceeding 40%. Darker color, low opacity, lower heights, larger diameters, and reduced flexibility after storage are associated with low amylose levels (Waniska et al 2002, Guo et al 2003b). Tortilla height and opacity are influenced by the retention of air bubbles. Amylose is probably involved in the retention of air bubbles in the hot dough system during and immediately after baking of tortillas (Waniska et al 2002).

The moisture content and weight of baked tortillas were similar between waxy blends and controls, even though the amount of water added to the different blends varied significantly. Lower amylose content produced fresh tortillas with higher extensibility, although the extensibility was not retained beyond three days of storage (Guo et al 2003b). Partial waxy wheats did not affect most quality parameters, except for tortilla height and opacity. Sufficient leavening reactions occurred early in baking to yield an opaque disc, although some baked tortillas became transparent after baking (Waniska et al 2002). Tortilla textural characteristics and shelf stability improved dramatically when 10–20% waxy wheat flour was added to wild-type flour, which correlated with a 24–26% amylose content (Guo et al 2003b).

Miscellaneous Applications

In the extrusion industry, the use of waxy wheat starch may result in puffed snacks with increased expansion, lower fat, and higher fiber contents. Another possible application is its use in "easy-to-cook" instant food products due to its rapid gelatinization at lower temperatures (Yasui et al 1996). Partial waxy wheat may be as effective as corn starch when used as a gelling agent in a wide range of soups, sauces, and confectionary products (Båga et al 1999). Finally, waxy wheat starch can most likely function as an alternative to chemically modified waxy corn starch in all present food and nonfood applications (Graybosch 1998). Waxy wheat starch has been reported to possess uniquely desirable properties that are not duplicated by waxy corn starch and may therefore be a desirable alternative for chemically modified starches (Deis 1998).

Acknowledgments

Ms. Karen Caswell is gratefully acknowledged for her editorial assistance. Financial support over the years from Saskatchewan Agriculture Development Fund, Saskatchewan Agriculture Food and Rural Revitalization Department, is gratefully acknowledged (RNC). The continual financial support and encouragement from the North Dakota Wheat Commission, and the State Board of Agricultural Research and Education (SBARE) are also gratefully acknowledged (MC).

References

Abdel-Aal, E. S., Hucl, P., Chibbar R. N., Han, H., and Demeke, T. 2002. Physicochemical and structural characteristics of flours and starches from waxy and nonwaxy wheats. Cereal Chem. 79:458-464.

Ainsworth, C., Clark, J., and Baldson, J. 1993. Expression, organization and structure of the genes encoding the *waxy* protein (granule-bound starch synthase) in wheat. Plant. Mol. Biol. 22:67-82.

Akashi, H., Takahashi, M., and Endo, S. 1999. Evaluation of starch properties of wheats used for Chinese yellow-alkaline noodles in Japan. Cereal Chem. 76:50-55.

Båga, M., Repellin, A., Demeke, T., Caswell, K., Leung, N., Abdel-Aal, E. S., Hucl, P., and Chibbar, R. N. 1999. Wheat starch modification through biotechnology. Starch/Stærke 51:111-116.

Baik, B. Y., and Lee, M. R. 2003. Effects of starch amylose content of wheat on textural properties of white salted noodles. Cereal Chem. 80:304-309.

Ball, S. B., van de Wal, M. H. B. J., and Visser, R. G. F. 1998. Progress in understanding the biosynthesis of amylose. Trends Plant Sci. 3:462-467.

Batey, I. L., Gras, P. W., and Curtin, B. M. 1997. Contribution of the chemical structure of wheat starch to Japanese noodle quality. J. Sci. Food Agric. 74:503-508.

Bettge, A., Giroux, J., and Morris, C. 2000. Susceptibility of waxy starch granules to mechanical damage. Cereal Chem. 77:750-753.

Bhattacharya, M., Erazo-Castrejon, S., Doehlert, D. C., and McMullen, M. S. 2002. Staling of bread as affected by waxy wheat flour blends. Cereal Chem. 79:178-182.

Biliaderis, C. G. 1992. Structures and phase transitions of starch in food systems. Food Technol. 46:98-109.

Boggini, G., Cattaneo, M., Paganoni, C., and Vaccino, P. 2001. Genetic variation for waxy proteins and starch properties in Italian wheat germplasm. Euphytica 119:111-114.

Briney, A., Wilson, R., Potter, R. H., Barclay, I., Crosbie, G., Appels, R., and Jones, M. G. K. 1998. A PCR-based marker for selection of starch and potential noodle quality in wheat. Mol. Breeding 4:427-433.

Chao, S., Sharp, P. J., Worland, A. J., Warham, E. J., Koebner, R. M. D., and Gale, M. D. 1989. RFLP-based genetic maps of wheat homoeologous group 7 chromosomes. Theor. Appl. Genet. 78:495-504.

Chibbar, R. N., and Båga, M. 2003. Genetic modification of primary metabolism—Carbohydrates. Pages 449-459 in: Encyclopedia of Applied Plant Sciences. B. Thomas, D. J. Murphy, and B. G. Murray, Eds. Elsevier, Oxford, U.K.

Clark, J. R., Robertson, M., and Ainsworth, C. C. 1991. Nucleotide sequence of a wheat (*Triticum aestivum* L.) cDNA clone encoding the *waxy* protein. Plant Mol. Biol. 16:1099-1101.

Crosbie, G. B. 1989. Wheat quality trends in Western Australia. In: Proc. 39th Annu. Conf. R. Aust. Chem. Inst., Cereal Chem. Div. Royal Australian Chemical Institute, Parkville.

Crosbie, G. B. 1991. The relationship between starch swelling properties, paste viscosity and boiled noodle quality in wheat flours. J. Cereal Sci. 13:145-150.

Davis, J. P., Netrphan, S., Khandelwal, R. L., and Chibbar, R. N. 2003. Synthesis of novel starches *in planta*: Opportunities and challenges. Starch/Stærke 55:107-120.

Deis, R. 1998. The new starches. Food Product Design. Online: http://www.foodproductdesign.com/archive/1998/0298CS.html

Demeke, T., Hucl, P., Nair, R. B., Nakamura, T., and Chibbar, R. N. 1997. Evaluation of Canadian and other wheats for waxy proteins. Cereal Chem. 74:442-444.

Demeke, T., Hucl, P., Abdel-Aal, E.-S. M., Båga, M., and Chibbar, R. N. 1999. Biochemical characterization of the wheat waxy A protein and its effect on starch properties. Cereal Chem. 76:694-698.

Demeke, T., Hucl, P., and Chibbar, R. N. 2000. Frequent absence of GBSS1 B isoprotein in endosperm starch of Canadian wheat cultivars. Starch/Stærke 52:349-352.

Dry, I., Smith, A., Edwards, A., Bhattacharya, M., Dunn, P., and Martin, C. 1992. Characterization of cDNAs encoding two isoforms of granule-bound starch synthase which show differential expression in developing storage organs of pea and potato. Plant J. 2:193-202.

Echt, C. S., and Schwartz, D. 1981. Evidence for the inclusion of controlling elements within the structural gene at the waxy locus in corn. Genetics 99:275-284.

Epstein, J., Morris, C. F., and Huber, K. C. 2002. Instrumental texture of white salted noodles prepared from recombinant inbred lines of wheat differing in the three granule bound starch synthase (waxy) genes. J. Cereal Sci. 35:51-63.

Fujita, S., Yamamoto, H., Sugimoto, Y., Morita, N., and Yamamori, M. 1998. Thermal and crystalline properties of waxy wheat (*Tritcum aestivum*) starch. J. Cereal Sci. 27:7-13.

Gale, K. R., Panozzo, J. F., Eagles, H. A., Blundell, M., Olsen, H., and Appels, R. 2001. Application of a high-throughput antibody-based assay for identification of the granule-bound starch synthase *Wx-B1b* allele in Australian wheat lines. Aust. J. Agric. Res. 52:1417-1423.

Grant, L. A., Vignaux, N., Doehlert, D. C., McMullen, M. S., Elias, E. M., and Kianian, S. 2001. Starch characteristics of waxy and nonwaxy tetraploid (*Triticum turgidum* L. var. durum) wheats. Cereal Chem. 78:590-595.

Graybosch, R. A. 1998. Waxy wheats: Origin, properties, and prospects. Trends Food Sci. Technol. 9:135-142.

Graybosch, R. A., Peterson, C. J., Hansen, L. E., Rahman, S., Hill, A., and Kerritt, J. H. 1998. Identification and characterization of U.S. wheats carrying null alleles at the *wx* loci. Cereal Chem. 75:162-165.

Graybosch, R. A., Schmmerhorn, K. J., and Skerritt, J. H. 1999. An enzyme-linked immunosorbent assay for the identification of wheats carrying null alleles at genetic loci encoding the granule-bound starch synthase. J. Cereal Sci. 30:159-163.

Graybosch, R. A., Guo, G., and Shelton, D. R. 2000. Aberrant falling numbers of waxy wheats independent of α-amylase activity. Cereal Chem. 77:1-3.

Graybosch, R. A., Souza, E., Berzonsky, W., Baenziger, P. S., and Chung, O. 2003. Functional properties of waxy wheat flours: Genotypic and environmental effects. J. Cereal Sci. 38: 69-76.

Guo, G., Jackson, D. S., Graybosch, R. A., and Parkhurst, A. M. 2003a. Asian salted noodle quality: Impact of amylose content adjustments using waxy wheat flour. Cereal Chem. 80:437-445.

Guo, G., Jackson D., Graybosch, R., and Parkhurst, A. 2003b. Wheat tortilla quality: Impact of amylose content adjustments using waxy wheat flour. Cereal Chem. 80:427-436.

Hayakawa, K., Tanaka, K., Nakamura, T., Endo, S., and Hoshino, T. 1997. Quality characteristics of waxy hexaploid wheat (*Triticum aestivum* L.): Properties of starch gelatinization and retrogradation. Cereal Chem. 74:576-580.

Hoshino, T., Yoshikawa, R., Ito, S., Hatta, K., Nakamura, T., Yamamori, M., Hayakawa, K., Tanaka, K., Akashi, H., Endo, S., Tago, S., and Ishigami, S. 2000. Flour blends for breads, cakes, or noodles, and foods prepared from flour blends. U.S. patent 6,042,867.

Hovenkamp-Hermelink, J. H. M., Jacobsen, E., Ponstein, S., Visser, R. G. F., Vos-Scheperkeuter, G. H., Bijmolt, E. W., DeVries, J. N., Withold, B., and Feenstra, W. J. 1987. Isolation of an amylose-free starch mutant of the potato. Theor. Appl. Genet. 75: 217-221.

Hucl, P., and Chibbar, R. N. 1996. Variation for starch concentration in spring wheat and its repeatability relative to protein concentration. Cereal Chem. 73:756-758.

Hug-Iten, S., Handschin, S., Conde-Petit, B., and Escher, F. 1999. Changes in starch microstructure on baking and staling of wheat bread. Food Sci. Technol. 32:255-260.

Jane, J., Chen. Y., Lee, L., McPherson, A., Wong, K., Radosavljevic, M., and Kasemsuwan, T. 1999. Effects of amylopectin branch chain length and amylose content on the gelatinization and pasting properties of starch. Cereal Chem. 76: 629-637.

Johnson, L. A., Hardy, C. L., Baumel, C. P., and White, P. J. 2001a. Identifying valuable corn quality traits for starch production. Cereal Foods World 46:417-423.

Johnson, L. A., Hardy, C. L., Baumel, C. P., Yu, T.-H., and Sell, J. L. 2001b. Identifying valuable corn quality traits for livestock feed. Cereal Foods World 46:472-481.

Kim, W., Johnson, J. W., Graybosch, R. A., and Gaines, C. S. 2003. Physicochemical properties and end-use quality of wheat starch as a function of waxy protein alleles. J. Cereal Sci. 37:195-204.

Kiribuchi-Otobe, C., Nagamine, T., Yanagisawa, T., Ohnishi, M., and Yamaguchi, I. 1997. Production of hexaploid wheats with waxy endosperm character. Cereal Chem. 74:72-74.

Kiribuchi-Otobe, C., Yanagisawa, T., Yamaguchi, I., and Yoshida, H. 1998. Wheat mutant with waxy starch showing stable hot paste viscosity. Cereal Chem. 75:671-672.

Klamczynski, A. P., and Czuchajowska, Z. 1999. Quality of flours from waxy and non-waxy barley for production of baked products. Cereal Chem. 76:530-535.

Klösgen, R. B., Gierl, A., Schwarz-Sommer, Z., and Saedler, H. 1986. Molecular analysis of the *waxy* locus of *Zea mays*. Mol. Gen. Genet. 203:237-244.

Kossmann, J., and Lloyd, J. 2000. Understanding and influencing starch biochemistry. Crit. Rev. Biochem. Mol. Biol. 35:141-196.

Krog, N., Olesen, S. K., Toernaes, H., and Joensson, T. 1989. Retrogradation of the starch fraction in wheat bread. Cereal Foods World 34:281-285.

Kuroda, A., Oda, S., Miyagawa, S., and Seko, H. 1989. A method for measuring amylose content and its variation in Japanese wheat cultivars and Kanto breeding lines. Jpn. J. Breed. 39:142-143.

Lee, M. R., Swanson, B. G., and Baik, B. K. 2001. Influence of amylose content on properties of wheat starch and breadmaking quality of starch and gluten blends. Cereal Chem. 78:701-706.

Loney, P. P., Jenkins, L. D., and Meredith, P. 1975. The developing starch granule. Part II. The role of amylose and amylopectin in the amylograph pasting properties of flour and starch of developing and mature wheats of diverse genetic origins. Starch/Stærke 27:145-151.

Lorenz, K. 1995. Physicochemical characteristics and functional properties of starch from a high β-glucan waxy barley. Starch/Stærke 47:14-18.

Mason-Gamer, R. J., Weil, C. F., and Kellog, E. A. 1998. Granule-bound starch synthase: Structure, function, and phylogenetic utility. Mol. Biol. Evol. 15:1658-1673.

McLauchlan, A., Ogbonnaya, F. C., Hollingsworth, B., Carter, M., Gale, K. R., Henry, R. J., Holton, T. A., Morell, M. K., Rampling, L. R., Sharp, P. J., Shariflou, M. R., Jones, M. G. K., and Appels, R. 2001. Development of a robust PCR-based DNA markers for each homoeo-allele of granule-bound starch synthase and their application in wheat breeding programs. Aust. J. Agric. Res. 52:1409-1416.

Messager, A., and Despre D. 2002. Flours and starches with a very high amylopectin content and methods for the production and uses thereof. U.S. patent application 20020037352.

Miura, H., and Sugawara, A. 1996. Dosage effects of the three *Wx* genes on amylose synthesis in wheat endosperm. Theor. Appl. Genet. 93:1066-1070.

Miura, H., and Tanii, S. 1994. Endosperm starch properties in several wheat cultivars preferred for Japanese noodles. Euphytica 72:171-175.

Miura, H., Araki, E., and Tarui, S. 1999. Amylose synthesis capacity of the three *Wx* genes of wheat cv. Chinese spring. Euphytica 108:91-95.

Miura, H., Wickramsinghe, M. H. A., Subasinghe, R. M., Araki, E., and Komae, K. 2002. Development of near-isogenic lines of wheat carrying different null *Wx* alleles and their starch properties. Euphytica 123:353-359.

Morita, N., Maeda, T., Miyazaki, M., Yamamori, M., Mura, H., and Ohtsuka, I. 2002. Dough and baking properties of high-amylose and waxy wheat flours. Cereal Chem. 79:491-495.

Morris, C. F., and Konzak, C. F. 2001. Registration of hard and soft homozygous waxy wheat germplasm. Crop Sci. 41:934-935.

Morris, C. F., King, G. E., and Rubenthaler, G. L. 1997a. Contribution of wheat flour fractions to peak hot paste viscosity. Cereal Chem. 74:147-153.

Morris, C. F., Shackley, B. J., King, G. E., and Kidwell, K. K. 1997b. Genotypic and environmental variation for flour swelling volume in wheats. Cereal Chem. 74:16-21.

Moss, H. J. 1980. The pasting properties of some wheat starches free of sprout damage. Cereal Res. Comm. 8:297-302.

Moss, H. J., and Miskelly, D. M. 1984. Variation in starch quality in Australian flour. Food Technol. Aust. 36:90-92.

Mua, J. P., and Jackson, D. S. 1997. Fine structure of corn amylose and amylopectin fractions with various molecular weights. J. Agric. Food Chem. 45:3840-3847.

Murai, J., Taira, T., and Ohta, D. 1999. Isolation and characterization of the three *Waxy* genes encoding the granule-bound starch synthase in hexaploid wheat. Gene 234:71-79.

Murata, T., Sugiyama, T., and Akazawa, T. 1965. Enzymic mechanism of starch synthesis in glutinous rice grains. Biochem. Biophys. Res. Comm. 18:371-376.

Myers, A. M., Morell, M. K., James, M. G., and Ball, S. G. 2000. Recent progress toward understanding biosynthesis of the amylopectin crystal. Plant Physiol. 122:989-997.

Nagao, S., Ishibashi, S., Imai, S., Sato, T., Kambe, T., Kaneko, Y., and Otsubo, H. 1977. Quality characteristic of soft wheats and their utilization in Japan. II. Evaluation of wheat from the United States, Australia, France, and Japan. Cereal Chem. 54:198-204.

Nakamura, T., Yamamori, M., Hirano, H., and Hidaka, S. 1993a. Decrease of waxy (Wx) protein in two common wheat cultivars with low amylose content. Plant Breed. 111:99-105.

Nakamura T., Yamamori, M., Hirano, H., and Hidaka, S. 1993b. Identification of three Wx proteins in wheat (*Triticum aestivum* L.). Biochem. Genet. 31:75-86.

Nakamura, T., Yamamori, M., Hirano, H., and Nagamine, T. 1995. Production of waxy (amylose-free) wheats. Mol. Gen. Genet. 248:253-259.

Nelson, O. E. 1968. The *waxy* locus in corn II. The location of the controlling alleles. Genetics 60:507-524.

Nelson, O. E., and Rines, H. W. 1962. The enzymatic deficiency in the *waxy* mutant of corn. Biochem. Biophys. Res. Comm. 9:297-300.

Oda, M., Yasuda, Y., Okazaki, S., Yamauchi, Y., and Yokoyama, Y. 1980. A method of flour quality assessment for Japanese noodles. Cereal Chem. 57:253-254.

Oda S., Kiribuchi, C., and Seko, H. 1992. A bread wheat mutant with low amylose content induced by ethyl methanesulphonate. Jpn. J. Breed. 42:151-154.

O'Farrell, P. H. 1975. High resolution two-dimensional electrophoresis of proteins. J. Biol. Chem. 250:4007-4021.

Otobe, K. C., Nagamine, T., Yanagisawa, T., Ohnishi, M., and Yamaguchi, I. 1997. Production of hexaploid wheats with waxy endosperm character. Cereal Chem. 74:72-74.

Park, C. S., Baik, B. K., Ha, Y. W., and Hong, B. H. 2001. End-use properties of Korean waxy wheat lines. Korean J. Crop Sci. 46:367-374.

Preiss, J., and Sivak, M. N. 1996. Starch synthesis in sinks and sources. Pages 63-96 in: Photoassimilate distribution in plants and crops, source-sink relationships. E. Zamski and A. A. Schaffer, Eds. Marcel Dekker, New York.

Rahman, S., Kosar-Hashemi, B., Samuel, M. S., Hill, A., Abbott, D. C., Skerritt, J. H., Preiss, J., Appels, R., and Morell, M. K. 1995. The major proteins of wheat endosperm starch granules. Aust. J. Plant Physiol. 22:793-803.

Rahman, S., Li, Z., Batey, I., Cochrane, M. P., Appels, R., and Morell, M. 2000. Genetic alteration of starch functionality in wheat. J. Cereal Sci. 31:91-110.

Rohde, W., Becker, D., and Salamamini, F. 1988. Structural analysis of the *waxy* locus from *Hordeum vulgare*. Nucleic Acids Res. 16:7185-7186.

Rodriguez-Quijano, M., Nieto-Taladriz, M. T., and Carrilo, J. M. 1998. Polymorphism of waxy proteins in Iberian hexaploid wheats. Plant Breed. 117:341-344.

Sayaslan, A., Seib, P. A., and Chung, O. K. 2001. Wet-milling properties of waxy wheat flours and breadmaking qualities of the gluten fractions. Proc. National Wheat Industry Research Forum 4:46.

Schofield, J. D., and Greenwell, P. 1987. Wheat starch granule proteins and their technological significance. Pages 407-420 in: Cereals in a European context. I. D. Morton, Ed. Ellis Horwood, Chicester, U.K.

Sears, E. R. 1966. Nullisomic-tetrasomic combinations in hexaploid wheat. Pages 29-45 in: Chromosome manipulations and plant genetics. R. Riley and K. R. Lewis, Eds. Oliver and Boyd, London, U.K.

Seib, P. 2000. Reduced-amylose wheats and Asian noodles. Cereal Foods World 45:504-512.

Shariflou, M. R., and Sharp, P. J. 1999. A polymorphic microsatellite in the 3′ end of 'waxy' genes of wheat, *Triticum aestivum*. Plant Breed. 118:275-277.

Shibanuma, Y., Takeda Y., and Hizukuri, S. 1996. Molecular and pasting properties of some wheat starches. Carbohydr. Polym. 29:253-261.

Shure, M., Wessler, S., and Fedoroff, N. 1983. Molecular identification and isolation of *waxy* locus in corn. Cell 35:225-233.

Smith, A. M. 1999. Making starch. Curr. Opin. Plant Biol. 2:223-229.

Tester, R. F., and Morrison, W. R. 1990. Swelling and gelatinization of cereal starches. I. Effects of amylopectin, amylose, and lipids. Cereal Chem. 67:551-557.

Thomas, J. D., and Atwell, W. A. 1998. Starch structure. Pages 1-11 in: Starches. Am Assoc. Cereal Chem., St. Paul, MN.

Toufeilli, I., Habbal Y., Shadarevian S., and Olabi, A. 1999. Substitution of wheat starch with non-wheat starches and cross-linked waxy barley starch affects sensory properties and staling of Arabic bread. J. Sci. Food Agric. 79:1855-1860.

Tsai, C. Y. 1974. The function of the *waxy* locus in starch synthesis in corn endosperm. Biochem. Genet. 11:83-96.

Wang, L., and Seib, P., A. 1996. Australian salt-noodle flours and their starches compared to U.S. wheat flours and their starches. Cereal Chem. 73:167-175.

Wang, Z., Wu, Z., Xing, Y., Zheng, F., Guo, X., Zhang, W., and Hong, M. 1990. Nucleotide sequence of rice *waxy* gene. Nucleic Acids Res. 18:5898.

Waniska, R., Graybosch, R., and Adams, J. 2002. Effect of partial waxy wheat on processing and quality of wheat flour tortillas. Cereal Chem. 79:210-214.

Yamamori, M., and Quynh, N. T. 2000. Differential effects of Wx-A1, -B1 and –D1 protein deficiencies on apparent amylose content and starch pasting properties in common wheat. Theor. Appl. Genet. 100:32-38.

Yamaguchi, I., Otobe, C., Ushiyama, T., Yanagisawa, T., Seko, H., Amano, Y., and Yoshida, H. 2000. Wheat starch with novel characteristics. U.S. patent 6,165,535.

Yamamori, M., Nakamura, T., and Kuroda, A. 1992. Variations in the content of starch-granule bound protein among several Japanese cultivars of common wheat (*Triticum aestivum* L.). Euphytica 64:215-219.

Yamamori, M., Nakamura, T., Endo, T. R., and Nagamine, T. 1994a. Waxy protein deficiency and chromosomal location of coding genes in common wheat. Theor. Appl. Genet. 89:179-184.

Yamamori, M., Nakamura, T., and Nagamine, T. 1994b. Production of waxy wheat by combining null alleles for the *wx* proteins. Jpn. J. Breed. 44:242.

Yan, L., and Bhave, M. 2000. Sequences of the *waxy* loci of wheat: Utility in analysis of waxy proteins and developing molecular markers. Biochem. Genet. 38:391-411.

Yan, L., and Bhave, M. 2001. Characterization of waxy proteins and waxy genes of *Triticum timopheevii* and *T. zhukovskyi* and implications for evolution of wheat. Genome 44:582-588.

Yan, L., Bhave, M., Fairclough, R., Konic, C., Rahman, S., and Appels, R. 2000. The genes encoding granule-bound starch synthases at the *waxy* loci of the A, B and D progenitors of common wheat. Genome 43:264-272.

Yasui, T., Matsuki, J., Sasaki, T., and Yamamori, M. 1996. Amylose and lipid contents, amylopectin structure, and gelatinisation properties of waxy wheat (*Triticum aestivum*) starch. J. Cereal Sci. 24:131-137.

Yasui, T., Sasaki, T., Matsuki, J., and Yamamori, M. 1997. Waxy endosperm mutants of bread wheat bread wheat (*Triticum aestivum* L.) and their starch properties. Breed. Sci. 47:161-163.

Yasui, T., Sasaki, T., and Matsuki, J. 1999. Milling and flour pasting properties of waxy endosperm mutant lines of bread wheat (*Triticum aestivum* L). J. Sci. Food Agric. 79:687-692.

Yoo, S. H., and Jane, J. 2002a. Molecular weights and gyration radii of amylopectins determined by high-performance size-exclusion chromatography equipped with multi-angle laser-light scattering and refractive index detectors. Carbohydr. Polym. 49:307-314.

Yoo, S., and Jane, J. 2002b. Structural and physical characteristics of waxy and other wheat starches. Carbohydr. Polym. 49:297-305.

Zallie, J., Trimble, R., and Bell, H. 1986. Bread containing wxsu.sub.2 genotype starch as an anti-stalent. U.S. patent 4,615,888.

Zhao, X. C., and Sharp, P. J. 1996. An improved 1-D SDS-PAGE method for the identification of three bread wheat 'waxy' proteins. J. Cereal Sci. 23:191-193.

Zhao, X. C., Batey, I. L., Sharp, P. J., Crosbie, G., Barclay, I., Wilson, R., Morell, M. K., and Appels, R. 1998. A single genetic locus associated with starch granule properties and noodle quality in wheat. J. Cereal Sci. 27:7-13.

Zhao, X. C., and Sharp, P. J. 1998. Production of all eight genotypes of null alleles at 'waxy' loci in bread wheat, *Triticum aestivum* L. Plant Breed.117:488-490.

Zobel, H. F., and Kulp, K. 1996. The staling mechanism. Pages 1-64 in: Baked Goods Freshness. R. E. Hebeda and H. F. Zobel, Eds. Marcel Dekker, New York.

CHAPTER 7

Hulless Barley for Food and Feed

C. W. Newman and R. K. Newman

Newman Associates Inc., Bozeman, MT 59715

"Barley is a grass plant whose seeds are useful to man." This simple but profound statement was made by Dr. Gus Wiebe, a prominent USDA barley researcher now deceased (Wiebe 1978a,b). Dr. Wiebe went on to say in his discussion that "naked or huskless (hulless) varieties are commonly used for human food, especially in countries with a primitive form of agriculture." Barley grain exists in many forms or types, including covered (hulled) or hulless. Archeological evidence indicates that barley is one of the most ancient of all the cereal grains; but even though extensive and voluminous literature exists on the subject, the true origin of barley is actually unknown according to J. R. Harlan (Harlan 1978).

The history and development of hulless barley in ancient and modern times is the same as that of hulled barley. The origin as currently accepted and the classification and morphology of barley have been thoroughly reviewed in other publications (Briggs 1978, Wiebe 1978b, Nevo 1992). Barley, including both hulless and hulled types, appeared under domestication in the Near and Middle East about 8,000 years ago, according to Nevo (1992), although remnants of barley grains have been dated back to 17,000 B.C. in the Nile valley (Wendorf et al 1979). Evidence indicates that this region may have been the site of barley's origin. Both hulled and hulless barleys were used by the people dwelling in the Nile valley in ancient times, as both types have been recovered there in archeological excavations. According to Zha and Wang (1992), as cited by Sun and Wang (1999), hulless barley has been used as food in China since the seventh century B.C., when the Tibetans started its cultivation. It is an accepted fact that hulless barley was a mainstay food item of ancient people and a raw material for various types of beverages. Now this grain is finding its way back into modern diets (Bhatty 1986a, 1995).

Relatively little hulless barley is produced today in comparison to hulled barley. The only significant production of hulless barley is in various areas of North Africa and Tibet, where barley is a dietary staple, and in the western United States and Canada for specialty-food markets and animal feed. The advantage of using hulless barley over hulled barley for human food is two-fold: (1) pearling is not required to make the grain edible, thus eliminating a processing procedure; and (2) by using the intact kernel, the full benefit of the kernel's nutritional components is achieved. In the pearling process, a significant portion (20–30%) of the outer layers of the caryopsis, containing a concentration of nutrients and other beneficial compounds, is removed along with the hull. Although hulless barley is ideal as a component for human diets, domestic farm animals and pets can utilize this grain as well. This is especially true for monogastric animals such as swine because the removal of the hull increases the available energy in the kernel (Bhatty et al 1979, Classen et al 1985).

Even though current usage of hulless barley in human diets and animal feeds is quite small, it has vast potential uses. Lack of acceptance by the food and feed industries and lack of consumer awareness are due partly to the lack of a sufficient volume of hulless barley production and partly to poor recognition of its food and feed value. Additionally, economic factors in North America such as reduced yields compared to those of hulled barley, lodging before harvest, kernel damage during harvesting, problems in maintaining postharvest identity, lack of end-product development, competition from hulled barley and other grains, and little demand by the food industry are major obstacles preventing wide acceptance of hulless barley by barley growers.

Hulless Barley Kernels

General Description

Hulless and hulled barleys share the same genetic background, except that the hulless gene, *nud*, is expressed in the hulless types. Hulless barley may be two- or six-rowed, have short or long awns, vary in straw height, and occur in hooded (awnless)-type barley. Kernels from two-rowed barleys are generally larger and more uniform in size than those from six-rowed types because of crowding on the spike in the latter. Kernels of six-rowed types are often twisted, also from crowding on the spike. However, kernel size also varies in two-rowed types, as kernels decrease in size with increased distance from the rachis. Environmental growing conditions have major influences on kernel size and composition. During drought conditions, the kernels do not "fill," resulting in an increased number of thin kernels or in reduced plumpness. This terminology refers to a reduction in starch deposition that results in higher levels of protein and other kernel components such as dietary fiber. Thin kernels produced under arid conditions or from late planting are generally high in fiber and protein and low in starch. Kernel size and shape are also genetically controlled characteristics; they may be elongated, short, or globular and can be various colors, including shades of red and purple, black, blue, or bronze. Color in the caryopsis results from anthocyanin pigment or from a black, melaninlike compound. When present, anthocyanin is red in the pericarp and blue in the aleurone layer (Pomeranz 1974b). The most common colors of hulless barley kernels are golden, tawny, or light tan, which may be influenced (dulled) by weather conditions before or during harvest.

The barley kernel consists of the caryopsis, the lemma, the palea, and the rachella. A detailed description of the morphology of the barley kernel is shown in Figure 1. In hulled barleys, the lemma and the palea (hulls) adhere to the caryopsis, whereas in hulless barley the caryopsis threshes free of the hull in the manner of common wheat. This characteristic is controlled by the single recessive gene (*nud*) located on chromosome 7H (Franckowiak and Konishi 1997). The cementing substance causing hull adherence in hulled barley is secreted by the caryopsis and appears 16 days after pollination

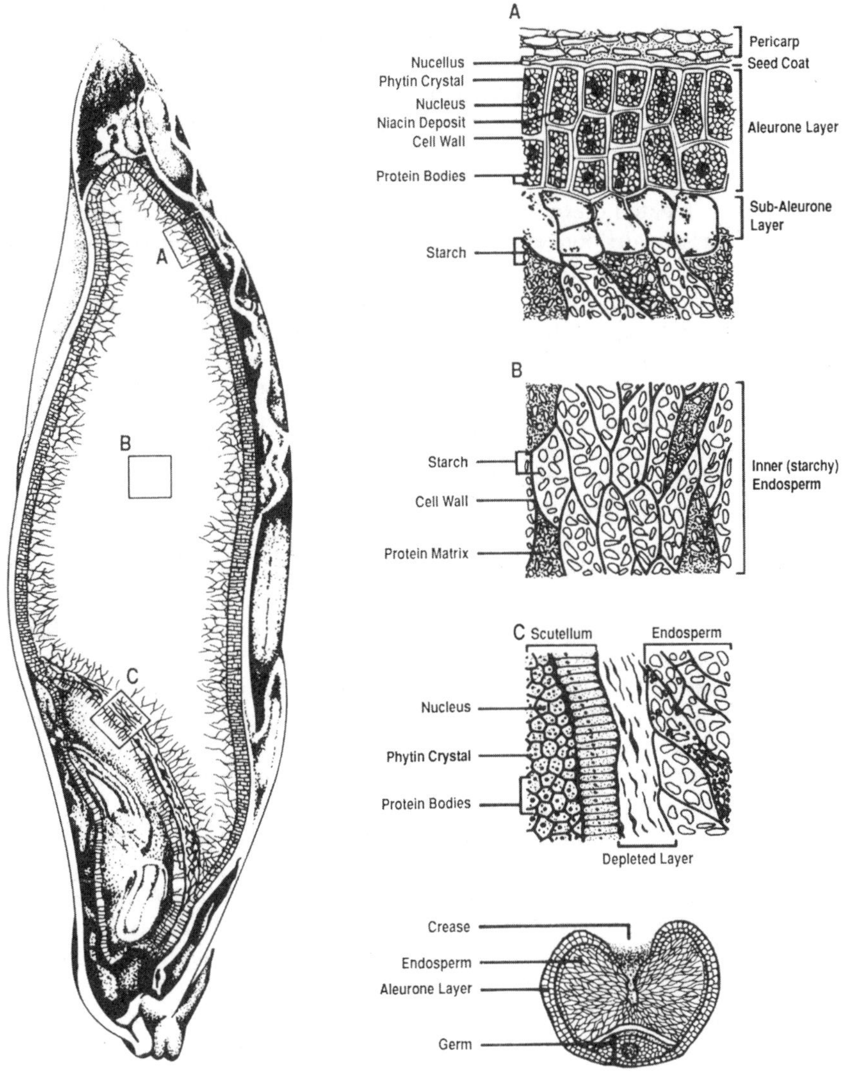

Fig. 1. Barley grain with enlarged cross sections. (Courtesy of R. G. Fulcher and S. I. Wong)

(Harlan 1920); it is lacking in hulless barley. The hull constitutes 9–13% of the kernel weight and is composed primarily of cellulose, lignin, arabinoxylans, and silica (Briggs 1978, Dickson 1978, Henry 1988). The amount of the hull varies according to type, variety, kernel size, and latitude of cultivation (Pomeranz 1974b). With the removal of the hulls, nutrients in the caryopsis increase in relative proportion because of reduction of fiber represented in the hulls (McGuire and Hockett 1981). The caryopsis consists of the pericarp, testa, aleurone layer, endosperm, and embryo. The pericarp is crushed during development in hulled barleys, whereas in hulless types the pericarp is less compressed and more robust. Pericarp tissue is not lignified, although some ligninlike material is found in the caryopsis of mature kernels. The testa and the aleurone layer lie below the pericarp and adjacent to the endosperm, the major storage area of protein and starch. The embryo or germ, a rudimentary plant containing the genetic information to produce a plant when the kernel germinates, is located on the dorsal side of the caryopsis at the end attached to the rachis. Lipids are concentrated in the embryo but are also found in the aleurone and endosperm tissue (Price and Parsons 1979).

As noted previously, hulless barley composition is influenced by genetics, environment, and the genetics by environment interactions. Starch and protein are almost always increased in hulless cultivars because of the removal of the diluting fibrous hull, but variations do occur. Hulless barleys, such as Prowashonupana (PWNP) (Eslick 1979) and the commercial product Barleyplus (D. Topping, *personal communication*) with shrunken endosperms are specific examples of such variability; these barleys contain significantly less starch and greater amounts of protein, dietary fiber, and low-molecular-weight sugars than do average hulled or hulless barleys (Åman and Newman 1986, D. Topping, *personal communication*). Three PWNP lines contain 20–30% starch, which is waxy (0.5–7% amylose). Barleyplus contains about 27% starch, which is 70% amylose; thus it is classified as a high-amylose barley. Protein content of these two barleys is high, around 20%, which corresponds to the low starch contents. Mixed-linked (1-3)-(1-4)-β-D-glucan (β-glucan) and total dietary fiber (TDF) levels in PWNP and Barleyplus barleys are 15 and 10%, and 30 and 25%, respectively. The shrunken endosperm syndrome in barley is created by a genetically controlled system that stops the synthesis of starch after a given period of time during kernel development. These barley types and their potential uses are discussed in a later section.

Barley breeding techniques have been used to produce near-isogenic or isolines of hulled and hulless barley in several barley varieties; these include Hulless Betzes and Hulless Compana, developed from Betzes (CI 6398) and Compana (CI 5438), respectively, now designated Nubet (CI 16557) and Nupana (CI 16185) (Hockett 1981). The procedure described by Hockett (1981) involves crossing barley having the hulless trait to hulled varieties followed by six back-crosses to the recurrent parents. Isoline hulled and hulless barleys have also been produced in different genotypes by other researchers (Bhatty et al 1979, Eslick 1979). Additionally, a number of hulless barley genotypes having superior agronomic characteristics have been developed in more recent times in Canada, China, the Czech Republic, Sweden, and the United States.

Chemical and Physical Composition

Data adapted from Xue (1992) and Xue et al (1997) shown in Table 1 illustrate the effect of the *nud* gene in the presence and absence of the waxy gene, *wax,* in barley isolines. The data shown were chosen because analyses for starch, soluble carbohydrates (low-molecular-weight sugars), total and soluble dietary fiber, and extract viscosity are presented in this work and are not completely available in earlier data. The effect of the *wax* gene is presented as it has become evident that the *wax* gene in barley has a major effect on increasing mixed-linkage β-glucan levels and extract viscosity. β-Glucans are a major part of the soluble dietary fiber (SDF) in barley, which is recognized as beneficial for a variety of health issues. The importance of β-glucans and viscosity in animal feed and human foods is discussed in a later section.

The *nud* gene had significant effects on most of the measurements shown in Table 1, although the higher protein level in the hulless types was not statistically significant. Ether extract was slightly but significantly increased in the hulless barleys, but the most obvious and important effects of the *nud* gene were the significantly lower TDF and higher starch and soluble sugar concentrations in the hulless types. All components of TDF, with the excep-

TABLE 1
Composition of Hulled and Hulless Barleys in Nonwaxy and Waxy Genotypes[a]

	Nonwaxy		Waxy	
Property	**Hulled**	**Hulless**	**Hulled**	**Hulless**
Protein, %	15.6[b]	16.3	16.1	16.9
Ether extract, %	2.0	2.1	2.3	2.6
Ash, %	2.7	2.1	2.8	2.1
Starch, %	55.9	61.3	51.5	58.5
Soluble carbohydrates, %	2.3	2.9	5.0	5.5
Fiber, %				
Total dietary fiber	17.0	13.2	19.6	13.8
Soluble dietary fiber	4.4	4.9	5.9	6.3
Arabinoxylans	6.2	4.4	6.7	4.6
Cellulose	3.8	2.1	4.4	1.9
Klason lignin	2.0	0.9	1.8	0.9
Total β-glucans	4.4	4.7	5.3	6.3
Soluble β-glucans	2.6	2.6	3.2	3.4
Viscosity, cP[c]	2.8	3.1	3.3	4.9
Test wt, kg/hl	67.8	74.5	66.4	73.0
Kernel wt, mg	43.3	38.4	43.1	38.2
Plump kernels, %	68.6	38.3	69.1	40.2
Thin kernels, %	14.5	33.6	14.2	31.3

[a] Adapted from Xue (1992) and Xue et al (1997).
[b] Each mean is an average of six observations for the hulled types and 12 observations for the hulless types.
[c] Centipoise units.

tion of SDF and β-glucans, were significantly lower in the hulless barleys. This was to be expected since Klason lignin, arabinoxylans, and cellulose, major components of insoluble dietary fiber, are concentrated in the hull, and β-glucans (a part of SDF) are not found in the hull, but occur principally in the aleurone and endosperm cell walls (Fastnaught 2001). Total β-glucan in the hulless barleys is increased and is primarily responsible for the significantly higher extract viscosity in these barleys, which agrees with data from other hulless genotypes (Ullrich et al 1986, Mori 1990, Wang et al 1992). Hulless barley had significantly lower levels of ash, due primarily to the silica that occurs in the hulls, principally in the outer lemma (Liu and Pomeranz 1975). The major minerals, calcium and phosphorus, were not significantly altered by the removal of the hull (data not shown), which is consistent with analytical data presented by Jood and Kalra (2001).

The data shown in Table 1 are consistent with that reported in six earlier studies comparing the composition of isolines of hulled and hulless barley (Newman et al 1968; Bhatty et al 1975, 1979; Åman and Newman 1986; Truscott et al 1988a; Wood et al 2003).

As noted earlier, composition of the waxy types is shown (Table 1) because of the effects of the *wax* gene on β-glucan content and viscosity of barleys. The data illustrate these effects and are consistent with other reports in that β-glucan levels and viscosity are significantly increased in waxy barleys regardless of genotype (Ullrich et al 1986, Bhatty et al 1991, Marlett 1991, Han and Froseth 1992, Ishikawa et al 1995, Swanston et al 1996, Ankrah et al 1999). However, the magnitude of β-glucan increase due to the waxy gene in barley depends on the background genotype (Fastnaught et al 1996, Xue et al 1997). Bhatty et al (1991) reported a correlation of +0.83 between acid-extract viscosity and total β-glucan in 13 barleys, 12 of which were hulless lines.

Although not limited to the hulless cultivars, soluble sugars (glucose, fructose, maltose, and sucrose) showed an increase in the waxy types. An increased level of soluble sugars other than maltose has been reported in waxy hulless barley (Hofer 1985, Åman and Newman 1986). The total starch level was 4.6% lower in the waxy hulless types compared to the nonwaxy types. A similar trend of lower starch content in waxy hulless barley was reported by Ankrah et al (1999), who compared six waxy cultivars with five nonwaxy cultivars. Researchers have suggested that high β-glucan levels in barley may be associated with reduced starch content due to genetic effects on partitioning of photosynthate (Smith et al 1987). Swanston et al (1996) postulated that the waxy gene may have a similar effect on reducing starch synthesis. A difference in starch and sugar deposition in waxy types was first noted by Harlan (1957). He stated that waxy barleys deposit amylodextrin (water-soluble starch) instead of normal starch during the final stage of carbohydrate synthesis and deposition in the kernel. Goering and Eslick (1976) reported higher α-amylase levels in waxy barleys, especially hulless types. Higher levels of α-amylase were confirmed in waxy hulless types by Xue et al (1997). These authors suggested that the increase in the maltose component of the free sugars in the waxy barleys may have happened when the kernel was being processed for analyses because of (1) increased amylase activity or (2) the presence of increased amounts of amylodextrin and not because of storage conditions (high moisture) conducive to malting. The authors concluded that because the nonwaxy and waxy types were harvested at the same stage of maturity and moisture levels and then stored under the same conditions, maltose increases in the waxy types were probably not due to harvesting and storage procedures.

Waxy barleys have been reported containing widely varying amounts (1–13%) of amylose (Morrison et al 1984, Bhatty and Rossnagel 1997). Bhatty and Rossnagel (1997) reported the development of zero-amylose lines of hulless barley by crossing two waxy hulless types. Ishikawa et al (1995) produced a zero-amylose waxy hulless barley mutant by treating nonwaxy hulless barleys with sodium azide. High-amylose hulless barleys containing ≥40% amylose in the starch are also known to contain higher-than-normal levels of β-glucans as with the waxy types (Swanston et al 1996, Sundberg et al 1998). Swanston et al (1996) reported that an inbred line from a cross of waxy Hector and a high-amylose line produced a barley with greater amounts of β-glucan (6.4%) than either a waxy (4.4%) or a high-amylose line (4.4%).

Using standard procedures that were developed for hulled barley to measure kernel size and other physical characteristics of hulless barley is misleading. However, the determination of comparative physical characteristics of hulled and hulless barleys is important to give a reference point for the latter. Decreased kernel weight and kernel plumpness with increased test weight and percentage of thin kernels in hulless barley compared to hulled types, as shown in Table 1, are consistent with reports from other authors (Hockett 1981, Truscott 1988a, Edney et al 1992, Baidoo and Liu 1998).

Amino Acid Composition

The comparative amino acid composition of hulled and hulless barley is shown in Table 2. The data were taken from Bhatty et al (1979), Truscott et al (1988a), and unpublished data from the Montana Agriculture Experiment Station and represented high, medium, and low protein levels, respectively. Within protein level, amino acid concentrations vary little in hulled and hulless types and represent values relatively consistent in barley. Similar findings have been reported by Mitchall et al (1976), Edney et al (1992), and Baidoo and Liu (1998). The composition and genetics of barley protein have been studied extensively since Osborne (1924) classified the proteins of barley by solubility. Amino acid composition in the protein of barleys is governed by the total protein content rather than by type of barley (Pomeranz 1974a, Edney et al 1992). Nitrogen fertilization generally increases protein level by increasing the hordeins, which are the storage proteins in barley. These proteins contain large amounts of the nonessential amino acids glutamic acid and proline, and very small amounts of lysine and threonine, the first and second most limiting essential amino acids. The latter two essential amino acids are concentrated in albumins and globulins, primarily located in the aleurone tissue. Thus, as protein level is increased in most barley, the biological value of the protein is decreased due to the shift in the relative amounts of essential versus nonessential amino acids.

Hiproly (CI 3947), a high-protein hulless barley cultivar found by Swedish researchers in the world barley collection (Munck et al 1969), does not follow normal protein accretion, in that the kernels of Hiproly contain almost normal levels of hordein and relatively high levels of albumins. Hiproly was the first high-lysine (≥4.0 g lysine/100 g protein) barley identified. A hulless sister-line to Hiproly (also high protein) was identified by the Swedish scientists, which they named Hiproly Normal (CI 4362), because the lysine level in the protein is that of normal barley. Hiproly kernels are characterized by a shrunken endosperm, whereas those of Hiproly Normal are relatively plump and smooth. The high-lysine characteristic of Hiproly is controlled by a single gene designated *lys1* located on chromosome 5HL. Sanshu is a high-protein, high-lysine, six-rowed hulless barley selected from a cross of Nanpuhadaka, a Japanese hulless variety with Hiproly (Seko et al 1998). The grain yield of Sanshu is reported to be 154% that of Hiproly, but grain yield was only 91% of the recurrent parent Nanpuhadaka. High-protein and high-lysine hulless barley lines, containing levels similar to those in Hiproly, have been identified in China (Sun and Wang, 1999). Several high-lysine barleys with lysine genes other than *lys1* have been identified since the discovery of Hiproly (Doll et al 1974, Tallberg 1981, Bang-

TABLE 2
Amino Acid Composition (%, w/w) of Hulled and Hulless Barley Isolines

	1[a]		2[b]		3[c]	
Amino Acid	**Hulled**	**Hulless**	**Hulled**	**Hulless**	**Hulled**	**Hulless**
Alanine	...[d]	...	0.44	0.47	0.35	0.38
Arginine	0.71	0.71	0.60	0.64	0.45	0.50
Aspartic acid	...	...	0.71	0.75	0.55	0.57
Cystine	0.35	0.35	0.28	0.31	0.20	0.20
Glutamic acid	...	...	2.98	3.24	2.28	2.44
Glycine	...	...	0.42	0.44	0.32	0.34
Histidine	0.27	0.35	0.26	0.28	0.20	0.22
Isoleucine	0.54	0.53	0.43	0.46	0.34	0.37
Leucine	1.11	1.16	0.79	0.84	0.67	0.71
Lysine	0.38	0.41	0.41	0.41	0.31	0.34
Methionine	0.39	0.40	0.20	0.28	0.15	0.17
Phenylalanine	0.83	0.86	0.68	0.73	0.51	0.53
Proline	...	...	1.32	1.43	0.96	0.98
Serine	...	...	0.54	0.57	0.41	0.45
Threonine	0.56	0.55	0.42	0.45	0.38	0.37
Tryptophan	...	...	0.22	0.23	0.14	0.15
Tyrosine	0.54	0.55	0.37	0.42	0.32	0.33
Valine	0.75	0.76	0.59	0.63	0.46	0.46
Protein	15.7	16.0	13.2	14.0	11.2	11.7

[a] Bhatty et al (1979), $n = 2$.
[b] Montana Agriculture Experiment Station, *unpublished data*, $n = 8$.
[c] Truscott et al (1988), $n = 6$.
[d] Not reported.

Olsen et al 1987). Although these barleys are hulled, it would be relatively simple to insert the *nud* gene into these genotypes to produce new, hulless, high-lysine cultivars. For more detailed information on barley protein and amino acid composition, the reader is referred to several reviews (Pomeranz 1974a, Newman and McGuire 1985, Newman and Newman 1992, Bhatty 1993). Also, the amino acid composition of several newer Canadian hulless barleys has been reported in recent studies (Li et al 1996, Yin et al 2001b).

Lipid Composition

Morrison (1993) presented a comprehensive review of the available literature on barley lipids that included similarities and differences between lipid composition of barley and wheat. The composition of lipids in hulled and hulless barley caryopses is assumed to be similar, if not identical. The data of Kim and Shin (1982), as shown in Morrison (1993), indicate this to be the case. Since barley hulls are reported to contain a small amount of lipid (Price and Parsons 1979), their removal results in slightly higher lipid levels in hulless barleys. Lipid is concentrated in the embryo, and although it represents only ≈3% of the kernel by weight, the embryo furnishes ≈20% of the total lipid in hulless barley. The bran-endosperm contains ≈3% lipid, but by virtue of size, furnishes ≈80% of the total lipid (Price and Parsons 1979).

The principal nonpolar lipid in barley is triacylglycerol, and the remainder is comprised of steryl esters, diacylglycerol, monoacylglycerol, and free fatty acids (Morrison 1993). Polar lipids consist of mainly phospholipids and are located in the membrane surrounding oil droplets or spherosomes. As in other cereals, barley lipids are classified as nonstarch and starch lipids. The principal fatty acids in barley nonstarch lipids are linoleic (50–60%), palmitic (20–30%), oleic (10–15%), and linolenic (4–9%), with small amounts of myristic and stearic. Starch lipids are found complexed inside starch granules of the endosperm, generally in proportion to amylose content. Waxy starches have little or no associated lipids, while high-amylose starches contain more lipids than normal grain starch. In starch lipids, the fatty acid composition shifts toward increased palmitic (46%) and lesser amounts of linoleic (34%) (Morrison 1993).

The tocols, comprised of tocopherols and tocotrienols, are important, nonsaponifiable lipid compounds occurring in cereal grains (Morrison 1978). The total tocol concentration in barley reportedly ranges from 30.5 mg/kg (Barnes 1983) to 80.6 mg/kg (Työppönen and Hakkarainen 1985). α-Tocopherol, commonly referred to as vitamin E, is an essential nutrient for certain metabolic functions in humans and animals. Combined tocopherol and tocotrienol is sometimes referred as the vitamin E isoform complex (Packer et al 2001). Tocotrienols are isomers of tocopherols, differing only in three double bonds in the isoprenoid chain. They have been reported to have a regulatory effect on lipid metabolism in birds and mammals (Qureshi et al 1986). Wang (1992) reported tocopherol and tocotrienol levels in nine barleys, six hulless cultivars, and three hulled cultivars grown at two locations in Arizona. The means for total tocotrienols and tocopherols were 39.8 ± 5 and 20.5 ± 4 mg/kg, respectively. The hulless cultivars contained 33% more tocotrienols than hulled cultivars, 43.4 ± 4 vs. 32.5 ± 4 mg/kg. α-Tocopherol was the predominant tocol in both hulless and hulled barleys, averaging 36.2 ± 4 and 27.0 ± 4 mg/kg, respectively. In a separate study, Wang et al (1993) reported that two waxy hulless barleys—Waxbar and Azhul—contained a combined average of 52.0 and 18.9 mg/kg total tocotrienol and tocopherol, respectively.

Minerals

The ash content of barley ranges from 2 to 3%, the major components of significance being phosphorus, potassium, and calcium, with lesser amounts of chlorine, magnesium, sulfur, and sodium (Owen et al 1977). Liu et al (1974) measured the minerals in hulless Himalaya barley and hulled Atlas barley after the grains were separated by abrasion and milling. Minerals were concentrated in the embryo, and the lowest concentration of minerals was found in the central endosperm. The aleurone layer was determined to have higher levels of all minerals than did the flour. Further studies by Liu and Pomeranz (1975) confirmed the concentration of minerals in the aleurone.

Phosphorus is the most abundant mineral in barley, ranging from 0.30 to 0.40% in hulled barley, with slightly higher levels in hulless types. Hofer (1985) reported an average phosphorus content of 0.39% in Compana, a hulled barley, and 0.43 and 0.42% in two hulless isolines of Compana. In this study, maximum phosphorus levels were attained in the kernels of the hulless barleys at about four weeks before maturity. Hiproly Normal and Hiproly hulless barleys are most noted for their high protein contents, and high lysine level in the latter; however, these barleys contain 10–20% more total phosphorus than other barleys, both hulled and hulless types (Newman et al 1974, Stobart 1977, Killen et al 1978). Newman et al (1974) reported phosphorus levels of 0.33, 0.53, and 0.56% in hulless Compana (Nupana), Hiproly Normal, and Hiproly, respecttively. Twenty pairs of Hiproly Normal and Hiproly grown at six locations in Montana and one location in Arizona averaged 0.49 ± 0.01 and 0.54 ± 0.01% phosphorus, respectively (*unpublished data*, Montana Agricultural Experiment Station). As in other cereals, a major portion of the phosphorus in barley is in phytic acid (Raboy 1990).

Bhatty (1997) reported the mineral content of flour milled from a hulless barley at a 70% extraction rate. Phosphorus and potassium levels were 0.21 and 0.25%, respectively, with smaller amounts of calcium (0.02%), sulfur (0.12%), magnesium (0.08%), copper (12.0 mg/kg), iron (49.9 mg/kg), manganese (13.9 mg/kg), zinc (24.4 mg/kg), and a trace amount of boron.

Compositional data on newer varieties of Canadian hulless barleys (Tupper, Phoenix, Falcon, Silky, Condor, and Buck) have been published in several recent reports (Bell and Keith 1993, Li et al 1996, Baidoo and Liu 1998, Yin et al 2001b).

Food Barley

What characteristics make a substance a food? A food must be *edible*, meaning that a substance capable of being consumed by humans without producing adverse effects such as injury, illness, or death. A food must also be *nutritional*, meaning that the substance supplies one or more nutrients required to nurture a metabolic system for growth, maintenance, and reproduction. These are the two most basic requirements of a food; however, the first humans who gathered seeds such as barley probably considered only the first of these two conditions (i.e., "Can this substance be eaten without hurting me, making me sick, or killing me?"). Taste, palatability, texture, mouthfeel, and satiety are other characteristics that influence the choice of a substance as a food. In addition, availability, abundance, ease of harvesting, storage life, and ease of preparation are important in the selection of a foodstuff.

Through trial and error over centuries, seeds of barley and other plants were discovered by our ancestors to be edible and tasty and to produce satisfying effects on their bodies. It is easy to rationalize why hulless barley was one the earliest "wild" seeds to be chosen and eventually cultivated as a crop by these early people. Reference is often made to Roman gladiators who consumed barley because they believed it gave them extra strength and stamina (Pomeranz 1974b). Hulless barley can be eaten raw or cooked, and it can be processed with relative ease through the use of simple tools such as stones. It can be fermented, roasted, boiled, or soaked in water to reduce hardness and can be stored for extended periods if kept dry. Barley was a naturally occurring, accessible plant where civilization began, obviously tasted good and satisfied hunger, and thus began a common bonding of humans and barley that has waxed and waned over time.

Processing

Hulless barley, like many foods, may be consumed with minimal processing. However, the application of various techniques or processing methods greatly enhances its acceptability and nutritional potential. A significant portion (10–25%) of the hulls of hulless barley remain loosely attached to the kernel or retained with the kernels at harvest. Therefore, the first processing procedure is to clean the barley of hulls and other foreign material. Once cleaned, the barley may be pearled or ground with various types of mills, roller milled, rolled (flaked), or cut to reduce particle size. Extrusion techniques have been applied to various forms of processed barley in laboratory situations. Hulless barley can be malted to produce various types of malt, malt extracts, and syrups for use in many food products.

Pearling

Pearling is the processing procedure most often applied to hulled barley to remove the fibrous hull. Pearling is an extension of a procedure called blocking, which is accomplished through the use of a coarse circular emery stone that is rotated on a horizontal axis and enclosed within a perforated metal container (Weaver et al 1981). In some instances, hulless barley is pearled for specific markets. This is done primarily to remove the "color" compounds contained in the aleurone and subaleurone tissue of the kernel, thereby producing a whiter product. Certain consumers believe that pearling removes undesirable taste factors such as tannin located in the pericarp, testa, aleurone, and subaleurone layers that make the remaining portion of the barley more palatable than the whole grain. The pearling process results in two products: (1) pearlings consisting of the fraction removed from the endosperm, and (2) the remaining endosperm, *pearl barley*.

Because of differences in the composition of the kernel, pearlings and pearl barley from hulless and hulled types differ considerably in chemical composition. Total dietary fiber and insoluble dietary fiber are reduced in pearl barley and concentrated in pearlings, whereas soluble dietary fiber is not greatly changed in pearl parley or pearlings compared to the whole kernel. β-Glucans and extract viscosity are increased in pearl barley (70–80% yield) and decreased in pearlings. If the pearling process continues beyond a 70% yield, β-glucan level and extract viscosity in pearlings are more representative of pearl barley. Protein, fat, and ash are decreased in pearl barley and increased in pearlings when pearl barley yields are maintained at or near 70% (Danielson 1994, Bhatty 1997). Bhatty (1997) concluded that the removal of 30% of the kernel of hulless barley (70% yield) produced pearlings that could be classed as true barley bran, similar to wheat bran produced in traditional roller milling of wheat. Since lysine and threonine are concentrated in the aleurone layers and the nonessential amino acids glutamic acid and proline are concentrated in the endosperm (Eggum 1973), the protein in pearlings is more nutritious than in pearl barley.

Pearl barley is currently the most accepted and widely used barley food product in North America, primarily consumed in soups and stews. For reasons already noted, however, the pearl barley most available to consumers is derived from hulled cultivars. In Japan, hulless barley is pearled to an approximate 30% yield and then split for use in numerous products. The split barley may be incorporated and cooked with rice for use in traditional Japanese foods (All Japan Barley Processors, *personal communication*). Although pearlings contain a variety of desirable nutrients for human consumption, they are generally limited to incorporation in livestock feeds or pet foods (Weaver et al 1981).

Milling

The term *milling* refers to two types of processing: grinding and roller milling. In the first instance, the whole grain is ground to various particle-size specifications, producing whole grain flour. Bhatty (1997) dry-milled non-waxy and waxy hulless barleys in a Quadrumat Jr. mill from which the reel was removed to produce a whole grain flour of 100% extraction. As expected, color and composition of the whole grain flour was nearly identical to that of the grains ground through a laboratory mill for analysis.

Traditional roller milling of barley, as with wheat, is not a routine practice in the cereal industry to produce refined flour, bran, and shorts. Nevertheless, numerous reports have been made of laboratory experiments on roller milling barley, both hulled and hulless. Cheigh (1979) compared the milling characteristics of hulless and hulled (two varieties of each) Korean barleys. The hulless varieties had a 10% higher extraction rate (71.9 vs. 61.0%), and were lower in ash (1.1 vs. 1.2%) and fat (1.7 vs. 2.1%) compared to the hulled varieties. Flour-extract viscosity was much higher for the hulless varieties. McGuire (1979) indicated wide variation in flour yield due to barley variety, and the lowest yield (50.5%) reported in this study was from a waxy hulless barley. He concluded that flour yield from hulless barleys can be improved because of the existing variability in this trait. Bhatty (1986b) demonstrated that two nonwaxy hulless barleys could be roller milled to obtain 70–74% flour yield, comparable to flour yields obtained from hard red spring and soft wheat. Two major problems were encountered in this study. Barley flour tended to be sticky and less free-flowing and was more difficult to separate from the bran and short fractions than was wheat flour. The bran was reported to be very fragile and quite unlike wheat bran in physical characteristics. In a more recent study, Bhatty (1997) presented roller-milling data for five hulless barley cultivars—three nonwaxy and two waxy. The barleys were milled at several moisture levels with a Buhler mill. Best results were obtained when hulless barley was dry-milled at moisture levels of 7–9%. Tempering the barleys with moisture reduced flour yields in both nonwaxy and waxy types, although yields were lower in waxy barleys than in nonwaxy barleys when milled at the same moisture level. Reduced flour yields were thought to be due to the higher β-glucan content of the waxy barleys and not to grain hardness. Unknown factors such as cell wall structure may have influenced yields. The higher β-glucan content of the waxy barley flour resulted in sticky flour that was less free-flowing and more difficult to separate from the bran and shorts fractions, as in the earlier report of Bhatty (1986b).

Roller milling hulless barleys that are currently available, using equipment designed for wheat and methods applied to wheat milling, presents a challenge to millers. However, if a demand for barley flour or other products produced by roller milling should develop, hulless barley should be more acceptable than hulled types. Because of the absence of hulls, the flour need not be sifted to remove hull fragments, the kernel is less abrasive, and more useful by-products for human foods can be produced. Essentially no selection pressure has been applied to barley populations to improve extraction rates of flour from barley grain, as has been done with wheat. For commercial flour production from hulless barley, milling would need to be optimized by selection of variety, mill flow, temper conditions, and roll settings (McGuire 1979). Barley variety selection and development for roller milling will follow as demand for milling products increases.

Flaking

The procedure used to produce barley flakes is not unlike the procedure used in producing oat flakes as described by Deane and Commers (1986). The kernel or groat is generally cut into two or more pieces with steel knives or corrugated rollers to produce the desired size and thickness of flakes. After cutting, the particles are passed through heavy metal rollers that apply pressure to produce the desired thickness of rolled or flaked barley. Moisture and heat in the form of steam are applied to soften the particles before they are passed through the rollers to enhance the process and inactivate enzyme systems.

Products and Product Testing

The baking potential of composite flour was investigated by Cheigh (1979) using hulless barley-wheat flour blends of 20, 30, and 40%. The composite flour, as compared to wheat flour alone, showed higher water absorption and a decrease in bread loaf volume with increased barley flour addition. At the level of 30% barley flour in the composite mixture, loaf volume decreased markedly, but loaf volume was significantly improved by the addition of 0.5% sodium stearoyl lactylate. External appearance of the breads showed a slight difference toward a darker color with the increase of barley flour content. Crumb color changed from a bright cream color in the all-wheat bread to somewhat dark with the inclusion of barley flour. Crumb grain became irregular, and stability decreased in the barley flour breads. The baking results were in agreement with farinograph data that indicated weaker dough properties for the composite flours than the wheat flour. The 20% barley-wheat flour composite produced a comparatively good bread product that was only slightly different from the all-wheat flour bread as measured in loaf volume, crumb quality characteristics, and appearance.

Bhatty (1997) concluded that not more than 5% hulless barley (Scout) flour could be added to wheat flour without seriously affecting loaf volume and appearance. Higher levels of barley flour brought about dilution of wheat gluten and impairment of its gas-retention capacity, resulting in undesirable loaf-volume reduction. At 5% barley flour, loaf volume was decreased by 14%, although bread was acceptable in other quality measurements.

Sensory scores and overall acceptability of bread containing 26% flour milled from waxy hulless barley (Wanubet) were not significantly different in comparisons with bread containing 26% whole wheat flour (Berglund et al 1992). The color score for the barley bread was lower than that of the wheat control but was not deemed unacceptable by the test panel. Barley flour bread was heavier than the wheat flour bread, suggesting that more moisture was retained by the barley flour.

Newman et al (1998) investigated the inclusion of the high-fiber shorts fraction obtained from roller milling waxy hulless barley (Shonkin) into bread (28%), biscuits (23%), cookies (30%), and muffins (23%), replacing wheat flour. Comparison of volume and dimension of the products with all-wheat-flour controls indicated that the only difference was a lower loaf volume in the bread, although the barley shorts products contained significantly more dietary fiber. Scores for overall quality and sensory characteristics for the products containing the barley milling fraction were similar to those for the standard wheat flour products. It was concluded in this report that barley milling fractions can make a substantial contribution to soluble dietary fiber in consumer diets.

Several reports have demonstrated successful replacement of wheat flour with varying amounts of hulless barley flour in products other than bread (i.e., buns, muffins, cookies, biscuits, noodles, pasta, spice and granola bars, extruded snacks, Chinese steamed bread, spaghetti, and porridge (Melland et al 1984, Berglund et al 1992, Newman et al 1994, Sundberg and Falk 1994,

Han 1996, Dudgeon-Bollinger et al 1997, Fastnaught et al 1997, Yokoyama et al 1997, Pick et al 1998, Seko et al 1998, Schlichting et al 2001, Ames et al 2002).

Hulless barley can be used to prepare diastatic malts having composition and enzyme activities comparable to those of brewer's and distiller's malts and superior to that of wheat malt (Bhatty 1996). According to Bhatty, advantages of hulless barley to produce food-grade malts over standard hulled malting barley were shorter steep time, ability to use the malt directly in food applications without preparing extracts and syrups, and no necessity for hull disposal. Bhatty also stated that nondiastatic hulless barley malts of desired color, composition, and enzyme activities may be prepared from hulless barley. Goering et al (1980) described a novel process for the production of ultra-high maltose (58–66%) syrup from waxy hulless barley (Washonupana). Various procedures have been researched and developed to produce β-glucan concentrates from hulless barley to enhance fiber levels and lipid components in food products (Wang et al 1993, Wu et al 1994, Yoon et al 1996, Yokoyama et al 1997).

Flour and milling fractions obtained from hulless barley have many uses in producing a variety of consumer-acceptable food products. High levels of barley flour in traditional wheat breads reduce loaf volume and increase loaf density; however, traditional flatbreads made with barley flour are tasty and nutritious. Loaf volume, appearance (color), crumb texture, and density are not considered important factors in the selection of baked goods by health-conscious consumers. Significant levels of hulless barley flour may be used to replace portions of wheat flour in breads and other cereal-based products to increase soluble dietary fiber levels. Malt and malt extracts, high-fructose syrups, and concentrates of barley fiber (β-glucan) and oil components may be added to many food products to enhance consumer acceptability and nutritional value. Health-related research, which is discussed in the following section, strongly supports the use of hulless barley in its various forms, including high-fiber barley flour and milling fractions in bakery products and other food applications.

Health Benefits of Hulless Barley

The relationship between diet and health is the subject of intense focus. Some chronic diseases, such as heart disease, diabetes, and metabolic syndrome, are increasing in the United States, and lifestyle practices including diet are considered to be causative factors. Changes in diet are promoted for prevention as well as control of these diseases. Modification of the quantity and the source of dietary fat is generally considered a basic or key factor in the prevention and control of heart disease. In addition, extensive evidence shows that certain components of hulless barley are powerful moderators for both heart disease and diabetes. These components are (1) starch type, (2) fiber, particularly a form of soluble fiber, β-glucan, and (3) phytochemicals such as tocotrienols, stanols, and ferulic acid that have less clearly defined health benefits.

Cereal grain starch generally contains a combination of amylopectin and amylose in a 3:1 ratio. Amylose is the starch component most likely to be altered during cooking or other heat treatment and to become resistant to digestive enzymes. It is then termed *resistant starch*, a very significant factor in modulating the response of blood glucose after a meal (Behall et al 1988). Normally, when available carbohydrate is ingested, blood glucose is elevated. Depending on the specific components of the food, the degree and duration of the glucose elevation can vary. Insulin is released and rises in the blood in response to the rise in glucose. Avoiding continual high spikes of glucose is desirable, particularly for persons who have diabetes or are prediabetic, because the corresponding insulin peaks can cause insulin resistance.

Foods are classified according to the degree of glucose response they elicit in experimental subjects. This relative response is called the glycemic index (GI). Foods that cause a rapid and steep rise in glucose have a high GI, whereas an attenuated, flattened rise has a low GI. Factors that may result in foods with a low GI include presence of resistant starch, soluble dietary fiber, and large particle size (Björck et al 1994). Barley is among the foods with a very low GI, particularly varieties high in amylose and β-glucan. The high-amylose characteristic in hulless Glacier barley is controlled by the *amol 1* gene located on chromosome 5L; however, the Australian barley commercial product Barleyplus, also a high-amylose cultivar, has a different genetic control of the amylose characteristic. This would be suspected since the starch contains significantly more amylose than barley where the *amol 1* gene is expressed.

Björck et al (1990) reported on the nutritional properties of barley genotypes containing different levels of amylose. Compared with waxy (5% amylose) and normal (25% amylose) starch barleys, high-amylose (40%) barley produced the most resistant starch and had the lowest rate of starch amylolysis after heat treatment by autoclave. Ikegami et al (1991) demonstrated that a barley diet reduced fasting blood glucose in rats with drug-induced diabetes, compared to diets of corn, brown rice, or wheat bran.

Glycemic response to barley products in humans was studied by Granfeldt et al (1994). Four genotypes of Glacier barley were selected, containing a range of amylose content from 7 to 44% and including hulless as well as hulled types. Products tested were boiled kernels and porridge made from ground kernels. The subjects consumed the products, and blood glucose and insulin were measured at intervals up to 180 min. Glycemic index was calculated using white wheat bread (GI = 100) as the reference. All barley products gave significantly lower GI values than white bread, and the intact boiled kernels gave lower values than the porridge. This study also included measure of a satiety score over the time period. Subjects experienced the greatest satiety after consuming the high-amylose barley products. This group (Liljeberg et al 1996) went on to investigate human glycemic responses to porridge and breads made from oats, wheat, and two barleys, one of which was Prowashonupana (PWNP), the waxy high-fiber hulless genotype developed by Eslick (1979). The lowest blood glucose concentrations were observed after consumption of the high-fiber barley products, and insulin responses followed the same pattern. In this study, the blunted glycemic and insulinemic responses were due not to the amylose content, but to the soluble fiber, β-glucan, concentration in the barley. Rendell and others (M. Rendell, J. Vanderhoof, M. Venn, M. A. Shehan, E. Arndt, C. S. Rao, and G. Geoffrey, *unpublished data*) compared PWNP barley flakes to a commercial product, Sustacal, a glucose source, and oatmeal as breakfast meals for patients with and without diabetes. The postprandial glycemic peak was substantially reduced following ingestion of PWNP barley compared to Sustacal or to oatmeal in patients both with and without diabetes. The insulin response to PWNP was quite flat and significantly less than the responses to Sustacal and oatmeal. This study demonstrated that eating a breakfast meal of PWNP did not substantially raise blood sugar or insulin levels in individuals who did not have diabetes.

A recent study by the Commonwealth Scientific and Industrial Research Organization in Australia, in which Barleyplus was compared with normal barley and glucose, produced blood glucose and insulin responses in individuals with and without diabetes that were almost identical to the responses reported by Rendell and others (see above, *unpublished data*) with PWNP (D. Topping, *personal communication*). The common factors between the two barleys are low starch levels (20–30%), and a high level of β-glucans (10–15%) and dietary fiber (25–30%). Lifschitz et al (2002) tested PWNP barley and a normal barley grown in a chamber into which ^{13}C-labeled CO_2 was injected. The barley was consumed by healthy adult humans and measured through breath CO_2 to test absorbable carbohydrate. Absorption of the high-fiber barley was significantly lower than that of the normal barley, indicating slower metabolism. This confirms the relationship of lowered glycemic response and slower carbohydrate absorption. A similar study was reported by Hallfrisch and Behall (2003), in which PWNP hulless barley and oat extracts were fed to subjects and breath hydrogen was measured as a test of colonic bacterial fermentation. Results showed increased hydrogen production, indicating fermentation of the fiber in the products, confirming the earlier results presented by Lifschitz et al (2002).

Extraction of β-glucan for inclusion in foods as a fiber supplement has been of interest. Yokoyama et al (1997) prepared such an extract from the hulless waxy barley Waxbar and incorporated it into durum wheat pasta at a 7.7% level of dry ingredients. Adult fasted subjects consumed the barley-wheat pasta and a control wheat pasta, each containing 100 g available carbohydrate. The barley-enriched pasta produced significantly lower glucose and insulin responses. The authors concluded that inclusion of barley fiber in wheat products may be a practical means of controlling blood sugar.

Further applications of waxy hulless barley in bread products in diets for diabetes subjects were reported by Pick et al (1998). Bread, buns, and muffins were made with 50% of a barley flour-cracked barley combination. Products contained 0.41–0.81 g of β-glucan per serving unit. A crossover design was used, with white wheat bread as a control product. Total dietary fiber in the barley period was 39 g/day, compared to 28 g/day in the white bread period. This was a long-term study in which 11 men with Type 2 diabetes consumed each type of bread for 12 weeks. Composite glucose response was 20% lower in the barley bread period than that in the white bread period. Insulinemic response improved, and some subjects were able to reduce their dosage of oral hypoglycemic medication after the barley period. This response compares favorably with a meta-analysis of glycemic response in diabetes, in which a 19% reduction in day-long blood glucose could be expected with incorporation of low-glycemic foods (Brand-Miller 1994).

Cardiovascular disease, the major cause of death in the United States and other industrialized countries, can often be prevented and controlled by diet. Elevated blood cholesterol, a major risk factor, is strongly related to lifestyle and to food choices in particular. Although total dietary fat, particularly saturated fat, and obesity are major factors, β-glucan, the soluble fiber in barley, can play a major role in modification of blood cholesterol and prevention of heart disease by a combination of mechanisms.

Probably the most significant mechanism of soluble fiber is the viscosity that occurs in the digestive tract (Wang et al 1992, Ankrah et al 1999), interfering with absorption of dietary fat and cholesterol. In addition, a portion of bile acids are bound to dietary fiber and excreted, resulting in conversion of circulating cholesterol into replacement bile acids (Story and Kritchevsky 1976). Although dietary fiber is not directly digested and absorbed in the stomach and small intestine, it passes on to the large intestine, where bacteria break it down to products that include short-chain fatty acids (SCFA). One theory relates the SCFA production to a feedback mechanism that reduces cholesterol synthesis in the liver (Chen et al 1984) by inhibiting HMG-CoA reductase.

In addition to the effects of β-glucan, lipid-associated components in barley may have a role in cholesterol control. The tocotrienols were investigated by Qureshi et al (1987) as being effective in suppressing cholesterol synthesis in the liver. α-Tocotrienol is also reported to be an antioxidant that blocks oxidation of low-density lipoproteins, the first step in development of arterial plaque (Packer et al 2001). Stanols, another plant component possibly effective in lowering cholesterol levels, are under investigation in hulless barley.

Numerous animal studies have documented the effectiveness of hulless barley in lowering plasma cholesterol (Fastnaught 2001). Fadel et al (1987) demonstrated that β-glucan was the responsible agent in reducing total and LDL cholesterol in hypercholesterolemic chicks fed Washonupana, a waxy hulless cultivar. Mori (1990) fed hulless barley-milled fractions to rats and showed that the feces of the rats fed barley contained increased amounts of fat related to plasma cholesterol reduction. This suggests that dietary cholesterol and fat were removed from the intestinal tract by the β-glucan in the barley.

Newman et al (1989a,b) conducted two human studies using the waxy hulless barley Azhul, which contained ≈10% β-glucan. In the first study, a variety of barley foods were compared to identical products made with wheat supplemented with wheat bran to equalize fiber. Healthy adult volunteers consumed the foods three times daily for four weeks. Subjects who ate wheat foods had significantly increased serum total and LDL cholesterol when compared to pretreatment levels. Those who ate hulless barley foods had lowered cholesterol, which was most significant in those with higher pretreatment cholesterol levels. The second study compared oat and hulless barley foods, since oats had been widely shown to be hypocholesterolemic. Adult men and women with elevated cholesterol (>250 mg/dL) were given nugget cereal, muffins, or flatbread made with Azhul barley or oat flour. The duration of the study was six weeks, and in both oats and barley groups, total and LDL cholesterol were reduced, with no significant difference between the two groups. These results indicated that the hulless barley Azhul was equivalent to oats in lowering serum cholesterol, a major risk factor for cardiovascular disease in humans.

Other human studies of barley have been reported demonstrating the reduction of serum cholesterol; however, the studies were conducted using available barley, not specifically hulless types. McIntosh et al (1991) compared foods made with wheat or barley fed to hypercholesterolemic men, wherein total and LDL cholesterol were decreased by barley. Ikegami et al (1996) combined pearled split barley with boiled rice, compared with all rice in a series of experiments with normal and high-cholesterol subjects. In all cases, cholesterol was decreased, but to a greater degree in persons with initial higher levels. Behall et al (2004) provided three levels of soluble fiber from barley to men on a low-fat diet. After five weeks, cholesterol levels were lower, in a stepwise fashion, according to the fiber level of the diets, compared to prestudy values.

Many acceptable food products can be made from hulless barley, either whole grain, milled in various ways, or pearled. These products can be produced to contain high levels of documented health-promoting compounds. Consumed on a regular basis, foods prepared from hulless barley are effective in reducing risk factors for cardiovascular disease and will moderate glycemic response in patients with Type 2 diabetes.

Feed Barley

Feed barley is often described as reject malt barley or barley that does not possess the characteristics necessary to make acceptable malt. Modern malt houses consider the attached hulls of barley an advantage or even necessary to ensure uniformity in water absorption during steeping, for protection of the sprout during germination, and as aids in filtering. Thus hulless barley does not enjoy wide acceptance for malt, although it can be successfully malted (Bhatty 1996). The most logical use of hulless barley is for human food or swine and poultry feed, since the largely indigestible fibrous hull remains in the field at harvest. Although the logic of utilizing hulless barley for animal feed has been recognized for many years (Joseph 1924), hulless barley has not been seriously considered as a feedstuff until the release of high-yielding varieties in the late 1980s and early 1990s.

Swine Feeding

For many years, barley has been fed to swine of all ages as the sole cereal grain. In parts of the world where barley can be cultivated, its value as feed was and is well recognized by the farming community. Joseph (1924) hypothesized that hulless barley was superior to hulled barley as a feed for swine on the basis of the known high-fiber content of the hull. Joseph postulated that there would be more total digestible nutrients (available energy) in barley with the hull removed. In 1983, Bell and co-workers published a classic study using simulated barleys containing 0, 10, 20, and 30% hulls, demonstrating decreasing digestible energy (DE) with increasing percentages of hulls. Regression equations were developed to predict DE of barley as influenced by the amount of hull. The data predicted 84.0, 77.4, 70.7, and 64.1% DE in barley at 0, 10, 20, and 30% hulls, representing 15.73, 14.48, 13.22, and 12.01 kJ/g DE. This study showed that protein digestibility was also decreased in the simulated barleys as the percentage of hulls was increased, although the magnitude of the effect on protein was much less than that on DE. Although data generated by Bell et al (1983) are useful and informative, most hulled barleys contain only 10–14% hull, and sometimes even lesser amounts. A similar study with Condor hulless barley in which hulls were added back to the barley was reported by Darroch et al (1996). The addition of hulls linearly decreased DE and protein content, and protein digestibility decreased in a curvilinear fashion. Condor barley with all hulls removed was reported to contain 17.6 kJ/kg and an energy digestibility of 87.4%.

Digestibility Studies

Trials with mice (Bhatty et al 1974, 1975) showed that hulless cultivars of barley had, on average, 8.2% more available energy than hulled barley: 16.39 vs. 15.18 kJ/g DE, respectively. Several digestibility studies using pigs indicated significantly higher levels of DE in hulless barley compared to those in hulled barley (Mitchall et al 1976, Bhatty et al 1979, Bell and Keith 1988, Thacker et al 1988a, Truscott et al 1988b). Mean values for DE taken from these studies were 80.8 and 75.5% for hulless and hulled barley, respectively. Newman et al (1968) reported a 5.2% increase in digestible, nitrogen-free extract (NFE) in hulless barley. Additionally, digestibility of NFE (Newman et al 1968) and DE (Wu et al 2000) of hulless barley was reported to be equal to that of corn for pigs. Baidoo and Liu (1998) concluded that the digestibility of energy (80–83%) and protein (70–76%) of the hulless barleys Condor, Falcon, and CDC Buck were comparable to that of wheat.

Feedlot Studies

Results of feeding trials comparing growth rate and feed efficiency of pigs fed hulless and hulled barleys have not been consistently in favor of the hulless types, as has been reported in digestibility trials. One of the earliest reports of feeding barley to swine was that of Joseph (1924). Joseph completed four trials in which he compared hulless Guy Mayle barley with unrelated hulled White Smyrna barley and to corn as basal grains for pigs fed from 22 to 90 kg live weight. In three of the four trials, rather large differences in rate of gain and improved feed efficiency favoring the hulless barley were apparent. However, in the fourth trial, rate of gain and feed efficiency were essentially equal for pigs fed hulled and hulless barleys. Gill et al (1966) reported that hulless Godiva barley was superior to an unrelated hulled barley, Hannchen, for growing-finishing pigs as measured by rate and efficiency of gain. Newman et al (1968) fed hulless and hulled Compana barley isogenic lines to early weaned pigs (8 kg initially) in two trials for three and four weeks, respectively. Pigs fed the hulless barley gained faster than those fed the hulled barley and had faster gains than those fed corn diets. Feed efficiency of hulless barley-fed pigs was also superior to that of pigs fed hulled barley or corn diets. In the same study, similar pigs were fed isogenic Glacier hulless and hulled barleys for eight weeks. Rate of gain, feed consumption, and feed-efficiency measurements were identical for the pigs fed these two barleys. In a follow-up study with the hulless and hulled Compana isogenic lines, Newman and Eslick (1970) compared the two barleys along with corn fed to pigs in starter diets (8–23 kg live weight), grower diets (20–45 kg live weight) and finisher diets (45–84 kg live weight). There were no differences in rates and efficiency of gains between the three grains in the starter and grower periods. However, during the finisher period, the performance of pigs fed the hulless barley and corn diets were identical and superior to those fed the hulled barley diet. Similar results were reported by Bell and Keith (1993) in that Tupper hulless barley was superior to Johnston hulled barley for pigs in the finishing period, but not in the growing period. Truscott et al (1988b) conducted two growing-finishing swine-feeding trials (19–94 kg live weight) comparing Betzes isogenic lines of hulless and hulled barleys. In the first trial, there were no differences in rate of gain; however, the hulless barley diets were more efficient. In the second trial with a second crop year of the same barleys, there were no differences in performance of the pigs due to barley type. Other reports also have observed inconsistent results along with little or no improvement in feeding performance of pigs fed hulless barleys compared to hulled barleys (Mitchall et al 1976; Aherne and Spicer 1986; Thacker et al 1988a,b; Bell and Keith 1993; Jensen et al 1998; Thacker 1999). Other studies have shown that hulless barley is equal to corn for young pigs (Newman et al 1968) and for older pigs (Mori and Newman 1989; Bell and Keith 1993; Wu et al 2000).

Processing

The majority of feed grains that are processed on farms and fed to pigs are ground with various types of machinery such as hammer mills to facilitate mixing or blending with other feed ingredients and to increase surface area of the grain, thereby aiding in nutrient utilization. Pelleting is a procedure primarily used by commercial feed companies to process many types of feeds, especially those fed to swine. In general, the process involves fine to medium grinding, followed by steaming and extrusion through a die to form a pellet. The greatest value of pelleting is found with high-fiber feeds such as hulled barley. Various types of extrusion processing other than pelleting are also used to prepare swine feeds, especially in combination with pelleting feedstuffs for very young pigs. Micronization is a thermal process that subjects a feed grain or food to infrared light, producing intensive heat in the product for a relatively short period of time. The application of heat and pressure through pelleting, extrusion, and micronizing are processing methods that have been applied to hulled and hulless barleys in efforts to improve the feed value of these grains.

Fadel et al (1988) reported that extrusion increased the DE of hulled barley (Pirolene), and a similar improvement in DE was reported due to baking Nupana hulless barley (Fadel et al 1989) and pelleting Waxbar, a waxy hulless barley (Graham et al 1989). The improvement was postulated to be due to rupture of endosperm cell walls of the barley and hydrolysis of starch, thereby increasing starch digestibility as well as nonstarch polysaccharides before the large intestine. Mori and Newman (1989) compared diets prepared from waxy hulless barley in three physical forms: ground, extruded, and pelleted to a ground corn diet for growing-finishing pigs (25–102 kg live weight). Pigs fed the pelleted barley gained slightly faster than those fed the ground barley, and feed efficiency was improved by nearly 7%. Extrusion without pelleting produced slightly slower pig gains compared to pigs fed ground or pelleted diets, but feed efficiency was improved by extrusion, as with the pelleted barley diet. The performance of pigs fed ground barley in that study were equal to those fed the ground corn, and pelleting and extrusion increased the feed value of the hulless barley over that of ground corn. In an earlier study (Newman et al 1968), young pigs fed ground hulless barley meal diets gained faster than pigs fed pelleted hulless barley diets in one of two trials, and feed efficiency tended to be best on meal diets. Newman and Heryford (1989) concluded that extrusion did not change the feed value of two hulless barleys (waxy Washonupana and nonwaxy Franubet) or hulled Hector barley for early weaned pigs (8 kg live weight) in contrast to the findings of Fadel et al (1988) for older pigs. Micronization of hulless barley (unknown variety) showed a positive effect on the digestibilities of energy and protein in young pigs (Huang et al 1998). Thacker (1999) reported that micronization of hulless barley (unknown variety) increased the percentage of gelatinized starch and improved the digestibility of protein for pigs. However, micronization of the barley severely reduced feed intake in a growing-finishing trial, leading to significant reduction in growth rate of pigs from 19 to 80 kg live weight, although feed efficiency was improved. It is well known that simply restricting intake of pigs will improve feed efficiency regardless of processing procedures used. In a second trial, Thacker and Campbell (1999) reported that micronization had no effect on protein and energy digestibility of hulless barley. Feed intake was reduced by micronization as in the first trial, although not as severely, allowing equal gains with improved feed efficiency due to micronization.

Enzyme Supplements

Starch and protein, the major nutrients in barley, are enclosed within aleurone and endosperm cell walls, which consist mainly of β-glucans and arabinoxylans. A bacterial diastase added to waxy and nonwaxy hulless barley isolines, Washonupana and Shonupana respectively, improved energy and nitrogen digestibility, rate of gain, and feed efficiency of growing-finishing pigs in one study (Newman et al 1983); but in an earlier trial, a similar product had no effect on pigs fed Washonupana (Newman et al 1980). β-Glucanase and xylanase supplementation of hulless barley diets have been shown to reduce intestinal viscosity and improve digestibilities of energy, protein, and amino acids in several trials with hulless barley (Thacker 1988b; Graham et al 1989; Li et al 1996; Thacker and Campbell 1999; Yin et al 2001a,b; Lindberg et al 2003). The magnitude of the responses depended on the type of carbohydrase (β-glucanase or xylanase) and the variety of hulless barley (Yin et al 2001b). Lindberg et al (2003) concluded that the impaired digestibility of hulless barley indicated that this grain had properties that limited its utilization and could not be alleviated by enzyme supplementation. In trials in which both enzymes were fed, β-glucanase had the greatest effect on improving nutrient digestibility and reducing intestinal viscosity. In those studies that included animal growth data, the improvements in digestibility of nutrients did not translate into faster and more efficient gains (Jensen et al 1998, Thacker et al 1988a, Thacker and Campbell 1999, Lindberg et al 2003). The results of these experiments support the contention that the potential for improvement of growth performance in pigs by supplementing hulless barley-based diets with cell wall-degrading enzymes is limited.

Digestibility studies confirm the expected greater DE of hulless barley compared to hulled barley in pig diets. However, a survey of literature indicates that the improved metabolic measurements are not consistently translated to faster and more efficient growth in pigs. This is somewhat of a paradox that has not been completely understood or explained. It has been suggested that incomplete removal of the hulls at harvest or before feeding hulless barley may be responsible in part for the observed lack of response. If this were true, the analytical values for fiber in the diets would have been indicative of such. In our work at the Montana station, every effort was made to remove the hulls before feeding trials, yet we saw equal performance of pigs fed covered and hulless barley in a number of trials even with isogenic lines. Additionally, the same diets fed in some of our digestibility trials showing improved digestibility values were the same diets fed in the feeding trials in which no differences were noted in pig performance. The pig's metabolic system may be able to adjust in some manner, thus compensating for the higher fiber levels in hulled barleys. It is also possible that some unknown factors may be associated with hulls that promote better performance, compensating for the lower digestibility. The barley hull may have been looked upon unjustly as a negative component in pig diets, especially in diets for young pigs. This concept is supported by data from a large cooperative study involving more than 1,200 weanling pigs fed at six research centers. The pigs were fed diets in which 0, 33, 67, or 100% of the corn as well as a portion of the soybean meal was replaced by hulled barley. Average daily gains (kg/day) and gain-feed (kg/kg) ratios of pigs fed the four diets for 28 days were not different: 0.41, 0.42, 0.41, 0.41 kg and 0.64, 0.62, 0.62, 0.63 kg, respectively

(Western Regional Research Project Committee W-166 1988). Perhaps the lack of consistency in improved performance of pigs fed hulless barley compared to covered barley and the equal performance of pigs shown in the corn-barley ratio study can be summed up as a possible prebiotic effect of the fiber or some other component of barley hulls. Age of pigs appeared to influence response to hulless barley. In several studies in which performance was measured separately in growing and finishing pigs, a more positive response to hulless barley was seen during the finishing phase, indicating that energy availability became limiting with age of pig.

Poultry Feeding

Barley has traditionally been recognized as a poor grain for poultry, which for many years was attributed to the high fiber content of the hull. Hulless barley, at first glance, would seem to have more productive value for poultry than hulled barley simply because of the lower fiber content. Many studies have failed to support this hypothesis (Anderson et al 1961, Eslick 1961, Coon 1979, Ullrich et al 1984, Classen 1985, Newman and Newman 1987, Scott et al 1998). Numerous investigations with broiler chickens have established that supplementation with β-glucanase preparations substantially improved the nutritive value of barley-based diets.

Broiler Chicks—Enzyme Studies

The true metabolizable energy (TME) of hulless barley was found to be significantly higher than that of hulled barley and similar to that of wheat for adult roosters. However, according to Sibbald (1982), the TME of hulless barley was no greater than that of hulled barley. Soaking in water followed by drying before feeding broiler chicks greatly improved the nutritive value of hulless barley (Anderson et al 1961, Eslick 1961). Eslick (1961) reported that soaking was more effective at improving the nutritive value of hulless barley for chicks than soaking a hulled variety. Classen (1985) found that the addition of cellulase, antibiotics, or gamma irradiation of the grain increased the growth rate of chicks fed hulless barley.

Burnett (1966) was perhaps the first researcher to demonstrate that mixed linked β-glucans were a major cause of the reduced feed value of barley. Newman and Newman (1987) demonstrated the beneficial effect of adding β-glucanase to both hulless and hulled isogenic cultivars when fed to broiler chicks. Additionally, hulless waxy barley (Washonupana), which had the highest extract viscosity of the barleys compared, had the lowest feed value of four isotype barleys. Subsequently, Fadel et al (1987) showed that waxy Washonupana and Franubet, a nonwaxy hulless barley, had similar levels of total β-glucans, although Washonupana had 35% more soluble β-glucans. Franubet was derived from Betzes barley and is characterized by angular starch granules that appear fractured (Chung 1982). Extract viscosity was nearly twice as great for the waxy hulless barley as that for the nonwaxy barley (2.65 vs. 1.35 cP). Broiler chicks fed Washonupana evidenced poor fat and dry matter digestibility along with poor growth performance that was significantly improved by supplemental β-glucanase. Chicks fed the nonwaxy hulless barley (Franubet) had greater retention of fats and greater dry matter digestibility than those fed the waxy type, and when fed with supplemental β-glucanase, chick performance was 92% that of chicks fed corn diets. Franubet was compared to hulled Ershabet, also derived from Betzes, and corn in a series of trials by Newman and Newman (1988). Chicks fed Franubet barley with or without supplemental β-glucanase had weight gains and feed efficiency values superior to the hulled barley and equal to those fed corn. It was postulated that Franubet was superior to Washonupana and hulled Ershabet because of the lower extract viscosity observed in this barley. This may be related to a reported difference in the type of starch granules in Franubet.

Scott et al (1998) conducted a large study comparing five hulled and 10 hulless barleys grown under different environmental conditions, using a broiler chick bioassay. These authors stated that the feeding value of hulled and hulless barleys were not different without enzyme (β-glucanase) supplementation. They suggested that this was because the higher fiber content of the hulled cultivars was counteracted by the higher (and possibly more soluble) β-glucan levels of the hulless cultivars. With enzyme supplementation, which reduced the negative effects of nonstarch polysaccharides (β-glucans), hulless cultivars were found to be superior to the hulled barleys. The authors concluded that the response to enzyme supplementation was a reflection of the value of the cereal grain without added enzyme.

Rotter et al (1989) compared hulless Scout barley and hulled Bedford barley supplemented with celluclast, a crude cellulase preparation, fed to broiler and Leghorn cockerels. Birds fed the hulless barley diets showed a dramatic response to the enzyme, whereas no response was observed with the hulled barley. The differential effects of enzyme supplementation of hulless Scout and hulled Bedford barleys was also found in a subsequent study (Friesen et al 1992). Campbell et al (1993) presented solid evidence of the negative impact of β-glucan content of hulless barleys. Hulless barley cultivars with high and low β-glucans levels exhibited high and low extract viscosities, respectively. Both high- and low-viscosity hulless barleys gave equivalent performance with β-glucanase supplementation. Comparisons made with hulled barley indicated that hulless barley diets gave higher body weight gain and improved feed conversion in chick diets when both barley types were supplemented with β-glucanase, which corresponds to the reports of Rotter et al (1989) and Friesen et al (1992).

Ankrah et al (1999) compared waxy and nonwaxy hulless cultivars for composition and feeding value for broiler chicks. Feeding waxy starch barley resulted in higher digesta viscosity than normal starch barley, which was attributed to the higher β-glucan content. Although there was a trend toward poorer growth performance of the chicks fed the waxy types, there were no statistical differences in body weight gain, feed intake, feed efficiency, or intestinal starch digestibility due to starch type. However, fecal digestibility of waxy starch was 10% higher than that of nonwaxy starch. β-Glucanase improved chick performance, which was attributed to increased starch digestibility and elimination of the high viscosity in the digesta. The reduction in digesta viscosity in broiler chicks fed waxy barley due to β-glucanase supplementation was also reported by Wang et al (1992). All negative trends were eliminated, and the waxy trait did not compromise chick performance when diets were supplemented with β-glucanase. The authors (Ankrah et al 1999) suggested that physical measurements made in this study indicated that waxy barley may offer advantages in feed processing (pelleting) associated with lower gelatinization temperature.

Layers vs. Broilers and Age of Birds

Hiproly and Hiproly Normal hulless barleys compared favorably in production criteria to wheat in layer diets, but wheat-fed birds were heavier after 18 weeks (Moss et al 1974). Rotter et al (1989) reported that broiler cockerels responded more positively to enzyme supplements in hulless barley than did Leghorn cockerels. Scott et al (2001) compared broiler and Leghorn chicks (4–21 days of age) fed hulless barley diets with and without supplemental β-glucanase. Response to the enzyme by broiler chicks was twofold that of Leghorn chicks for growth and feed intake. Broilers subjected to feed restriction had a lower growth response to enzyme supplementation compared to birds allowed ad libitum feed intake. The authors postulated that restricting feed intake reduced digesta viscosity in broilers; however, digesta viscosity in Leghorn chicks consuming enzyme-treated diets was twice as high as that in broiler chicks fed the same diet. These results suggest a difference between broilers and layer chicks in their ability to cope with high digesta viscosity created by the hulless barley. Hulless barley was evaluated by Classen et al (1988) as a replacement for wheat or hulled Harrington barley for laying hens. These authors concluded that hulless barley was equivalent to wheat and superior to hulled barley as a cereal grain for laying hens. Salih et al (1991) presented evidence that age of broiler and Leghorn chicks has a marked effect on the ability to cope with β-glucans in both hulled and hulless barley. Both broiler and Leghorn chicks fed hulless barley diets without supplemental β-glucanase had poorer gain and feed conversion, higher digesta viscosity, lower rate of food passage, and lower fat digestibility than chicks fed enzyme-supplemented diets. The effects were largely confined to the early growth period (0–4 weeks) and, with the exception of higher digesta viscosity, disappeared with aging. Similar results with broiler-type turkeys were reported by Stevens et al (1988). Birds fed hulless barley diets (variety unknown) supplemented with β-glucanase had higher body weights than birds fed hulless barley without enzymes or wheat diets at four weeks of age, but not by 12 weeks.

The negative impact of β-glucans in hulled and hulless barley when included in diets fed broiler chicks is well documented. The somewhat higher levels of β-glucans found in hulless types increases the problem, but the depressing effects appear to be greater than would be expected. It is possible that the hulls have some sort of mediating effect on the negative effect of β-glucans. It has been postulated that increased digesta viscosity created by β-glucans is the primary cause of reduced growth of broiler chicks fed hulless barley diets; however, the increased digesta viscosity does not seem to be the same problem in Leghorn chicks. Age of bird as well as genotype must be considered. The major negative effects of hulless barley β-glucans are seen only in the chick before three weeks of age, and older birds are much less negatively affected. In spite of the problems seen when hulless barley is fed to poultry, it is an excellent feed grain when supplemented with β-glucanase or β-glucanase and pentosanase.

Summary

Hulless barley, an ancient grain with modern applications, has much potential. Its first and foremost future success is anticipated in human food because of its potential health benefits. Optimal processing techniques and widely acceptable product development have not yet been fully achieved. Modern consumer interest in health promotion should provide optimum market opportunities.

In the animal-production industry, hulless barley is totally acceptable as a feed grain. For swine, it compares very favorably with hulled barley, corn, and other feed grains. In climates where barley grows well, there is an economic advantage to hulless barley because of its protein level and balance of essential amino acids. In the past, barley of any type was considered undesirable for poultry. However, modern use of specialized enzyme supplements makes barley, including hulless barley, totally appropriate for broilers or laying hens.

There are many markets as yet unexplored, such as pet foods, farmed fish food, and human infant food. The future of hulless barley is promising, with the development of new, more-productive genotypes with improved nutritional potential.

References

Aherne, F. S., and Spicer, H. 1986. An evaluation of the nutritive value of hulless barley for young pigs. Pages 107-108 in: Annual Feeders Day Rep., University of Alberta, Edmonton, Canada.

Åman, P., and Newman, C. W. 1986. Chemical composition of some different types of barley grown in Montana. J. Cereal Sci. 4:133-141.

Ames, N., Cliff, M., and Rhymer, C. 2002. Consumer acceptance of barley tortilla products. Presented at the Am. Assoc. Cereal Chem. annual meeting. Online: http://www.aaccnet.org/meetings/2002/abstracts/a02ma403.asp

Anderson, J. O., Wagstaff, R. K., and Dobson, D. C. 1961. Studies on the value of hulless barley in chick diets and means of increasing this value. Poult. Sci. 40:1571-1584.

Ankrah, N. O., Campbell, G. G., Tyler, R. T., Rossnagel, B. G., and Sokhansanj, S. R. T. 1999. Hydrothermal and β-glucanase effects on the nutritional and physical properties of starch in normal and waxy hull-less barley. Livestock Prod. Sci. 81:205-219.

Baidoo, S. K., and Liu, Y-G. 1998. Hull-less barley for swine: Ileal and faecal digestibility of proximate nutrient, amino acids and non-starch polysaccharides. J. Sci. Food Agric. 76:397-403.

Bang-Olsen, K., Stilling, B., and Munck, L. 1987. Breeding for yield in high-lysine barley. Pages 865-870 in: Barley Genetics V, Proc. 5th International Barley Genetics Symposium. S. Yasuda and T. Konishi, Eds. Sanyo Press Co., Okayama, Japan.

Barnes, P. J. 1983. Non-saponifiable lipids in cereals. Pages 33-55 in: Lipids in Cereal Technology. P. J. Barnes, Ed. Academic Press, New York.

Behall, K. M., Scholfield, D. J., and Canary, J. 1988. Effect of starch structure on glucose and insulin responses in adults. Am. J. Clin. Nutr. 47:428-432.

Behall, K. M., Scholfield, D. J., and Hallfrisch., J. G. 2004. Lipids significantly reduced by diets containing barley in moderately hypercholesterolemic men. J. Am. Coll. Nutr. 23:55-62.

Bell, J. M., Shires, A., and Keith, M. O. 1983. Effect of hull and protein contents of barley on protein and energy digestibility and feeding value for pigs. Can. J. Anim. Sci. 63:201-211.

Bell, J. M., and Keith, M. O. 1988. Comparisons of HY-320 wheat, Tupper hulless barley and yellow corn in feeding grower-finisher pigs. Annual Report. Prairie Swine Centre, University of Saskatchewan, Saskatoon, Canada.

Bell, J. M., and Keith, M. O. 1993. Effects of combinations of wheat, corn or hulless barley with hulled barley supplemented with soybean meal or canola meal on growth rate, efficiency of feed utilization and carcass quality of market pigs. Anim. Feed Sci. Technol. 44:129-150.

Berglund, P. T., Fastnaught, C. E., and Holm, E. T. 1992. Food uses of waxy hull-less barley. Cereal Foods World 37:707-714.

Bhatty, R. S. 1986a. The potential of hull-less barley—A review. Cereal Chem. 63:97-103.

Bhatty, R. S. 1986b. Physiochemical and functional (bread-making) properties of hull-less barley fractions. Cereal Chem. 63:31-35.

Bhatty, R. S. 1993. Nonmalting uses of barley. Pages 355-417 in: Barley Chemistry and Technology. A. W. MacGregor and R. S. Bhatty, Eds. Am. Assoc. Cereal Chem., St. Paul, MN.

Bhatty, R. S. 1995. Hull-less barley bran: A potential new product from an old grain. Cereal Foods World 40:819-824.

Bhatty, R. S. 1996. Production of food malt from hull-less barley. Cereal Chem. 73:75-80.

Bhatty, R. S. 1997. Milling of regular and waxy starch hullless barleys for the production of bran and flour. Cereal Chem. 74:693-699.

Bhatty, R. S., and Rossnagel, B. G. 1997. Zero amylose lines of hulless barley. Cereal Chem. 74:190-191.

Bhatty, R. S., Christison, G. I., Sosulski, F. W., Harvey, B. L., Hughes, G. R., and Berdahl, J. D. 1974. Relationship of various physical and chemical characters to digestible energy in wheat and barley. Can. J. Anim. Sci. 54:419-427.

Bhatty, R. S., Berdahl, J. D., and Christison, G. I. 1975. Chemical composition and digestible energy of barley. Can. J. Anim. Sci. 55:759-764.

Bhatty, R. S., Christison, G. I., and Rossnagel, B. G. 1979. Energy and protein digestibility of hulled and hulless barley determined by swine feeding. Can. J. Anim. Sci. 59:585-588.

Bhatty, R. S., MacGregor, A. W., and Rossnagel, B. G. 1991. Total and acid soluble β-glucan content of hulless barley and its relationship to acid-extract viscosity. Cereal Chem. 68:221-227.

Björck, I., Eliasson, A-C, Drews, A., Gudmundsson, M., and Karlsson, R. 1990. Some nutritional properties of starch and dietary fiber in barley genotypes containing different levels of amylose. Cereal Chem. 67:327-333.

Björck, I., Granfeldt, Y., Liljeberg, H., Tovar, J., and Asp, N-G. 1994. Food properties affecting the digestion and absorption of carbohydrates. Am. J. Clin. Nutr. 59(Suppl): 6995-7055.

Brand-Miller, J. C. 1994. Importance of glycemic index in diabetes. Am. J. Clin. Nutr. 59(Suppl): 7475-7525.

Briggs, D. E. 1978. Barley. Chapman and Hall Ltd., London, UK.

Burnett, G. S. 1966. Studies of viscosity as the probable factor involved in the improvement of certain barleys for chickens by enzyme supplementation. Br. Poult. Sci. 7:55-75.

Campbell, G. L., Rossnagel, B. G., and Bhatty, R. 1993. Evaluation of hull-less barley genotypes varying in extract viscosity in broiler chick diets. Anim. Feed Sci. Technol. 41:191-197.

Cheigh, H. S. 1979. Rheological baking and noodle making properties of barley-wheat flour blends. Pages 48-71 in: Proc. Joint Barley Utilization Seminar. Korean Sci. Eng. Foundation, Suweon, Korea.

Chen, W.-J., Anderson, J. W., and Jennings, D. 1984. Propionate may mediate the hypocholesterolaemic effects of certain soluble plant fibers in cholesterol-fed rats. (Abstr.) Fed. Proc. Soc. Exp. Biol. Med. 75:215.

Chung, T. Y. 1982. Isolation, description, inheritance, associated traits and possible uses of three barley (*Hordeum vulgare* L.) starch mutants. Ph.D. thesis, Montana State University, Bozeman, MT.

Classen, H. L., Campbell, G. L., Rossnagel, B. G., Bhatty, R., and Reichert, R. D. 1985. Studies on the use of hulless barley in chick diets: Deleterious effects and methods of alleviation. Can. J. Anim. Sci. 65:725-733.

Classen, H. L., Campbell, G. L., Rossnagel, B. G., and Bhatty, R. S. 1988. Evaluation of hulless barley as replacement for wheat or conventional barley in laying hen diets. Can. J. Anim. Sci. 68:1261-1266.

Coon, C. N., Shepler, R., McFarland, E., and Nordheim, J. 1979. The nutritional evaluation of barleys selections and cultivars from Washington State. Poult. Sci. 58:913-918.

Danielson, A. D. 1994. Chemical composition, physical properties and physiological responses of whole barley and barley fractions. M.S. thesis, Montana State University, Bozeman, MT.

Darroch, C. S., Aherne, F. X., Helm, J., Sauer, W. C., and Jaikaran, S. 1996. Effects of dietary level of barley hulls and fibre type on protein and energy digestibilities of Condor hulless barley in growing swine. Anim. Feed Sci. Technol. 61:173-182.

Deane, D., and Commers, E. 1986. Oat cleaning and processing. Pages 371-412 in: Oats Chemistry and Technology. F. H. Webster, Ed. Am. Assoc. Cereal Chem., St. Paul, MN.

Dickson, A. D. 1978. Barley for malting and food. Pages 136-146. in Barley: Orgin, Botany, Clulture, Winter Hardness, Genetics, Utilization, Pest. Handbook 338. U.S. Department of Agriculture, Washington, DC.

Doll, H., Koie, B., and Eggum, B. O. 1974. Induced high-lysine mutants in barley. Radiat. Bot. 14:73-80.

Dudgeon-Bollinger, A. L., Fastnaught, C. E., and Berglund, P. T. 1997. Extruded snack products from waxy hulless barley. Cereal Foods World 42:762-766.

Edney, M. J., Tkachuk, R., and MacGregor, A. W. 1992. Nutrient composition of the hull-less barley cultivar, Condor. J. Sci. Food Agric. 60:451-456.

Eggum, B. O. 1973. Biological availability of amino acid constituents in grain protein. Pages 391-408 in: Nuclear Techniques for Seed Protein Improvement. (Panel proc.) International Atomic Energy Agency, Vienna, Austria.

Eslick, R. F. 1961. Is barley just "barley" in a feed ration? Pages 43-52. in: Proc. Montana Nutrition Conference. O. O. Thomas, Ed. Montana State University Press, Bozeman, MT.

Eslick, R. F. 1979. Barley breeding for quality at Montana State University. Pages 2-25 in: Proc. Joint Barley Utilization Seminar. Korean Sci. Eng. Found., Suweon, Korea.

Fadel, J. G., Newman, R. K., Newman, C. W., and Barnes, A. E. 1987. Hypocholesterolemic effects of β-glucans in different barley diets fed to broiler chicks. Nutr. Rep. Int. 35:1049-1058.

Fadel, J. G., Newman, C. W., Newman, R. K., and Graham, H. 1988. Effects of extrusion cooking of barley on ileal and fecal digestibilities of dietary components in pigs. Can. J. Anim. Sci. 68:891-897.

Fadel, J. G., Newman, R. K., Newman, C. W., and Graham, H. 1989. Effects of baking hulless barley on the digestibility of dietary components as measured at the ileum and in the feces in pigs. J. Nutr. 119:722-726.

Fastnaught, C. E., Bergland, P. T., Holm, E. T., and Fox, G. J. 1996. Genetic and environmental variation in β-glucan content and quality parameters of barley for food. Crop Sci. 36:941-946.

Fastnaught, C. E., Bond, J. M., and Berglund, P. T. 1997. Oil reduction in muffins using waxy hulless barley β-glucan. Cereals Food World 42:666.

Fastnaught, C. E. 2001. Barley fiber. Pages 519-542 in: Handbook of Dietary Fiber. S. S. Cho and M. L. Dreher, Eds. Marcel Dekker, Inc., New York.

Franckowiak, J. D., and Konishi, T. 1997. BGS 7, naked caryopsis, *nud*, revised. Barley Genet. Newsl. 26:51-52.

Friesen, O. D., Guenter, W., Marquardt, R. R., and Rotter, B. A. 1992. The effect of enzyme supplementation on the apparent metabolizable energy and nutrient digestibilities of wheat, barley, oats, and rye for the young broiler chick. Poult. Sci. 71:1710-1721.

Gill, D. R., Oldfield, J. E., and England, D. C. 1966. Comparative values of hulless barley, regular barley, corn and wheat for growing pigs. J. Anim. Sci. 25: 34-36.

Goering, K. J., and Eslick, R. F. 1976. Barley starch VI. A self-liquefying waxy barley starch. Cereal Chem. 53:174-180.

Goering, K. J., DeHaas, B. W., Chapman, D. W., Eslick, R. F., and Gramera, R. E. 1980. New process for production of ultra high maltose syrup from special genetically derived barley. Starch/Stærke 32:349-332.

Graham, H., Fadel, J. G., Newman, C. W., and Newman, R. K. 1989. Effect of pelleting and β-glucanase supplementation on the digestibility of a barley-based diet in the pig gastrointestinal tract. J. Anim. Sci. 67:1293-1298.

Granfeldt, Y., Liljeberg, H., Drews, A., Newman, R., and Björck, I. 1994. Glucose and insulin responses to barley products: Influences of food structure and amylose-amylopectin ratio. Am. J. Clin Nutr. 59:1075-1082.

Hallfrisch, J., and Behall, K. M. 2003. Physiological responses of men and women to barley and oat extracts (Nu-trimX). I. Breath hydrogen, methane, and gastrointestinal symptoms. Cereal Chem. 80:76-79.

Han, X. 1996. Noodle-making quality from Australian standard white wheat and Montana wheat and barleys. M.S. thesis, Montana State University, Bozeman, MT.

Han, M. S., and Froseth, J. A. 1992. Composition of pearling fractions of barleys with normal and waxy starch. Proc. West. Sec. Am. Soc. Anim. Sci. 43:155-158.

Harlan, H. V. 1920. Daily development of kernels of Hannchen barley from flowering to maturity at Aberdeen, Idaho. J. Agric. Res. 19:393-429.

Harlan, H. V. 1957. Pages 168-169 in: One Man's Life with Barley—The Memories and Observations of Harry V. Harlan. J. R. Harlan, Ed. Exposition Press, New York.

Harlan, J. R. 1978. On the origin of barley. Pages 10-36 in: Barley: Origin, Botany, Culture, Winter Hardness, Genetics, Utilization, Pest. Handbook 338. U.S. Department of Agriculture, Washington, DC.

Henry, R. J. 1988. The carbohydrates of barley grain—A review. J. Inst. Brew. 94:71-78.

Hockett, E. A. 1981. Registration of hulless and short-awned spring barley germplasm. Crop Sci. 21:146-147.

Hofer, P. J. 1985. The composition and nutritional value of a high lysine, high sugar barley (*Hordeum vulgare* L.). M.S. thesis, Montana State University, Bozeman, MT.

Huang, S. X., Sauer, W. C., Pickard, M. Li, S., and Hardin, R. T. 1998. Effect of micronization on energy, starch and amino acid digestibility in hulless barley for young pigs. Can. J. Anim. Sci. 78:81-87.

Ikegami, S., Tsuchihashi, F., Nakamura, K., and Innami, S. 1991. Effect of barley on development of experimental diabetes in rats. J. Jpn. Soc. Nutr. Food Sci. 44:447-454.

Ikegami, S., Tomita, M., Honda, S., Yamaguchi, M., Mizukawa, R., Suzuki, Y., Ishii, K., Ohsawa, S., Kiyooka, N., Higuchi, M., and Kobayashi, S. 1996. Effect of boiled barley-rice-feeding in hypercholesterolemic and normolipemic subjects. Plant Foods Human Nutr. 49:317-328.

Ishikawa, N., Ishihara, J., and Masamitsu, I. 1995. Artificial induction and characterization of amylose-free mutants of barley. Barley Genet. Newsl. 24:49-53.

Jensen, M. S., Knudsen Bach, K. E., Inborr, J., and Jakobsen, K. 1998. Effect of β-glucanase supplementation on pancreatic enzyme activity and nutrient digestibility in piglets fed diets based on hulled and hulless barley varieties. Anim. Feed Sci. Technol. 72:329-345.

Jood, S., and Kalra, S. 2001. Chemical composition and nutritional characteristics of some hull less and hulled barley cultivars grown in India. Nahrung/Food 45:35-39.

Joseph, W. E. 1924. Feeding pigs in drylot. Bull. No. 169. Montana State University, Mont. Agric. Exp. Stn. Bozeman, MT.

Killen, G. J., Newman, C. W., Eslick, R. F., and El-Negoumy, A. M. 1978. The effect of nitrogen fertilizer on the nutritional quality of barley. Proc. West. Sec. Am. Soc. Anim. Sci. 29:169-172.

Kim, H. K., and Shin, H. S. 1982. Lipids and fatty acid composition of free and bound lipids in barley grain. Han'guk Sikp'um Kwahakhoechi 14:382-387.

Li, S., Sauer, W. C., Huang, S. X., and Gabert, V. M. 1996. Effect of β-glucanase supplementation to hulless barley- or wheat-soybean meal diets on the digestibilities of energy, protein, β-glucans, and amino acids in young pigs. J. Anim. Sci. 74:1649-1656.

Lifschitz, C. H., Grusak, M. A., and Butte, N. F. 2002. Carbohydrate digestion in humans from a β-glucan-enriched barley is reduced. J. Nutr. 132:2593-2596.

Liljeberg, H. G. M., Grandfeldt, Y. E., and Björck, I. M. E. 1996. Products based on a high fiber barley genotype, but not on common barley or oats, lower postprandial glucose and insulin responses in healthy humans. J. Nutr. 126:458-466.

Lindberg, J. E., Arvidsson, A., and Wang, J. 2003. Influence of naked barley cultivar with normal, amylose-rich or amylopectin-rich starch and enzyme supplementation on digestibility and piglet performance. Anim. Feed Sci. Technol. 104:121-131.

Liu, D. J., and Pomeranz, Y. 1975. Distribution of minerals in barley at the cellular level by x-ray analysis. Cereal Chem. 52:620-629.

Liu, D. J., Robbins, G. S., and Pomeranz, Y. 1974. Composition and utilization of milled barley products. IV. Mineral components. Cereal Chem. 51:209-216.

Marlett, J. A. 1991. Dietary fiber content and effect of processing on two barley varieties. Cereal Foods World 36:576-578.

McGuire, C. F. 1979. Roller milling and quality evaluation of barley flour. Pages 89-93 in: Proc. Joint Barley Utilization Seminar. Korean Sci. Eng. Found., Suweon, Korea.

McGuire, C. F., and Hockett, E. A. 1981. Effect of awn length and naked caryopsis on malting quality of "Betzes" barley. Crop Sci. 21:18-21.

McIntosh, G. H., Whyte, J., McArthur, R., and Nestel, P. J. 1991. Barley and wheat foods: Influence on plasma cholesterol concentrations in hypercholesterolemic men. Am. J. Clin. Nutr. 53:1205-1209.

Melland, R., Newman, R. K., McGuire, C. F., and Eslick, R. F. 1984. The effects of bleach treatment on pasta made from a series of barley genotypes. Cereal Res. Comm. 12:201-207.

Mitchall, K. G., Bell, J. M., and Sosulski, F. W. 1976. Digestibility and feeding value of hulless barley for pigs. Can. J. Anim. Sci. 56:505:511.

Mori, T. 1990. Chemical characterization and metabolic function of soluble dietary fiber from select milling fractions of a hulless barley and its waxy starch mutant. M.S. thesis, Montana State University, Bozeman, MT.

Mori, T., and Newman, C. W. 1989. Influence of extrusion and pelleting of barley diets on performance of growing-finishing swine. Proc. West. Sect. Am. Soc. Anim. Sci. 40:206-208.

Morrison, W. R. 1978. Cereal lipids. Pages 221-343 in: Advances in Cereal Science and Technology, Vol. II. Y. Pomeranz, Ed. Am. Assoc. Cereal Chem. St. Paul, MN.

Morrison, W. R. 1993. Barley lipids. Pages 199-246 in: Barley: Chemistry and Technology, A. W. MacGregor and R. S. Bhatty, Eds. Am. Assoc. Cereal Chem., St. Paul, MN.

Morrison, W. R., Milligan, T. P., and Azudin, M. N. 1984. A relationship between the amylose and lipid contents from diploid cereals. J. Cereal Sci. 2:257-271.

Moss, B. R., Beeckler, A., Hari, R., and Newman, C. W. 1974. Nutritional value of barley for poultry. Proc. West. Sec. Am. Soc. Anim. Sci. 25:162-165.

Munck, L., Karlsson, K-E., and Hagberg, A. 1969. Selection and characterization of a high-protein, high-lysine variety from the world barley collection. Pages 544-558 in: Barley Genetics II. Proc. 2nd Intl. Barley Genet. Symp. R. A. Nilan, Ed. Washington State University Press, Pullman, WA.

Nevo, E. 1992. Origin, evolution, population genetics and resources for breeding of wild barley, *Hordeum spontaneum* in the fertile crescent. Pages 19-43 in: Barley: Genetics, Biochemistry, Molecular Biology and Biotechnology. P. R. Shewry, Ed. C. A. B. International., Wallingford, U.K.

Newman, C. W., and Eslick, R. F. 1970. Barley varieties for swine diets. Proc. West Sect. Am. Soc. Anim. Sci. 21:111-116.

Newman, C. W., and Heryford, A. G. 1989. Influence of extrusion of barley diets on starter period performance of growing/finishing swine. Pages 7.1-7.6 in: Proc. Montana Nutrition Conference. R. Brownson, Ed. Montana State University Press, Bozeman, MT.

Newman, C. W., and McGuire, C. F. 1985. Nutritional quality of barley. Pages 403-456 in: Barley. D. C. Rasmusson, Ed. Am. Soc. Agron., Soil Sci. Soc. Am., Madison, WI.

Newman, C. W., and Newman, R. K. 1992. Nutritional aspects of barley seed structure and composition. Pages 351-368 in: Barley: Genetics, Biochemistry, Molecular Biology and Biotechnology. P. R. Shewry, Ed. C. A. B. International, Wallingford, U.K.

Newman, C. W., Thomas, O. O., and Eslick, R. F. 1968. Hulless barley in diets for weanling pigs. J. Anim. Sci. 27: 981-984.

Newman, C. W., Eslick, R. F., and Rasmuson, R. C. 1974. Effect of barley variety on protein quality and nutritional value for rats. J. Anim. Sci. 38:71-74.

Newman, C. W., Eslick, R. F., Pepper, J. W., and El-Negoumy, A. M. 1980. Performance of pigs fed hulless and covered barleys supplemented with or without a bacterial diastase. Nutr. Rep Int. 22:833-837.

Newman, C. W., Eslick, R. F., and El-Negoumy, A. M. 1983. Bacterial diastase effect on the feed value of two hulless barleys for pigs. Nutr. Rep. Int. 28:139-146.

Newman, R. K., and Newman, C. W. 1987. β-Glucanase effect on the performance of broiler chicks fed covered and hulless barley isotypes having normal and waxy starch. Nutr. Rep Int. 36:693-699.

Newman, R. K., and Newman, C. W. 1988. Nutritive value of a new hull-less barley cultivar in broiler chick diets. Poult. Sci. 67:1573-1579.

Newman, R. K., Lewis, S. E., Newman, C. W., Boik, R. J., and Ramage, R. T. 1989a. Hypocholesterolemic effect of barley foods on healthy men. Nutr. Rep. Int. 39:749-760.

Newman, R. K., Newman, C. W., and Graham, H. 1989b. The hypocholesterolemic function of barley β-glucans. Cereal Foods World 34:883-886.

Newman, R. K., Newman, C. W., McGuire, C. F., and Han, X. 1994. Preparation of Chinese steamed bread with hard white winter wheat and waxy barley flours. Pages 118-121 in: Proc. 1994 International Symposium and Exhibition on New Approaches in the Production of Food Stuffs and Intermediate Products from Cereal Grains and Oil Seeds. X. Guifang and M. Zhongdeng, Eds. Chinese Cereals and Oils Association, Beijing.

Newman, R. K., Ore, K. C., Abbott, J., and Newman, C. W. 1998. Fiber enrichment of baked products with a barley milling fraction. Cereal Foods World 43:23-25.

Osborne, T. B. 1924. The vegetable proteins, 2nd ed. Longmans, Green and Co., London, U.K.

Owen, B. D., Sosulski, F., Wu, K. K., and Farmer, J. J. 1977. Variation in mineral content in Saskatchewan feed grains. Can. J. Anim. Sci. 57:679-687.

Packer, L., Weber, S. U., and Rimbach, G. 2001. Molecular mechanisms of protective effects of vitamin E in atherosclerosis. J. Nutr. 131:369s-373s.

Pick, M. E., Hawrysh, J., Gee, M. I., and Toth, E. 1998. Barley bread products improve glycemic control of type 2 subjects. Int. J. Food Sci. Nutr. 49:71-78.

Pomeranz, Y. 1974a. Proteins and amino acids of barley, oats and buckwheat. Pages 13-78 in: Protein Nutritional Quality of Foods and Feeds. 2. Quality Factors—Plant Breeding, Composition, Processing and Antinutrients. M. Friedman, Ed. Marcel-Dekker, New York.

Pomeranz Y. 1974b. Food uses of barley. CRC Crit. Rev. Food Technol. 4(Jan.):377-394.

Price, P. B., and Parsons, J. G. 1979. Distribution of lipids in embryonic axis, bran-endosperm and hull fractions of hulless barley and hulless oat grain. J. Agric. Food Chem. 27:813-815.

Qureshi, A. A., Burger, W. C., Peterson, D. M., and Elson, C. E. 1986. The structure of an inhibitor of cholesterol biosynthesis isolated from barley. J. Biol. Chem. 261:10544-10550.

Qureshi, A. A., Crenshaw, T. D., Abuirmeileh, N., Peterson, D. M., and Elson, C. E. 1987. Influence of minor plant constituents on porcine hepatic lipid metabolism. Atherosclerosis 64:109-115.

Raboy, V. 1990. The biochemistry and genetics of phytic acid synthesis. Pages 52-73 in: Inositol Metabolism in Plants. D. J. Morke, W. Boss, and F. Loewus, Eds. Wiley-Liss, New York.

Rotter, B. A., Neskar, M., Guenter, W., and Marquardt, R. R. 1989. Effect of enzyme supplementation on the nutritive value of hulless barley in chicken diets. Anim. Feed Sci. Technol. 24:233-245.

Salih, M. E., Classen, H. L., and Campbell, G. L. 1991. Response of chickens fed on hull-less barley to dietary β-glucanase at different ages. Anim. Feed Sci. Technol. 33:139-149.

Schlichting, L. M., Dexter, J. E., Izydorczyk, M. S., Rossnagel, B. G., and Marchylo, B. A. 2001. Effect of hulless barley addition on colour and texture of spaghetti. Presented at the Am. Assoc. Cereal Chem. annual meeting. Online: http://www.aaccnet.org/meetings/2001/abstracts/a01ma400.htm

Scott, T. A., Silversides, F. G., Classen, H. L., Swift, M. L., and Bedford, M. R. 1998. Effect of cultivar and environment on the feeding value of western Canadian wheat and barley samples with and without enzyme supplementation. Can. J. Anim. Sci. 78:649-656.

Scott, T. A., Leslie, M. A., and Karimi, A. 2001. Measurements of enzyme response with hulless barley-based diets full-fed to Leghorn and broiler chicks or restricted-fed broiler chicks. Can. J. Anim. Sci. 81:403-410.

Seko, H., Ito, M., and Doi, Y. 1998. Breeding of naked barley for improved protein quality. Pages 140-144 in: Proc. Cereals for Human Health and Preventive Nutrition. K. Vaculová and J. Ehrenbergerová, Eds. Mendel Univ. Agric. Forestry, Brno, Czech Republic.

Sibbald, I. R. 1982. The effect of grinding on the true metabolizable energy value of hull-less barley. Poult. Sci. 61:2509-2511.

Smith, D. B., Gill, A. A., and Ahluwalia, B. 1987. Cultivar differences in the concentration of β-D glucans in developing and mature barley grains and their significance for malting quality. Asp. App. Biol. 15:105-113.

Stevens, V. I., Salmon, R. E., Classen, H. L., and Campbell, G. L. 1988. Effects of dietary β-glucanase, vitamin D3 and available phosphorus of the utilization of hulless barley by broiler turkeys. Nutr. Rep. Int. 38:283291.

Stobart, J. E. 1977. Nutritional evaluation of selected high-lysine grains. M.S. thesis, Montana State University, Bozeman, MT.

Story, J. A., and Kritchevsky, D. 1976. Comparison of binding of various bile acids and bile salts in vitro by several types of fiber. J. Nutr. 106:1292-1997.

Sun, L., and Wang, X. 1999. Genetic diversity of Chinese hull-less barley and germplasm and its utilization. Plant Genet. Resour. Newsl. 120:55-57.

Sundberg, B., and Falk, H. 1994. Composition and properties of bread and porridge prepared from different types of barley flour. Am. J. Clin. Nutr. 59(Suppl):7080S.

Sundberg, G., Xue, Q., Newman, R. K., and Newman, C. W. 1998. Glycaemic responses and hypercholesterolaemic effects of high-amylose barley diets on broiler chicks. J. Sci. Food Agric. 76:457-463.

Swanston, J. S., Ellis, R. P., and Tiler, S. A. 1996. Effects of the waxy and high amylose genes on total β-glucan and extractable starch. Barley Genet. Newsl. 27:72-74.

Tallberg, A. 1981. Characterization of high-lysine barley genotypes. Ph.D. thesis, Lund University, Lund, Sweden.

Thacker, P. A. 1999. Effect of micronization on the performance of growing/finishing pigs fed diets based on hulled and hulless barley. Anim. Feed Sci. Technol. 79:29-41.

Thacker, P. A., and Campbell, G. L. 1999. Performance of growing/finishing pigs fed untreated or micronized hulless barley-based diets with or without β-glucanase. J. Anim. Feed Sci. 8:157-170.

Thacker, P. A., Bell, J. M., Classen, H. L., Campbell, G. L., and Rossnagel, B. G. 1988a. The nutritive value of hulless barley for swine. Anim. Feed Sci. Technol. 19:191-196.

Thacker, P. A., Campbell, G. L., and GrootWassink, J. W. D. 1988b. The effect of β-glucanase supplementation on the performance of pigs fed hulless barley. Nutr. Rep. Int. 38:91-99.

Truscott, D. R., Newman, C. W., and Roth, N. J. 1988a. Effects of hull and awn type on the feed value of Betzes barley. I. Chemical and physical characteristics of the kernels. Nutr. Rep. Int. 37:681-693.

Truscott, D. R., Newman, C. W., and Roth, N. J. 1988b. Effects of hull and awn type on the feed value of Betzes barley III. Growth performance, carcass characteristics and nitrogen and energy digestibility by pigs. Nutr. Rep Int. 38:221-230.

Työppönen, J. T., and Hakkarainen, R. V. J. 1985. Thermal stability of vitamin E in barley. Acta Agric. Scand. 35:136.

Ullrich, S. E., Coon, C. N., Mahs, J. R., Lance, R. C. M., Seaman, T. M., Sever, J. M., and Blake, T. M. 1984. Assessment of barley quality. Pages 131-135 in: Proc. 2nd Int. Summer School in Agriculture. Cereal Production. M. E. E. Gallagher, Ed. The Royal Dublin Society, Butterworth, Stoneham, UK.

Ullrich, S. E., Clancy, J. A., Eslick, R. F., and Lance, R. C. M. 1986. β-Glucan content and viscosity of extracts from barley. J. Cereal Sci. 4:279-285.

Western Regional Research Project Committee W-166. 1988. Substitution of barley for corn and soybean meal in starter diets for weanling swine. J. Anim. Sci. (Suppl. 1):66:319.

Wang, L. 1992. Influences of oil and soluble fiber of barley grain on plasma cholesterol concentrations in chicks and hamsters. M.S. thesis, Montana State University, Bozeman, MT.

Wang, L., Newman, R. K., Newman, C. W., Hofer, P. J., and Fengler, A. I. 1992. Barley β-glucans alter intestinal viscosity and reduce plasma cholesterol concentrations in chicks. J. Nutr. 122:2292-2297.

Wang, L., Xue, Q., Newman, R. K., and Newman, C. W. 1993. Enrichment of tocopherols, tocotrienols, and oil in barley fractions by milling and pearling. Cereal Chem. 70:499-501.

Weaver, C. M., Chen, P. H., and Rynearson, S. L. 1981. Effect of milling on trace element and protein content of oats and barley. Cereal Chem. 58:120-124.

Wendorf, F., Schild, R., Hadidi, E., Close, A. E., Kobusiewicz, M., Wieckowska, H., Issawi, B., and Haas, H. 1979. Use of barley in the Egyptian late Paleolithic. Science 205:1341-1347.

Wiebe, G. A. 1978a. Introduction. Page 1 in: Barley: Origin, Botany, Culture, Winter Hardness, Genetics, Utilization, Pest. Handbook 338. U.S. Department of Agriculture, Washington, DC.

Wiebe, G. A. 1978b. Introduction of barley into the new world. Pages 2-9 in: Barley: Origin, Botany, Culture, Winter Hardness, Genetics, Utilization, Pest. Handbook 338. U.S. Department of Agriculture, Washington, DC.

Wood, P. J, Weisz, J., Beer, M. U., Newman, C. W., and Newman, R. K. 2003. Structure of (1-3)-(1-4)-β-D-glucan in waxy and nonwaxy barley. Cereal Chem. 80:329-332.

Wu, J.-F., Cheng, C.-S., Yu, I.-T., and Hsyu, J.-N. 2000. Hulless barley as an alternative energy source for growing-finishing pigs on growth performance, carcass quality, and nutrient digestibility. Livestock Prod. Sci. 65:155-160.

Wu, V. Y., Stringfellow, A. C., and Inglett, G. E. 1994. Protein- and β-glucan enriched fractions from high-protein, high β-glucan barleys by sieving and air classification. Cereal Chem. 71:220-223.

Xue, Q. 1992. Influence of waxy and high-amylose starch genes on the composition of barley and the cholesterolemic and glycemic responses on chicks and rats. Ph.D. thesis, Montana State University, Bozeman MT.

Xue, Q., Wang, L., Newman, R. K., Newman, C. W., and Graham, H. 1997. Influence of the hulless, waxy starch and short-awn genes on the composition of barleys. J. Cereal Sci. 26:251-257.

Yin, Y.-L., Baidoo, S. K., Schulze, H., and Simmins, P. H. 2001a. Effects of supplementing diets containing hulless barley varieties having different levels of non-starch polysaccharides with β-glucanase and xylanase on the physiological status of the gastrointestinal tract and nutrient digestibility of weaned pigs. Livestock Prod. Sci. 71:97-107.

Yin, Y.-L., Baidoo, S. K., Jin, L. Z., Liu, Y. G., Schulze, H., and Simmins, P. H. 2001b. The effect of different carbohydrase and protease supplementation on apparent (ileal and overall) digestibility of nutrients of five hulless barley varieties in young pigs. Livestock Prod. Sci. 71:109-120.

Yokoyama, W. H., Hudson, C. A. Knuckles, B. E., Chiu, M.-C. M., Sayre, R. N., Turnlund, J. R., and Schneeman, B. O. 1997. Effect of barley β-glucan in durum wheat pasta on human glycemic response. Cereal Chem. 74:293-296.

Yoon, S. H., Berglund, P. T., and Fastnaught, C. E. 1996. Evaluation of selected barley cultivars and their fractions for β-glucan enrichment and viscosity. Cereal Chem. 72:187-190.

Zha, S., and Wang, X. 1992. Tibetan barley cultivar and ecological region. Pages 194-195 in: Ecological Regions of Barley in China. Zhejiang Press for Technology and Science, Hangzhou, China.

CHAPTER 8

Hairless Canary Seed: A Potential Food Crop

E.-S. M. Abdel-Aal[1] and P. Hucl[2]

[1]Agriculture and Agri-Food Canada, Food Research Program, Guelph, ON, Canada N1G 5C9; [2]Crop Development Centre, Department of Plant Sciences, University of Saskatchewan, Saskatoon, SK, Canada N7S 5A8

Canary seed or annual canarygrass is a cereal crop that is used almost solely in food mixtures for caged birds. The grain, however, has a unique composition and characteristics that make it a promising cereal crop for food and industrial uses. Most canary seed cultivars are not safe for food consumption because the attached hulls are covered by small siliceous trichomes or hairs that can contaminate the dehulled grain or canary groat during harvesting and subsequent handling. The trichomes are potential carcinogens and have been linked to esophageal cancer when present as a contaminant in wheat flour used in baking bread (O'Neill et al 1980). The trichomes also cause severe skin irritation to operators during harvesting and transportation of canary seed. Thus, elimination of hairs is necessary and a crucial requirement for expanding production and uses of canary seed.

Because of the hazards associated with the presence of hairs on the surface of canary seed, several attempts to remove them were conducted using traditional breeding programs as well as chemical and mechanical processing technologies (Abdel-Aal et al 1997a). In Canada, a hairless glabrous canary seed cultivar was developed by mutagenesis (Hucl et al 2001b). The hairless cultivar was registered under the name CDC Maria. Because canary seed has no history of human consumption in Canada, it is considered a "novel food" by Health Canada, the Canadian federal department responsible for ensuring the health and safety of drugs, food, chemicals, pesticides, etc. Canary seed is currently being assessed by Health Canada as a potential food crop as regards its safety and grain quality. This kind of assessment requires multidisciplinary input and is a lengthy process. The availability of hairless (nonitchy) canary seed cultivars will help promote the development of canary seed as a food and feed crop. Robinson (1978) concluded that no toxicity problem exists with canary seed grain because generations of caged birds have survived on the grain as a major part of their diet. However, the birds dehull the seeds before consumption, and the seeds are also polished to remove trichomes before they are marketed as birdseed. Additionally, a German monograph published in 1885 reported that canary seed has been used for human consumption and in flour blends for making bread (Körnicke and Werner 1885).

The present chapter is designed to highlight the properties and unique characteristics of canary seed components (i.e., starch, protein, and lipids) and their potential food and nonfood uses. The development of the commercial hairless canary seed and its agronomic properties and production are also discussed.

Origin and Classification

Annual canarygrass (*Phalaris canariensis* L.) is grown primarily for the production of grain as a source of bird seed and is known in the trade as canary seed. In French and Spanish, canary seed goes by the name *alpiste*, and in German it is referred to as *Kanariensaat*. The genus *Phalaris* belongs to the botanical family Poaceae (Gramineae) and subfamily Pooideae. Thus, annual canarygrass is somewhat genetically related but completely reproductively isolated from common cereal crops such as wheat (*Triticum aestivum* L.), barley (*Hordeum vulgare* L.), and oat (*Avena sativa* L.). Anderson (1961) reviewed the literature and described what he considered to be 15 separate species within the genus *Phalaris*. Annual canarygrass is the only annual species in the genus that has been domesticated as a grain crop. Another annual species (*Phalaris angusta*) is used as a fodder crop. The remaining annual species are not domesticated, some being weeds (Anderson, 1961), primarily in other cereal crops. A number of perennial *Phalaris* species (e.g., *P. arundinaceae*; reed canarygrass) are cultivated as forage crops. Annual canarygrass is of Mediterranean origin. Weedy species of *Phalaris* (e.g., *P. minor*) are found around the Mediterranean basin and farther east (Anderson 1961). The *P. minor* species (littleseed canarygrass) is a problem weed in wheat fields in Pakistan and India (Singh et al 1999, Qureshi and Bhatti 2001) and in Mediterranean climates, including California. Littleseed canarygrass biotypes have developed resistance to a number of herbicides (Malik and Singh 1995, Tal et al 1996), making this species a more problematic weed. Short-spiked canarygrass (*P. brachystachys*) is another problem weed in cereal crops in the Mediterranean basin (Afentouli and Eleftherohorinos 1996). Paradoxagrass (*P. paradoxa*) is a major weed in winter wheat production in Australia (Walker et al 2001).

Annual canarygrass is a diploid with ($2n = 12$), whereas most other *Phalaris* species (annual and perennial) have a basic chromosome number of $x = 7$. The only other species with $2n = 12$ are the weedy annual *P. brachystachys* and the perennial *P. truncata* (Anderson 1961). Based on isozyme and morphological analyses, *P. canariensis* and *P. brachystachys* are closely related (Matus and Hucl 1999, Matus-Cádiz and Hucl 2002). Taking into account the chromosome number homology between the two species, one can infer that *P. brachystachys* is probably the ancestral species from which annual canarygrass is derived.

Canary seed was first domesticated in the Mediterranean region. However, no evidence currently exists to indicate specifically where this domestication took place. Anderson (1961) quotes a number of seventeenth- and eighteenth-century references that allude to canary seed or to a morphologically similar species originating in the Canary Islands, in Spain, or in both areas, and being used to feed birds. Körnicke and Werner (1885) indicate that canary seed was assumed to originate in the Canary Islands. It is not clear whether the crop is named after the islands or after the birds (*Serinus canarius*) that originated there. In any case, the grain was fed to canaries, and the spread of the two outward from Spain to countries such as Belgium was linked (Körnicke and Werner 1885). A mid-1700 dictionary indicates that *alpiste* is a Basque word, suggesting that canary seed has a long history on the Iberian peninsula.

Production

Canary seed is produced primarily in Canada and Argentina (FAO 2000), and to a lesser extent in Australia, the United States, North Africa, and the Middle East (Putnam et al 1996). Canada accounts for 65% of the global production (Putnam et al 1996). Canary seed production on a global scale has ranged between 167,000 and 307,000 metric tonnes (MT) (McVicar et al 2002). Canadian production of canary seed fluctuates quite widely, averaging 155,800 MT per annum from 157,500 ha in recent years (Saskatchewan Agriculture and Food 1997). The province of Saskatchewan accounts for more than 90% of the Canadian production (McVicar et al 2002). Major importers of canary seed are Mexico, Brazil, the United States, Belgium, Spain, and Italy. Highly urbanized countries tend to carry higher populations of small, caged birds and are thus markets for canary seed (McVicar et al 2002).

Canary seed was initially grown in the northern Great Plains in the Red River valley of North Dakota and Minnesota starting after World War II. Production subsequently shifted to Manitoba, reaching that province by 1963 (Manitoba Agriculture and Food 1999) and subsequently shifting to central Saskatchewan starting in the early 1970s. Currently, more than 1,000 Canadian growers produce the crop. During the 1970s, up to 700 growers produced canary seed in Minnesota and North Dakota (Robinson 1978). By the late 1980s, the area sown to canary seed there had decreased to fewer than 1,200 ha (Putnam et al 1990). The area sown to canary seed in Argentina annually varies between 19,000 and 125,000 ha (Bodega et al 1996). Australian production varies between 3,000 and 10,000 MT annually (Norton and Ford 2001).

Nine *Phalaris* canariensis cultivars are currently eligible for seed certification according to the Organization for Economic Co-operation and Development (OECD 2002). Six cultivars are registered in Hungary and one each in the Netherlands, Yugoslavia, and the United States. Three pure-line selections from the USDA germ plasm collection were released as cultivars in the United States. Two of those cultivars, Keet (Robinson 1979) and Elias (Robinson1983), are still widely grown.

The canary seed grains are polished to remove the hairs before packaging for consumption by birds. Birds tend to remove the hulls before ingestion.

Canario

Annual canarygrass was assigned the genus designation *Phalaris* by Linnaeus, the eighteenth-century taxonomist who devised the nomenclature system (genus species) (Anderson 1961). The dictionary (Oxford English Dictionary 1971) definition of the term *Phalarism* is as follows:

> like that of Phalaris the tyrant of Agrigentum, who caused those condemned to death by him to be roasted alive in a brazen bull, the maker himself being the first victim. Inhuman cruelty; pleasure in the infliction of torture.

The same dictionary also refers to the noun *Phalaric* (from the Etruscan *falaric*):

> a javelin or dart wrapped in tow and pitch, set on fire and thrown by the catapult or by hand, in order to set fire to a fortified place, a ship, etc.

A brief historical description of Phalaris's exploits is presented elsewhere (Wikipedia 2002). Why did Linnaeus select the genus name in question for canarygrass? Canary seed is one of two species initially assigned to the genus (Anderson 1961).

The hulls (paleae, lemmae, and glumes) of canary seed are covered in microscopic trichomes (hairs). These trichomes break off during harvesting and subsequent grain handling and make canary seed dust very irritating to the skin (Alberta Agriculture, Food and Rural Development 1998). Those combine harvesting the crop are urged to wear dust masks when dealing with canary seed (McVicar et al 2002). Grain handlers generally do not like dealing with the crop because of its extremely irritating properties (Putnam et al 1996). The mineral content of the canary seed trichomes is 98% silicon. This is higher than the silicon content of either asbestos (60%) or glass fiber (O'Neill et al 1980). The trichomes become silicified after the panicle emerges from the boot (Sangster et al 1983). The dimensions of the trichomes, a length of 500 μm and a tip radius of 0.3 μm (Newman and MacKay 1983) are similar to those of potentially carcinogenic mineral fibers (O'Neill et al 1980) such as asbestos. O'Neill et al (1980) linked wild canary seed trichomes to esophageal cancer in a region of Iran where the annual *Phalaris* was a weed in wheat fields. The canary seed grain contaminated the harvested wheat, and the trichomes persisted intact through the milling process to the baked product. The trichomes also survived when heated at temperatures up to 550°C for 5 hr (Abdel-Aal et al 1997a). The blending of wheat flour with canary seed flour may be linked to esophageal cancer in Brazil (O'Neill et al 1986). In a controlled study, Bhatt et al (1984) demonstrated that the canary seed trichomes could promote benign skin tumors in mice.

The skin-irritating properties of canary seed coupled with potentially serious health risks provide a basis for eliminating the trichomes via genetic means. This was achieved by the selection of an induced genetic variant (Hucl et al 2001a). The initial glabrous cultivar, CDC Maria, lacks trichomes on the paleae, lemmae, and glumes of the panicle. The absence of trichomes increases the test weight by 12% and produces a cleaner harvested sample. The glabrous cultivar yields, on average, 10% less than the cultivar Keet from which it was derived. The net effect of the increased test weight, reduced chaffiness, and grain yield is a reduction of 30% in harvest volume.

The glabrous trait in canary seed is controlled by a single gene (Matus-Cádiz et al 2003), with the glabrous phenotype being recessive to the pubescent condition. In addition to the glabrous trait, a yellow-seeded genetic variant has been isolated in canary seed (Matus-Cádiz et al 2003). Yellow seed color is recessive to the wild-type brown color present in commercial cultivars.

Agronomic Properties

The long-term average commercial grain yield of canary seed in Saskatchewan is 1,100 kg/ha (McVicar et al 2002). The average yields vary widely (697–1,267 kg/ha) from one crop district to the next in any given year (Saskatchewan Agriculture and Food 1997). On average, canary seed achieves 34–50% of the yield obtained by Canada Western Red Spring wheat cultivars grown under uniform conditions (Miller 2000). The canary seed plant is shallow rooted and thus sensitive to high temperature and drought stress. Under such stresses, the crop will suffer extensive tiller mortality, panicle blasting, or both (McVicar et al 2002). Panicle blasting refers to the abortion of florets, starting at the apex of the panicle. The degree of blasting varies with the magnitude of the crop stress. Annual canarygrass evolved as a winter annual in a Mediterranean climate. Thus the crop is classified as a cool-season crop and does best in a crop-growing regime that includes cooler conditions during the vegetative stage of the plant.

Because of its sensitivity to environmental stress, canary seed is best adapted to heavier-textured, moisture-retaining soils in regions where wheat is also grown. Canary seed produces excessive vegetative growth under conditions of excessive moisture and soil fertility, resulting in a very low harvest index. Canary seed is generally characterized by low harvest indices ranging from 12 to 24% (Holt and Hunter 1987; Bodega et al 1996, 1998; Norton and Ford 2001). In comparison, the harvest index for spring wheat varies between 35 and 45%. In an attempt to reduce straw production, Bodega et al (1996, 1998) treated the crop with chemical growth regulators such as chlormequat. These treatments had no effect on straw length, grain yield or harvest index.

To keep canary seed economically competitive with other crops, plant-breeding efforts will need to emphasize increased grain yields and increased harvest indices.

Canary seed is later maturing than wheat and has a tough straw that slows down combine harvesting. It is recommended that canary seed be sown early, particularly in environments characterized by terminal drought (Miller 2000). On average, an early or mid-May seeding date is optimal for canary seed grain yield in Saskatchewan (May et al 2001). The crop may have a slight vernalization requirement (Miller 2000), which means that delayed seeding is likely to aggravate its tendency to mature late. Miller (2000) and Norton and Ford (2001) detected a mild vernalization requirement in canary seed. Norton and Ford (2001) concluded that annual canarygrass is a long-day plant (photoperiod-sensitive).

Canary seed has a relatively strong seed dormancy and requires two to four weeks of after-ripening to ensure satisfactory germination levels (Matus-Cádiz et al 2001).

The seeding rate for canary seed can vary widely (15–60 kg/ha), without significantly affecting yield. The lack of a seeding rate response has been reported in both the United States and Canada (Holt 1989, Putnam et al 1990, May et al 2001). Canary seed can tiller profusely and can thus compensate for lower plant populations. Similarly, canary seed yields are generally not affected by row spacing in the 23–30-cm range (Holt 1989). A seeding rate of 30 kg/ha is recommended as this may help compensate for poor seedling emergence and improve competition with weeds during the early stages of crop development (Putnam et al 1996). The small seed size and weak seedling growth of canary seed require that the crop not be sown too deeply. Seeding depths of greater than 5 cm are not recommended.

The fertilizer requirement of canary seed is thought to be similar to that of wheat, taking into account its lower grain yield potential. Canary seed grain yield increased in response to increased nitrogen fertilizer rates in each year of a six-year study conducted in eastern Saskatchewan (Holt 1988), with an optimum of 50–75 kg ha^{-1} of applied nitrogen. The nitrogen source was ammonium nitrate for three years and urea for the subsequent three years of the study. Averaged over six years, grain yield increased by 76% when 75 kg of nitrogen was applied relative to the control of 0.0 kg ha^{-1}. The N-response was observed in both low- and high-yielding years. Increased nitrogen fertilization increased plant height, had no effect on seed weight, and reduced test weight (Holt 1988). A more recent study conducted at four sites in Saskatchewan detected small yield responses to nitrogen fertilization in five of nine trials (May et al 2001). In the United States, canary seed response to nitrogen fertilization was not consistent (Putnam et al 1990). Grain yield response to potassium and sulfur was evaluated in a one-year study at five sites (May et al 2001). There is currently no information on the effect of micronutrients on canary seed plant growth.

Canary seed has a slow-growing seedling, which results in slow canopy closure and very poor competition against weeds. It is thus essential that weeds be controlled early during crop development. Currently eight herbicides are registered for weed control in canary seed in Canada (McVicar et al 2002). Canary seed is very sensitive to a number of herbicides with residual activity in the soil, requiring a minimum 24-month break before planting.

Crop Diseases

Septoria leaf mottle caused by the fungal pathogen *Septoria triseti* was first reported in Saskatchewan in 1987 (Berkenkamp et al 1989) and was the most widespread disease in canary seed in 1988. Since its first appearance, canary seed leaf mottle has been of economic significance, particularly in wet years. The disease can be very destructive in that most of the leaf area is destroyed before it is detected in the upper canopy. The canary seed plant tends to have small flag and penultimate leaves compared to leaves formed in the lower canopy. Once the pathogen has destroyed the lower leaves, little photosynthetic area is left to maintain grain yield potential in the crop. The use of fungicides to control leaf mottle has resulted in yield increases of 20–40%, depending on the severity of the disease (May et al 2001). Canary seed seedlings are susceptible to *Fusarium graminearum* infection under controlled testing conditions (Chongo et al 2001), with a 60% reduction in emergence, a level similar to that obtained for wheat, rye, and triticale. No reports exist on the impact of *Fusarium* on canary seed under field conditions. The causal agent of common root rot in wheat and barley, *Bipolaris sorokiniana*, forms conidia on the crowns of canary seed plants, but the sporulation levels are 12–20% of those observed in spring wheat (Duczek et al 1996). Ergot infestations can occur in canary seed under high rainfall conditions (McVicar et al 2002).

Dehulling Process

Canary seed produces small, elliptical grains with lengths and widths of approximately 4.0–5.1 and 1.5–2.0 mm, respectively (Abdel-Aal et al 1997a). The grain weighs approximately 7 mg, with an average hulled test weight of 63 kg/hL (Hucl et al 1997). The test weight of hulled canary seed is lower than that of hard red spring wheat by about 15%. Removal of the hulls increases test weight to levels similar to those of common wheat. After hull removal, the dehulled canary seed grain is called a groat, or more precisely, a canary groat, as suggested by Abdel-Aal et al (1997a). The canary groat is approximately two-thirds the length of a common wheat kernel length and one-half its width, and about one-sixth the wheat kernel weight.

The shape and size of seed are crucial factors in selecting and designing equipment for cleaning and dehulling processes. The elliptical shape and small size of canary seed require certain equipment in cleaning and dehulling processes. A cone-type dehuller was designed and constructed by the Department of Agricultural and Bioresource Engineering, University of Saskatchewan, to separate the hulls and to produce dehulled canary seed or canary groat (Hucl et al 2001a). This dehuller consists of a hopper, a guillotine-type seed-flow regulator, a shroud section, a rubber-lined screen section, a rubber-coated aluminum cone mounted on a splined shaft, a height-adjustment rod, a bucket collection system, a cyclone for dust collection, a shaft receiver/bearing permitting vertical shaft movement, a motor-and-pulley drive system, and an inverter speed control. The efficiency of the dehulling device is evaluated by manual inspection of a subsample obtained from the aspirated seed. The subsample is separated into three categories, including seed with hull, seed without hull, and broken or damaged seed. Each category of seed is assessed using the following criteria:

$$\% \text{ broken seeds} = \frac{\text{mass of broken or damaged seeds}}{\text{mass of aspirated subsample}}$$

$$\% \text{ hulled seeds} = \frac{\text{mass of seeds retaining hulls}}{\text{mass of aspirated subsample}}$$

$$\% \text{ dehulled seeds} = \frac{\text{mass of seeds without hulls}}{\text{mass of aspirated subsample}}$$

A dehulling effectiveness index is calculated using the following equation:

$$D_{\text{eff}} = \frac{1}{m_{\text{s}}}[(m_{\text{c}} + m_{\text{hr}}) - (m_{\text{ud}} + m_{\text{br}})]$$

where D_{eff} is dehulling effectiveness index; m_s is mass of the original sample; m_c is mass of dehulled seeds; m_{hr} is mass of hull recovered by aspiration; m_{ud} is mass of hulled seed; and m_{br} is mass of broken seeds.

The presence of broken or damaged seeds is undesirable and hence must be minimized, whereas the percentage of successfully dehulled seeds should be maximized. The dehulling-effectiveness index (D_{eff}) is a performance index that penalizes operations resulting in excessive breakage or incomplete dehulling (Sokhansanj 1997). The theoretical range of D_{eff} is from –1 (complete destruction of seed) to +1 (perfect dehulling without waste).

The variation in dehulling effectiveness is a function of machine speed and seed-flow rate. The cone-type dehulling machine speed of 1,100 rpm and feed rate of 0.95 kg/min resulted in the highest dehulling effectiveness (0.85), with 91.3% of the seeds dehulled and only 2.4% of seeds retaining hulls. The percentage of broken seeds in the aspirated seed sample with the same operation conditions was 6.1%. Tempering of canary seed to 12, 14, and 16% moisture content or heating the seeds to 250°C for 1 min (10% moisture) followed by fluidized bed heating to 90°C for 3 min before dehulling did not significantly improve dehulling effectiveness as compared with the non-pretreated seeds. The percentage of broken seeds was not reduced when compared with the control sample. Passing the seeds twice through the dehuller significantly reduced the percentage of seeds retaining hulls to 0.29%, compared with 2.4% for a single pass. In general, the cone-type dehulling machine equipped with rubber dehulling surfaces performed well using a single pass without pretreatment. After aspiration, fewer than 2.5% of seeds contained hulls.

Milling Performance

The milling performance of canary groat was evaluated by roller milling to separate canary groat into flour (starchy endosperm) and bran (outer layers and germ) fractions (Abdel-Aal et al 1997a). Flour yield of canary groat is significantly affected by tempering moisture level with or without additional sifting (Hucl et al 2001a). As the tempering moisture is increased, canary groat flour yield decreased because of the very soft endosperm, which is broken down into small pieces attached to the seed coat. Soaking and drying at 50°C to 14.0% moisture content before milling resulted in an increase in flour yield. Drying at higher temperature, however, produced a lower flour yield. The same finding was observed when canary groat was roasted. Despite the differences in flour yield resulting from using different tempering moisture levels, slight differences in Hunterlab color scores (*L*, *a*, and *b*) were found between canary groat flours. Slight changes due to soaking, drying, or roasting were also observed in the colors of the flours.

The microstructure of canary groat flour appears as aggregates of starch granules that are embedded in a protein matrix and are clearly dissimilar to those of wheat flour (Abdel-Aal et al 1997a). The particle size of the aggregates ranges from 25 to 35 μm. The bran fraction consists of thin flakes 0.3–1.0 mm in their longest magnitude. The flour and bran fractions do not exhibit any evidence of the presence of trichomes. The results suggest that roller milling can be used to fractionate canary groat into flours at various extraction rates (50–75%) for a diverse range of food and nonfood applications.

Components of Canary Seed

Starch

Little information is available about the structure and composition of carbohydrates in canary seed. Canary groat is a cereal grain containing starch as the major component, averaging 61% db, which is comparable to common wheat (Abdel-Aal et al 1997a). By fractionating the groat into flour and bran (flour yield of about 75%), starch is concentrated in the flour fraction to approximately 67%. Other carbohydrate components found in canary groat are sucrose and dietary fiber. Sucrose averages approximately 0.8%, accounting for about 47% of total soluble sugars (1.7%), whereas fructose and glucose are present at very low concentrations (<0.1%). The concentration of total soluble sugars in canary groat is too low to have a major effect on storage or utilization. Canary groat is found to have relatively low concentrations of soluble and insoluble dietary fiber, approximately half that in common wheat (Abdel-Aal et al 1997a).

The starch extracted from canary groat by the alkali steeping isolation process ranges from 46.6 to 52.3 g per 100 g, with an average of 49.7 ± 2.9 g/100 g (Abdel-Aal et al 1997b). This yield is higher than that obtained from common wheat (46.8 g/100 g), even though wheat grain contains a slightly higher level of starch. The mean extraction efficiency of 77% for canary groat is significantly higher than the 72% obtained for wheat. Canary seed starches are relatively low in amylose content, ranging from 16.2 to 19.5% in three samples, compared to 22.7% in wheat and 24.5% in corn starch. The average diameter of canary seed starch granules (n > 1,000 readings) is 2.0 μm (more than 95% of the granules have a diameter in the range of 1.5–3.5 μm and about

48% in the range of 1.5–2.5 μm), which falls within the range (0.5–3.0 μm) usually considered small (Wilhelm 1992). In an earlier study, Goering and Schuh (1967) reported a granule size range of 2.5–5.0 μm for starch isolated from canary seed. The granule sizes of amaranth and quinoa starches are comparable to those of canary seed starch. The small and uniform granule size of canary seed starch relative to potato, corn, and wheat starches is a feature that may hold promise because many applications benefits from a uniform small granule size.

Canary seed starch had a high pasting temperature and intermediate peak viscosity compared to wheat and corn starch when slurries (8%, pH 5.5) were heated in a Brabender viscoamylograph (Abdel-Aal et al 1997b). During the cooking period at 95°C for 30 min, the viscosity of canary seed starch was consistent, indicating high shear and heat stability. On cooling, the canary seed starch pastes showed higher setback viscosity compared with wheat and corn starches. When canary seed starch gel was stored in a refrigerator at 4°C or in a freezer at –15°C for seven days, the degree of syneresis was lower than for wheat and corn starch gels by about 3.0%, showing a higher gel stability. The microstructure (SEM) of canary seed starch granules, pastes, and gels obtained at specific points of the amylograph cycle are presented in Figure 1.

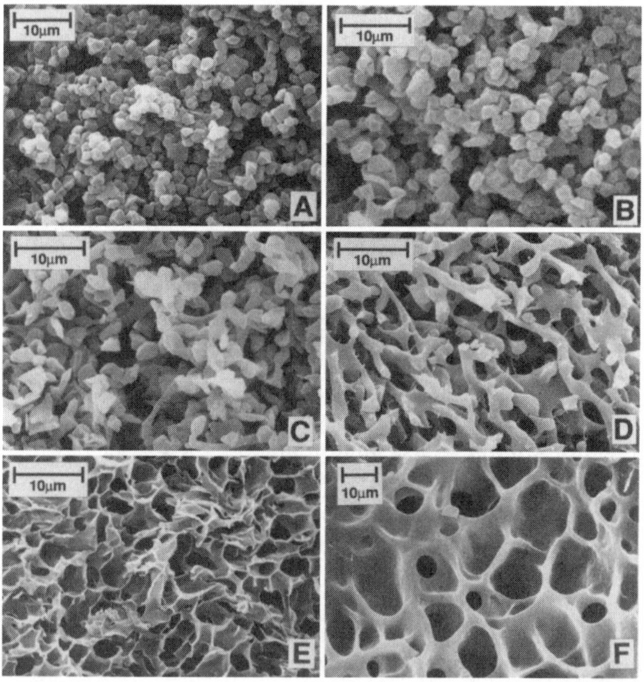

Fig. 1. SEM photomicrographs of canary seed native starch and starch slurries (8%) sampled from viscoamylograph: **(A)** native starch, **(B)** at 60°C, **(C)** at 90°C, **(D)** at 95°C, **(E)** at peak viscosity (after 10 min of holding at 95°C), and **(F)** after cooling to 50°C. (Adapted from Abdel-Aal et al 1997b)

The native starch granules have a polygonal shape and uniform size (Figure 1A). At 60°C, the granules start to swell but remain intact (Figure 1B). At 90°C, the granule swelling is much more extensive and the granules exhibit more extended flat linear structures (Figure 1C). When the temperature reaches 95°C, almost all the granules associate into linear composite structures (Figure 1D). After reaching the peak viscosity temperature (during the holding period at 95°C), the linear structures disappear and a three-dimensional network is formed (Figure 1E). The gel structure continues to develop and becomes more rigid after cooling to 50°C (Figure 1F). Abdel-Aal et al (1997b) suggested that the amylose and amylopectin chains in canary seed starch granules are associated through relatively strong bonding forces that hold the linear structures together during the initial heating and shearing treatments and after cooling.

The average DSC onset, peak, and completion gelatinization temperatures of canary seed starches (55, 65, and 76°C, respectively) are higher than those

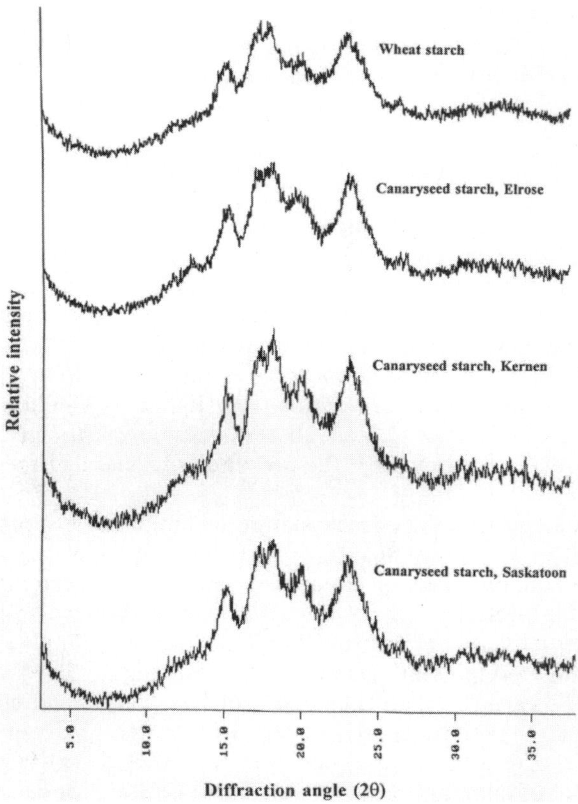

Fig. 2. X-ray diffraction patterns of canary seed and wheat starches. (Adapted from Abdel-Aal et al 1997b)

of wheat (55, 59, and 70°C, respectively) (Abdel-Aal et al 1997b). The greater enthalpy of gelatinization of canary seed starch compared to that of wheat further supports the suggestion that stronger molecular associations exist within the canary seed starch granule's macromolecular complex than in a wheat starch granule. These results also support the amylograph data showing high granule stability in canary seed starch and may relate to the formation of the linear polymeric structures when peak viscosity is achieved.

X-ray diffraction of canary seed starches shows major peaks near *d*-spacings of 5.9, 5.2, 4.8, and 3.8 Å, as does wheat (Figure 2). Zobel (1988) reported that X-ray *d*-spacings of 5.8, 5.2, and 3.8 Å are characteristics of the A-type starch crystal that is common to most cereal starches. Canary seed starch granules possess the three *d*-spacings and thus are considered A-type starch. The *d*-spacing of 4.4 Å, which is characteristic of the amylose-lipid complex (Zobel 1988), is found in two canary seed starch samples, suggesting the presence of amylose-lipid complex in at least some canary seed starch.

In general, canary seed starch consists of granules that are uniformly small with a low amylose content. Canary seed starch has the characteristics of an A-type starch crystal that is common to most cereal starches. The starch forms rigid gels with high stability on cooling and freezing. These features make canary seed starch distinct from wheat or corn starch, and they may allow development of canary seed as a source of specialty starch, such as in cosmetic applications.

Protein

Canary seed is exceptionally high in protein for a cereal crop. The average protein content in canary groat is 18.7% (N × 5.7) or 20.5% (N × 6.25), which exceeds that of high-protein hard red spring wheat by about 25% (Abdel-Aal et al 1997a). Earlier studies also showed that canary seed contains higher levels of protein than do other cereal grains (Robinson 1978, Holt 1988, Putnam et al 1996). The protein distribution in the groat appears to be relatively uniform because the bran and flour fractions are similar in protein concentration, exceeding 20%. With greater than 20% protein in canary groat flour, this component would have a major influence on nutritional and functional properties.

Using the classic solubility fractionation technique of Osborne with some modifications as outlined by Sosulski and Bakal (1969), canary seed proteins were found to contain levels of albumins (water-soluble proteins) and globulins (salt-soluble proteins), which were well below the levels found in common wheat (Abdel-Aal et al 1997a). Prolamins (alcohol- soluble proteins) are the major storage proteins in canary groat, averaging 45.5% of total protein, compared to 37.1% in wheat. The total prolamins and glutelins (dilute base soluble proteins) constitute approximately 78% of the total canary seed proteins. The ratio of prolamins to glutelins in canary seed proteins is 1.4, much higher than that of common wheat (1.0). This indicates that canary seed flour may have the potential to produce viscous, not elastic, dough that may be similar to that produced from ancient wheats. The high prolamin content in canary seed proteins would not be predicted from its low proline content, and further studies are needed on this protein fraction.

Among the essential amino acids, canary seed proteins are found to be deficient in lysine and threonine for human and animal requirements, as are most cereal proteins. Canary seed proteins contain only two-thirds of the lysine found in wheat protein, but canary seed is comparable to wheat in threonine level. The methionine concentration in canary seed proteins is comparable to that of wheat, which in turn is only one-half of the level found in casein and the FAO standard. The deficiency in this sulfur-containing amino acid is ameliorated by the presence of high concentrations of cystine, which is methionine-sparing during protein synthesis. Tryptophan is another essential amino acid that is commonly deficient in dietary protein sources. The tryptophan level in canary seed protein is exceptionally high. At 2.8 g/100 g protein, canary seed would be an excellent supplement or blending protein for other cereal (wheat at 1.1 g/100 g) or animal (casein at 1.0 g/100 g) protein sources that barely meet the FAO pattern of 1.1 g/100 g protein. Of the limited data available on tryptophan concentrations in canary seed, Robinson (1978) reported 3.3 g/100 g protein and Holt (1988) reported 2.0 g/100 g protein. The high concentrations of cystine, tryptophan, phenylalanine, and arginine combined with low levels of lysine and proline suggest a unique protein composition and functionality in canary seed. The low concentration of lysine and high concentration of arginine provide a low lysine-to-arginine ratio that was found to be hypocholesterolemic in soybean protein (Kritchevsky 1979). The ratio is 0.9 in soybean protein but only 0.2 in canary seed protein, which suggests that a hypocholesterolemic effect might be provided by canary seed proteins.

Lipid

The purified total lipid content in canary groat averages about 11.0% compared to 2.6% in common wheat (Abdel-Aal et al 1997a). Thus, the total lipids in canary seed groat are a major component, a high proportion of which is polar lipids that were not extracted with the nonpolar solvents such as diethyl ether, which extracts only 8.7% crude fat. This level, however, is about four times that in common wheat. In an earlier study, Robinson (1978) reported that canarygrass caryopses are much higher in oil, nitrogen, ash, phosphorus, and potassium than other grain crops, but lower in fiber. Canary seed oil is highly unsaturated, consisting mainly of linoleic (54%), oleic (32%), and palmitic (12%) acids (Malik and Williams 1966). However, the crude oil exhibits an excellent antioxidant activity; sterol and triterpene alcohol esters of caffeic acid are the major effective antioxidant components in the crude oil (Takagi and Iida 1980).

The fatty acid composition of canary seed total lipid is somewhat similar to that of crude oil. In general, the canary seed fatty acid profile is 55% linoleic, 29% oleic, 11% palmitic, 2.5% linolenic, and 1% stearic acid, compared with 62% linoleic, 17% oleic, 16% palmitic, 4% linolenic, and 1% stearic acid in wheat grown side by side with canary seed (Abdel-Aal et al 1997a). This profile is similar to that reported by Malik and Williams (1966) for canary seed oil. The results showed that canary seed and wheat lipids are highly unsaturated and potentially subject to rapid rancidity, but because of the high antioxidant activity in canary seed oil, the oil can last for a relatively long time without developing rancidity. Additionally, canary seed lipid has a higher ratio (7.5) of unsaturated to saturated fatty acids, compared to 5.0 obtained for wheat lipids, but it contains less polyunsaturated fatty acids (57%) than the 68% contained in wheat lipid. The lower levels of polyunsaturated fatty acids, particularly linolenic, might be another reason for the longer shelf life of canary seed oil.

Biologically Active Components

Phytate, phenols, tannins, enzyme inhibitors, glucosides, and alkaloids are natural metabolic compounds found in cereals. The genus *Phalaris* was found to contain a wide range of indole alkaloids such as tryptamine, β-carboline, gramine, and their derivatives and phenolic alkaloid (e.g., hordenine). These alkaloids are found mainly in the plant leaves, but dhurrin, a toxic cyanogenic glucoside, was found in the seedlings of sorghum. The functions of these naturally occurring compounds in plants are still questionable, but most likely they provide protection against predation. The effects of these compounds on human health are debatable, and although some certainly are toxic in sufficient amounts, recently some of these compounds have been considered as health promoters with some evidence for a role in reducing the risk of chronic diseases and in protecting cells and tissues against body free radicals.

Phytate is considered anitnutritional because it may chelate minerals such as calcium and zinc in the human body. However, beneficial effects such as ability to lower blood glucose response to starchy foods, reduce plasma levels of cholesterol and triacylglycerols, and reduce cancer risk have also been observed (Rickard and Thompson 1997). Phytic acid is mainly concentrated in the cotyledon of legumes and oilseeds but in the outer layers of cereal grains. Canary groat was found to contain relatively high levels of phytate compared to common wheat, averaging about 18.8 mg/g versus 10.7 mg/g in wheat (Hucl et al 2001a). Removal of the outer layers on a roller mill significantly reduced phytic acid content in the flour fractions and concentrated it in the bran, at 32.9 mg/g compared to 21.7 mg/g in wheat bran.

Phenolic compounds exist in several chemical forms in many plants. These compounds possess antioxidant properties, which play an important role in human nutrition and health as well as in preserving the quality of food products by controlling lipid oxidation. Canary seed oil was found to contain sterol and triterpene alcohol esters of caffeic acid with high antioxidant properties (Takagi and Iida 1980). The content of total phenolics in canary groat is similar to that of common wheat, averaging 0.84 mg/g (Hucl et al 2001a). After milling, the phenolic compounds are concentrated mainly in the bran fractions, particularly in the wheat bran. The flour fractions of canary groat, however, still contain higher concentrations of total phenolic compounds compared with the flour of common wheat.

Low levels of trypsin inhibitor were detected in both canary groat and common wheat, averaging about 0.51 trypsin inhibitor units (TIU)/mg compared to 30.26 TIU/mg in soybean, a rich source of trypsin inhibitor (Hucl et al 2001a). Removal of the branny material from the grains reduced trypsin inhibitor activity by about one-third, but it increased in the bran fraction by about 18%. Canary groat and common wheat had similar α-amylase inhibitor activities (Hucl et al 2001a). After milling, however, the two grains behave slightly differently. In the case of canary groat, an α-amylase inhibitor is concentrated in the flour fraction, while in wheat it is concentrated in the wheat bran fractions.

Alkaloids are nitrogen-containing organic compounds that can be potentially toxic. They are found in some species and families of higher plants, particularly in leguminosae as by-products of plant metabolism, as a reservoir for protein synthesis, or as protective agents. Several types of alkaloids have been found in reed canarygrass (forage crop), which are grouped into phenol (e.g., hordenine), indole (e.g., gramine, tryptamine), and β-carbolines (Østrem 1987). These alkaloids were determined in canary groat and its milled products by gas liquid chromatography as described by Duynisveld et al (1990). Canary groat and its milling fractions are found to have no detectable levels of the above-mentioned alkaloids (Hucl et al 2001a). These results were confirmed by using high-performance liquid chromatography techniques as outlined by Muir et al (1992). A standard mixture of gramine, tryptamine, and β-carboline containing 5 mmol was used for calibration and quantification. Again, no alkaloids were detected in canary groat or in any milling product (Hucl et al 2001a). Additionally, selected samples of canary groat products were spiked with pure alkaloids and analyzed by both methods. There was no evidence that canary groat products contain hordenine, gramine, tryptamine, or β-carboline. Also, there was no detectable concentration of dhurrin in canary groat or its milled products (Hucl et al 2001a), using the method described by Gorz et al (1986). The absence of alkaloids in canary seed products can be considered crucial for the development of canary seed for human consumption.

Potential Value of Canary Seed Components

The chemical composition of canary groat makes it a potential source of not only one or two, but three main ingredients: starch (61%), protein (19%), and oil (11%). Thus, canary seed holds promise as a crop suitable for fractionation, with potential for total utilization. Additionally, each of these three primary constituents of commerce show distinct compositional and structural properties, enhancing added-value potential (Abdel-Aal et al 1997a,b). The novel combination of characteristics of canary seed starch of high extraction efficiency, uniform and small granule size, gel formation, and stability could provide the basis of a valuable specialty starch supply for both food and nonfood uses. The elevated content of tryptophan in canary seed proteins would make canary seed an excellent supplement or blending protein with plant and animal proteins that barely meet the human requirement for tryptophan. The very low ratio of lysine to arginine in canary seed protein compared to soybean protein suggests that some health benefits could be provided by the canary seed protein fraction, since in soybean, a low ratio of lysine to arginine in the protein is associated with hypocholesterolemic activity in animals and humans (Kritchevsky 1979). Given the prominence of heart disease associated with high cholesterol levels in many developed nations, additional modes for dietary control of cholesterol levels as opposed to drug use are urgently needed. The high content of oil in canary seed with a distinct fatty acid composition (e.g., high ratio of unsaturated to saturated fat, less polyunsaturated fat) and inherent antioxidant properties could make canary seed oil useful in specific uses. These chemical compositions and characteristics should be addressed during the development of canary seed as a food and as an industrial crop.

Conclusions

The distinctive chemical composition of canary seed associated with the development of hairless cultivars and the absence of naturally occurring toxic constituents could help promote the development of canary seed for human consumption and industrial uses. Further trials on canary groat products are required to ensure safety. Preliminary feeding trials suggested that the nutritive value of canary seed is similar or superior to that of common wheat (Hucl et al 2001a). Additionally, there did not appear to be any significant adverse toxic effects in rats fed canary groat (Hucl et al 2001a). As is usual in such testing, the 50% level of canary seed in the test diets was far beyond what would be expected in a normal human diet. These findings are crucial and should help in promoting canary seed as a food crop. Nevertheless, a larger number of trials is required to confirm these findings and ensure safety.

Once there is a sufficient level of confidence in the acceptance of canary seed as human food, processing technologies for fractionation and novel utilization in foods and nonfoods should be developed to keep apace with the development and promotion of canary seed as a food crop. A wide range of fractionated canary seed commodities are feasible on the basis of its composition and grain characteristics, including intact canary groat, flour, bran, starch, protein, and oil, but these need much more characterization and evaluation in the appropriate food and nonfood applications. Several canary seed food prototypes have been evaluated and explored (e.g., as low-fat sesame substitute in bakery products and as a flour blend for making bread and cookies) (Hucl et al 1997). The present lack of data, relative to mainstream resources, is a constraint to the development of canary seed as a specialty cereal. This can change, of course, only if more funding becomes available for appropriately directed research.

References

Abdel-Aal, E.-S. M., Hucl, P., and Sosulski, F. W. 1997a. Structural and compositional characteristics of canary seed (*Phalaris canariensis* L.). J. Agric. Food Chem. 45:3049-3055.

Abdel-Aal, E.-S. M., Hucl, P., and Sosulski, F. W. 1997b. Characteristics of canary seed (*Phalaris canariensis* L.) starch. Starch/Stärke 49:475-480.

Afentouli, C. G., and Eleftherohorinos, I. G. 1996. Littleseed canarygrass (*Phalaris minor*) and short-spiked canarygrass (*Phalaris brachystachys*) interference in wheat and barley. Weed Sci. 44:560-565.

Alberta Agriculture, Food and Rural Development. 1998. Canary seed. Agri-fax. Agdex 147/20-1.

Anderson, D. E. 1961. Taxonomy and distribution of the genus *Phalaris*. Iowa State J. Sci. 36:1-96.

Berkenkamp, B., Jesperson, G. D., and Bisset, J. 1989. Leaf mottle, a new disease of canarygrass caused by *Septoria triseti*. Plant Dis. 73:859.

Bhatt, T. S., Coombs, M. M., and O'Neill, G. H. 1984. Biogenic silica fibre promotes carcinogenesis in mouse skin. Int. J. Cancer. 34:519-528.

Bodega, J. L., de Dios, M. A., and Pereyra Iraola, M. 1996. Evaluation of two growth regulators on development, stem bending and seed yield of canarygrass (*Phalaris canariensis* L.). Test of agrochemicals and cultivars 17. Ann. Appl. Biol. 128(suppl.):46-47.

Bodega, J. L., de Dios, M. A., and Pereyra Iraola, M. 1998. Evaluation of a growth regulator on development, stem bending and seed yield in canarygrass (*Phalaris canariensis* L.). Test of agrochemicals and cultivars 19. Ann. Appl. Biol. 132(suppl.):34-35.

Chongo, G., Gossen, B. D., Kutcher, H. R., Gilbert, J., Turkington, T. K., Fernandez, M. R., and Mclaren, D. 2001. Reaction of seeding roots of 14 crop species to *Fusarium graminearum* for wheat heads. Can. J. Plant Pathol. 23:132-137.

Duczek, L. J., Jones-Flory, L. L., Reed, S. L., Bailey, K. L., and Lafond, G. P. 1996. Sporulation of *Bipolaris sorokiniana* on the crowns of crop plants grown in Saskatchewan. Can. J. Plant Sci. 76:861-867.

Duynisveld, G. W., Slominski, B. A., Wittenberg, K. M., and Campbell, L. D. 1990. Alkaloid content of reed canarygrass (*Phalaris arundinaceae* L.) as determined by gas-liquid chromatography. Can. J. Plant Sci. 70:1097-1103.

FAO. 2000. Production Year Book. Food and Agriculture Organization, Rome.

Goering, K. J., and Schuh, M. 1967. New starches. III. The properties of the starch from *Phalaris canariensis*. 44:532-538.

Gorz, H. J., Haskins, F. A., and Vogel, K. P. 1986. Inheritance of dhurrin content in mature sorghum leaves. Crop Sci. 26:65-67.

Holt, N. W., and Hunter, J. H. 1987. Annual canarygrass (*Phalaris canariensis* L.) tolerance and weed control following herbicide application. Weed Sci. 35:673-677.

Holt, N. W. 1988. Effect of nitrogen fertilizer on the agronomic performance and seed quality of annual canarygrass. Can. Plant Sci. 68:41-45.

Holt, N. W. 1989. Effects of row spacing and seeding rate on the agronomic performance of annual canarygrass. Can. Plant Sci. 69:1193-1198.

Hucl, P., Abdel-Aal, E.-S. M., Sosulski, F. W., Vandenberg, A., and Hughes, G. 1997. Development of canary seed as a food crop. ADF Project 94000082. Online: http://www.agr.gov.sk.ca

Hucl, P., Han, H. L., Abdel-Aal, E.-S. M., and Hughes, G. 2001a. Development and quality of glabrous canary seed. AFIF Project 96000287. Online: http://www.agr.gov.sk.ca.

Hucl, P., Matus-Cádiz, M., Vandenberg, A., Sosulski, F. W., Abdel-Aal, E.-S. M., Hughes, G. R., and Slinkard, A. E. 2001b. CDC Maria annual canarygrass. Can. J. Plant Sci. 81:115-116.

Körnicke, F., and Werner, H. 1885. *Phalaris canariensis L.* Das Kanariengras. Pages 238-244 in: Handbuch des Getreidebaues. Verlag von Paul Parey, Berlin, Germany.

Kritchevsky, D. 1979. Vegetable protein and atherosclerosis. J. Am. Oil. Chem. Soc. 56:135-140.

Malik, R. K., and Singh, S. 1995. Littleseed canarygrass (*Phalaris minor*) resistance to isoproturon in India. Weed Technol. 9:419-425.

Malik, M. Y., and Williams, W. D. 1966. Composition of the seed oil of *Phalaris canariensis*. J. Sci. Food Agric. 17:174-175.

Manitoba Agriculture and Food. 1999. Manitoba specialty and forage crops industry profiles 1999. Canary seed sector. Online: http://www.gov.mb.ca/agriculture/statistics.

Matus, M., and Hucl, P. 1999. Isozyme variation within and among 143 accessions of annual *Phalaris* L. species in North American germplasm collections. Crop Sci. 39:1222-1228.

Matus-Cádiz, M., and Hucl, P. 2002. Morphological variation within and among five annual *Phalaris* species. Can. J. Plant Sci. 82:85-88.

Matus-Cádiz, M., Hucl, P., and Munasinghe, G. 2001. Seed dormancy and germination in three annual canarygrass (*Phalaris canariensis* L.) cultivars relative to spring wheat (*Triticum aestivum* L.). Seed Sci. Technol. 29:523-531.

Matus-Cádiz, M., Hucl, P., and Vandenberg, A. 2003. Inheritance of hull pubescence and seed color in annual canarygrass. Can. J. Plant Sci. 83:729-735.

May, W. E., Gan, Y., and Lafond, G. L. 2001. The effect of seeding date, seeding rate and applied nitrogen on the yield of canary seed. Pages 162-168 in: Soils and Crops Workshop. University of Saskatchewan, Saskatoon.

McVicar, R., Hartley, S., Brenzil, C., Pearse, P., Panchuk, K., Hucl, P., and May, B. 2002. Canary seed in Saskatchewan. (Factsheet.) Saskatchewan Agriculture, Food and Rural Revitalization, Regina, SK, Canada.

Miller, P. R. 2000. Effect of varying seeding date on crop development, yield and yield components in canary seed. Can. J. Plant. Sci. 80:83-86.

Muir, A. D., Westcott, N. D., and Hinks, C. F. 1992. New quantitative high-performance liquid chromatography method for analysis of gramine in cereal leaf tissue. J. Agric. Food Chem. 40:1836-1838.

Newman, R. H., and MacKay, A. L. 1983. Silica spicules in canarygrass. Ann. Bot. 52:927-929.

Norton, R. M., and Ford, J. F. 2001. Canary seed-industry development for south-eastern Australia. Publ. 01/179, Nov., p. 89. Rural Industries Research and Development Corporation, Kingston, ACT.

Organization for Economic Co-operation and Development (OECD). 2002. OECD List of varieties eligible for Certification 2002/2003. Online: http://www. oecd.org/pdf/M00037000/M00037693.

O'Neill, C. H., Hodges, G. M., Riddle, P. N., Jordan, P. W., Newman, R. H., Flood, T. J., and Toulson, E. C. 1980. A fine fibrous silica contaminant of flour in the high oesophagial cancer area of north-east Iran. Int. J. Cancer 26:617-628.

O'Neill, C. H., Jordan, P., Bhatt, T. S., and Newman, R. H. 1986. Silica and oesophaogeal cancer. CIBA Found. Symp. Proc. 121:214-230.

Østrem, L. 1987. Studies on genetic variation in reed canarygrass, *Phalaris arundinacea* L. 1. Alkaloid type and concentration. Hereditas 107:235-248.

Oxford English Dictionary. 1971. The compact edition of the Oxford English Dictionary. Oxford University Press, Oxford.

Putnam, D. H., Miller, P. R., and Hucl, P. 1996. Potential for production and utilization of annual canarygrass. Cereal Foods World 41:75-83.

Putnam, D. H., Oelke, E. A., Oplinger, E. S., Doll, J. D., and Peters, J. B. 1990. Annual canarygrass. Online: http://www.hort.purdue.edu/newcrop/afcm/cangrass.html

Qureshi, R., and Bhatti, G. R. 2001. Determination of weed communities in wheat (*Triticum aestivum* L.) fields of district Sukkur. Pak. J. Bot. 33:109-115.

Rickard, S. E., and Thompson, L. U. 1997. Interactions and biological effects of phytic acid. Pages 294-312 in: Antinutrients and Phytochemicals in Foods. Symposium Series 662. F. Shahidi, Ed. American Chemical Society, Washington, DC.

Robinson, R. G. 1978. Chemical composition and potential uses of annual canarygrass. Agron. J. 70:797-800.

Robinson, R. G. 1979. Registration of 'Keet' annual canarygrass. Crop Sci. 19:562.

Robinson, R. G. 1983. Registration of 'Elias' annual canarygrass. Crop Sci. 23:1011.

Sangster, A. G., Hodson, M. J., Parry, D. W., and Rees, A. J. 1983. A developmental study of silification in the trichomes and associated epidermal structures of the inflo-resence bracts of the grass *Phalaris canariensis* L. Ann Bot. 52:171-187.

Saskatchewan Agriculture and Food. 1997. Specialty Crop Report. Statistics Branch. Saskatchewan Agriculture and Food. Regina, SK, Canada.

Singh, S., Kirkwood, R., and Marshall, G. 1999. Biology and control of *Phalaris minor* Retz. (littleseed canarygrass) in wheat. Crop Prot. 18:1-16.

Sokhansanj, S. 1997. Separation processing of canola, peas and lentils. ADF Project 94000092. Online: http://www.agr.gov.sk.ca/apps/adf

Sosulski, F. W., and Bakal, A. 1969. Isolated proteins from rapeseed, flax and sunflower meals. Can. Inst. Food Sci. Technol. J. 2:28-32.

Takagi, T., and Iida, T. 1980. Antioxidant for fats and oils from canary seed: Sterol and triterpene alcohol esters of caffeic acid. J. Am. Oil. Chem. Soc. 57:326-330.

Tal, A., Zarka, S., and Rubin, B. 1996. Fenoxaprop-P resistance in *Phalaris minor* conferred by insensitive acetyl-coenzyme A carboxylase. Pesticide Biochem. Physiol. 56:134-140.

Walker, S. R., Robinson, G. R., and Medd, R. W. 2001. Management of *Avena ludoviciana* and *Phalaris paradoxa* with barley and less herbicide in subtropical Australia. Aust. J. Exp. Agric. 41:1179-1185.

Wikipedia. 2002. *Phalaris*. Wikipedia the Free Encyclopedia. Online: http://www.wikipedia.org/wiki/Phalaris

Wilhelm, E. C. 1992. Properties of small starch granules and their application in paper coatings. Pages 180-190 in: Plant Polymeric Carbohydrates. F. Meuser, D. J. Manners, and W. Seibel, Eds. The Royal Society of Chemistry, Cambridge.

Zobel, H. F. 1988. Starch crystal transformations and their industrial importance. Starch/Stärke 40:1-7.

CHAPTER 9

Hulless Oats

Vernon D. Burrows

Agriculture and Agri-Food Canada, Eastern Cereal and Oilseed Research Centre, Ottawa, Canada K1A 0C6

In most oat-growing regions of the world, the covered-seeded oat (*Avena sativa L.*) is the traditional oat of choice, and breeders have continuously bred new improved varieties. These oats were used on the farm to feed domestic animals, especially the work horse and some ruminants. In spite of all the successful breeding efforts, the area devoted to growing oats has declined steadily during the past 100 years because the work horse, the principal user, was replaced with mechanical equipment powered by petroleum products. A relatively small portion of the crop produced each year was used by processors to prepare human food. Interest in oats for human food has increased in recent years because of its recognized nutritional and health benefits, but the number of hectares required for this purpose is much smaller than what was required in former years to service the work horse. With the demise of the work horse, the covered oat lost its major client, and this client was not replaced by nonruminant animals such as pigs and poultry because these animals were unable to digest the hulls. The role of the covered oat has thus been reduced to that of a minor utility, or specialty, crop, which is unfortunate because the oat groat is one of nature's most nutritious and functional cereal grains. It is also a cool-season crop that is broadly adapted and of great value to farmers in northern regions to design proper crop rotations.

The successful breeding and processing of hulless oats represents, in the opinion of this author, an opportunity to return oats to its former greatness. Once the hull is removed genetically, the groat represents a grain that can be used to great advantage in the feed, food, and industrial sectors. It becomes a multipurpose grain and can be used to generate many new niche markets and to replace or complement crops such as corn (*Zea mays* L.) and soybeans (*Glycine max* (L.) *Merr.*) in nonruminant feeding. Heat-demanding corn and soybeans cannot be grown with certainty in traditionally cool regions. Feed grains must be imported, and this adds to the cost of animal production.

Morphology of Hulless and Covered-Seeded Oats

Hulless or naked oat seeds differ from hulled or covered-seeded oats because each floret has a thin, papery hull (lemma and palea) that breaks free from the true caryopsis, or groat, when the crop is threshed (Figure 1). The hulls of covered oats are thick; they are retained by the groat and form part of the harvested yield. They make up approximately 250–330 g kg^{-1} of kernel weight, and they have essentially kept the oat anchored to the farm because of added transportation costs. The hulls of hulless oats are separated from the groats in the combine harvester and are left in the field when the grains are threshed. Consequently, the gross yield of hulless oats is approximately 25–30% less than that of covered oats, but the yield of groats for the two types of oats may be equal (Burrows et al 2001a). This latter conclusion was determined by comparing the groat yields of near-isogenic lines of covered and hulless oats. If the groat yield of a good hulless variety is less than that of a good, standard covered-seeded variety, the difference in yield potential can probably be ascribed to factors other than the genes determining the hulless condition.

The hulless oat is closely related to the covered oat, and both are hexaploids (42 chromosomes) and can be hybridized readily. They both belong to *A. sativa* L. The trait is conditioned by one major gene (Jenkins and Hanson 1976), but several modifier genes have been reported (Moule 1972) that affect the degree of hullessness. In many hybrid populations, it is difficult to isolate varieties that are completely hulless. The typical hulless oat spikelet is multifloreted, with the groats in the primary, secondary, and possibly the tertiary florets hulless. The uppermost fourth floret is often covered. Sometimes the

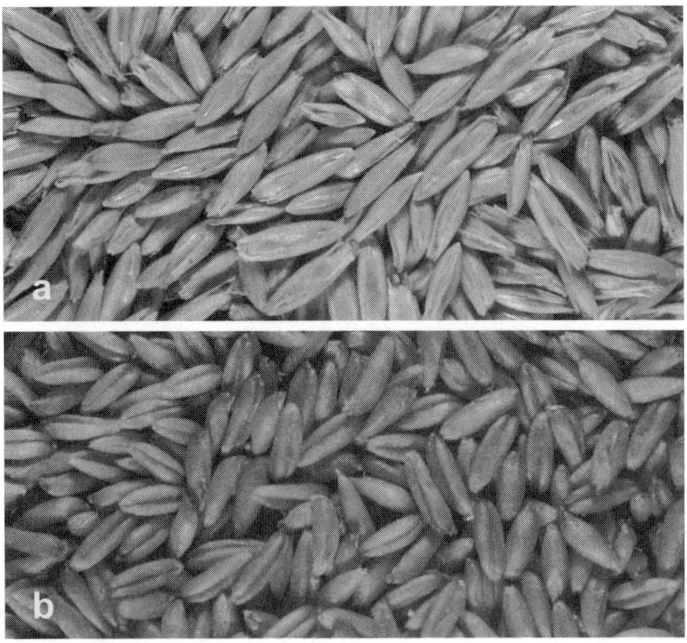

Fig. 1. Threshed samples of covered (AC Rigodon) oat kernels **(a)** and hulless (CN 19197) oat kernels **(b)**.

tertiary kernel at the apex of the panicle branches is also covered. The degree of hulless expression is conditioned by both genetic and environmental factors, and some parents give rise to varieties that have more covered seeds than others. However, some varieties are almost completely hulless, and the presence of any covered seed in the threshed sample may be due to inefficient threshing or exposure of the developing plants to cool temperatures at the time of floral differentiation (Lawes and Boland 1974). Spraying the crop with certain herbicides at the wrong stage of growth (Marshall et al 1992) can also lead to large numbers of covered seeds in threshed grain samples.

The florets in spikelets of different hulless strains are quite variable in their arrangement. Spikelets may be determinate (with two to four florets) or indeterminate (with as many as 8–12 florets), and rachilla length varies greatly (Figure 2). Short rachilla length results in a compact spikelet, which may occur in strains of both determinate and indeterminate ("chevron") spikelets (Burrows 1986a, Burrows et al 2002). Separate genetic systems probably condition both rachilla length and the determinate and indeterminate conditions. A single recessive gene *sr-1* (Burrows et al 2002) was found to be responsible for the very short rachillas of the mutant hulless oat CN 19018. The genetics of the determinate and indeterminate traits have yet to be elucidated. It is very difficult to breed hulless oat varieties that are completely hulless. This represents a problem for seed inspectors in the field because they are unable to determine whether the hulless crop is mixed with covered-seeded varieties. It is also a problem for food processors, who must remove the covered seed before processing. Usually the problem arises most frequently with awnless hulless varieties such as AC Frégeau (CN 99048). In

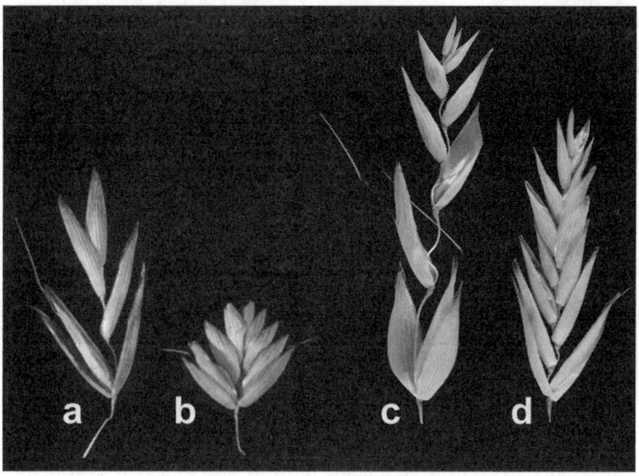

Fig. 2. Determinate spikelets with long rachillas **(a)** and and intermediate spikelets with very short **(b)**, long **(c)**, and short **(d)** rachillas. Spikelets b and d are referred to as "chevron spikelets."

the field, inspectors find it difficult to distinguish between covered-seeded "off-types" and covered-seeded variants. Covered seeds can be present in any hulless variety caused by accidental mixing with seed of covered-seeded varieties. Covered-seeded variants sometimes occur because the variety was not completely homozygous before being distributed to growers. Some covered-seeded variants arise in "pure breeding" varieties as the result of unfavorable environmental conditions, but they usually give rise to hulless progeny in the next generation.

Improving the Expression of Hulless Genes

Two strategies have been followed by the author to solve the problem of incomplete expression of hullessness. The method that has proved to be quite efficient is to breed varieties that are hulless fatuoids such as AC Baton (CN 99047), AC Ernie (CN 99046), and AC Navan (CN 19199). Hulless fatuoids retain their grain at maturity. In comparison, a covered-seeded fatuoid resembles the wild oat (*A. fatua* L.) in its gross morphology and shattering behavior. In both the wild oat and covered-seeded fatuoid (Figure 3a and b), an abscission zone forms at the base of each kernel and, when ripe, the seed shatters or breaks free from the spikelet and falls to the soil. Shattering in the field is an important trait for the weedy wild oat, but it constitutes a loss of grain yield for covered-seeded varieties. Varieties having a high incidence of this trait are discarded by breeders. When the fatuoid trait is combined with the hulless trait (Hoekstra et al 2003), an important interaction occurs

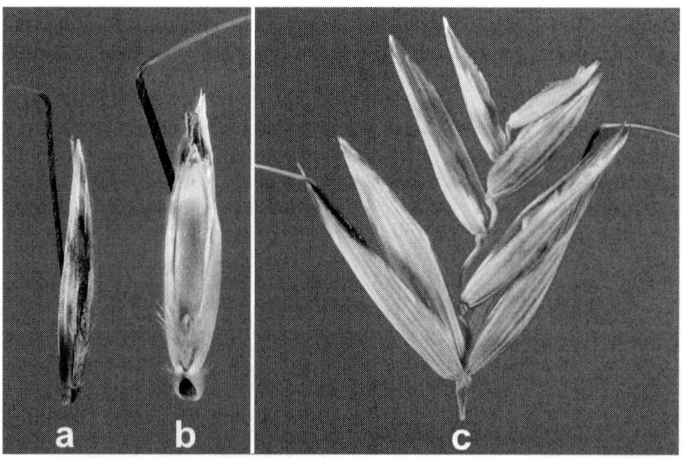

Fig. 3. *Avena fatua* L. wild seed **(a)** and *Avena sativa* L. fatuoid covered seed with heavy geniculate awns **(b)**. Hulless seeded fatuoid spikelet **(c)** with heavy geniculate awns. Both (a) and (b) have an abscission ("sucker mouth") kernel base, and the seeds shatter when ripe, whereas (c) has a fracture base and the groats are released by threshing.

between the two traits that leads to a better expression of the hulless condition throughout the panicle, and shattering is largely prevented (Fig. 3c). Either the abscission zone (commonly called the "sucker mouth") does not form in the presence of hulless genes or, if it forms, it does not separate when the grain is ripe (Hoekstra et al 2001). Superficially, the plant panicle resembles a large, seeded, wild oat because it has heavy geniculate awns on the lemma of each primary and secondary floret and occasionally on the tertiary floret of each spikelet. The groats are captured when harvested, but the awns are lost along with the thin, papery hulls during the threshing operation. In some hybrid populations where one parent was covered and the other hulless, the hulless expression in the progeny is not as complete as just described. In this situation, the uppermost seeds in each spikelet may be covered and have a "sucker-mouthed" base, in which case, they may shatter at maturity. It is possible that such segregates lack one or more of the minor modifying genes referred to earlier, but this has not yet been proven. Any strains exhibiting this behavior are discarded. It is not clear why the combination of the fatuoid and hulless traits leads to a better expression of the hulless genes, but it may be related to natural hormonal conditions within the plant. There is no proof for this supposition, but, as already stated, hormones such as those in commercial herbicides often play a role in hulless expression.

A second strategy to reduce hull content in hulless oat is to breed varieties with "chevron-type" (Burrows 1986a) spikelets (Fig. 2). These spikelets are multiflorous and indeterminate. The florets have short rachillas. Each spikelet may contain as many as 8–10 florets. The lower-ranked florets are usually fairly fertile, and they set seed. However, the uppermost florets are usually sterile, which eliminates the possibility of producing covered seeds at the tip of the spikelet, where they usually occur in traditional nonfatuoid varieties.

Breeding Oat Groats with Reduced Trichomes

The groats of most varieties of hulless oats sold today possess surface-borne hairs (trichomes) that break free during threshing and handling and act as skin, eye, and respiratory irritants (Figure 4b). In fact, some farmers refuse to grow hulless varieties because of this problem. The trichomes also develop an electrostatic charge that attracts fungal spores, leading to diseases or blemishes on the groat that interfere with acceptance in food markets. The trichomes of covered-seeded varieties are not a problem to farmers because they are trapped beneath the hull and are released into the air only when the seed is dehulled in a processing plant. The released trichomes are separated from the groats by aspiration. This constraint for hulless varieties has been removed by identifying a "bald" conditioning gene *Gt-1* in CN 18943 (Fig 4a) bred at Ottawa (Burrows et al 2001b). Burrows has introgressed this gene into several hundred new bald-seeded strains, which are at various levels of homozygosity. Two such bald strains, which are hulless fatuoids, are the value-added oats VAO-2 (CN 19196) and VAO-8 (CN 19197). These strains are not completely glabrous (bald), but when they are harvested with a combine, most of any residual trichomes are rubbed off as the groats pass through the machine, and the trichomes are discarded with the straw and leaf material. VAO-2 is daylength sensitive, and VAO-8 carries the *Di-1* gene (Burrows 1986a), making it daylength insensitive and early in maturity. VAO-8 is the most trichome-free, hulless oat produced to date at Ottawa (Fig. 1b). Both strains thresh very well, and the test weights of each are almost equal to that of wheat (*Triticum aestivum* L.), which is an important quality factor. In addition to solving the grain dust problem for farm producers, the grains of bald groats do not stick together and cause "bridging" in seeders and conveyance systems. When seeds "bridge" in seeders, the supply of seed from the drill box to the disc openers in the soil is prevented, causing missing rows in the field and thus providing open space for weeds to flourish.

In the breeding process, selecting seeds for baldness is a long and tedious procedure. One cannot thresh single panicles, or panicles of a single plant, with conventional threshing equipment because the procedure rubs many trichomes off the seed surface. This interferes with the accuracy of the selection process. Two techniques have been found useful to isolate undamaged groats from florets so the seeds can be accurately classified as bald or hairy. The first is to gently squeeze the groats out of a number of florets with one's fingers before examining for the presence of trichomes. This is a satisfactory procedure to use in advanced generations, where most of the seeds in the panicle are fairly uniform. The second technique involves the use of a custom-

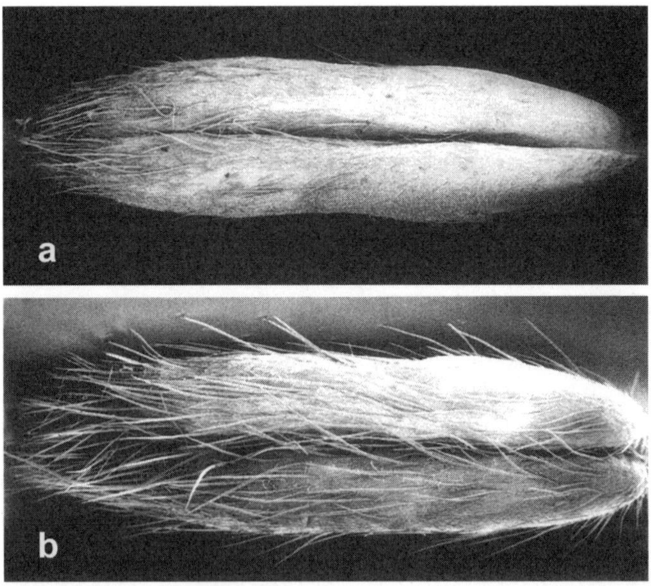

Fig. 4. Electron microscope photos showing the trichome coverage of a bald oat groat **(a)** and a typical pubescent oat groat **(b)**.

made machine (Figure 5a) that acts like an wringer on an old-fashioned washing machine. Passage of a panicle through the slow-rotating wringer (with the base of the panicle first) squeezes out all the groats (Fig. 5b and c). This technique is useful in early-segregating generations, where the panicle contains both bald and hairy seeds. Both of these techniques are labor intensive, but they do not remove trichomes, so the seeds can be scored for trichome coverage with the aid of an illuminated magnifying lens. It is a simple matter to select bald seeds from a segregating population or to select lines that are breeding true for the bald condition, using either of these procedures. The trait is highly heritable, and progress can be made quite rapidly.

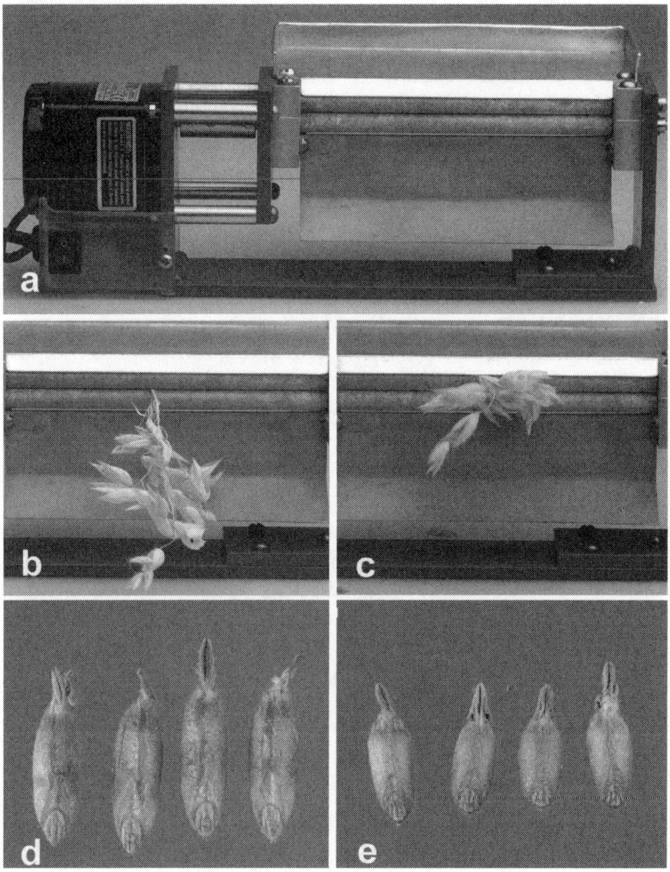

Fig. 5. Custom-made motorized roller **(a)** designed to "squeeze out" ripe groats from florets; **b,** panicle being drawn into slowly rotating (10 rpm) closely gapped, knurled rollers; **c,** threshing operation almost complete; **d,** threshed groats with adhering trichomes, brush end, and vestigial anthers; and **e,** thresh-bald seeded groats with reduced brush end and vestigial anthers.

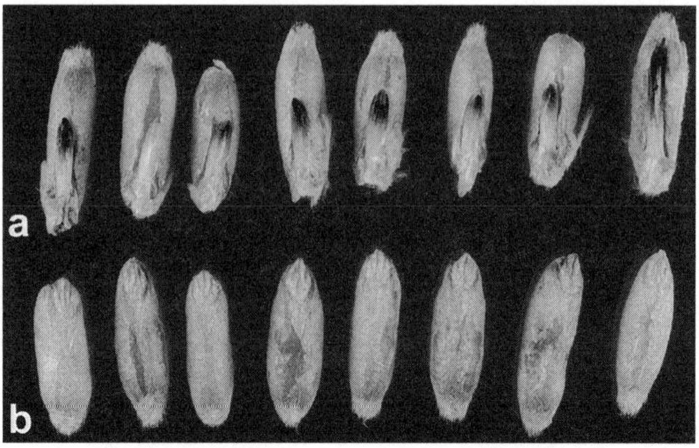

Fig. 6. Preharvest sprouting of field-grown AC Frégeau (CN 99048) seed **(a),** and sprout resistant (dormant) seed of hulless "dormoat" breeding stock (CN 19198) **(b).**

Preharvest Sprouting

Preharvest sprouting of oats (Figure 6a) usually occurs in seasons when the ripe crop is not harvested on time because of prolonged wet weather. Seed sprouting is especially common in the panicles of oats if the crop has been swathed and is lying on the stubble. Moisture is retained by a swathed crop longer than by a standing crop. The yield and quality losses experienced by farmers in some years can be very large.

Breeding for sprouting resistance in oats has not received the high priority that has been given to the white wheats because oats are not as sensitive as wheat to sprouting. When sprouting does occur, the grains do not enter the high-quality food market but are usually fed to animals on the farm. However, genes that provide resistance to sprouting are available in the experimental crop "dormoats" (Burrows 1970, 1986a) and in genetic stocks of sprouting-resistant hulless oats (CN 19198), as well as in any accession bearing a CN number. They are available to researchers and can be obtained from the Plant Gene Resources of Canada Office, Agriculture and Agri-Food Canada, Saskatoon, SK. This resistance had its origin in *A. fatua L.* and was first transferred from the wild oat by Burrows (1986a) to covered-seeded strains of *A. sativa* L. Now the author has transferred the gene(s) governing dormancy from covered to hulless oats (Fig. 6b).

Embryo Damage and Reduced Germination

Care must be exercised when threshing hulless oats compared to threshing covered oats, wheat, barley (*Hordeum vulgare* L.) or rye (*Secale cereale* L.) because oat groats are fairly fragile. The embryo of the oat groat of standard hulless varieties protrudes slightly and is very easily damaged. If this happens, the primary roots are destroyed and the seedling either fails to germinate or

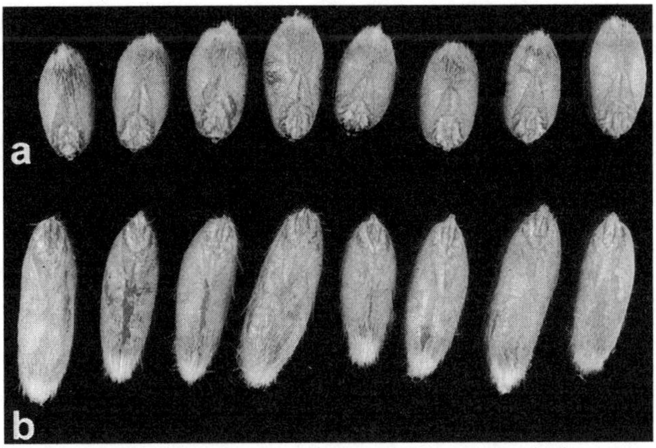

Fig. 7. Short groats of VAO-7 (CN 19200) with recessed embryos that are not easily damaged **(a)** and long groats of AC Baton (CN 99047) with protruding embryos that are commonly damaged during threshing and handling **(b)**.

evelops abnormally. The embryos of wheat and rye kernels are recessed, thus avoiding this problem. To avoid damaging the oat embryo during threshing, farmers are advised to reduce the combine cylinder speed and narrow the gap between the concaves so that the straw cushions the seed as it passes through. Operators must carefully monitor the seed periodically and make adjustments to the combine as air moisture conditions change during the day.

Damage to the embryo can also occur when the grain is cleaned after harvest, usually during winter in Canada and the northern United States. After storage, the groats are usually dry and brittle and there is a danger of causing chips and cracks, especially if the grain is moved quickly using a pneumatic system with bends in the pipe. Hulless oats should never be processed through a debearder if the grain is to be used for seed purposes because this leads to extensive embryo damage, causing greatly reduced germination.

Progress has been made in breeding the small-seeded hulless oat groats VAO-7 (CN 19200), with recessed embryos (Figure 7a). The small size makes the groat less vulnerable to damage. This seed also has less mass, which makes it less likely to suffer breaks and cracks when threshed and cleaned.

Diseases

Hulless and covered-seeded oats are both plagued by the same spectrum of disease organisms. However, the absence of the hull in hulless oats increases the vulnerability of the oat plant to loose smut, *Ustilago avenae* (*Pers.*) *Rostr.* The incidence of smutted plants in susceptible hulless varieties, compared to that in susceptible covered varieties, can be very large. The hull of covered-seeded varieties offers a partial barrier to the penetration of fungal hyphae, but the hulless groat is completely exposed to fungal attack. Smut spores are carried on the surface of the groat, germinating and infecting the seedling at the time of germination. Seed treatments are effective in controlling smut, but breeding resistant varieties is the best strategy to follow both from an economic and an environmental standpoint. When breeding for resistance, it is easy to innoculate the seed with the spores of the common races of smut to identify resistant plants. Many sources of genetic resistance are available to breeders in gene banks.

Grain Storage

Moisture content is critical to proper storage of hulless oats, and the harvested seed should be stored in aerated bins. Groats containing 12% moisture or less will store properly and will germinate well when sown. If moisture is above 12%, the grain should be aerated to prevent it from heating and developing molds. During long-term storage, fans may be turned on periodically to keep the seed in good condition. The bins must be rodent proof and free of insects before filling, because storage insects and mice have a great affinity for hulless oats.

Abrasion Milling of Groats

Oat bran is commonly made from groats by grinding them into flour and separating the bran from the flour by sieving. An alternative method is to remove the bran from the outside of the kernel by abrasive milling using the grinding wheel(s) in a "Satake mill" or in a mill that performs the same function. Satake milling of unprocessed groats results in two fractions: groats with a greatly reduced bran layer (except what is left in the crease) and a bran fraction. The bran produced by abrasion has a very fine texture, and the groat remains more or less intact, although some breakage occurs during the process. The amount of breakage is a function of several factors, including variety, groat moisture content, kernel length and weight, and the duration of exposure to abrasion. Long groats break easily, and the broken ends are further abraded, which adds finely divided endosperm flour to the bran. If the debranned groats are to be cooked alone or mixed with polished rice, the broken kernels should be removed because they cook faster than the intact grains. To avoid breakage, the ideal groat shape for abrasive milling is short and as close to spherical as possible. The author has found seed types that meet these short-seeded specifications in segregating populations of hulless oats—CN 72574 (VAO-3), CN 72575 (99VB-22-2N), and CN 72576 (VAO-9)—derived from hybrids between a bald-seeded Canadian and a Chinese hulless-oat parent (CN 18945). Burrows was also able to isolate long (CN 72577) and short (CN 72578) groat strains with shallow creases that permit a greater extraction of bran when milled. A comparison of shallow- and deep-creased groats and a cross section of each is illustrated in Figure 8. The use of these special small-seeded oats is discussed below.

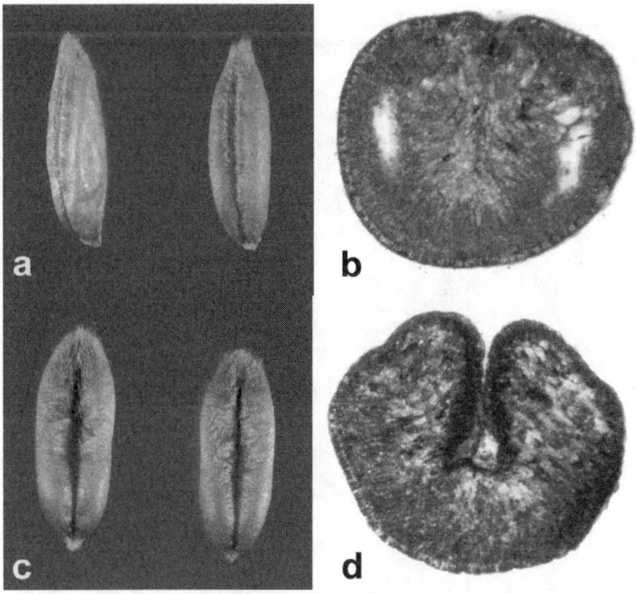

Fig. 8. Intact groats of CN 72577 with shallow crease **(a),** a cross section of a single seed showing a shallow crease **(b),** deep-creased groats of AC Frégeau (CN 99048) **(c),** and a cross section of a single seed showing a deep crease **(d)**.

Use of Hulless Oats in Food Preparations

Intact or debranned groats can be cooked separately like rice or can be mixed with rice (Figure 9) and used whole in a variety of food products (*personal communication*, Jianquang Zhou, Eastern Cereal and Oilseed Research Centre, Agriculture and Agri-Food Canada, Ottawa, ON), including breakfast cereals, desserts, puddings, cookies, pies, side dishes, soups, casseroles, pilafs, tabula, snack bars, salads, and fish and poultry stuffings. The groats may be ground and used in breakfast cereals, batters, gravies, drinks such as oat "milk" or soy-oat drink, tofu, noodles, dumplings, steam breads, bread loaves, and extruded products. The recipes that use rice to prepare a wide range of food products may also use oat groats or oat flour. Debranned groats absorb water faster than intact groats, which reduces the cooking time from 45 min to approximately 10–15 min. The cooking time of intact groats is close to that of brown rice and that of debranned oats is about equal to that of polished rice. The author has discovered that debranned groats absorb approximately an equal volume of water, but polished rice absorbs twice its volume. The addition of oat groats to rice increases the protein, lipid, and soluble fiber content of the product. The oats also contribute a better flavor to processed foods.

Hulless oats have their origin in China, where they have been cultivated since the fifth century. They are grown widely in Shanxi Province, where the grain is used to make porridge and a traditional food called *kaonao*. This food

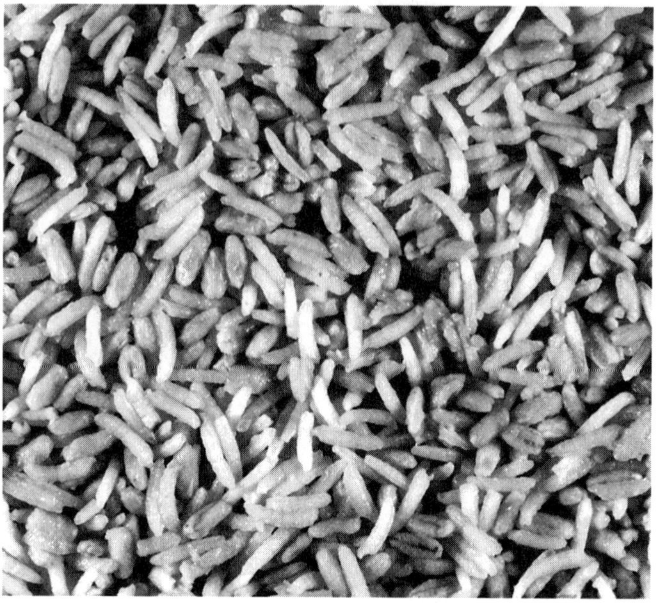

Fig. 9. Side dish prepared by boiling Basmati polished rice mixed together with abrasively milled oat groats (50:50 w/w) in water for 15 min.

has a history of more than 1,000 years, dating from the Yuan Dynasty. Roasted hulless oats are milled, and the resulting flour is mixed with boiling water, forming a loose dough that is rolled into rough strips. These are cut into pieces and worked by hand into bucket shapes called hulless *kaonao*. After steaming for 10–15 min, the *kaonao* is seasoned with a condiment sauce and eaten. A hulless oat *kaonao* is white to yellow in color and has good flavor. Virtually all of the oats grown in China are hulless varieties, and the grain is used for both food and animal feed.

Celiac Disease and Gluten Sensitivity

The human diet has changed dramatically over several million years from a dependence on hunted meats and wild fruits and vegetation to the consumption of agricultural products, including cereals such as wheat, rice, barley, rye, oats, corn, millet, sorghum, and triticale. Dependence on several of these cereal grains has led to some serious medical problems for celiac patients, variously numbered as from one in 100 (Maki et al 2003) to one in 250 (Berti et al 2000), who are sensitive to the gluten proteins in wheat, barley, rye, and triticale. Celiac disease is an immunologically mediated small-intestinal injury defined by histological appearance on biopsy. It is triggered by the ingestion of gluten-containing grains in genetically predisposed individuals, and it responds to dietary restriction of gluten. People with celiac disease cannot process gluten satisfactorily. The gliadin protein fraction of gluten is thought to be the offending protein. Cereals such as rice and maize (corn) are safe to consume because these grains lack the prolamin gliadin and pose virtually no risk to patients unless the grains have become contaminated with the offending cereals during processing (Størsrud et al 2003b). The oat kernel is also free of gliadin and is safe for celiac patients, but, unfortunately, commercial oats are commonly mixed, or contaminated, with gluten-type cereals, which are almost impossible to separate from oat groats. Mixtures occur on the farm or somewhere in the pooling, cleaning and transportation steps leading to delivery to the processing plants. At the present time, oat products are not considered safe and are not recommended for patients suffering from gluten sensitivity.

Braly and Hoggan (2002) have authored an excellent and thought-provoking book on this subject entitled *Dangerous Grains*, which describes gluten sensitivity and celiac disease. They make reference to 200 chronic illnesses and conditions caused by the consumption of gluten. Celiac disease is a special case of gluten sensitivity. Braly and Hoggan (2002) describe how gluten is digested into amino acids and peptides and how some of these peptides pass through the small intestinal wall of celiac patients and act as antigens, causing immune and autoimmune responses. The vast majority of celiac patients have silent (nonspecific, nonabdominal) symptoms. These affected individuals develop specific antibodies against gluten that travel in the bloodstream and may cause serious damage to a variety of organs, body systems, and tissues. Individuals with the silent form of celiac disease can be diagnosed employing a battery of blood tests, but often a proper diagnosis is not made until real damage occurs.

Shan et al (2002) identified a 33-mer gliadin peptide in wheat, barley, and rye that resists digestion in celiac patients. It interacts with the intestinal wall villi and initiates an autoimmune reaction, which results in a malformation of the villi, thus preventing the absorption of digested food and minerals such as calcium and iron. They also report in the same article that they failed to find this 33-unit peptide sequence in the prolamin fractions of rice, maize, and oats. Several authors have concluded that pure oats are a safe grain for celiac patients to consume (Janatuinen et al 1995, Srinivasan et al 1996, Hardman et al 1997, Picarelli et al 2001, Janatuinen et al 2002, Størsrud et al 2003a,b). Janatuinen et al (2002) reported that adult celiac patients fed pure oats for a period of five years suffered no ill effects. Størsrud et al (2003a), reported that celiac patients in remission were able to tolerate large amounts (93 g/day) of pure oats for an extended period without adverse effects. Srinivasan et al (1996) stated, "our results suggest that oats cereal is neither toxic nor immunogenic in celiac disease." This is in contrast to the commonly held historic view in North America and elsewhere that oat and oat products are not safe for celiac patients.

As stated earlier, the number of patients with celiac disease in North America is estimated to be from one in 100 to one in 250 people. If this percentage is similar in other regions of the world, the potential number of people requiring pure oats to consume would be between 24 and 60 million. If all silent, or nonspecific, celiac patients could be tested and identified, celiac numbers may even be much higher. Medical practitioners are gradually becoming more acquainted with the knowledge that sensitivity to gluten should be checked as the primary cause of a host of seemingly unrelated conditions. The use of diagnostic antibody blood tests and tissue biopsies should be employed earlier rather than later in diagnosing difficult patient conditions. The disease has recently been linked to neurological diseases such as peripheral neuropathy and "small fiber neuropathy," which affect 20 million people in the United States alone (Chin et al 2003). Five percent of patients suffering from peripheral neuropathy and 16% of those suffering small fiber neuropathy were positively diagnosed as celiac patients and are sensitive to gluten. Unfortunately, it may take several years of suffering before patients are evaluated for celiac disease. Celiac patients must follow a gluten-free diet for the remainder of their lives. Pure oats may find a place in this diet, but special procedures and standards must be followed to render them safe.

Pure Oats for Celiac Patients

Any strategy devised to supply pure oats for celiac patients will likely involve establishing a dedicated production, cleaning, grading, inspection, and processing system for oats. In Canada, the existing production system must be modified for oats to make certain that the grains entering the processing plants are of food-grade quality and of high purity. It is important that they meet or exceed the foreign-seed tolerances established by the Canadian Seeds Act for the various classes of pedigreed seed and those stated by the medical profession. Existing foreign-seed contamination standards for the various classes of pedigreed seed (Breeder, Select, Foundation, Registered, and Certified) and Common seed were established primarily for the benefit of producers, processors, exporters, and consumers. The purest seed is Breeder seed, and the most contaminated seed belongs to the Certified and Common seed classes, which are the most commonly grown and delivered to food processors by farmers. Common seed may contain as many as 50 or more foreign seeds per kilogram. These seed lots must be cleaned by food processors, but it is virtually impossible to reduce the wheat, barley, and rye seed content to tolerable levels for celiac patients because the seed size is in the same range as that of oat groats. Different seed shipments will contain different levels of offending grains, and the products made from these different shipments will produce products with different levels of offending grains. This is probably the reason why some oat products or brands are less safe for celiac patients than others and may explain some of the discrepancies on oat safety reported in the literature. When a purchaser, or researcher, buys oats in the marketplace, the oats may contain various levels of wheat, barley, rye, or triticale because such contamination cannot easily be determined by visual inspection.

A safer strategy to follow is to obtain oats from professional oat seed growers who are willing to dedicate their land, seeding, harvesting, transportation, seed cleaning, and packaging equipment and storage facilities to oats. In Canada, these are the Select Seed Growers, belonging to the Canadian Seed Growers

Association, who have learned how to produce pure oat seed and have graduated from a probationary period as seed growers. They buy and grow pedigreed seed and rogue it by hand to remove any impurities. They grow Select and Foundation seed plots, which are all inspected in the field by government inspectors. For this dedicated system to work, government inspectors would also have to inspect the seed derived from the inspected fields before it is bagged and tagged. The amount of contamination with foreign seeds permitted for Foundation no. 1 status is very low (1/kg). This represents about one wheat, barley, or rye seed per 30,000–40,000 oat groats. The number of oat groats per kilogram depends upon their seed weight. If this dedicated protocol is followed, one could expect that the amount of contamination would even be lower than that demanded by the Canadian Seeds Act regulations. To aid the seed grower, it would be recommended that he or she follow a three-year cropping rotation involving pure oats and two other crops that are naturally free of gluten.

For the total system to be effective, food processors would have to be identified who are willing to operate existing processing plants, or construct new ones, that are dedicated to using pure oats only. As a matter of policy, these facilities must be kept free of existing commercial oats and of offending cereals. The costs of using only pedigreed oat seed would be much higher than the cost of buying commercial grain grown by ordinary farmers, but the seed would open up a new market that does not exist today. Celiac patients would have to pay more for pure oats than for the commercial oats that are now on the market. The Select grower would be responsible for cleaning the grain; it would be his/her responsibility to obtain the proper inspection certificate and tag; and the processor would have to keep the processing facility essentially free of offending grains.

Pedigreed seed oats that meet or exceed the purity standards of Foundation no. 1 seed should probably be sold to patients, both nationally and internationally, under a different class name such as "Cavena" (Canadian *Avena*). Oat products bearing the Cavena label would guarantee a high and acceptable level of purity that would readily distinguish them from products made from commercial, contaminated oats.

Choice of Oat Varieties to Serve Celiac Patients

Both covered-seeded and hulless oat varieties could be used to produce pure oats for celiac patients, but certain new bald-seeded hulless oat varieties, as described earlier in this chapter, may be the best choice to service this market. Covered-seeded oats must be dehulled and sorted before the groats can be used, which is a very long and tedious process requiring much sorting equipment. Dehulling is not an efficient process as grains that are not dehulled in the first or second pass through the dehullers must either be returned to the dehulling machine or be discarded as feed. Dehulling is also a violent process, and many groats are broken, which lowers the yield of whole groats and increases the risk of oil rancidity.

In addition, select seed growers are usually not equipped to conduct a dehulling operation, which means the dehulling must be done by food processors, who then have to dispose of the hulls. Hulls have a low or negative market value and are considered a nuisance by most oat processors. Approximately 35–45% of the grain weight is lost in the dehulling process as hulls and broken groat fragments. Wheat, barley, rye, or triticale grains, because of their weight, can remain in the groat sample after the oats are dehulled, so the frequency of these offending grains increases in the dehulled grain, which may then not grade Foundation no. 1.

Hulless oat varieties lend themselves to this program because food processors would not have to clean the grain, and the seeds would be ready immediately for conditioning and processing. Processors could contract with seed growers to deliver grains of specific sizes because small- and large-seeded varieties can be made available for specific processing requirements. Small seeds can be obtained by choosing a small-seeded variety to grow (such as VAO-7) or by sieving out larger-seeded varieties such as VAO-2 or VAO-8 to obtain only secondary or tertiary kernels for special flours or baby foods. These small seeds would be smaller than any of the offending grains containing gluten. The larger groat could be processed as oat flakes or debranned in an abrasion mill to provide groats to mix and cook with rice. It is the opinion of the author that producing pure oat groats for celiac patients would best be served by choosing, and working with, modern, bald-seeded, hulless oat varieties.

Use of Groats in Feeds

The rearing of animals, in many regions of the world today, is usually accomplished in large production facilities where the emphasis is placed on efficiency. This was not true in the past, when most of the covered-seeded oats produced on the farm never left the farm because farmers were in charge of feeding horses, ruminants, and poultry. Today, the scale for producing beef, milk and milk products, pork, and poultry products such as broiler meat, eggs, roaster chicken, and turkey meat has increased dramatically, and diet formulation decisions are made by nutrition specialists assisted by many other professionals. Crops are considered as ingredients, and the ones chosen and the amounts used in any diet depend upon nutritional requirements and cost. Welch (1995) has presented a thorough description of the chemical composition of both covered and hulless oats, which is of use to both food and feed diet formulators.

Schrickel et al (1992) and Cudderford (1995) have reviewed the feeding of both covered and hulless oats to domestic animals.

Feed formulators have made increasing use of the combination of corn and soybeans, with corn as the metabolizable energy source and soybean meal as a source of protein. Other sources of energy are often substituted for corn in certain geographical regions if corn is too expensive and barley, wheat, or sorghum (*Sorghum bicolor* L.) grains are more available and less expensive. Similarly, other protein sources such as fish meal, cotton seed meal (*Gossypium hirsutum* L.), canola *(Brassica napus*) meal, and alfalfa (*Medicago sativa* L.) may be substituted for soy meal.

In many cool regions of the world, corn and soybeans cannot be grown reliably, and these grains must be imported from warmer regions, which adds to diet cost. Barley and wheat are not as ideally suited as corn for animal diets, especially for nonruminants, because they contain less metabolizable energy. They have less fat (lipid) content than corn, and the barley hull dilutes the total energy. Hulless barley may overcome this latter problem. Barley and wheat also have a higher protein content than corn, but this is not necessarily a desirable feature because the protein is not well balanced with essential amino acids such as lysine and must be supplemented with high-quality meal or with authentic amino-acid chemicals.

The problems with wheat and barley can be overcome by replacing these grains with hulless oats. The hulless oat, as represented by the variety Tibor (Burrows 1986b), contains approximately the same metabolizable energy as corn (Table 1) because the oil content of the groat is much higher than that of wheat or barley and is comparable to that of corn. The protein quality of hulless oats is better balanced with essential amino acids than is the protein of either corn, wheat, or barley, which means it requires less balancing. The

TABLE 1
Chemical Composition and Energy Content of Tibor Hulless Oat and Corn[a]

Characteristics	Tibor Grain	Corn Grain
Gross energy, MJ kg^{-1} of DM[b]	19.8	18.8
True metabolizable energy, rooster, MJ kg^{-1} of DM	16.9	16.4
True metabolizable energy, chick, MJ kg^{-1} of DM	16.2	16.4
Fat, ether extract, g kg^{-1} of DM	55.4	44.0
Fatty acids, g kg^{-1} of fat		
C 16:0	180	120
C 18:0	20	20
C 18:1	400	290
C 18:2	370	560
C 18:3	10	10
Fiber, crude g kg^{-1} of DM	25	29
β-Glucan, g kg^{-1} of DM	42	0
Ash, g kg^{-1} of DM	23	15
Protein, crude, g kg^{-1} of DM	184	62
Amino acids, g kg^{-1} of DM		
Arginine	11.7	5.5
Histidine	3.7	3.3
Isoleucine	5.7	3.6
Leucine	12.4	13.8
Lysine	6.5	3.4
Methionine + cystine	7.8	5.0
Phenylalanine + tyrosine	13.8	9.5
Threonine	5.0	3.7
Valine	7.8	4.8

[a] N. A. Cave and D. W. Friend (*personal communication*, 1989, Animals Research Centre, Research Branch, Agriculture and Agri-Food Canada, Ottawa, ON).
[b] DM = dry matter.

protein composition of the oat groat is not perfect, but it is more complete than those of corn, wheat, or barley.

Experiences with Feeding Oat Groats to Domestic Animals

Poultry

More and more evidence is accumulating to support the conclusion that oat groats, whether they are obtained by dehulling covered oats or feeding hulless varieties, represent a good grain for broilers, laying hens, turkeys, or wild birds. Hulan et al (1981) concluded that groat levels up to 600 g kg^{-1} in starter diets (1–21 days) and 800 g kg^{-1} in finishing diets (22–42 days) had no significant adverse effect on biological performance or monetary returns compared to control diets. Cave and Burrows (1985) fed, from 28 to 42 days, an experimental hulless oat strain PGR 8646 at 0, 300, and 600 g kg^{-1} and concluded that there was no significant difference in weight gains compared to those from the corn-soy diet control. Feed efficiency was reduced at the 600 g kg^{-1} but not at the 300 g kg^{-1} level. Inclusion of the oats had no effect on mortality or carcass quality of dressed birds. Hulless oats were concluded to be a suitable replacement for corn and soybean meal in broiler-grower diets. When fed to chicks one to four weeks of age, feed intake and weight gains were depressed for diets with oat contents of >200 g kg^{-1} (Cave and Burrows 1985). Maurice et al (1985) fed broilers (from one day to seven weeks of age) diets containing hulless oat levels of 0–600 g kg^{-1} of diet. They concluded that levels of 200–400 g kg^{-1} could be added to diets, but at 600 g kg^{-1}, weight gain and bone strength were depressed, which led to leg deformities. These problems were ascribed to P deficiency caused by the phytic acid content of the diet. A reduction in true amino acid availability was identified by Hsun et al (1986) as an additional cause of low weight gain of chicks fed hulless oat diets.

The mixed linkage β-D-glucans in oat groats (Wood 1986), like those in barley (Broz and Frigg 1986), are thought to be mainly responsible for reducing feed efficiency of young chicks fed hulless oats. These gums are natural cell wall constituents in oat groats and barley kernels. They are thought to interact with microorganisms in the alimentary tract and reduce the absorption of certain essential nutrients. Degradation of the gums by β-glucanase treatment (Broz and Frigg 1986, Cave et al 1990), gamma radiation (Campbell et al 1986), autoclaving or addition of antibiotic to feed (Cave et al 1990) all resulted in increased growth and feed efficiency. They demonstrated that the addition of β-glucan or oat bran to corn-soybean meal diets reduced growth and feed efficiency in proportion to the amount of gum added. By supplementing the hulless oat diet with antibiotic (neomycin), bile salt (Na taurocholate), and fat-soluble vitamins (A, D_3, and E) in factorial combination, Cave et al (1990) demonstrated that the absorption of lipids, including fat-soluble vitamins, may be the factors limiting energy intake and growth of the chicks fed Tibor (Burrows 1986b) hulless oat. Campbell et al (1986) found that the degradation of the gum in oat groats by gamma-irradiation also resulted in increases in fat absorption and the bone mineral content of chicks.

Egg size was reported to be increased by feeding hens oat pellets or oat groats (Herstad 1980, Karunajeewa and Tham 1987, Cave et al 1989). Higher levels of linoleic acid in oat oil were thought to be responsible. The content of linolenic and arachidonic acids in egg yolk were also increased, which may have improved the eggs' nutritional value. Cave et al (1989) concluded that Tibor hulless oats can replace 600 g kg^{-1} of the corn in layer diets without detrimental effects on hen performance. The addition of lysine and methionine to diets in which hulless oat made up 870 g kg^{-1} of the total, and to canola meal in which hulless oat made up 690 g kg^{-1} of the diet, resulted in hen performance equal to that resulting from the corn-soy control diet. No significant difference was observed in mortality, specific gravity, or shell quality, or in the organoleptic eating quality of the eggs as determined by trained taste panelists (*personal communication*, L. Poste, Food Res. Inst., AAFC, Ottawa, ON, Canada). Feed efficiency was improved, but yolk color was reduced when the hens were fed oat groats. This may be a problem when the eggs are to be prepared for table use. Yolk color can be intensified by adding carotenoid pigment to the rations, which is commonly done in noncorn diets. In Australia, Karunajeewa and Tham (1987) were able to replace all or part of the wheat in a laying diet with oat groats. Feed intake was reduced and feed conversion was improved without the loss of performance due to the higher oil content of the ration from oats. Unlike the results of Cave et al (1989), yolk color was improved, but this may have been due to fats from meat and bonemeal that were included in the oat diet.

Swine

Grower-Finishing Diets

Hulless oats have been found to be an excellent high-energy grain to incorporate into hog diets. Morris and Burrows (1986) fed several levels of Tibor hulless oat (0,300, 600, and 967 g kg^{-1} of diet) to hogs starting when they were 32 kg and ending when they were 97 kg live weight. The crude protein values were 168, 177, 175, and 195 kg^{-1} of dry matter (DM), respectively, for the oat diets. All diets contained 32.5 g kg^{-1} of mineral and vitamin premix. The control diet consisted of 762.5 g of shelled corn and 200 g of soybean meal kg^{-1} (486 g of protein kg^{-1} of DM). Total live weight gains, carcass backfat, and quality index values were not significantly different at the end of the 72-day growth period. As the amount of oat in the diet increased, feed conversion was progressively improved. This was probably due to the fact that the energy content of the diets increased in proportion to the lipid concentration (80–100 g kg^{-1} of DM). Higher levels of oat also produced better carcass yields or "dressing percentage" than the control diet. The researchers concluded that Tibor oat at 195 g kg^{-1} of crude protein was a suitable replacement for all, or part, of the grain corn and soybean meal in the grower-finishing ration.

Friend et al (1988, 1989) concluded, from both feeding and metabolism experiments, that Tibor hulless oat is a suitable dietary ingredient for grower-finishing pigs. Weight gains and feed conversions as good as, or better than, those of the corn-soybean meal control diet were obtained with Tibor contents up to 970 g kg^{-1} of diet when the diet was supplemented with the amino acid lysine. The addition of lysine reduced the time to market weight by eight days, ensured high weight gain, improved feed conversion, and prevented excess carcass fat accumulation, which may be a problem with an all-hulless-oat diet. Presumably the addition of lysine permitted the animal to grow and produce meat tissue rather than producing fat during the latter stages of the finishing phase. The experiments of Friend et al (1989) provide support for the inclusion of at least 48% hulless oats as a replacement for corn and soybean meal in the diet of grower-finishing pigs, while providing evidence of satisfactory performance by pigs fed up to 95% hulless oats in their diet. This was a remarkable result because it is rare to discover a rather inexpensive grain that, when added to a well-researched control diet, will perform or outperform that control diet.

Azain and Jones (1995) performed two experiments on the use of hulless oats in swine diets. In the first experiment, hulless oats were added at 0, 22, or 44% of a nursery diet and replaced half or all of the corn in the diet. They fed the diets for four weeks, and performance results indicated no difference between the control corn-based diet and either of the oat diets. In the second experiment, oats were used to replace corn and soybean meal and were fed at 0, 60, and 95% of the finisher diet. The growth rate of pigs fed the 60% oat and 40% corn-soybean diet showed a trend of being greater than that of the control group or the group on the 95% oat diet. This is a confirmation of the results reported by Friend et al (1989). The researchers also concluded that hulless oats can substitute for corn and soybean meal in nurser and finishing hog diets. From these experiments (Azain and Jones 1995, Friend et al 1989), one may conclude that hulless oats can be added at the 50–60% level to hog diets to improve commercial feeds that use corn as a source of energy and soybean meal as a source of protein.

Trained sensory evaluation panelists concluded that the flavor of loin roasts taken from the gilts and barrows (Friend et al 1988) and the barrows and boars (Friend et al 1989) fed the all-hulless-oat diet, or diets supplemented with lysine, had significantly greater flavor intensity than those from the control diet or the diet composed of 50% hulless oat plus 50% corn-soybean meal. In both experiments, meat juiciness was superior in the all-hulless-oat diet, but the addition of lysine returned the rating to the control level, presumably because of a reduction of fat content. Tenderness scores ranked higher for the oat diets than for the control in both experiments, but only one value was significantly higher than the control. It is clear that hulless oats can replace both corn and soybean meal in pig diets, which is important to oat and hog producers operating in cool geographical regions to which corn and soybeans are not adapted. There appears to be no upper limit to the amount of high-quality hulless oats that can be added to hog diets, provided the diet is supplemented with an adequate supply of authentic lysine or meal that is rich in lysine. It can also be concluded that the addition of hulless oats to hog diets opens the possibility of manufacturing "designer pork," or "branded meat," for market. The replacement of corn with hulless oats leads to pork with white fat, which is a good selling point in some markets such as the Japanese market.

Weaner Diets

Davies (1987) fed the Welsh hulless oat variety Rhiannon to young pigs and found that this hulless oat can be used as an alternative to flaked oats in a diet for early weaned piglets. A creep feed containing hulless oats, however, reduced the food intake and performance of suckling pigs. Probably very young pigs react in the same way as young chicks to the β-D-glucan in hulless oat diets. The amount of oats incorporated into weaner diets should be reduced and monitored carefully, or the β-D-glucan in the feed should be modified by adding glucanase enzymes or by employing some other means such as short-term germination or irradiation to change the integrity before feeding very young pigs. Probably the best solution would be for oat breeders to produce varieties with seed having a very low β-D-glucan content for both young and older animals and other varieties with a high content of β-D-glucan for human use because of its health benefits.

Recreational Horses

Fibrous forages are the natural food for horses, but as owners increase the horses' work load, grains are added to the diet to provide extra energy. The amount of grain added is dependent upon the animal's age, its weight, and the duration and intensity of the workload. A high-energy grain should not exceed 50% of the diet; otherwise, there is a risk of contributing to obesity, diarrhea, cholic, or founder. The covered-seeded oat has traditionally been the grain of choice to feed horses. It contains both insoluble fiber in the hull and metabolizable energy and soluble fiber in the groat. The hull has very low nutritional value, but it does add to the insoluble fiber provided by the forage. Insoluble fiber keeps the horse's alimentary tract healthy and functioning efficiently. Since hulless oats are available, the question must be asked, "Why would anyone pay grain prices for the insoluble fiber in oat hulls when this fiber could easily be replaced by feeding inexpensive fiber from forage?"

Determination of the energy value of covered oats is complicated because covered oats vary greatly in quality as a result of weather conditions and the incidence of viral, fungal, and bacterial diseases. Quality is usually measured by grain test weight (kg/hl): the higher the test weight, the higher the proportion of groat to hull. Oats with low test weight have groats that are thin or shriveled and contain a reduced amount of energy. From test weight values of covered seed, the feed formulator can get only an approximate value of the grains' energy content. The test weight values of a hulless oat are a much more reliable measure of the grain's energy content because the hull percentage is not a factor.

Hulless oats typically have a higher concentration of all the major and minor constituents in the grain than covered oats because the hull contains very little nutritive value. Groats contain 14–19% protein (Peterson and Brinegar 1986, Valentine 1995), which supplies most of the essential amino acids required by the horse. Feed formulators who prepare horse diets, like the ones who prepare pig and poultry diets, commonly add the amino acids lysine and methionine, or another feed source rich in these amino acids, to horse diets to balance any deficiencies of oat protein. What they choose to add is a function of availability and cost. The groat also contains between 6 and 9% lipid (oil or fat), which contains approximately 20% saturated and 78% unsaturated fatty acids (Youngs 1986). With this concentration of oil, the common procedure of adding messy oil to the formulated feed to provide added energy for racehorses is unnecessary. The water-soluble B vitamins such as thiamin, riboflavin, niacin, and pantothenic acid are in good supply in oat groats, as well as some fat-soluble tocopherols and tocotrionols, which make up vitamin E activity.

Some feed formulators prefer to roll or crimp oats, including hulless oats, to increase digestibility, but the practice is not thought to be necessary since whole groats rarely have been found in horse feces. If rolling or crimping is followed, the shelf life of the oat flake is reduced greatly because the flakes develop rancidity quickly after the groat is damaged.

Hulless oats are gaining popularity as a feed grain for recreational horses. In Canada, Semican Seed Company, Plessisville, PQ, is selling hulless oats under the trademark Equavena (www.equavena.com). It is rather ironic that the decline of interest in oats worldwide was caused primarily by the replacement of the workhorse with machines powdered by petroleum, but the removal of the hull genetically has begun to stimulate the use of groats in many new niche markets, including the recreational horse market.

Dairy and Beef Animals

In spite of a long history of feeding covered oats to cattle, the hull can limit the amount of protein and energy an animal can ingest before its satiety level is satisfied. This is very important in the case of high-producing dairy cattle. Covered oats have been replaced by corn silage, grain corn, and barley in dairy and beef animal diets. In recent years, some dairy producers in Canada and the United States have provided this author with testimonials stating that they are using and benefitting from feeding hulless oats to their dairy cattle because the oats are cheaper than corn and soybean meal and milk production remains unaffected. Anderson et al (1997) evaluated reciprocal levels of hulless oats and barley in diets for growing and finishing steers. They concluded that "hulless oats appears to be a very useful feed when fed in combination with barley for growing steers but shows more pronounced and positive response in finishing diets."

Marx (1997) studied the usefulness of hulless oats in grain starter rations for calves. Hulless oats should benefit young calves because these animals function more like a monogastric animal since their rumen is underdeveloped for digestion as a ruminant. He concluded that

> no problems were observed with feed intake or palatability and no unusual health problems were observed in either the preweaned or weaned groups. Results indicate that the newly developed hulless/naked oat cultivar (Paul) is satisfactory as an ingredient in grain starters for both nonweaned and weaned dairy calves.

The amount of hulless oat used in cattle diets depends upon economic considerations.

Lambs

Haugen and Limesand (1998) fed fall- and spring-born purebred Hampshire, Suffolk Columbias lambs plus crossbred lambs diets consisting of 0, 20, and 40% hulless oats for 63 days and concluded that there was no significant difference in average daily gain, daily feed intake, or feed efficiency among the three diets.

Rabbits

Extensive experiments were conducted (D. E. Drevjany and L. A. Drevjany, *unpublished data*, 1988) on the suitability of hulless oats as the only grain source in diets for rabbits. These studies were conducted on their own farm while L. A. Drevjany (now retired) was employed as an animal scientist and teacher at the Kemptville College of Agricultural Technology, Kemptville, ON, Canada.

Tests with breeding, lactating, and growing rabbits indicated that hulless oats could be used as the main source of concentrated energy and protein for all categories of rabbits and thus could replace the need for purchased feed. They felt that rabbit growers needed a source of "home grown feed" and concluded that hulless oats fit this objective. In their report to this author, they answered the question, "What properties of hulless oats make it ideal as rabbit feed?" their answer stated:

> Its high content of energy and protein removes the need for mixing it with other concentrated sources of energy and protein.
>
> Physical properties of hulless oats ideally suit the rabbits. There is no need for any processing (rolling, grinding or pelleting).
>
> The ether extract fraction of hulless oats has a positive effect on color and consistency of body fat.
>
> Hulless oat is highly palatable to young rabbits and, as such, it speeds up the possibility of early weaning. Similarly, it is liked by all classes of rabbits.
>
> Because of the seeds' glossy surface, fine particles of supplement, supplying the missing vitamins, minerals and, if needed growth promoting factors, attach themselves nicely to the surface of the hulless oats, assuring acceptable uniformity of distribution of such components in the ration. Hulless oats thus fully replace pelleted feed, however, without the expense of grinding and pelleting.
>
> The need for supplementation of hulless oats with vitamins, amino acids, minerals and growth and health improving factors is relatively minimal but supplementation produced seemingly healthier animals and shortened the time to slaughter by approximately 10 days.
>
> In combination with good quality hay, hulless oats provide an inexpensive and very suitable home grown ration especially on farms supplying the organic rabbit meat markets.

Hulless Oats for Other Animals

Many domestic and wild animals can tolerate, or can thrive on, the inclusion of oat groats or flour in their diet. Animals such as sheep, goats, turkeys, geese, ducks, domestic cats, dogs, mice, rats, exotic and native birds, racing camels, bison, deer, and even fish that eat vegetation can utilize hulless oats. Deer should be fed only small portions of hulless oats at one time; otherwise they gorge themselves, which may lead to death (*personal communication*, J. Beauchesne, Semican Seed Co., Plessisville, PQ, Canada).

Nonfood Uses for Hulless Oats

Hulless oats can be used to advantage by the cosmetic, pharmaceutical, and fermentation industries because they do not have to be dehulled. Dehulling of covered oats rapidly shortens the shelf life of the groats, as stated earlier. Dehulling is a violent process, and groats are damaged in the operation, which leads to the rapid development of rancidity. The dehulled groats may be stabilized by the application of heat and steam, but this may lead to a decline in the functionality of components of importance to the industries listed above. Hulless oats that are stored at the proper moisture content and protected from insects, birds, and rodents will not develop short-term rancidity and can be delivered to processors as needed.

Cosmetics

Oat flakes and whole oat flour made from groats of dehulled or hulless oats have been used for many years to treat a wide range of skin conditions ranging from minor itching to soothing the itchiness from poison ivy, oak, or sumac as well as insect bites. Soap containing colloidal oatmeal is used by some individuals with sensitive skin. In more recent times, alcoholic extracts from groats have been marketed and used in products to treat the same skin irritations or used as sun screens to protect skin from UV damage (*personal communication*, D. Fielder, Ceapro, Inc., Edmonton, AB, Canada).

Oat starch is fine grained and can be used in eye shadow and to replace talcum powder in body powders and corn starch in latex gloves. It can also be fermented to make ethanol (gasohol), which produces valuable by-products such as distillers' grains for animal feed or oat proteins, oils, and β-glucan.

Hydrolyzed oat protein is used by some manufactures to make hair care products. β-Glucan forms a basis for making shampoos or can be added to surgical dressings to promote wound healing. Oat oil contains some unique antioxidants, including the avenanthramides (Collins 1986), which have been identified as the anti-itch factor in oats.

Pharmaceuticals

Oat groats and materials extracted from them are rapidly becoming known as health-promoting agents. Oat bran helps reduce the level of low-density lipoprotein (LDL) cholesterol in the blood serum of hypercholesterolemic patients (Anderson et al 1984, Anderson and Chen 1986, Anderson and

Gustafson 1988, Braaten et al 1994). The β-glucan was identified as the active principle, and it has also been found (Jenkins et al 1978, Anderson 1980, Wood et al 2000) to help type II diabetics control their blood sugar level.

Summary

It is the opinion of the author that, if covered oats represent the past, hulless oats represent the future for the crop. It may take time to achieve this result, but if interest continues to mount as it has in recent years, the hulless oat will lead the way to a renaissance of the crop. The change of emphasis will likely be led by the interest now being shown by the recreational horse and racehorse industries, although it could come from food companies that wish to serve the celiac customer or to exploit the nutritional and health-promoting value of oats. It is also interesting to note that this redesigning of oats has been made possible by the use of only one major and a few minor genes to convert covered to hulless varieties. Transforming the crop to the hulless condition was the first step in overcoming most of the deficiencies of the old hulless oat varieties, which were in a state of disrepair due to lack of plant breeding effort. The overbearing presence of covered varieties has acted as a major constraint to the development of new uses and the identification of new markets and clients for oats. Now hulless oats are being used to advantage by all classes of livestock and domestic pets because research has recognized their superior nutritional value and because oat is a relatively inexpensive grain. The main factor preventing acceptance is the lack of well-established markets for hulless oats, although this situation is changing with the passage of time and the positive experiences of producers and users. As more hulless oats become available, both small and large businesses may process the grain to create the new products required to develop niche markets in the food, feed, and industrial sectors.

The hulless oat could also play a major role in preventive medicine because of its chemical content, including both major and minor components. It is a healthy food and can be prepared in many novel ways to be consumed at all meals of the day as well as in drinks and snack foods. Its role in lowering the LDL cholesterol in the blood of hypercholesterolemic patients is well documented and well known. The avenantheramides, which are unique to oats, are important antioxidants, and recent research (*personal communication*, B. Collins, Eastern Cereal and Oilseed Research Centre, AAFC, Ottawa, ON, Canada) has indicated that they help keep cholesterol in a desirable, chemically reduced state. Also, the role of oats in helping people with type II diabetes control their blood sugar level and also presenting nondiabetic people with a grain of low glycemic index (Wood et al 2000) is considered a major benefit. The more frequent consumption of oats could play a very useful role in helping to reduce the medical costs caused by a number of diseases. In addition, the development of a pure-oats industry would solve the problem that celiac patients now have in locating pure oats, which are considered safe for them to consume.

New hulless varieties have opened the possibility of adding groats to the diets of many domestic and wild animal species that cannot digest oat hulls in an efficient manner. The oat groat contains approximately the same metabolizable energy as corn and enough good-quality protein to replace the traditional corn-soybean meal ration. Oat protein quality is not perfect, so adding lysine or combining oats with soybean meal (50:50 by weight) produces a more balanced diet for pigs, one that is superior to feeding oats alone or feeding the standard corn-soybean meal diet.

The cosmetic, pharmaceutical, and nonfood industries are able to use hulless oats to make many value-added products. Oat starch, which is fine grained, is used to make eye shadow and face and body powders to replace the mineral talc. The protein can be hydrolyzed to make hair-care products. The β-glucan is used to make shampoos and surgical dressings. The oil is largely polyunsaturated and contains some unique antioxidants, including the avenanthramides, which have several merits when taken internally or used for their anti-itch properties on skin.

If the demand and usefulness of hulless oats continues for both human and animal consumption, no longer will the hulls of covered-seeded varieties take up valuable storage space, cost excessive amounts of money to transport from producer to food processors and feed formulators, and limit the inclusion of oat groats into human and animal diets.

Even if the crop is converted from the covered to the hulless condition, breeders will still have access to the vast array of oat germ plasm available in international gene banks. As new specifications for oats are requested by entrepreneurs to better serve newly discovered markets, oat accessions will usually be found in gene banks to act as parental material to initiate new breeding programs. Many of the deficiencies in old hulless oat varieties have been overcome by a host of breeders located in various regions of the world. The deficiencies of the old varieties are low yield, lodging susceptibility, low test weight, improper maturity, poor groat shape, preharvest seed sprouting, groat hairiness, incomplete hullessness, protruding embryos that make the seed susceptible to mechanical damage, unsatisfactory chemical composition, poor milling quality, and disease susceptibility. The agronomic performance of hulless varieties has been improved greatly so that the new hulless oats have been bred to produce the same or higher yield of groats per hectare as covered varieties. The grain can now be used for more purposes, especially by small processors who do not have the expensive equipment to dehull and sort oat groats. In the opinion of the author, removal of the hull genetically is the last major step in the domestication and evolution of the oat crop.

References

Anderson, J. W. 1980. Dietary fiber in diabetes. Pages 193-221 in: Medical Aspects of Dietary Fiber. G. A. Spiller and R. M. Kay, Eds. Plenum Press, New York.

Anderson, J. W., and Chen,W. L. 1986. Cholesterol-lowering properties of oat products. Pages 309-334 in: Oats: Chemistry and Technology. F. H. Webster, Ed. Am. Assoc. Cereal Chem., St. Paul, MN.

Anderson, J. W., and Gustafson, N. J. 1988. Hypocholesterolemic effects of oat and bean products. Am. J. Clin. Nutr. 40:1146-1155.

Anderson, J. W., Story, L., and Sieling, B. 1984. Hypocholesterolemic effects of oat bran or bean intake for hypocholesterolemic men. Am. J. Clin. Nutr. 40:1146-1155.

Anderson, V. L., Bauer, M. L., Canton, J. S., Berg, P., and Dhuyvetter, D. H. 1997. An evaluation of reciprocal levels of hulless oats and barley in diets for growing and finishing steers. (http://www.ag.ndsu.nodak.edu/carringt/97research/carr97_reciprocal.htm)

Azain, M. J., and Jones, R. D. 1995. Hulless oats in swine diets. Annual Report of the University of Georgia Department of Animal and Dairy Science, pp. 245-249. Online: http://www.ads.uga.edu/annrpt/1995/95_245.htm

Berti, I., Horvath, K., Green, P. H. R., Sblattero, D., Not, T., and Fasano, A. 2000. Prevalence of celiac disease among risk groups and the general population in U.S.A. J. Invest. Med. 48:206-220A.

Braaten, J. T., Wood, P. J., Scott, F. W., Wolynetz, M. S., Lowe, M. K., Bradley-White, P., and Collins, M. W. 1994. Oat β-glucan reduces serum cholesterol concentration in hypercholesterolemic subjects. Eur. J. Clin. Nutr. 48:465-474.

Braly, J., and Hoggan, R. 2002. Dangerous Grains: Why Gluten Cereal Grains May Be Hazardous to Your Health. Avery Penguin Putnam, New York.

Broz, J., and Frigg, M. 1986. Effects of beta-glucanase on the feeding value of broiler diets based on barley or oats. Archiv. Gefluegelkd. 50(1):41-47.

Burrows, V. D. 1970. Yield and disease escape potential of fall-sown oats possessing seed dormancy. Can. J. Plant Sci. 50:371-377.

Burrows, V. D. 1986a. Breeding oats for food and feed: Conventional and new techniques and materials. Pages 13-46 in Oats: Chemistry and Technology. F. H. Webster, Ed. Am Assoc. Cereal Chem., St. Paul, MN.

Burrows, V. D. 1986b. Tibor oat. Can. J. Plant Sci. 66:403-409.

Burrows, V. D., Molnar, S. J., Tinker, N. A., Marder, T., Butler, G., and Lybaert, A. 2001a. Groat yield of naked and covered oat. Can. J. Plant Sci. 81:727-729.

Burrows, V. D., McDiarmid, G., and Marder, T. 2001b. Gene controlling reduced trichomes on oat groats. Can. J. Plant Sci. 81:413-414.

Burrows, V. D., Konzak, C. F., McDiarmid, G., and Deyl, J. 2002. A naked oat mutant with very short rachillas. Can. J. Plant Sci. 82:83-84.

Campbell, G. L., Classen, H. L., and Ballance, G. M. 1986. Gamma irridiation treatment of cereal grains for chick diets. J. Nutr. 116:560-569.

Cave, N. A., and Burrows, V. D. 1985. Naked oats in feeding the broiler chicken. Poult. Sci. 64:771-773.

Cave, N. A., Hamilton, R. M. G., and Burrows, V. D. 1989. Naked oats (cv. Tibor) as a feedstuff for laying hens. Can. J. Anim. Sci. 69:789-799.

Cave, N. A., Wood, P. J., and Burrows, V. D. 1990. The nutritive value of naked oats for broiler chicks as affected by dietary additions of oat gum, enzymes, antibiotics, bile salts and fat-soluble vitamins. Can. J. Anim. Sci. 70:623-633.

Chin, R. L., Sander, H. W., Brannagan, T. H., Green, P. H., Hays, A. P., Alaedini, A., and Latov, N. 2003. Celiac neuropathy. Neurology 60:1581-1585.

Collins, F. W. 1986. Oat phenolics: Structure, occurence, and function. Pages 227-296 in: Oats: Chemistry and Technology. F. H. Webster, Ed. Am. Assoc. Cereal Chem., St. Paul, MN.

Cudderford, D. 1995. Oats for animal feed. Pages 279-320 in: The Oat Crop: Production and Utilization. W. Welch, Ed. Chapman and Hall, London.

Davies, O. D. 1987. Naked oats in the diets of young pigs. Anim. Prod. 44:487-488.

Friend, D. W., Fortin, A., Poste, L. M., Butler, G., Kramer, J. K. G., and Burrows, V. D. 1988. Feeding and metabolism trials, and assesment of carcass and meat quality for growing finishing pigs fed naked oats (*Avena nuda*). Can. J. Anim. Sci. 68:511-521.

Friend, D. W., Fortin, A., Butler, G., Poste, L. M., Kramer, J. K. G., and Burrows, V. D. 1989. The feeding value of naked oats (*Avena nuda*) for boars and barrows: Growth, carcass, meat quality, and energy and nitrogen metabolism. Can. J. Anim. Sci. 69:765-778.

Hardman, C. M., Garioch, J. J., Leonard, J. N., Thomas, J. W., Walker, M. M., Lortan, J. E., Lister, A., and Fry, L. 1997. Absence of toxicity of oats in patients with dermatitis herpetiformis. New Engl. J. Med. 337:1884-1887.

Haugen, R., and Limesand, W. 1998. The utilization of naked oats (hulless oats) in growing rations of early weaned lambs. (Website: http://www.ag.ndsu.nodak.edu/hettinge/sheepday/nakedoat.htm)

Herstad, O. 1980. Kombinet foring av verpehoener med kraftforblanding og havrepellets. (Combined feeding of laying hens with concentrate mixture and pelled oats.) Meld. Nor. Landbrukshoegsk. 59(24):8.

Hoekstra, G. J., Darbyshire, S. J., and Mather, D. E. 2001. Anatomical features at the disarticulation zone in florets of fatuoid and non fatuoid oat (*Avena sativa* L.). Can. J. Bot. 79:1409-1416.

Hoekstra, G., Burrows, V. D., and Mather, D. E. 2003. Inheritance and expression of the naked-grained and fatuoid characters in oat. Crop Sci. 43:57-62.

Hsun, C. L., Jones, J. E., and Maurice, D. W. 1986. True amino acid availability (TAAA) of naked oats (*Avena nuda* L.) and performance of broiler chicks. Poult. Sci. 65:51-59.

Hulan, H. W., Proudfoot, F. G., and Zarkadas, C. G. 1981. Nutritive value and quality of oat groats for broiler chickens. Can. J. Anim. Sci. 61:1013-1021.

Janatuinen, E. K., Pikkarainen, P. K., Kemppainen, T. A., Kosma, V. K., Järvinen, M. K., Uusitupa, M. I. J., and Julkunen, R. J. K. 1995. A comparison of diets with and without oats in adults with celiac disease. New Engl. J. Med. 333:1033-1037.

Janatuinen, E. K., Kemppainen, T. A., Julkunen, R. J. K., Koona, V. M., Maki, M., and Hulkinen, M. 2002. No harm from five years of oats in coelic disease. Gut 50:332-335.

Jenkins, G., and Hanson, P. R. 1976. The genetics of naked oats (*Avena nuda* L.). Euphytica 25:167-174.

Jenkins, D. J. A., Wolever, T. M. S., Leeds, A. R. 1978. Dietary fibres, fibre analogues and glucose tolerance: Importance of viscosity. Br. Med. J. 1:1392-1394.

Karunajeewa, H., and Tham, S. H. 1987. The influence of oat groats and dietary level of lysine on the laying performance of crossbred hens. Anim. Feed Sci. Technol. 17:271-283.

Lawes, D. A., and Boland, P. 1974. Effect of temperature on the expression of the naked grain character in oats. Euphytica 23:101-104.

Maki, M., Mustalahti, K., Kokkonen, J., Kulmala, P., Haapalahti, M., Karttunen, T., Ilonen, J., Laurila, K., Dahlbon, I., Hansson, T., Hopfl, P., and Knip, M. 2003. Prevalence of celiac disease among children in Finland. N. Engl. J. Med. 348:2517-2524.

Marshall, H. G., McDaniel, M. E., and Creggar, L. M. 1992. Cultural practices for oat: Weed and pest control. Pages 209-210 in: Oat Science and Technology. H. G. Marshall and M. E. Sorrells, Ed. Agron. Monogr. 33. American Society of Agronomy, Madison, WI.

Marx, G. D. 1997. Utilization of hulless oats in dairy calf grain starter rations. J. Dairy Sci. 80(Suppl. 1).

Maurice, D. W., Jones, J. E., Hall, M. A., Castaldo, D. J., and Whesenhunt, J. E. 1985. Chemical composition and nutritive value of naked oats (*Avena nuda* L.) in broiler diets. Poult. Sci. 64:529-535.

Morris, J. R., and Burrows, V. D. 1986. Naked oats in grower-finisher pig diets. Can. J. Anim. Sci. 66:833-836.

Moule, C. 1972. Contribution à l'etude de l'hérádité du caractère 'grain nu' chez l'avoine cultiveé. Ann. Amelior. Plant. 22:335-361.

Peterson, D. M., and Brinegar, A. C. 1986. Oat storage proteins. Pages 153-203 in : Oats: Chemistry and Technology. F. H. Webster, Ed. Am. Assoc. Cereal Chem., St. Paul, MN.

Picarelli, A., Di Tola, M., Sabbatella, L., Gabrielli, F., Di Cello, T., Anania, M. C., Mastracchio, A., Silano, M., and De Vincenzi, M. 2001. Immunologic evidence of no harmful effect of oats in celiac disease. Am. J. Clin. Nutr. 74:137-140.

Schrickel, D. J., Burrows, V. D., and Ingemansen, J. A. 1992. Harvesting, storing and feeding of oat. Pages 223-245 in: Oat Science and Technology. H. G. Marshall and M. E. Sorrells, Ed. Agron. Monogr. 33. American Society of Agronomy, Madison, WI.

Shan, L., Molberg, O., Parrot, I., Hausch, F., Filiz, F., Gray, G. M., Sollid, L., and Khosla, C. 2002. Structural basis for gluten intolerance in celiac sprue. Science 297:2275-2279.

Srinivasan, U., Leonard, N., Jones, E., Kasarda, D. D., Weir, D. G., O'Farrelly, C., and Feighery, C. 1996. Absence of oats toxicity in adult coeliac disease. Br. Med. J. 313:1300-1301.

Størsrud, S., Olsson, M., Arvidsson, L. R., Nilsson, L. A., Nilsson, O., and Kilander, A. 2003a. Study confirms oat tolerance in CD adults. Eur. J. Clin. Nutr. 57:163-169.

Størsrud, S., Yman, I. M., and Lenner, R. A. 2003b. Gluten contamination in oat products and products naturally free from gluten. Eur. Food Res. Technol. 217:481-485.

Valentine, J. 1995. Naked oats. Pages 504-532 in: The Oat Crop: Production and Utilization. W. Welch, Ed. Chapman and Hall, New York.

Welch, R. W. 1995. The chemical composition of oats. Pages 279-320 in: The Oat Crop: Production and Utilization. W. Welch, Ed. Chapman and Hall, New York.

Wood, P. J. 1986. Oat β-glucan: Structure, location, and properties. Pages 121-152 in: Oats: Chemistry and Technology. F. H. Webster, Ed. Am. Assoc. Cereal Chem., St. Paul, MN.

Wood, P. J., Beer, M. U., and Butler, G. 2000. Evaluation of role of concentration and molecular weight of oat β-glucan in determining the effect of viscosity on plasma glucose and insulin following an oral glucose load. Br. J. Nutr. 84:19-23.

Youngs, V. L. 1986. Oat lipids and lipid-related enzymes. Pages 205-226 in: Oats: Chemistry and Technology. F. H. Webster, Ed. Am. Assoc. Cereal Chem., St Paul, MN.

CHAPTER 10

Rye for Improved Food and Feed

Sanaa Ragaee[1] and Graham Scoles[2]

[1]Department of Food Sciences, College of Food Systems, United Arab Emirates University, Al Maqam Campus, Al-Ain, United Arab Emirates; [2]Department of Plant Sciences, College of Agriculture, University of Saskatchewan, Saskatoon, SK, Canada, S7N 5A8

Origin and History

Like all crops, rye was originally a wild species. It has undergone the process of domestication to become what we now recognize as a crop. Crop domestication refers to the changes that occur when a plant is exposed to the influence of agricultural practices such as seeding and harvesting: accelerated evolution under the influence of human beings. These changes, which have a genetic base, come about as a result of the selection pressures imposed by the agricultural practices and also by deliberate human selection of certain types. Rye and its close relatives are Old World species, and in the Old World, crop domestication probably first occurred in southwest Asia around 10,000 BC (Deodikar 1963). Rye, wheat, and barley all have their origins in this area. Compared to wheat and barley, rye might be considered less domesticated because (1) unlike wheat and barley, rye retains the cross-pollinating habit of its wild relatives, and (2) rye shows a greater tendency than wheat or barley to shatter (shed its seeds at maturity).

Archeological evidence suggests that wheat and barley were among the first crops to be domesticated in southwestern Asia. Rye may well have been a weed in those early fields of wheat and barley, but the first evidence of rye as a crop comes from ancient northern European writings rather than earlier evidence from Greek or Roman times (Bushuk 2001). Thus it is most likely that rye underwent the transition from a weed to a crop in its own right in northern Europe because of its ability to tolerate inferior soils and cold temperatures. Rye was transported by European settlers to other parts of the world.

In medieval times, in parts of Europe and western Asia, rye was a much more important crop than it is today, probably accounting for 40% of bread grain production (Horsley 1969). At some point, wheat became the preferred grain in many of these areas because its flour made a lighter and whiter loaf of bread. For those reasons, rye is now a minor grain compared to wheat and the two other major grain crops, rice and corn, with world production at about

5% of each of those three crops. In most of the world, with the exception of northern and eastern Europe and western Asia, rye bread now tends to be regarded as a specialty product.

Production

As indicated, world production of rye is about 5% of the major cereal grains. Given its origins in southwestern Asia along with wheat and barley, rye, like those two crops, is primarily a crop of temperate regions, although it may be used as a forage or pasture in semitropical regions. In 2001, world rye production was almost 23 million tonnes (FAO 2001). Russia, Germany, and Poland each produced 6.6, 5.1, and 4.9 million tonnes, respectively, with two other major producers (Ukraine, 1.8 and Belarus, 1.3 million tonnes). In 2001, the combined production of these five countries represented 87% of world production. A number of European countries, along with China and Argentina, produce more than 100,000 tonnes.

Like many crops, rye can be grown as either a fall-seeded or a spring-seeded crop. Given the major areas of production and the advantages of growing a fall-seeded crop, most of the rye grown for grain is fall-seeded. This requires that the crop survive the cold temperatures of winter; in fact, a cold period is required by fall-seeded cultivars to induce flowering the following summer. Rye is the most cold-hardy of the common cereal crops, and this tends to favor its production over the other cereals in some areas of Canada, Scandinavia, and Siberia.

Rye is often said to be the cereal with the widest adaptation to various soil types (Deodikar 1963). It is considered to be the most drought tolerant of the cereals and as a result is often planted in light, sandy soils. Such soils tend to be low in fertility and hence to produce low yields, and because of this rye is sometimes characterized as being low yielding. However, numerous experiments have shown that under similar fertility regimes, rye yields can equal or even exceed those of wheat and barley. Rye is also the cereal that best tolerates acid soils because of its ability to grow under the high levels of aluminum that occur in such soils. As a result, in some areas of the world (e.g., South America and Australia), rye may be grown on such soils rather than wheat.

Rye is generally regarded as a relatively disease-resistant crop, particularly to the leaf diseases that infect other cereals (Czembor and Sowa 2001). In fact, resistance to diseases such as rust has been successfully transferred from rye to wheat through interspecific crosses. The major exception to rye's good disease resistance is the disease ergot. Rye is particularly susceptible to ergot infection because of its cross-pollinating habit. This results in florets that remain open for an extended period of time, which allows entry of the disease spores. Ergotism—poisoning as a result of consumption of ergot-infected grain or flour—is well known from medieval times when it was referred to as St. Anthony's Fire. Wheat and barley are as susceptible to ergot as rye, but ergot infection is minimal because of their closed flowering habit. Under good agronomic conditions, resulting in a high pollen load and minimal periods of flower opening, problems with ergot in rye are also minimized. Rye's susceptibility to ergot and the fact that rye is often grown under less-than-ideal agronomic conditions with low pollen loads account for past problems of ergot in rye. However, the perception that rye is always contaminated with ergot and that this may be the cause of feeding problems is often inaccurate.

Breeding and Genetics

The cross-pollinating habit of rye has a profound effect on breeding and genetic studies (Scoles et al 2001). As a cross-pollinated crop, rye cannot tolerate any level of inbreeding without undergoing significant inbreeding depression (low vigor and yield). Thus, unlike wheat and barley, the pedigree method of plant breeding cannot be used. Various methods of breeding cross-pollinating crops, usually variations on the technique of mass selection, must be used to produce new cultivars. These techniques tend to be slow in the rate of advance that is made. Given decline in acreage and lack of interest in rye in many areas of the world, rye breeding has generally declined. The exception is in northern Europe and western Asia, where the continued importance of rye has resulted in a sustained breeding effort. In both Germany and Poland, much of the rye that is grown is now hybrid rye. The hybrid production system is based on cytoplasmic male sterility. Hybrid cultivars tend to be higher yielding than other cultivars and also more uniform. However, hybrid production requires significant investment and is feasible in those areas only because of the interest and acreage. Although they are higher yielding, hybrid cultivars are unlikely to be produced in the many areas of the world with relatively low production, where breeding will instead continue to rely on a combination of mass selection and introduction from other rye-growing areas.

Rye is a diploid species and has the basic seven pairs of chromosomes found in many of the grasses. As a cross-pollinated species, rye is not ideally suited to traditional inheritance studies. Most recently, genetic studies have been performed within inbred lines that have been produced through enforced inbreeding. Because of its many unique characteristics that are also of agronomic importance and because of its close relationship to wheat, genetic studies have been performed and the genetics of many traits are understood. This is particularly true for disease resistance, cold hardiness, and aluminum tolerance. The significant difference in the breadmaking quality of wheat and rye and the economic significance of breadmaking quality have led to considerable genetic research to understand these differences. These accumulated studies have resulted in a detailed genetic map of rye.

Rye has also been the subject of considerable cytogenetic investigation. Because of its relatively large chromosomes and its economic importance, rye was often studied by early cytogeneticists. Through cytogenetic manipulation, a trisomic series of rye was produced (Kamanoi and Jenkins 1962) that is useful in genetic studies. (A trisomic is a plant that carries three copies of a chromosome rather than the normal two.) In addition, because of its ability to cross with wheat, entire rye chromosomes and parts of rye chromosomes have been transferred to wheat for genetic studies and for agronomic purposes. These studies have led to an understanding that each chromosome of rye is homologous (ancestrally related) to a wheat chromosome and that under certain situations such chromosomes could pair. More recently, this homology has been confirmed through molecular genetic work by demonstrating that the chromosomes of rye show strong synteny (gene order) with those of wheat and of other close relatives. Recent studies have shown that some stretches of rye chromosomes are also syntactic to rice, and given the fact that the DNA sequence of the rice genome is available, this will allow rye genes to be cloned and possibly used in crop improvement.

Utilization

Most of the world's rye grain is consumed by humans as bread; however, many so-called rye breads may contain only a low percentage of rye. Rye grain can also be used as an animal feed, but in this use, rye grain often constitutes only a portion of the ration because of feeding problems associated with higher levels in the diet (Seibel and Weipert 2001). The extent to which this is a problem depends on the animal. Poultry appear to be the most susceptible to these problems. Also the age of the animal plays a role, younger animals being the most susceptible. The cause of these problems remains elusive. High-molecular-weight (HMW) NSP (pentosans) seem to play a significant role. The entire rye plant can also be used as animal feed, either as harvested forage or grazed as pasture. A small part of the rye crop is utilized in distillation for the manufacture of rye whisky. Similarly, rye grain could be used as feedstock to produce ethanol as a renewable energy source where supply and economics dictate this as being appropriate.

During the last few decades, attention has been paid to the possibility of enhancing the quality of rye in terms of viscosity. High- and low-extract-viscosity ryes could have different applications in food and feed industries. High-extract-viscosity rye would be preferred in fiber-enriched human foods, or its water-extractable arabinoxylan (WEAX) could be useful in pharmaceutical or cosmetic products. Low-extract-viscosity rye would be preferred for animal feed and by the distilling industry. This chapter provides more details on these newly developed ryes.

Grain Structure

The rye kernel is a small, one-seeded fruit or caryopsis ranging from 6 to 8 mm in length and from 2 to 3 mm in width (Simmonds and Campbell 1976). The ripe grain is free-threshing and normally grayish, although a number of color variants occur. As with wheat, the grain consists of the embryo attached via a scutellum to the endosperm, the outer layer of which is the aleurone.

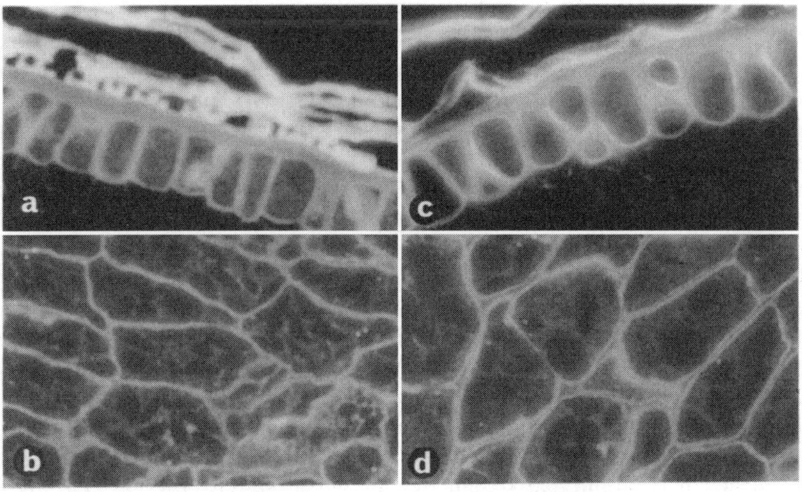

Fig. 1. Fluorescence micrographs of representative cross-sections from low- (R5; left), and high- (R95; right) extract-viscosity rye kernels showing aleurone layers (top) and endosperm cell walls (bottom); 400× magnification. (Source: Ragaee 2001)

These are enclosed by the remnants of the nucellar epidermis, the testa (seed coat), and the pericarp (fruit coat). The latter layers surround the seed and adhere to it tightly. The grain possesses a crease that extends the full length of the ventral side.

Using fluorescence microscopy to compare the microstructure of rye grains with wheat grains, Autio et al (1997) examined cell walls in both kernels. The rye endosperm cell walls were of fairly even thickness throughout the endosperm, unlike wheat, in which the inner endosperm cell walls are thinner than the outer endosperm and aleurone walls, and thinner than the rye cell walls. This would account for the higher dietary fiber content of rye compared to that of wheat. Using fluorescence microscopy, Ragaee (2001) observed that the aleurone was slightly larger with thicker walls in a high-viscosity (R95) compared to a low-viscosity (R5) rye (Fig. 1). There were no obvious differences in the shape of endosperm cells between the two samples. Although endosperm cells were slightly larger in R95 than in R5, both exhibited the same types of endosperm cells (peripheral, prismatic, and central) having different shapes and sizes (Simmonds and Campbell 1976).

Nutrient Composition

In a mature dry rye grain, carbohydrates (starch, fiber, sugar) make up 80% of the kernel weight, protein accounts for 15%, and fat and ash account for 2% each (Vinkx and Delcour 1996). The content of the major nutrients in rye, wheat, and triticale (which has a rye parent) are shown in Table 1. Starch is the main carbohydrate, followed by dietary fiber. The starch content of the rye grain ranges from 55.5 to 64.5% (Pettersson and Åman 1987, Harkonen et al 1997) and does not differ greatly from that of wheat (62.4%) (Abdel-Aal et al 1995). Wheat starch granules have a bimodal size distribution, with about 3–4% (50–75% by weight) being lenticular (15–40 μm in length) and the remainder being small, spherical granules (1–10 μm in diameter). Rye starch granules also occur in two similarly distinctive populations. However, rye starch granules have a mean particle diameter greater than that of wheat, and the size distribution covers a wider range (Berry et al 1971, Klassen and Hill 1971).

Like other cereal starches, rye starch granules show birefringence in polarized light and exhibit an A-type X-ray diffraction pattern. According to Matz (1991), rye and wheat starches were similar in their birefringence endpoint temperature and gelatinization temperature ranges. Also the chemical composition of rye starch resembled that of wheat, durum, and triticale starches (Berry et al 1971, Klassen and Hill 1971), except for phosphorus content, which was about half that of the other starches (0.025%). The absolute density of rye starch (1.42 g/mL) was slightly less than that of wheat starch (1.47 g/mL), and the water-binding capacity (86.5%) was slightly higher than that of wheat (85.0%) (Berry et al 1971, Klassen and Hill 1971).

The α-amylase activity in rye flour is much higher than in wheat flour, as indicated by amylograph viscosity (Klassen and Hill 1971) and falling number (FN) determinations (Ragaee et al 2001b). In the latter study, the authors observed significant differences in FN among commercial cultivars of rye and

TABLE 1
Comparison of Nutrient Composition of Rye with Wheat and Triticale (g/100 g, db)

Constituent	Rye[a]	Wheat[b]	Triticale[c]
Starch	64.6	62.4	62.1
Crude protein (N × 6.25)	9.5	16.8	14.3
Total soluble sugars	6.6	3.3	5.5
Crude fat	2.4	2.1	2.2
Ash	1.9	1.7	2.0
Dietary fiber	16.5	12.5	16.8
Arabinoxylan	7.6	6.7[d]	7.6[d]
β-Glucan	2.3	0.6[e]	...[f]
Cellulose	2.6	2.5[g]	2.8[h]
Klason lignin	3.0	1.2[i]	3.9[h]

[a] Bengtsson and Aman (1990).
[b] Abdel-Aal et al (1995).
[c] Grela (1996).
[d] Saini and Henry (1989).
[e] Henry (1985).
[f] Not determined.
[g] Lineback and Rasper (1988).
[h] Theander and Westerlund (1986).
[i] Jedel and Salmon (1994).

wheat flours and among new experimental lines of rye flours. When the flours were treated with enzyme inhibitor (0.2% mercuric acetate), the differences became more obvious. The wheat flour exhibited a slight increase in the FN with the addition of the inhibitor, which indicated that the enzyme activity in the original flour is very low. Among the new experimental rye flours, there was a positive correlation between FN and extract viscosity of rye flour in the presence ($r = 0.73$, $P < 0.05$) or absence ($r = 0.65$, $P < 0.05$) of the enzyme inhibitor. The authors concluded that the new ryes exhibited lower α-amylase activity than the commercial rye cultivar even when extract viscosities were comparable or lower.

The main constituents of the cell walls of parenchymatous and lignified tissues in cereals are nonstarch polysaccharides (NSP) (Fincher and Stone 1986), the primary component of dietary fiber. These macromolecules impart a variety of properties based on the nature of the fiber (e.g., viscosity of soluble fiber and rigidity of insoluble fiber). Rye is unique among cereals in its high content of soluble and insoluble dietary fibers, which constitute 15–17% (Bengtsson and Åman 1990, Girhammar 1992, Ragaee et al 2001a). Most of the fiber is insoluble, but 3–5% is soluble (Girhammar 1992, Ragaee et al 2001a), depending on cultivar. Bengtsson and Åman (1990) categorized the fiber in a rye sample (cv. Kungs II) containing 15.5% dietary fiber (db) into arabinoxylan (7.6%), Klason lignin (3%), cellulose (2.6%), and mixed linked (1→3),(1→4)-β-glucan (2.3%). In addition, rye contains arabinogalactan (Vinkx and Delcour 1996); the ratio of WEAX to arabinogalactan was reported to be 4.5 (Meuser et al 1986). According to recent definitions of dietary fiber, fructan is included in dietary fiber. Rye fructan is water-soluble and easily retrieved in the water extract. A water-extractable concentrate of rye bran contained as much as 23% of fructan (Karppinen et al 2003).

Arabinoxylan plays a key role in determining the quality and processing characteristics of cereal grains (Fincher and Stone 1986, McCleary et al 1986, Meuser and Suckow 1986, Kühn and Grosch 1989, Bengtsson et al 1992a,b, Ragaee et al 2001b). It may have a positive or a negative role, depending on the application, affecting milling behavior, starch-gluten separation, dough handling, loaf volume, and crumb and crust characteristics of breads. In brewing and baking, it limits the accessibility of starch granules to enzyme attack (Weipert 1997). Harkonen et al (1997) and Ragaee et al (2001b) demonstrated that WEAX is concentrated in the flour fraction of rye because of its primary location in the cell walls of the starchy endosperm. This was confirmed in the higher-extract viscosity of the rye flour fraction compared to that of the whole meal (Fig. 2).

The soluble and highly viscous arabinoxylan is recognized as the major antinutritive factor in rye grain for animal feeds. It has a detrimental effect in monogastric animals, chicks in particular, by interfering with the digestion and absorption of all nutrients (GrootWassink et al 1989, Bedford and Classen 1992, McLeod et al 1996, Ragaee et al 2001b). While this limits the value for animal feed where the economic considerations of rate of gain and feed conversion are paramount, it may be beneficial in human diets, at least in Western countries, where undernutrition is not a primary health concern.

The protein concentration in the rye grain ranges from 9.5 to 14.7% (Pettersson and Åman 1987, Harkonen et al 1997), depending on cultivar, growing conditions, and climate. The higher values usually occur in North America, where the level of nitrogen fertilizer applied is generally high. A unique characteristic of rye protein is the comparatively high (compared to wheat, barley, and most other cereals) proportion of water- and salt-soluble proteins, both fractions of which have high levels of the first limiting essential amino acid (lysine). As a result, the biological value of rye protein is considered to be superior to that of wheat and most other cereal proteins. However, its availability is reduced by other factors that restrict its true digestibility (Boros et al 1985).

The crude fat content of rye ranges between 1.5 and 2.5%, resembling the amount in other cereals such as wheat, barley, and triticale (Simmonds and Campbell 1976, Harkonen et al 1997). The linolenic acid (C18:3) concentration tends to be higher in rye oil (10.4%) compared to wheat (5.7%) (Simmonds and Campbell 1976, Matz 1991).

The ash content of rye grain ranges from 1.9 to 2.1% (Harkonen et al 1997), which is similar to that of wheat (1.7%) (Abdel-Aal et al 1998) and triticale (2.0%) (Munck 1972). Ash is concentrated in the outer pericarp, aleurone layer, and endosperm cell walls of cereal kernels. It is particularly high in the aleurone layer of rye, primarily because of the presence of phytin granules or aleurone bodies, a mixture of potassium and magnesium salts of

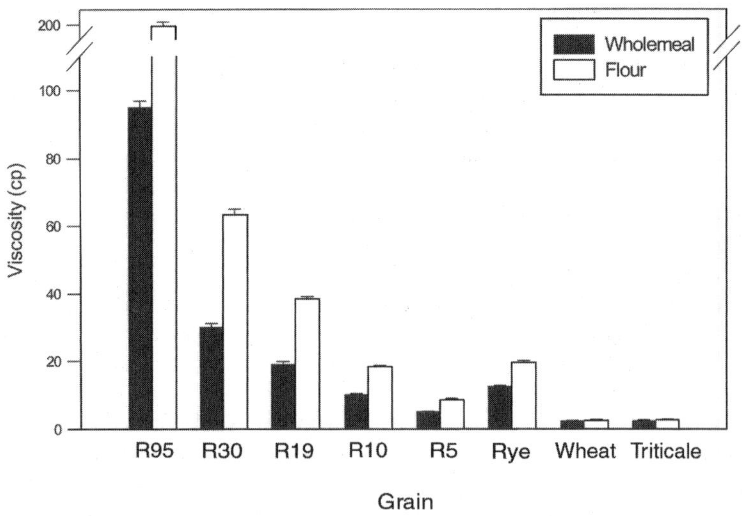

Fig. 2. Extract viscosity of whole meals and flours from rye, wheat, and triticale. (Reprinted, by permission, from Ragaee et al 2001b; ©American Chemical Society)

myoinositol hexaphosphate (Jacobsen et al 1971, Pomeranz 1973) surrounded by a protein-containing envelope (Lui and Altschul 1967). The mineral composition of rye ash is similar to that of other cereals (Matz 1991). Like other cereals, rye is an important source of B vitamins such as thiamin, nicotinic acid, riboflavin, pyridoxine, and pantothenic acid, as well as vitamin E. These components occur mainly in the embryo, scutellum, and aleurone layer (Simmonds and Campbell 1976).

In summary, rye differs in composition from wheat (less so from triticale), and these differences, such as those in the structure of the protein, starch, and fiber, have important effects on behavior during baking and brewing.

Extract Viscosity in Rye

Viscosity is a measure of the resistance to flow shown by a fluid under shear stress. Extract viscosity, the viscosity of a water extract of rye whole meal, has been developed as the single most important functional characteristic associated with both the baking (Weipert 1997, Ragaee et al 2001b) and the feeding quality of rye (Campbell and Bedford 1992, Marquardt et al 1994). The viscosity of rye, wheat, and triticale extracts is attributed to their content of WEAX (Bengtsson and Åman 1990), which has the ability to bind large amounts of water (McCleary et al 1986, Meuser and Suckow 1986). WEAX is the predominant water-extractable NSP in the endosperm of rye and is considered responsible for the high viscosity of rye.

Ragaee et al (2001a) studied the relationship between extract viscosity (EV) (1:10 w/v whole meal to water) and dietary fiber composition (both soluble and insoluble) of new rye lines (Table 2) varying in their baking and feeding characteristics. The results indicated that EV of rye whole meal was weakly correlated with total dietary fiber and total arabinoxylan content, and strongly correlated with soluble dietary fiber ($r = 0.90$, $P < 0.05$) and WEAX ($r = 0.89$, $P < 0.05$) content. No significant association was evident between EV and β-glucan content of the rye lines. When WEAX was calculated as a percentage of the total arabinoxylan (Table 2), the differences among ryes became more obvious. The viscosity of the water extracts ranged between 5 and 95 cP, indicating different concentrations and different molecular weights of the WEAXs among the rye lines. Water-unextractable arabinoxylan (WUAX), although not dissolving, does also bind water (Neukom 1976).

Addition of xylanase (from *Trichoderma reesei*) to either rye extracts or pure arabinoxylan decreased viscosity significantly (Harkonen et al 1995), confirming that the viscosity of rye extracts was attributable to arabinoxylan. Ragaee et al (2001a) studied the effect of different enzyme treatments (α-amylase, protease, β-glucanase, and xylanase) on the water extract from a high-viscosity rye whole meal (Fig. 3). Neither α-amylase nor β-glucanase significantly reduced the viscosity of the extract, indicating the small contribution of starch and β-glucan to rye extract viscosity. A slight reduction in the viscosity was observed after treating the extract with protease, which

TABLE 2
Nonstarch Polysaccharide Contents of Rye and Wheat Grains (% of dry whole meal)[a]

Grains	TDF[b] (%)	SDF[c] (%)	TAX[d] (%)	WEAX[e] (%)	WEAX[f] (% of TAX)	β-Glucan[g] (%)
Rye cultivars						
R95[h]	16.98 ± 0.11[i]	5.20 ± 0.04	7.31 ± 0.04	2.46 ± 0.02	33.65	1.94 ± 0.01
R30	16.19 ± 0.25	4.01 ± 0.04	6.77 ± 0.08	2.04 ± 0.02	30.13	2.48 ± 0.01
R19	16.76 ± 0.51	4.62 ± 0.13	6.73 ± 0.23	2.02 ± 0.01	30.01	1.90 ± 0.06
R10	14.67 ± 0.18	4.04 ± 0.02	5.59 ± 0.03	1.31 ± 0.01	23.43	1.98 ± 0.01
R5	16.45 ± 0.21	3.80 ± 0.17	6.73 ± 0.01	1.49 ± 0.01	22.14	1.76 ± 0.08
Prima rye (12.5)	15.20 ± 0.10	4.10 ± 0.20	7.00 ± 0.20	1.80 ± 0.01	25.20	2.10 ± 0.08
HRS[j] wheat (2.5)	11.56 ± 0.16	1.43 ± 0.11	4.88 ± 0.14	0.99 ± 0.02	20.30	0.60 ± 0.01

[a] Source: Ragaee et al (2001a); used by permission. ©American Chemical Society.
[b] Total dietary fiber.
[c] Soluble dietary fiber.
[d] Total arabinoxylan.
[e] Water-extractable arabinoxylan.
[f] Water-extractable arabinoxylan as % of total arabinoxylan.
[g] Total β-glucan in the whole meal.
[h] Figures represent extract viscosity of whole meals.
[i] Mean ± standard deviation ($n = 3$).
[j] Hard red spring.

may be due to hydrolysis of peptide bridges between WEAX and protein. A very marked reduction in the viscosity of the extract was obtained from the xylanase treatment, confirming previous results (Boros et al 1993, Vinkx et al 1993).

Both genetics and environment influence the extract viscosity of rye grain. Scoles et al (1993) identified genetic variability in extract viscosity among inbred rye lines. Gan et al (1996, 1997) found substantial variability in extract viscosity among individual rye plants within an open-pollinated cultivar and among cultivars and lines. These authors found that a cultivar and a line with higher mean extract viscosity exhibited larger variability in viscosity across environments and were more sensitive to environment than were those with low extract viscosity. This may simply reflect the nature of the influence of concentration and molecular weight (MW) on viscosity, where small changes in the former can lead to greater changes in the latter. Plaami et al (1989) found that environmental factors also affected total dietary fiber (TDF) content. These authors studied TDF in 15 rye cultivars from Finland and in 10 cultivars from Canada, Sweden, the United States, and the former USSR. High precipitation increased TDF content, whereas a high mean temperature during the growing period reduced TDF. A cold, wet season resulted in a high arabinoxylan content (Saastamoinen et al 1989). In contrast, Gan et al (1997)

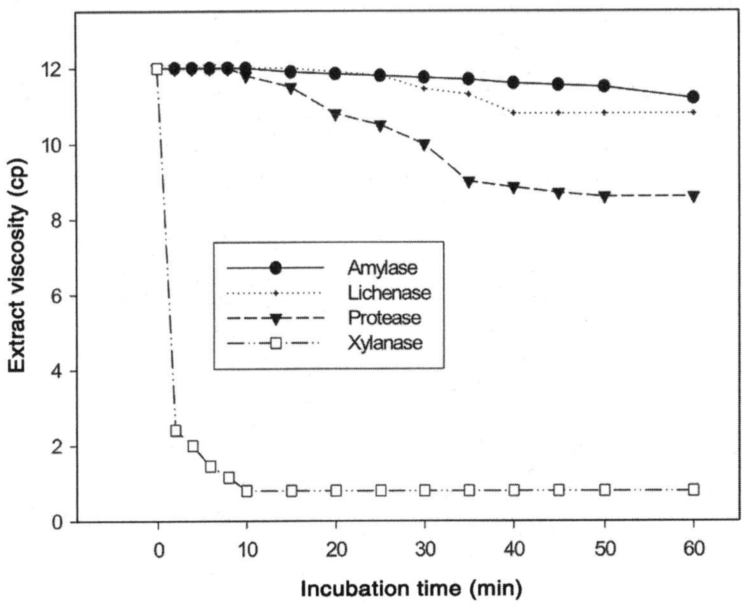

Fig. 3. Effect of α-amylase, lichenase, protease, and xylanase treatment on the viscosity of a water extract from high-extract viscosity rye (R95) whole meal. The ratio of whole meal to water was 1:10, w/v. (Reprinted, by permission, from Ragaee et al 2001a; ©American Chemical Society)

reported greater extract viscosity with grain maturing under hot, dry conditions, suggesting higher WEAX.

When seed numbers are too limited for viscosity analysis in early generations, kernel weight could be used as a nondestructive selection criterion, although it would not be equivalent to direct selection based on EV (Gan et al 1996). The authors reported that EV was negatively correlated with kernel weight, positively correlated with FN, and not correlated with test weight. Other seed characteristics such as color, plumpness, and starch content did not appear to be related to EV or to the level of HMW arabinoxylan in rye grain (Scoles et al 1993).

Oxidative Gelation of Arabinoxylan

An important property of arabinoxylan is its ability to form gels. Oxidative cross-linking has been suggested to be responsible for arabinoxylan gel formation, and this might change the rheological properties of a dough and influence bread volume (Hoseney 1984, Meuser and Suckow 1986). Oxidative gelation occurs when free-radical-generating agents (e.g., hydrogen peroxide/peroxidase, ammonium persulfate, ferric chloride, linoleic acid/-lipoxygenase) induce interchain covalent linkages through oxidative coupling of ferulic acid residues attached to the arabinoxylan (Fig. 4) (Neukom and Markwalder 1978, Vinkx and Delcour 1996), resulting in a three-dimensional network of gel. The influences of structure and MW on the gelation capacity of arabinoxylan have been studied (Izydorczyk and Biliaderis 1992a,b). Only arabinoxylan fractions having a high ferulic acid content, high molecular weight, and a relatively unsubstituted xylan backbone structure were capable of extensive cross-linking to yield well-developed gel networks.

Ferulic acid, attached through ester linkage to the L-arabinofuranose substituents of the xylan chain, is considered primarily responsible for oxidative gelation (Izydorczyk et al 1990, Vinkx et al 1991, Vinkx and Delcour 1996).

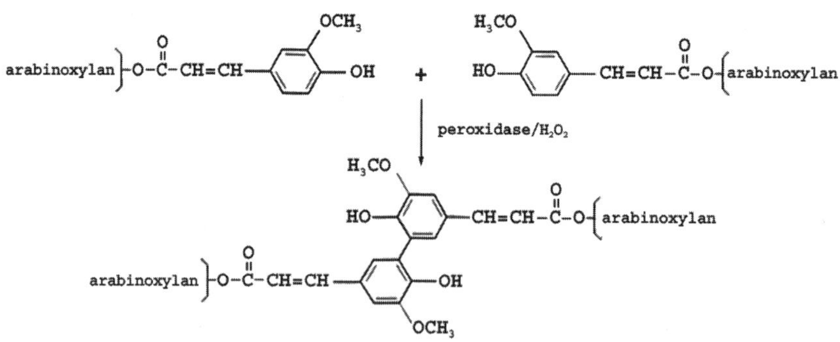

Fig. 4. Cross-linking of arabinoxylan by formation of diferulic acid during oxidative gelation. (Source: Vinkx and Delcour 1996)

Ferulic acid has three potential reactive sites that could participate in cross-linking of arabinoxylan chains by the formation of diferulic acid bridges, two on the aromatic ring and one at the double bond. Moore et al (1990) demonstrated that the aromatic ring of ferulic acid rather than the double bond (Hoseney and Faubion 1981) served as a cross-linking center for arabinoxylan polymers. Because the presence of feruloyl groups is essential for cross-linking, their relative amounts and distribution along the chain will influence the gelling potential of arabinoxylan (Izydorczyk et al 1991, Izydorczyk and Biliaderis 1992a,b, Rattan et al 1994). The higher gelling potential of less-substituted arabinoxylan is thought to be due to the greater flexibility of the chain, which promotes the establishment of cross-links by facilitating the initial contact between feruloyl groups of neighboring arabinoxylan chains (Izydorczyk and Biliaderis 1992a,b). The hydration capacity of arabinoxylan is greatly increased upon oxidative gelation (Izydorczyk et al 1990), and cross-linked arabinoxylan chains hold up to 100 times their weight of water.

A role for protein has been proposed in oxidative gelation. Neukom et al (1962) observed that a pure, protein-free arabinoxylan would not gel, indicating that glycoprotein was involved in the reaction. Vinkx et al (1991) found that the pentosan in a water extract from rye was necessary for oxidative gelation and that the protein moiety was of much less importance with respect to both the viscous properties of the extracts and the increase in viscosity upon gelation. Geissmann and Neukom (1973) concluded that oxidative gelation occurred as a result of oxidative phenolic coupling of ferulic acid residues, causing cross-linking of the polysaccharide molecules. In the presence of proteins, ferulic acid reacted with the N-terminal of an amino group or with tyrosine residues (Neukom and Markwalder 1978).

Rye in Human Diets

In a large-scale epidemiological study on elderly Finnish men, the fiber complex in rye (in Finland, mainly consumed in food as whole-meal rye flour) was shown to be of possible help in defending against heart attack and coronary death (Pietinen et al 1996). Several factors in rye grain and baked rye products may contribute to a healthy diet, but dietary fiber is recognized as one of the most important. The beneficial effect of soluble fiber in rye is attributed to its water-binding capacity and its inhibition of the absorption of saturated fatty acids and sodium (Åman et al 1997), whereas insoluble fiber is beneficial in improving colon health.

Comparing the dietary fiber composition of whole-meal rye bread with that of white wheat bread, Bach Knudsen et al (1997) found that the dietary fiber composition was similar in both breads, but their contents were different. The dietary fiber content of whole-meal rye bread was almost four times higher than that of white wheat bread (Table 3), because 98–100% extraction flour was used for making rye bread compared to the 70–80% extraction flour used in the white wheat bread. However, even at the same extraction rate, the dietary fiber content was higher in whole-meal rye flour than in whole-meal wheat flour (Nyman et al 1984).

Studies on the digestibility of cereal starch (Bach Knudsen et al 1997) and NSP (Englyst and Cummings 1985, Åman et al 1995, Pettersson et al 1996) in humans indicated that digestibility of cereal starch is high, with values mostly above 97%, whether the cereal product is served as raw starch (e.g., oat) or as breads (Table 4). Degradation of NSP occurred in the human small intestine and depended on the type of polysaccharide. The digestibility of NSP (arabinoxylan) from rye bread was 5.5%, while the digestibility of NSP (β-glucan) from oat was 15.2%. The authors concluded that the lower degradation of arabinoxylans is undoubtedly due to their branched structure, which makes them less susceptible to microbial degradation compared with β-glucan.

TABLE 3
Dietary Fiber Composition (g/100 g dry matter) of Wholemeal Rye Bread and White Wheat Bread[a]

Constitutent	Wholemeal Rye Bread	White Wheat Bread
NSP[b]		
Cellulose	1.4	0.4
NCP[c]	11.4 (4.9)[d]	3.3 (1.6)
Arabinose	2.7 (1.1)	0.8 (0.4)
Xylose	4.2 (1.8)	1.1 (0.6)
Mannose	0.3 (0.1)	0.3 (0.2)
Galactose	0.6 (0.3)	0.2 (0.2)
Glucose	3.0 (1.3)	0.7 (0.1)
Uronic acids	0.6 (0.3)	0.1 (0.1)
Total NSP	12.8	3.7
Klason lignin	2.2	0.3
Dietary fiber	15.0	4.0

[a] Source: BachKnudsen et al (1997); used by permission.
[b] Nonstarch polysaccharides.
[c] Noncellulosic polysaccharides.
[d] Values in parentheses are soluble NSP.

TABLE 4
Digestibility of Starch and NSP[a] in the Small Intestine of Humans with Ileostomies[b]

	Starch			NSP		
	Amount Fed (g/day)	Amount Recovered (g/day)	% Digested	Amount Fed (g/day)	Amount Recovered (g/day)	% Digested
White bread	61.9	1.6	97.4	2.3	2.3	0.0
Oat	57.8	1.2	97.9	6.7	6.3	5.2
Wheat bread	278.0	3.5	98.7	22.4	19.0	15.2
Rye bread	256.0	4.1	98.4	49.3	46.6	5.5

[a] Nonstarch polysaccharides.
[b] Data from Englyst and Cummings (1985); Åman et al (1995); and Pettersson et al (1996).

Inulin and fructo-oligosaccharides have been reported to improve gut function and to selectively stimulate the growth of bifidobacteria (Bouhnik et al 1999, Brighenti et al 1999, Kruse et al 1999). Karppinen et al (2003) reported that rye is an important natural fructan source in human nutrition, as indicated by the high fructan concentration in rye bread. The authors reported that one slice of soft rye bread (25 g) contains 0.3–0.4 g of fructan, and one slice of rye crisp bread (12 g) contains 0.3 g of fructan. Bach Knudsen et al (1997) studied the degradation of fructans in the small intestine of humans. The results indicated that most fructans were recovered in the ileal effluent.

Relative to white wheat bread, rye bread provides more stimulation of microbial growth in the large intestine. This results in increases in short-chain fatty acid production and in the rate of passage, reductions in pH and dehydroxylation of bile acids, dilution of the colonic content, and alteration of nitrogen metabolism (Englyst and Cummings 1985, Åman et al 1995, Pettersson et al 1996). According to current knowledge, these effects are considered positive for human health. Furthermore, rye bran was shown to be more effective than oat bran or barley flakes in lowering plasma and liver cholesterol levels in hamsters and was claimed to be a useful source of soluble fiber (Rieckhoff et al 1999).

The development of rye lines exhibiting high-extract viscosity compared to the available commercial cultivars would be of use in the development of various healthful value-added food products. Scoles et al (1993) identified ryes having extract viscosity up to 95 cP (viscosity of whole meal-water extract at a ratio of 1:10 w/v meal-water) compared to 12 cP for the commercial cultivar Prima. When this rye whole meal was baked into bread and fed to broiler chicks (Ragaee et al 2001b), it increased digesta viscosity. These results indicated that a significant proportion of the WEAX survived the baking procedure and exerted its effect on the digesta viscosity, suggesting a beneficial effect on human health of high-extract-viscosity rye compared to the commercial rye cultivars.

Plant lignans in the form of matairesinol and secoisolariciresinol are found in whole-meal rye flour at levels of 0.33–0.52 and 0.27–0.45 mg/kg of dry matter, respectively (Nilsson et al 1997). These components are found in high levels in flaxseed (Thompson et al 1996) and have been associated with health effects such as inhibiting cancer development. The highest levels of rye lignans were found in fractions enriched in pericarp/testa and aleurone tissues; the lowest levels were in the endosperm. Juntunen et al (2000) reported a significant increase in daily excretion of enterolactone when human subjects consumed rye bread for four weeks, compared to when they consumed wheat bread. The enterolactone was 5- and 10-fold higher in men and women, respectively, in comparison with the amount of plant lignan precursor measured in the rye bread. These data indicated the possible role of fiber in enhancement of the formation of mammalian lignans from their plant precursor in the gut.

Rye bran also provides a source of dietary phenolic antioxidants such as hydroxycinnamates, ferulic acid, sinapic acid, and *p*-coumaric acid (Andreasen et al 2001). These substances may have potential health effects by protecting low-density lipoprotein from oxidation and therefore helping to prevent atherosclerosis and coronary heart disease, and protecting against other oxidative damage of tissues.

Rye in Animal Diets

Several compounds such as alkylresorcinol and other phenolic compounds, trypsin inhibitors, phytic acid, and NSP have been implicated as having potentially deleterious effects on the utilization of nutrients by animals (Rakowska 1994). Recent studies, however, have shown that these constituents can also have health benefits for humans as antioxidants and antidisease factors (Rieckhoff et al 1999, Juntunen et al 2000). Alkylresorcinol is a common name for alkyl and alkenyl derivatives of dihydroxybenzene. The toxicity of isolated alkylresorcinol was found to decrease with chain length and increase with the number of double bonds. Fortunately, low-molecular-weight homologues with alkyl chain lengths up to 13, which are the most toxic, are absent from cereal grains. The chain length of the alkylresorcinol in rye and wheat varies from 15 to 31. The total content of alkylresorcinol in rye grains varies from 0.9 to 2.0 mg/g, which is higher than that in wheat (0.2–0.6 mg/g) (Rakowska 1994). The alkylresorcinol in rye was found not to harm either poultry (Fernandez et al 1973) or swine (Honeyfield et al 1983). This is the basis for the current view that alkylresorcinol in rye is not a serious concern.

Trypsin inhibitors occur at a relatively high level in rye (4.0 U/g) compared to other cereals (wheat <1.0 U/g, triticale 1.5–3.0 U/g) (Rakowska et al 1992). The trypsin inhibitors isolated from rye or triticale had no effect on protein digestibility in rats and chickens when the dietary concentration was 1.4 U/g diet, but when it was added at higher levels (2.64 U/g diet), protein digestibility was depressed in rats by about 5.0%.

Phytic acid (myoinositol hexaphosphoric acid) and its salts are present in the aleurone cells of rye and other cereals (Kent-Jones and Amos 1967). The antinutritional effect of phytic acid is based on its ability to form highly insoluble and indigestible salts of various cations (Fennema 1985) and thus render some essential minerals poorly available to monogastric animals (Deshpande and Damodaran 1990). Phytate also interacts with proteins, resulting in reduced protein solubility and availability (Sathe et al 1984), and it inhibits several enzymes such as pepsin (Camus and LaPorte 1976), α-amylase (Deshpande and Cheryan 1984), and trypsin (Singh and Krikorian 1982). The endogenous enzyme phytase is able to hydrolyze phytic acid and its salts to inositol and phosphoric acid. The phytase activity of rye has been reported to be higher than that of wheat (Gontzea and Sutzescu 1968).

Cell walls and their dietary fiber are largely or completely indigestible by alimentary enzymes in monogastric animals (Fennema 1985) and tend to remain intact during digestion, although the water-soluble fraction is at least partially digestible. The 3–5% soluble dietary fiber in rye, which consists mainly of arabinoxylan (Vinkx and Delcour 1996, Åman et al 1997, Ragaee et al 2001a) has a significant impact on the nutritive value of rye in animal feed (Jones 1997).

WEAX is recognized as the major factor responsible for depressed feed intake and impaired nutrient digestibility in chicks (Campbell and Bedford 1992, Marquardt et al 1994). Inclusion of 20% rye in a broiler chick diet decreased weight gain by 25% (Friesen et al 1991). Rybka et al (1993) determined that the level of total indigestible components (NSP plus indigestible protein) in rye averaged 197 mg/g, which is considered an intermediate value compared to barley (257 mg/g) and triticale and wheat (169 mg/g). The amount of indigestible protein associated with the soluble and insoluble fiber that was not utilized by animals was found to be approximately 13–22% of the total protein in rye (Raczynska-Bojanowska and Rybka 1994).

The problems observed with rye in animal diets are mainly associated with the amount and MW of WEAX. Fengler and Marquardt (1988b) showed that the high viscosity of the gut contents of chicks fed rye was related to the concentration of WEAX. Bedford and Classen (1992) demonstrated that high viscosity in the gut was not correlated with total arabinoxylan content or with the content of WEAX, but only with the content of the HMW fraction of WEAX. Purified pentosan (arabinoxylan + arabinogalactan) preparations retained the majority of the antinutritional effects (Fengler and Marquardt 1988a,b). Recently, Ragaee et al (2001b) reported that chicks fed diets containing high-extract-viscosity rye (R95) that was rich in both WEAX and the HMW fraction of WEAX exhibited the poorest body-weight gains and feed conversion compared to those fed diets containing low-viscosity rye (R5) or wheat. These results were consistent with other data (Campbell and Bedford 1992, McLeod et al 1996). Ward and Marquardt (1983) demonstrated that fat retention was affected when rye was fed to chicks, with malabsorption of saturated and long-chain fatty acids being particularly severe.

The problems associated with rye-based animal feeds can be at least partially overcome by several means. Campbell et al (1983) depolymerized arabinoxylan using gamma irradiation, which increased the nutritive value of the rye. Numerous studies have shown a beneficial response to enzyme supplementation of rye diets, with improvements noted in growth and feed conversion, as well as in digestibility (Campbell and Bedford 1992). GrootWassink et al (1989) demonstrated that the principal activity required was endoxylanolytic; however, a purified xylanase was less effective than a crude preparation. Pawlik et al (1990) improved the nutritive value of rye by water soaking, enzyme treatment, or both, which reduced the viscosity of rye extracts. This was attributed to endogenous or exogenous enzymes partially hydrolyzing the viscous WEAX. Synergism has been reported between endoxylanase and arabinosidase, xylosidase, or acetyl-xylan esterase (Seeta et al 1989, Tenkanen et al 1991) in model systems. However, the beneficial effect of xylanase could be affected by the structure of the arabinoxylan, which varies among cereals, and the degree of substitution of the arabinofuranosyl residues (Antoniou et al 1981, Henry 1985). The phenolic residues associated with arabinoxylan may also interfere with xylanase activity (Renard et al 1990). Employing breeding programs to improve the nutritive value of rye for monogastric animals is another way to overcome the antinutritional effects of rye for animal feed. Scoles et al (1993) and McLeod et al (1996) developed new ryes exhibiting low extract viscosity (viscosity of whole meal-water extract at a ratio of 1:10, w/v, was 5.0 cP). These ryes exhibited better feeding quality, lower digesta viscosity, and a high rate-of-gain and feed conversion when fed to broiler chicks (Ragaee et al 2001b).

Rye Bread, Arabinoxylan, and Breadmaking

In traditional rye bread, rye whole meal is used as the raw material. In North America, most rye breads use rye flour in a blend with wheat flour to produce rye-flavored, light-textured breads. The proportion of rye flour varies from 10 to 90% (Drews and Seibel 1976, Poutanen 1997). Rye bread produced in North America usually contains 50% or more wheat flour, unlike European rye bread, which is often made from 100% rye flour (Hoseney 1984). The traditional method of preparing rye bread uses the sourdough formula. This procedure has the advantage that slightly damaged (sprouted) rye with increased α-amylase activity is usable, and the method produces flavorful bread with a long shelf life (Rychlik and Grosch 1995). Additionally, the quality of rye bread is mainly dependent on the physical characteristics of the crumb rather than on loaf volume, which is the principal quality parameter in wheat bread.

In spite of being a relatively minor constituent in wheat and rye flours, arabinoxylan has a major impact on bread quality. The ability to bind large quantities of water and to form viscous solutions or gels is a significant attribute that has important implications for mixing, dough development, and bread quality (loaf volume, crumb texture, and staling characteristics) (Amado and Neukom 1985, Meuser and Suckow 1986). WEAX and WUAX have different functional roles in rye dough. WEAX forms a sticky gel that keeps the dough together (Pomeranz 1985, Holas et al 1992) and also can affect the rate of starch degradation (Gudmundsson et al 1991). WUAX has a high water-binding capacity and a capacity to swell (Pomeranz 1985, Meuser and Suckow 1986) and has important deleterious influences on the breadmaking properties of rye flour, such as dark gray color, dull surface, and bitter taste (Meuser and Suckow 1985, 1986; Kühn and Grosch 1989; Weipert 1993).

Despite the recognition that water absorption, viscosity enhancement, and gelling properties of arabinoxylan have considerable effect upon the rheological behavior of dough, loaf volume, and crumb texture, interpretation of experimental results is not always straightforward, as the method of isolation, degree of purity, composition, MW, and level of supplementation of arabinoxylan or pentosan preparations and the baking system employed all affect the results and impact of arabinoxylan on breadmaking (Hoseney 1984, Lineback and Rasper 1988).

Arabinoxylan has the ability to retain gas in the dough (Hoseney 1984) and protect protein foams against thermal disruption (Izydorczyk et al 1992b). It is thought that the high viscosity of arabinoxylan adds to the strength and elasticity of gluten-starch films surrounding gas bubbles in dough and thus slows the rate of CO_2 diffusion from dough during baking. The fineness and homogeneity of crumb texture was found to be directly related to the extent to which gas cells combine and collapse during heating (Izydorczyk and Biliaderis 1995).

When added to wheat flour, arabinoxylan clearly competes with other dough constituents for water. Significant increases in farinograph water absorption and dough-development time were evident when pentosans or purified arabinoxylan were added to wheat flour dough (Michniewicz et al 1991, Vanhamel et al 1993, Biliaderis et al 1995). Addition of crude (Delcour et al 1991, Michniewicz et al 1992) or purified (Biliaderis et al 1995) arabinoxylan to wheat flour enhanced loaf volume. The beneficial effect of arabinoxylan on loaf volume is not a linear relationship with respect to concentration; low levels are beneficial, but higher than optimal concentrations cause excessive viscosity in the dough and may even decrease the volume of the final baked product (Delcour et al 1991, Biliaderis et al 1995). On the other hand, when wheat flour was treated with a highly purified xylanase (McCleary et al 1986), it yielded sticky doughs and breads of low loaf volume and soggy texture.

High- and low-viscosity rye flours were evaluated in breadmaking and compared with commercial cultivars of rye and wheat as control checks (Ragaee et al 2001b). The results showed that the high water-binding capacity of WEAX in rye flour resulted in high water absorption and short dough-development time compared to the values for the control wheat flour (Table 5). Extract viscosity of rye flour was negatively correlated ($r = -0.65$, $P < 0.05$) with farinograph mixing tolerance index (MTI) and positively correlated ($r = 0.64$, $P < 0.05$) with dough stability, thus showing a positive impact of extract viscosity of rye flour on dough strength. No relationship was observed between extract viscosity and water absorption, arrival time, or dough-development time. In the same study, two different rye (R10 and R95) flours varying in their extract viscosities (20 and 199 cP, respectively) were blended with wheat flour in various ratios (from 10 to 70%, in 10% increments). Despite the differences in extract viscosity of the rye flours, loaf volume declined in a similar fashion as the level of each rye flour increased in the blend (Fig. 5), which was expected as a result of dilution of the wheat gluten, but R95 flour depressed loaf volume more than R10. Beyond 30% rye flour in the blend, loaf volume and other bread characteristics (including crust smoothness and crumb stickiness and density) became progressively less satisfactory. Accordingly, 30:70 rye-wheat blends were considered suitable for producing rye-wheat bread having good quality.

When each of six rye flours that exhibited different extract viscosities (10, 20, 39, 63, and 199 cP) were mixed with wheat flour at the same ratio (30:70,

TABLE 5
Farinograph Characteristics of Rye and Wheat Flours, Individually and in Blends with Wheat Flour[a]

	Water Absorption (%)	Arrival Time (sec)	DDT[b] (sec)	MTI[c] (BU)	Stability[d] (sec)
Ryes[e]					
R95	73.3 ± 0.1[f]	55.0 ± 2.5	92.5 ± 3.5	125.0 ± 7.1	97.5 ± 4.0
R30	68.1 ± 0.2	30.0 ± 0.1	52.5 ± 2.5	122.5 ± 3.5	117.5 ± 3.5
R19	72.8 ± 0.4	45.0 ± 0.1	87.5 ± 3.5	165.0 ± 7.1	60.0 ± 0.1
R10	66.3 ± 0.4	42.5 ± 1.5	63.5 ± 2.9	157.5 ± 3.5	47.5 ± 0.5
R5	72.3 ± 0.4	67.5 ± 3.0	80.0 ± 3.4	172.5 ± 3.5	47.5 ± 1.5
Prima rye	66.1 ± 0.2	57.5 ± 2.5	87.5 ± 3.5	127.5 ± 3.5	62.5 ± 2.5
LSD	0.8	9.5	11.3	10.1	13.8
Rye/wheat blends (30:70, w/w)					
R95	70.3 ± 1.1	157.5 ± 6.6	322.5 ± 10.6	20.0 ± 0.1	540.0 ± 22.4
R30	69.3 ± 0.4	127.5 ± 5.6	345.0 ± 15.2	47.5 ± 1.5	465.0 ± 21.2
R19	70.0 ± 0.1	180.0 ± 0.6	332.5 ± 3.5	37.5 ± 1.5	382.5 ± 10.6
R10	67.8 ± 0.4	157.5 ± 6.6	315.0 ± 21.2	22.5 ± 1.0	472.5 ± 10.6
R5	67.3 ± 0.4	175.0 ± 7.1	322.5 ± 10.6	52.5 ± 2.5	322.5 ± 10.6
Prima rye	66.3 ± 1.1	127.5 ± 5.6	315.0 ± 0.1	20.0 ± 0.1	450.0 ± 20.4
Hard red spring wheat	66.7 ± 0.4	115.5 ± 5.1	315.0 ± 4.2	5.0 ± 0.0	1,155.0 ± 21.2
LSD	2.3	13.4	23.9	6.8	51.1

[a] Source: Ragaee et al (2001b); used by permission. ©American Chemical Society.
[b] Dough development time.
[c] Mixing tolerance index (in Brabender Units).
[d] Dough stability (in seconds).
[e] Each line is designated as R (rye) followed by its whole meal extract viscosity (in cP).
[f] Mean ± standard deviation ($n = 3$).

rye-wheat), a significant positive correlation ($r = 0.85$, $P < 0.05$) was observed between extract viscosity of the rye-wheat blends and their farinograph water absorptions. The arrival time increased for all blends compared to that of wheat flour or individual rye flours, which was explained by a reduction in the dough-forming ability of the wheat flour when mixed with any of the rye flours. The baking characteristics of the rye flours indicated that extract viscosity of rye flours was negatively correlated with loaf volume ($r = -0.68$, $P < 0.05$), with the lowest loaf volume obtained for bread produced from wheat-rye R95.

The greater depressing effect of the high-extract-viscosity rye flour (R95) on loaf volume was explained by studies of the structure of the purified WEAX isolated from R95, R30, and R5 rye whole meals using proton nuclear magnetic resonance and high-performance size-exclusion chromatography equipped with a triple detector system (Ragaee et al 2001a). High-viscosity rye (R95) had a high proportion of an HMW fraction (39%), and its pure arabinoxylan exhibited higher average MW (~500 kD) (Table 6) compared to the other samples (~280 and 199 kD for R30 and R5, respectively). The pure arabinoxylan from R95 had an extended molecular structure with a large radius of gyration (Rg) and hydrodynamic radius (Rh), and a high degree of monosubstituted xylopyranosyl residues. These features would facilitate more hydrogen bonding (in the dough system) between the gluten protein (in the wheat flour) and the unsubstituted region on the arabinoxylan (in the rye flour). Hydrogen bonding would enhance the strength of the dough, as indicated by the relatively high farinograph stability of the R95-wheat blend

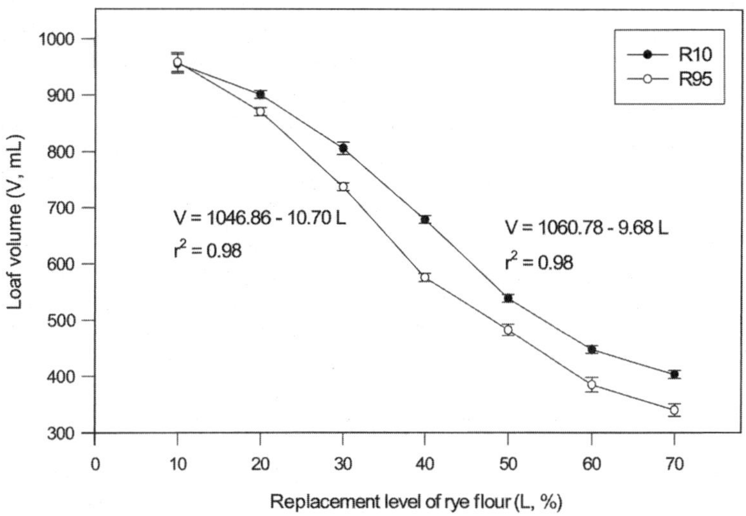

Fig. 5. Effect of level of replacement of wheat flour by low- (R10) and high- (R95) extract-viscosity rye flour on bread volume. (Reprinted, by permission, from Ragaee et al 2001b; ©American Chemical Society)

TABLE 6
Fine Structure of Purified Water-Extractable Arabinoxylan Isolated from High- (R95), Intermediate- (R30), and Low- (R5) Extract-Viscosity Rye Whole Meals, as Determined by H-NMR and High-Performance Size-Exclusion Chromatography/Triple Detection[a]

Parameter	R95[b]	R30	R5
Unsubstituted Xylp (%)	34	24	23
Monosubstituted Xylp (%)	51	59	49
Disubstituted Xylp (%)	15	18	28
$Xylp_{disub}/Xylp_{monsub}$[c]	0.29	0.31	0.35
MW[d]	494,950 ± 2,3971[e]	280,400 ± 18,809	199,050 ± 5,162
Rg (nm)[f]	54.5 ± 1.2	37.1 ± 1.2	29.1 ± 0.5
Rh (nm)[g]	41.9 ± 0.9	28.5 ± 1.0	22.4 ± 0.4
IV (dL/g)[h]	10.2 ± 0.2	6.2 ± 0.3	4.3 ± 0.2
"a" value[i]	0.57 ± 0.01	0.72 ± 0.02	0.67 ± 0.02

[a] Source: Ragaee et al (2001a); used by permission. ©American Chemical Society.
[b] Each line is designated as R (rye) followed by its wholemeal extract viscosity (in cP).
[c] Ratio of disubstituted xylose residues to monosubstituted xylose residues.
[d] Weighted average molecular weight.
[e] Mean ± standard deviation ($n = 2$).
[f] Weighted average radius of gyration.
[g] Weighted average hydrodynamic radius.
[h] Intrinsic viscosity.
[i] Slope of Mark-Houwink plot.

(Table 5). The relatively low loaf volume obtained with the R95-wheat blend suggests, however, that hydrogen bonding between arabinoxylan and gluten was disrupted during baking, which may result in a loss of gas-retentive strength and consequently reduced loaf volume. More excessive dehydration of gluten by the high concentration and HMW of arabinoxylan in R95 flour would also contribute to the inferior loaf volume obtained with R95-wheat blend. Conversely, the lower concentration of WEAX in flour from low (R5) or intermediate (R30) extract viscosity ryes along with higher degrees of di- and monosubstitution of xylopyranosyl residues, and lower MW (Rg and Rh) would lead to less effective formation of hydrogen bonds with the dough gluten (reducing dough strength) and lesser competition with gluten for moisture (which would enhance loaf volume). Udy (1956) similarly observed that the degree of interaction between gluten proteins and water-soluble pentosans of flour (in the dough system) was dependent on the molecular size (degree of polymerization), branching, and shape of the pentosans.

Future of Rye in North America

People are becoming increasingly aware of the relationship between diet and health. This awareness is slowly leading to improved eating habits, and it is predicted that, in the future, people will increasingly make food choices based on what is beneficial for their health and well-being. Therefore, designing a new generation of foods that reduce reliance on drug therapy is a worthwhile goal for food scientists and plant breeders. Rye could clearly play a role in this new generation of foods. In countries such as Finland, the average rye intake of 43 g/day (Anonymous 2001) corresponding to a daily intake of 7.7 g of dietary fiber or 2.0 g of fructan should have beneficial health effects.

In view of the above as well as exceptional winter hardiness, low demand for pesticides, and the ability to make efficient use of limited nutrients and soil moisture reserves, rye could be a most promising value-added sustainable cereal crop for North America, particularly in the northern Great Plains. These considerations might encourage the development of breeding programs for fall rye with either low extract viscosity (for animal feed and distilling) or high extract viscosity (for human food). Long-term breeding programs are needed for such developments and may require greater incentives than exist at present.

References

Abdel-Aal, E-S. M., Hucl, P., and Sosulski, F. W. 1995. Compositional and nutritional characteristics of spring einkorn and spelt wheat. Cereal Chem. 72:621-624.

Abdel-Aal, E-S. M., Sosulski, F. W., and Hucl, P. 1998. Origins, characteristics, and potential of ancient wheats. Cereal Foods World 43:708-715.

Amado, R., and Neukom, H. 1985. Minor constituents of wheat flour: The pentosans. Page 249 in: New Approaches to Research on Cereal Carbohydrates. R. D. Hill and L. Munch, Eds. Elsevier Science Publishers, Amsterdam.

Åman, P., Nilsson, M., and Andersson, R. 1997. Positive health effect of rye. Cereal Foods World 42:684-688.

Åman, P., Pettersson, D., Zhang, J.-X., Tidehag, P., and Hallmans, G. 1995. Starch and dietary fiber components are excerted and degraded to variable extents in ileostomy subjects consuming mixed diets with wheat and oat-bran bread. J. Nutr. 125:2341-2349.

Andreasen, M. F., Kroon, P. A., Williamson, G., and Garcia-Conesa, M. T. 2001. Esterase activity able to hydrolyze dietary antioxidant hydroxycinnamates is distributed along the intestine of mammals. J. Agric. Food Chem. 49:5679-5684.

Anonymous. 2001. Food balance sheet for food commodities 1999 and 2000. Information Center of the Ministry of Agriculture and Foresty, Helsinki.

Antoniou, T. C., Marquardt, R. R., and Cansfield, P. E. 1981. Isolation, partial characterization, and antinutritional activity of a factor (pentosans) in rye grain. J. Agric. Food Chem. 29:1240-1247.

Autio, K., Parkkonen, T., and Fabritius, M. 1997. Observing structural differences in wheat and rye breads. Cereal Foods World 42:702-705.

Bach Knudsen, K. E., Johansen, H. N., and Glitsø, V. 1997. Rye dietary fiber and fermentation in the colon. Cereal Foods World 42:690-694.

Bedford, M. R., and Classen, H. L. 1992. Reduction of intestinal viscosity through manipulation of dietary rye and pentosanase concentration is affected through changes in carbohydrate composition of the intestinal aqueous phase and results in improved growth rate and feed conversion efficiency of broiler chickens. J. Nutr. 122:560-569.

Bengtsson, S., and Åman, P. 1990. Isolation and chemical characteristics of water-soluble arabinoxylans in rye grain. Carbohydr. Polym. 12:267-277.

Bengtsson, S., Åman, P., and Andersson, R. 1992a. Structural studies on water-soluble arabinoxylans in rye grain using enzymatic hydrolysis. Carbohydr. Polym. 17:277-284.

Bengtsson, S., Andersson, R., Westerlund, E., and Åman, P. 1992b. Content, structure and viscosity of soluble arabinoxylans in rye grain from several countries. J. Sci. Food Agric. 58:331-337.

Berry, C. P., D'Appolonia, B. L., and Gilles, K. A. 1971. The characterization of triticale starch and its comparison with starches of rye, durum and HRS wheat. Cereal Chem. 48:415-427.

Biliaderis, C. G., Izydorczyk, M. S., and Rattan, O. 1995. Effect of arabinoxylans on bread-making quality of wheat flours. Food Chem. 53:165-171.

Boros, D., Marquardt, R. R., Slominski, B. A., and Guentor, W. 1993. Extract viscosity as an indirect assay for water-soluble pentosan content in rye. Cereal Chem. 70:575-580.

Boros, D., Rakowska, M., Raczynska-Bojanowska, K., and Kozaczynski, K. 1985. The response of Japanese quails and chicks to the water-soluble antinutritive compounds from rye grain. Nutr. Rep. Int. 32:827-836.

Bouhnik, Y., Vahedi, K., Achour, L., Attar, A., Salfati, J., Pochart, P., Marteau, P., Flourie, B., Bornet, F., and Rambaud, J. C. 1999. Short-chain fructo-oligosaccharide administration dose-dependently increases fecal bifidobacteria in healthy humans. J. Nutr. 129:113-116.

Brighenti, F., Casiraghi, M. C., Canzi, E., and Ferrari, A. 1999. Effect of consumption of ready-to-eat breakfast cereal containing inulin on the intestinal milieu and blood lipids in healthy male volunteers. Eur. J. Clin. Nutr. 53:726-733.

Bushuk, W. 2001. Rye—History, World Distribution, Production and Marketing. Pages 1-7 in: Rye, Production, Chemistry and Technology, 2nd ed. W. Bushuk, Ed. Am. Assoc. Cereal Chem., St. Paul, MN.

Campbell, G. L., and Bedford, M. R. 1992. Enzyme applications for monogastric feed: A review. Can. J. Anim. Sci. 72:449-466.

Campbell, G. L., Classen, H. L., Reichert, R. D., and Campbell, L. D. 1983. Improvement of the nutritive value of rye for broiler chickens by gamma irradiation-induced viscosity reduction. Br. Poult. Sci. 24:205-212.

Camus, M. C., and LaPorte, J. D. 1976. Inhibition de la proteolyse pepsique in vitro par le ble role de l'acide phytiquedes issues. Ann. Biol. Anim. Biochim. Biophys. 16:719-729.

Czembor, H. J., and Sowa, W. 2001. Diseases and pests of rye. Pages 37-52 in: Rye, Production, Chemistry, and Technology, 2nd ed. W. Bushuk, Ed. Am. Assoc. Cereal Chem., St. Paul, MN.

Delcour, J. A., Vanhamel, S., and Hoseney, R. 1991. Physicochemical and functional properties of rye non-starch polysaccharides. II. Impact of a fraction containing water soluble pentosans and proteins on gluten-starch loaf volumes. Cereal Chem. 68:72-76.

Deodikar, G. B. 1963. *Secale cereale* Linn. Indian Council of Agricultural Research, New Delhi.

Deshpande, S. S., and Cheryan, M. 1984. Effects of phytate, divalent cations, and their interactions on alpha-amylase activity. J. Food Sci. 49:516-519.

Deshpande, S. S., and Damondaran, S. S. 1990. Food legumes: Chemistry and technology. Pages 147-241 in: Advances in Cereal Science and Technology, Vol. 10. Y. Pomeranz, Ed. Am. Assoc. Cereal Chem., St. Paul, MN.

Drews, E., and Seibel, W. 1976. Bread baking and other uses around the world. Pages 127-178 in: Rye: Production, Chemistry and Technology, 1st ed. W. Bushuk, Ed. Am. Assoc. Cereal Chem., St. Paul, MN.

Englyst, H. N., and Cummings, J. H. 1985. Digestion of polysaccharides of some cereal foods in the human small intestine. Am. J. Clin. Nutr. 42:778-787.

Fennema, O. R. 1985. Food Chemistry, 2nd ed. Marcel Dekker, New York.

Fengler, A. I., and Marquardt, R. R. 1988a. Water-soluble pentosans from rye: I. Isolation, purification and characterization. Cereal Chem. 65:291-297.

Fengler, A. I., and Marquardt, R. R. 1988b. Water-soluble pentosans from rye: II. Effect on rate of dialysis and on the retention of nutrients by the chick. Cereal Chem. 65:298-302.

Fernandez, R., Lucas, E., and McGinnis, J. 1973. Fractionation of a chick growth depressing factor from rye. Poult. Sci. 52:2252-2259.

Fincher, G. B., and Stone, B. A. 1986. Cell walls and their components in cereal grain technology. Pages 207-295 in: Advances in Cereal Science and Technology, Vol. 8. Y. Pomeranz, Ed. Am. Assoc. Cereal Chem., St. Paul, MN.

FAO. 2001. Yearbook of Food and Agricultural Statistics, Production and Trade. Food and Agricultural Organization, Rome.

Friesen, O. D., Guenter, W., Rotter, B. A., and Marquardt, R. R. 1991. The effect of enzyme supplementation on the nutritive value of rye grain (*Secale cereale*) for young broiler chicks. Poult. Sci. 70:2501-2508.

Gan, Y., McLeod, J. G., Scoles, G. J., and Campbell, G. L. 1996. Genetic and environmental influence on the extract viscosity of winter rye. Plant Breed. Seed Sci. 40:93-102.

Gan, Y., McLeod, J. G., Scoles, G. J., and Campbell, G. L. 1997. Extract viscosity of winter rye: Variation with temperature and precipitation. Can. J. Plant Sci. 77:555-560.

Geissmann, T., and Neukom, H. 1973. On the composition of the water soluble wheat flour pentosans and their oxidative gelation. Lebensm. Wiss. Technol. 6:59-62.

Girhammar, U. 1992. Water-soluble non-starch polysaccharides from cereals. Their properties in solution, dough and bread. Ph.D. thesis, Lund University, Lund, Sweden.

Gontzea, I., and Sutzescu, P. 1968. Natural anti-nutritive substances in foodstuffs and forages. Karger, Basel, Switzerland.

Grela, E. R. 1996. Nutrient composition and content of antinutritional factors in spelt (*Triticum spelta* L.) cultivars. J. Sci. Food Agric. 71:399-404.

GrootWassink, J. W. G., Campbell, G. L., and Classen, H. L. 1989. Fractionation of crude pentosanase (arabinoxylanase) for improvement of the nutritional value of rye diets for broiler chickens. J. Sci. Food Agric. 46:289-300.

Gudmundsson, M., Eliasson, A. C., Bengtsson, S., and Åman, P. 1991. The effects of water soluble arabinoxylan on gelatinization and retrogradation of starch. Starch/Stærke 43:5-10.

Harkonen, H., Lehtinen, P., Suortti, T., Parkkonen, T., Siikaaho, M., and Poutanen, K. 1995. The effects of a xylanase and a β-glucanase from *Trichoderma reesei* on the non-starch polysaccharides of whole meal rye slurry. J. Cereal Sci. 21:173-183.

Harkonen, H., Pessa, E., Suortti, T., and Poutanen, K. 1997. Distribution and some properties of cell wall polysaccharides in rye milling fractions. J. Cereal Sci. 26:95-104.

Henry, R. J. 1985. A comparison of the non-starch carbohydrate in cereal grains. J. Sci. Food Agric. 36:1243-1253.

Holas, J., Prihoda, J., and Kratochvil, J. 1992. Rye flour and bread. Pages 121-127 in: A Long Past and a Bright Future. B. Fellet, Ed. Institute de Resherches Technologiques Agroalimentaires des Cereals, Paris.

Honeyfield, D. C., Proseto, J. A., and McGinnis, J. 1983. Comparative feeding value of rye for poultry and swine. Nutr. Rep. Int. 28:1253-1260.

Horsley, B. 1969. Rye—A casualty of our affluent society. Foreign Agric. VII(12):2-4.

Hoseney, R. C. 1984. Functional properties of pentosans in baked foods. Food Technol. 38:114-117.

Hoseney, R. C., and Faubion, J. M. 1981. A mechanism for the oxidative gelation of wheat flour water-soluble pentosans. Cereal Chem. 58:421-424.

Izydorczyk, M. S., and Biliaderis, C. G. 1992a. Effect of molecular size on physical properties of wheat arabinoxylan. J. Agric. Food Chem. 40:561-568.

Izydorczyk, M. S., and Biliaderis, C. G. 1992b. Influence of structure on the physicochemical properties of wheat arabinoxylan. Carbohydr. Polym. 17:237-247.
Izydorczyk, M. S., and Biliaderis, C. G. 1995. Cereal arabinoxylans: Advances in structure and physicochemical properties. Carbohydr. Polym. 28:33-48.
Izydorczyk, M. S., Biliaderis, C. G., and Bushuk, W. 1990. Oxidative gelation studies of water-soluble pentosans from wheat. J. Cereal Sci. 11:153-169.
Izydorczyk, M. S., Biliaderis, C. G., and Bushuk, W. 1991. Comparison of structure and composition of water-soluble pentosans from different wheat varieties. Cereal Chem. 68:139-144.
Jacobsen, J. V., Knox, R. B., and Pyliotis, N. A. 1971. The structure and composition of aleurone grains in the barley aleurone layer. Planta 101:189-209.
Jedel, P. E., and Salmon, D. F. 1994. Forage potential of Wapiti triticale mixtures in central Alberta. Can. J. Plant Sci. 74:515-519.
Jones, J. M. 1997. Fiber, saccharides, and health. Cereal Foods World 42:713-716.
Juntunen, K. S., Mazur, W. M., Liukkonen, K. H., Uehara, M., Poutanen, K. S., Adlercreutz, H. C. T., and Mykkanen, H. M. 2000. Consumption of wholemeal rye bread increases serum concentrations and urinary excretion of enterolactone compared with consumption of white wheat bread in healthy Finnish men and women. Br. J. Nutr. 84:839-846.
Kamanoi, M., and Jenkins, B. C. 1962. Trisomics in common rye, *Secale cereale* L. Seiken Ziho 13:118-123.
Karppinen, S., Myllymaki, O., Forssell, P., and Poutanen, K. 2003. Fructan content of rye and rye products. Cereal Chem. 80:168-171.
Kent-Jones, D. W., and Amos, A. J. 1967. Modern Cereal Chemistry, 6th ed. Food Trade Press, London.
Klassen, A. J., and Hill, R. D. 1971. Comparison of starch from triticale and its parental species. Cereal Chem. 48:647-654.
Kruse, H. P., Kleesen, B., and Blaut, M. 1999. Effect of inulin on fecal bifidobacteria in human subjects. Br. J. Nutr. 82:375-382.
Kühn, M. C., and Grosch, W. 1989. Baking functionality of reconstituted rye flours having different non-starch polysaccharide and starch contents. Cereal Chem. 66:149-153.
Lineback, D. R., and Rasper, V. F. 1988. Wheat carbohydrates. Pages 277-372 in: Wheat, Chemistry and Technology, 3rd ed., Vol. I. Y. Pomeranz, Ed. Am. Assoc. Cereal Chem., St. Paul, MN.
Lui, N. S. T., and Altschul, A. M. 1967. Isolation of globoids from cottonseed aleurone grain. Arch. Biochem. 121:678-684.
Marquardt, R. R., Boros, D., Guenter, W., and Crow, G. 1994. The nutritive value of barley, rye, wheat and corn for young chicks as affected by use of a *Trichoderma reesei* enzyme preparation. Anim. Feed Sci. Technol. 45:363-378.
Matz, S. A. 1991. The Chemistry and Technology of Cereals as Food and Feed, 2nd ed. Pan-Tech International, McAllen, TX.
McCleary, B. V., Gibson, T. S., Allen, H., and Gams, T. C. 1986. Enzymic hydrolysis and industrial importance of barley β-glucans and wheat flour pentosans. Starch/Stærke 38:433-437.
McLeod, J. G., Gan, Y., Scoles, G. J., and Campbell, G. L. 1996. Extract viscosity and feed quality of rye. Int. Symp. on Rye Breeding and Genetics. University of Hohenheim, Stuttgart, Germany.
Meuser, F., and Suckow, P. 1985. Non-starch polysaccharides. Pages 42-46 in: Chemistry and Physics of Baking. J. M. V. Blanshard, P. J. Frazier, and T. Gilliard, Eds. Royal Society of Chemistry, London.
Meuser, F., and Suckow, P. 1986. Non-starch polysaccharides. Pages 42-61 in: Chemistry and Physics of Baking. J. M. V. Blanshard, P. J. Frazier, and T. Galliard, Eds. Royal Society of Chemistry, London.

Meuser, F., Suckow, P., and Abdel-Gawad, A. 1986. Chemisch-physikalische charactersisierung von Roggenpentosanen. Getreide Mehl Brot 40:198-204.

Michniewicz, J., Biliaderis, C. G., and Bushuk, W. 1991. Effect of added pentosans on some physical and technological characteristics of dough and gluten. Cereal Chem. 68:252-258.

Michniewicz, J., Biliaderis, C. G., and Bushuk, W. 1992. Effect of added pentosans on some properties of wheat bread. Food Chem. 43:251-257.

Moore, A. M., Martinez-Munoz, I., and Hoseney, R. C. 1990. Factors affecting oxidative gelation of wheat water solubles. Cereal Chem. 67:81-84.

Munck, L. 1972. Improvement of nutritional value in cereals. Hereditas 72:1-128.

Neukom, H., Kündig, W., and Deuel, H. 1962. The soluble wheat flour pentosans. Cereal Sci. Today 7:112-115.

Neukom, H. 1976. Chemistry and properties of the non-starchy polysaccharides (NSP) of wheat flour. Lebens. Wiss. Technol. 9:143-148.

Neukom, H., and Markwalder, H. U. 1978. Oxidative gelation of wheat flour pentosans: A new way of cross-linking polymers. Cereal Foods World 23:374-376.

Nilsson, M., Åman, P. Harkonen, H., Hallmans, G., Bach Knudsen, K. E., Mazur, W., and Adlercreutz, H. 1997. Content of nutrients and lignans in roller milled fractions of rye. J. Sci Food Agric. 73:143-148.

Nyman, M., Siljestrom, M., Pedersen, B., Bach Knudsen, K. E., Asp, N. G., Johansson, C. G., and Eggum, B. O. 1984. Dietary fiber content and composition in six cereals at different extraction rates. Cereal Chem. 61:14-19.

Pawlik, J. R., Fengler, A. I., and Marquardt, R. R. 1990. Improvement of the nutrition value of rye by the partial hydrolysis of the viscous water-soluble pentosans following water-soaking or fungal enzyme treatment. Br. Poult. Sci. 31:525-538.

Pettersson, D., and Åman, P. 1987. The variation in chemical composition of triticale grown in Sweden. Acta Agric. Scand. 37:20-26.

Pettersson, D., Åman, P., Bach Knudsen, K. E., Zhang, J.-X., Hallmans, G., Harkonen, H., and Adlercreutz, H. 1996. Intake of rye bread by ileostomists increases ileal excretion of fiber polysaccharide components and organic acids but does not increase plasma or urine lignans and isoflavonoids. J. Nutr. 126:1594-1600.

Pietinen, P., Rimm, E., Korhonen, P., Hartman, A., Willett, W., Albanes, D., and Virtamo, J. 1996. Intake of dietary fiber and risk of coronary heart disease in a cohort of Finnish men. The alpha-tocopherol, beta-carotene cancer prevention study. Circulation 94:2720-2726.

Plaami, S., Saastamoinen, M., and Kumpulainen, J. 1989. Effect of variety and environment on dietary fiber content of winter rye in Finland. J. Cereal Sci. 10:209-215.

Pomeranz, Y. 1973. Structure and mineral composition of cereal aleurone cells as shown by scanning electron microscopy. Cereal Chem. 50:504-511.

Pomeranz, Y. 1985. Carbohydrates: Starch. Pages 25-119 in: Functional Properties of Food Components. Y. Pomeranz, Ed. Academic Press, New York.

Poutanen, K. 1997. Rye bread: Added value in the world's bread basket. Cereal Foods World 42:682-683.

Raczynska-Bojanowska, K., and Rybka, K. 1994. Rye dietary fiber. Hodowla Roslin Aklimatyzacija Nasiennictwo. 38:43-65.

Ragaee, S. M. 2001. Physicochemical and structural characteristics of water-extractable arabinoxylan from rye lines varying in extract viscosity and its relationship to end-use characteristics. Ph.D. thesis, University of Saskatchewan, Canada.

Ragaee, S. M., Campbell, G. L., Scoles, G. J., McLeod, J. G., and Tyler, R. T. 2001a. Studies on rye (*Secale cereale* L.) lines exhibiting a range of extract viscosities. I. Composition, molecular weight distribution of water extracts and biochemical characteristics of purified water-extractable arabinoxylan. J. Agric. Food Chem. 49:2437-2445.

Ragaee, S. M., Campbell, G. L., Scoles, G. J., McLeod, J. G., and Tyler, R. T. 2001b. Studies on rye (*Secale cereale* L.) lines exhibiting a range of extract viscosities. II. Rheological and baking characteristics of rye and rye/wheat blends and feeding value for chicks of wholemeals and breads. J. Agric. Food Chem. 49:2446-2453.

Rakowska, M., Kupiec, R., and Rybka, K. 1992. Studies on antinutritive compounds in rye grain. VI. Effect of dietary fiber fractions on protein digestibility in rats. Pol. J. Food Nutr. Sci.1:103-107.

Rakowska, M. 1994. Antinutritive compounds in rye grain. Hodowla Roslin Aklimatyzacija Nasiennictwo. 38:21-41.

Rattan, O., Izydorczyk, M. S., and Biliaderis, C. G. 1994. Structure and rheological behaviour of arabinoxylan from Canadian bread wheat flours. Lebensm. Wiss. Technol. 27:550-555.

Renard, C. M. G. C., Rouau, X., and Thibault, J. F. 1990. Structure et proprietes de pentosanes hydrosolubles de la farine de ble. Sci. Aliments. 10:283-292.

Rieckhoff, D., Trautwein, E. A., Malkki, Y., and Erbersdobler, H. F. 1999. Effect of different cereal fibers on cholesterol and bile acid metabolism in the Syrian golden hamster. Cereal Chem. 76:788-795.

Rybka, K., Sitarski, J., and Raczynska-Bojanowska, K. 1993. Ferulic acid in rye and wheat grain in grain dietary fiber. Cereal Chem. 70:55-59.

Rychlik, M., and Grosch, W. 1995. Flavour of toast bread. Lebensmittelchemie 49:105-108. [In German]

Saastamoinen, M., Plaami, S., and Kumpulainen, J. 1989. Pentosans and α-glucan content of Finnish winter rye varieties as compared with rye of six other countries. J. Cereal Sci. 10:199-207.

Saini, H. S., and Henry, R. J. 1989. Fractionation and evaluation of triticale pentosans: Comparison with wheat and rye. Cereal Chem. 66:11-14.

Sathe, S. K., Deshpande, S. S., and Salunkhe, D. K. 1984. Dry beans of *Phaseolus*. A review. Part 1. Crit. Rev. Food Sci. Nutr. 20:1-46.

Scoles, G. J., Campbell, G. L., and McLeod, J. G. 1993. Variability for grain extract viscosity in inbred lines and an F2 population of rye (*Secale cereale* L.). Can. J. Plant Sci. 73:1-6.

Scoles, G. J., Gustafson, J. P., and McLeod, J. G. 2001. Rye—Genetics and breeding. Pages 9-35 in: Rye, Production, Chemistry and Technology, 2nd ed. W. Bushuk Ed. Am. Assoc. Cereal Chem., St. Paul, MN.

Seeta, R., Deshpande, V., and Rao, M. 1989. Role of α-xylosidase in hemicellulose hydrolysis by xylanase from *Pencillium funiculosum*. Biotechnol. Appl. Biochem. 11:128-132.

Seibel, W., and Weipert, D. 2001. Rye—Animal feed and industrial uses. Pages 213-233 in: Rye, Production, Chemistry and Technology, 2nd ed. W. Bushuk, Ed. Am. Assoc. Cereal Chem., St. Paul, MN.

Simmonds, D. H., and Campbell, W. P. 1976. Morphology and chemistry of the rye grain. Pages 63-105 in: Rye: Production, Chemistry and Technology, 1st ed. W. Bushuk, Ed. Am. Assoc. Cereal Chem., St. Paul, MN.

Singh, M., and Krikorian, A. D. 1982. Inhibition of trypsin activity in vitro by phytate. J. Agric. Food Chem. 30:799-800.

Tenkanen, M., Schuseil, J., Puls, J., and Poutanen, K. 1991. Production, purification and characterization of an esterase librating phenolic acids from lignocellulosics. J. Biotechnol. 18:69-84.

Theander, O., and Westerlund, E. 1986. Studies on dietary fiber. 3. Improved procedure for analysis of dietary fiber. J. Agric. Food Chem. 34:330-336.

Thompson, L. U., Rickard, S. E., and Siedl, M. M. 1996. Flaxseed and its lignan and oil components reduce mammary tumor growth at a late stage of carcinogenesis. Carcinogenesis 17:1373-1376.

Udy, D. C. 1956. The intrinsic viscosity of the water-soluble components of wheat flour. Cereal Chem. 33:67-74.

Vanhamel, S., Cleemput, G., Delcour, J. A., Nys, M., and Darius, P. L. 1993. Physicochemical and functional properties of rye non-starch polysaccharides. IV. The effect of high molecular weight water soluble pentosans on wheat-bread quality in straight-dough procedure. Cereal Chem. 70:306-311.

Vinkx, C. J. A., and Delcour, J. A. 1996. Rye (*Secale cereale* L.) arabinoxylans: A critical review. J. Cereal Sci. 24:1-14.

Vinkx, C. J. A., Van Nieuwenhove, C. G., and Delcour, J. A. 1991. Physicochemical and functional properties of rye non-starch polysaccharides. III. Oxidative gelation of a fraction containing water-soluble pentosans and proteins. Cereal Chem. 68:617-622.

Vinkx, C. J. A., Reynaert, H. R., Grobet, P. J., and Delcour, J. A. 1993. Physicochemical and functional properties of rye non-starch polysaccharides. V. Variability in the structure of water-soluble arabinoxylan. Cereal Chem. 70:311-317.

Ward, A. T., and Marquardt, R. R. 1983. The effect of saturation, chain length of pure triglycerides, and age of bird on the utilization of rye diets. Poult. Sci. 62:1054-1062.

Weipert, D. 1993. Sprouting damage and processing value of rye. Effects of alpha-amylase activity and pentosan content. Pages 448-454 in: Pre-Harvest Sprouting in Cereals. M. K. Walker-Simmons and J. L. Reid, Eds. Am. Assoc. Cereal Chem., St. Paul, MN.

Weipert, D. 1997. Processing performance of rye as compared to wheat. Cereal Foods World 42:706-712.

CHAPTER 11

Specialty Sorghums for Healthful Foods

Lloyd W. Rooney and Joseph M. Awika

Cereal Quality Lab, Soil and Crop Sciences Department, Texas A&M University, College Station, TX 77843-2474

Overview

Sorghum is a major crop used for food, feed, and industrial purposes worldwide. In the Western Hemisphere, sorghum is used mainly as a livestock feed and has not been considered a significant ingredient in foods. With more than 40,000 accessions in the world collection, tremendous diversity exists in sorghum in both composition and processing properties. The kernel varies in size, shape, color, density, hardness, composition, processing properties, taste, texture, and nutritional value.

In this chapter, we review information on new food sorghums and other special sorghums with unique properties that could be used in producing a wide variety of food products for specialty markets and health foods. We emphasize white food sorghum hybrids and special tannin and black sorghums with high levels of phytochemicals. These special sorghum varieties are an excellent source of nutraceuticals that can compete effectively with fruit and vegetable sources. In addition, we indicate other opportunities for producing healthful foods from sorghum.

Sorghum Production

Sorghum is the fifth most important cereal crop grown in the world. It is a major food grain in Africa and in parts of India and China. In 2003, 42.1 million hectares of sorghum were harvested worldwide, with a total production of 54.7 million metric tons. The United States, India, and Nigeria are the largest producers of sorghum, representing approximately 19.2, 14.5, and 14.5% of the total world production, respectively, in 2003. Mexico and Sudan are also major producers, accounting for 10.2 and 8.0%, respectively, of world sorghum production in 2003. In yield, the United States averages approximately 3,181 kg/ha, while Africa and India average 920 and 808 kg/ha, respectively (USDA 2004). In the United States, sorghum production is concentrated in Kansas, Texas, Nebraska, Oklahoma, and Missouri, in order of decreasing importance. Sorghum is a drought-tolerant crop that does well in harsh environments with limited water. It does not develop significant levels of aflatoxins and fumonisins in the field prior to harvest.

Recently in the United States, significant research and development has led to the production of food sorghums in significant quantities. Food sorghums are defined as white-pericarp, tan-plant sorghums with a clean, bright grain. Actual food sorghum production occurs on 8,100 hectares (20,250 acres), with a production of 10,000 tons. Some are grown under identity-preserved production schemes, while others are collected at harvesttime and held for marketing. They are sold for use in feeds if sufficient food markets are unavailable.

Growing niche markets are major outlets for these white food-type sorghums, which have excellent properties for pet foods and poultry rations and for ethnic and dietary products (e.g., gluten-free foods for celiac-sprue patients who are intolerant of wheat and some other cool-season cereals). Companies are marketing dry mixes and other products containing sorghum, including high-antioxidant bread, gluten-free foods, flours, snacks, and related products. The bottom line is that food sorghums are available for those who want them and are willing to contract production ahead of time.

Tannin sorghums are not grown in the United States because they cause reduced feed efficiency and have been discriminated against in commercial markets. However, commercial tannin hybrids with good grain yields exist, so tannin sorghum can be grown easily for specialty markets under identity-preserved systems. They would not be grown unless a contract were available to ensure their use in special foods, since the grain would be reduced in price for use in feeds.

The black sorghum is available only in an open-pollinated variety, which does not have outstanding grain yields. So it would cost more to produce and would be grown only under contract. The waxy and heterowaxy hybrids are available but would need to be grown under contract-production schemes. The heterowaxy hybrids have excellent yields of grain, while the waxy hybrids have slightly reduced grain yields and would require additional premiums for production.

Sorghum Utilization

Many populations in Africa and India have consumed sorghum for thousands of years. Sorghum is used in many traditional foods, including porridges, fermented and nonleavened breads, ricelike products such as couscous, alcoholic and nonalcoholic beverages, snacks, and many baked products. Industrial production of sorghum beer, nonalcoholic beverages, and porridges occurs in Africa, especially in Nigeria, South Africa, and Botswana (Taylor and Dewar 2000). Malt extracts are used extensively for nonalcoholic beverages and for commercial products like Bournevita and Milo in Africa. *Nini Nanini* is a stabilized opaque beer made in South Africa that has a long shelf life.

African and Indian cultures, in general, have demonstrated preferences for white kernels, preferably with a tan plant and glume color. The soft white sorghums grown under dry conditions during grain maturation and harvesting are often preferred. In India, *Rabbi* (dry season) sorghums of the Maldandi 35 type are often preferred over wheat for milling into whole grain flour for *roti* or chapattis. They are used in many foods, including rice substitutes, thick and thin porridges, snacks, and other products. Nearly all of the Rabbi sorghums are used for human foods, and they command premium prices, while the wet season (*Kharife*) sorghums are used only for livestock feed or for commercial alcohol production, since the grain is often damaged by grain molds and turns black. Other improved hybrids produce grains of inferior quality, and the Indian markets discount the prices of these significantly.

Darker sorghums are usually avoided for these traditional products. However, in southern and East Africa, soft-endosperm tannin sorghums are grown to escape losses from birds and molds. Often these tannin sorghums are preferred for certain foods. For example, farmers doing field work prefer tannin sorghum porridges because the feeling of fullness remains longer. The slower digestibility of the tannin sorghums probably relates to the binding that occurs between the condensed tannins, proteins, and other grain components. Often tannin sorghum foods are fed to new mothers and people with digestive problems. Dark-colored sorghums are preferred for use in beer and alcoholic beverages in Africa. In East Africa, special procedures, including cooking in alkali or malting, are used to process tannin sorghums into foods.

The composition and structure of sorghum is similar to that of corn, with minor differences (Rooney and Waniska 2000, Waniska and Rooney 2000). Sorghum grain has less oil with slightly more starch and protein than corn. The nutrients are distributed in the kernel similarly to those of corn. The sorghum kernel contains up to 0.3% waxes as a thick layer on the pericarp surface. These waxes have some valuable components, including phytosterols and policosanols. Sorghums differ dramatically in that some varieties contain high levels of condensed tannins and other phenolic compounds.

Sorghum is more slowly digested than other cereals. It has been considered more filling; its slower digestibility may be advantageous for people with diabetes. Being more filling and less digestible than other cereals, it may have some role in reducing obesity. The sorghum proteins contain more cross-linked prolamins than do other cereals. These affect the processing properties and digestibility of the grain. A higher proportion of the kernel (corneous endosperm) contains significantly larger amounts of protein surrounding the starch granules, which makes the starch more difficult to solubilize.

Proper processing converts sorghum into highly digestible foods and feeds. However, the processes must disrupt the kernel structure, especially that of the peripheral endosperm, to increase digestibility. Steam flaking, micronizing, reconstitution, and fine grinding are used to increase digestibility. Most food-processing methods in Africa and Asia thoroughly alter the sorghum structure through attrition grinding and other methods.

Sorghum Types

Two types of sorghum are grown worldwide: open-pollinated varieties, found primarily in developing countries, and hybrids, grown predominately in developed countries. Most sorghum hybrids grown in the Western Hemisphere are red with a normal (nonwaxy) white or heteroyellow endosperm, and lack pigmented testas. The dark red color of the pericarp adversely affects the acceptability of the grain in many food ingredients where a light color is required. However, modern breeding programs have developed an array of special sorghums ranging from white food sorghums to sorghums with high levels of condensed tannins and anthocyanins.

Sorghum Endosperm Types

The composition of the endosperm can greatly affect the properties of sorghum in food-production systems. Several types of endosperm exist and are summarized below.

Yellow Endosperm

These cultivars contain high levels of carotenoid pigments in the endosperm. Caryopses appear yellow when the pericarp is thin and colorless, the testa is absent, and the endosperm is yellow. A thick mesocarp and colorless pericarp cause a white or chalky appearance. Heteroyellow endosperm sorghum results when sorghums with yellow and nonyellow endosperm colors are hybridized (Rooney and Miller 1982). Bronze sorghums contain a thicker, red pericarp with yellow endosperm color, while cream sorghums contain a thicker, white pericarp with yellow endosperm. The levels of carotenoid pigments in yellow endosperm sorghums are not as high as in yellow corn. In addition, the carotenoids are bleached during and after maturation because the kernel is exposed to sunlight. Sorghums can have a bright yellow pericarp color (*rrYY*) that is lost upon maturation because the pigments are bleached by the sun.

Waxy Endosperm

These cultivars contain three genes (*wx*) in the recessive form. Heterowaxy genotypes contain one or two of these genes in the dominant form, whereas normal or nonwaxy endosperm sorghums contain all three genes in the dominant form. Waxy cultivars contain nearly 100% amylopectin, and the endosperm looks like candle wax (Rooney and Miller 1982).

The waxy sorghums have excellent expansion during extrusion and produce tender, crisp extrudates. They also produce steamed flakes and micronized flakes with significantly greater expansion and significantly more tender flakes than those of normal food sorghums (Rusnak et al 1980, Cruz-Celis et al 1996, McDonough et al 1998). In addition, the waxy sorghums have improved digestibility and feed efficiency when fed to feedlot cattle on high-concentrate rations since they are more easily fermented (Rooney and Pflugfelder 1986). Current waxy hybrids do not have as high a yield as their nonwaxy counterparts. However, heterowaxy hybrids have excellent yields and modified processing properties. Special waxy or heterowaxy hybrids are available for contract production.

Other Endosperm Types

The high-lysine sorghums from Ethiopia have a soft, floury endosperm texture and a shriveled kernel structure and are very susceptible to deterioration in humid environments during and after caryopsis development (Rooney and Miller 1982). The improved-protein-digestibility sorghum (Weaver et al 1998) and high-lysine sorghums have intermediate to soft endosperm textures, which cause reduced grain yield and increased deterioration from molds and weathering. Attempts to modify this highly digestible type into harder endosperm kernels continue. These highly digestible types of sorghum will most likely find applications in areas of the world where sorghums mature in dry, low-humidity environments. In such cases, they could provide a significant improvement in lysine and digestibility. Areas where these types might be adapted are Ethiopia, Sudan, and India during *Rabbi.*

Sugary endosperm sorghums exist and are used for roasting in the dough stage in Africa and India. These types have higher levels of free amino acids in addition to reducing sugars. During roasting, they produce excellent aromatic flavors and are mixed with other sorghums to enhance their flavor.

Appearance and Genetics of Sorghum

Several interacting factors affect the color and overall appearance of sorghum caryopses. Appearance is affected mainly by pericarp color and thickness, presence of pigmented testa, and endosperm color (Rooney and Miller 1982). Secondary plant and glume colors, as well as deterioration from the environment, insects, and molds, complicate the evaluation of pericarp color and other properties. Immature pericarp tissues, when damaged, respond by producing phenolic compounds that form pigments that stain the pericarp and endosperm. Insect and mold damage of the pericarp commonly occurs when caryopses mature in hot, humid environments.

Pericarp color is genetically controlled by the *R* and *Y* genes. The combination of these genes produces white or colorless (*R_yy* or *rryy*), lemon yellow (*rrY_*), or red (*R_Y_*) color. The intensifier (*I_*) gene increases the intensity of the red pericarp color. The *Z* gene controls pericarp thickness. Sorghums with homozygous recessive (*zz*) genes possess a thick mesocarp. A thick pericarp contains small starch granules, which cause a chalky appearance that masks the colors of the testa and endosperm (Rooney and Miller 1982, Earp et al 1983). A pigmented seed coat or testa is present when both *B1_* and *B2_* genes are dominant. The *tptp* genes control testa color, which can be brown or purple. Caryopses with a pigmented testa (*B1_B2_*) and a recessive spreader gene (*ss*; type II) or a dominant spreader gene (*S*; type III) contain condensed tannins and are called "brown" or "tannin" sorghums (Hahn and Rooney 1986, Earp et al 2004). Type III sorghum tannins are easier to extract than type II sorghum tannins, whereas type I sorghums (without a pigmented testa) do not contain tannins (proanthocyanidins).

Grading and Classification in the United States

Sorghum is marketed according to U.S. grain standards (Rooney and Waniska 2000) in four classes: sorghum, white sorghum, tannin sorghum, and mixed sorghum. The sorghum class cannot contain more than 3% sorghum with a pigmented testa or undercoat. The white grade contains sorghum with a white pericarp without a pigmented testa and cannot contain more than 2% sorghum with colored pericarp or testa.

Tannin sorghums have a pigmented testa beneath the pericarp (Figure 1). The pigmented testa is seen as a dark layer between the light endosperm and the pericarp when the caryopsis is scraped to remove the pericarp. Bleaching using the chlorine bleach test causes the constituents in the pericarp and testa to oxidize and gives a pronounced black color to the bleached kernels, while nontannin sorghums have a white appearance. The bleach test, however, can produce many false positives, especially with molded or weathered grain (Dykes et al 2002) and should be used judiciously. Mixed sorghum contains sorghum with and without pigmented testa.

Sorghum in South Africa is graded into classes for feed, malting, and tannin sorghums. The grain is tested quite similarly to the tests used in the U.S. grading system. Taylor (*personal communication*) developed some simple methods to use in grading and classifying sorghum in southern Africa.

White Food Sorghums in the United States

U.S. food-grade white sorghum has a white kernel with tan plant and glume characteristics (white/tan/tan) and excellent quality for food use. The tan plant and light-colored glumes reduce the amount of anthocyanin pigments that cause off-colors in the otherwise similar white grains that have

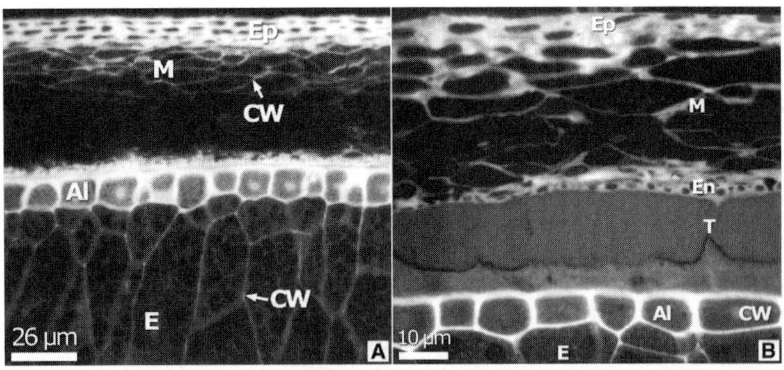

Fig. 1. Fluorescence photomicrograph of sorghum kernel cross-section, showing structural differences between a nontannin sorghum without a testa (left) and a tannin sorghum with a pigmented testa (right). Al: aleurone layer, CW: cell wall, E: endosperm, En: endocarp, Ep: epicarp, M: mesocarp, T: pigmented testa. (Adapted from Earp et al, 2004)

purple or red glumes. The tan plant and straw color glumes provide grain with excellent properties for processing into whole grain foods or for milling into meal, flour, and grits for use in foods. The white food sorghums do not contain genetically modified organisms; are gluten-free (as is all sorghum), bland in flavor, and light colored; and have excellent processing properties. Decorticated white sorghum compares favorably with rice for extrusion into bland extrudates that will carry mild flavors. It has a definite advantage over corn products because of its bland flavor.

Identity-preserved production of food sorghums occurs in the sorghum belt, where highly adapted hybrids are produced. Yearly production figures have increased to levels that are adequate for large-scale production of food products, as presented earlier. It is possible to obtain large quantities of food sorghums by contracting with farmer groups. Grain yields are comparable to those for red sorghum hybrids, so the premium is for maintaining the identity and quality specifications of food-grade sorghum.

Food sorghum is currently being used in production of high-quality, gluten-free sorghum flour in the United States and is exported to Japan for use in a variety of foods, including snacks, baked products, porridges, ricelike products, and other food ingredients. The cost of food sorghums is competitive and in some cases lower than rice in some countries. Consequently, it can be substituted for rice in snacks and breakfast foods to lower the cost.

Processing Properties of White Food Sorghums

The white food sorghum hybrids typically have harder kernels with a thin pericarp (Table 1) compared to commercial hybrids with red or white grain and purple plants. The data in Table 1 represent the means of selected hybrids grown at four locations in Texas, Nebraska, and Kansas for each of three years. Both environment and hybrids significantly affect the composition as well as the physical and processing properties of the grains. However, the white tan sorghum hybrids were harder, more dense, and lighter in color than grain of white purple or red purple hybrids.

The milling yields of white food sorghums are markedly better than those of red-pericarp hybrids (Figures 2 and 3), especially when the yield of decorticated grain is adjusted to comparable color of decorticated grain or flour (Awika et al 2002). The data for 11 white tan hybrids compared to three commercial red sorghum hybrids illustrate the tremendous advantage of white sorghums for milling into light-colored milled products. They also show that there is significant variation among different white tan hybrids.

The hardness, pericarp thickness, and ease of removal, size, and shape of the kernel affect the decortication procedure. In our studies of milling properties during the last 15 years, ATx635 (Miller et al 1992) hybrids always have excellent decortication properties (Table 1). This hybrid was selected for improved kernel hardness and density and is useful for whole grain extrusion (Acosta 2003). Variations of it are in commercial hybrid production, although the hybrids are too tall and late for widespread adoption. Other commercially available hybrids have good milling properties.

TABLE 1
Physical Properties and Composition of Food and Feed Sorghum Hybrids Grown Over Four Years at Four Locations in Texas, Kansas, and Nebraska[a,b]

Pedigree	Type[c]	Hardness Index	Decortication Yield (%)	Grain *L* Value[d]	Grit *L* Value	TKW[e] (g)	Diameter (mm)	Density (g/cc)	Protein[f] (%)	Fat[f] (%)
ATx378*RTx430	RP	83.4 bc	75.9 cd	47.7 d	65.3 b	30.0	2.22	1.376 cd	11.5	3.8
ATx623*RTx430	WP	83.0 c	74.9 cd	59.5 c	68.2 a	29.0	2.17	1.373 cd	10.0	3.5
AOK11*RTx2741	WP	70.6 e	70.7 d	60.4 bc	68.2 a	25.9	1.97	1.368 d	9.5	3.5
ATx635*RTx436	WT	94.9 a	85.8 a	63.1 a	68.2 a	23.2	1.97	1.396 a	11.0	3.8
888Y	WT	90.3 ab	86.4 a	59.5 c	67.8 ab	25.8	1.92	1.396 a	11.2	3.9
ATx631*RTx436	WT	89.9 ab	79.1 bc	63.8 a	69.6 a	25.6	2.07	1.381 bc	11.1	3.9
ATxArg-1*RTx436	WT	91.5 a	82.7 ab	62.6 ab	69.6 a	22.6	1.83	1.389 ab	10.8	3.6
LSD ($P < 0.05$)		7.2	5.9	2.3	2.4	4.0	0.22	0.011	1.3	0.3

[a] Means with same letters not significantly different.
[b] The first three sorghums are feed sorghums typical of the commercial production of sorghum in the United States. The last four samples of grain are hybrids that produce food-type sorghums.
[c] RP: red grain, purple plant; WP: white grain, purple plant; WT: white grain, tan plant.
[d] *L* value indicates brightness.
[e] Thousand-kernel weight.
[f] Expressed on dry weight basis.

White-pericarp, purple-plant hybrids are more adversely affected by weathering and molds than are white tan hybrids. A small amount of moisture during maturation moves the purple or red anthocyanins from the glumes into the pericarp and endosperm, which reduces milling yields or causes off-colored products. These types of sorghum are not recommended for food production in the United States, although they have excellent properties when they mature and are harvested under dry conditions.

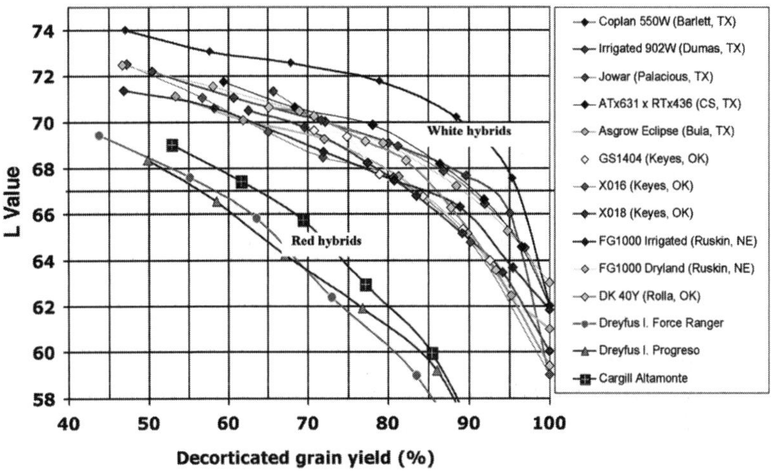

Fig. 2. Relationship between *L* color value and decorticated yields of food and nonfood sorghums. Note the reduced yield of the nonfood sorghums (Cargill Alt. and Dreyfus I. varieties) relative to the food sorghums at comparable lightness value. (*Unpublished data*, Cereal Quality Lab, Texas A&M Univ.)

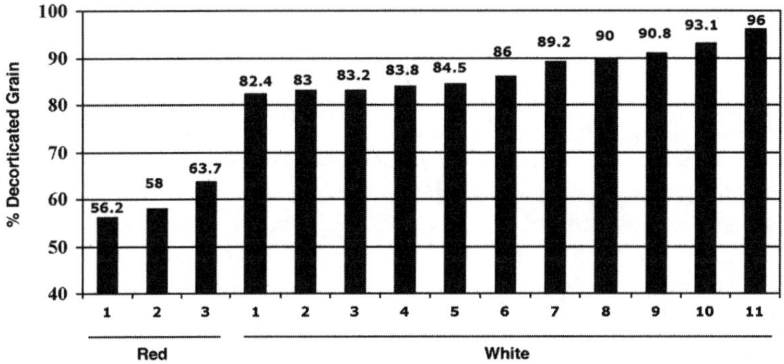

Fig. 3. Decorticated grain yield of food (white) and commercial feed (red) sorghums adjusted to an *L* color value of 67 (CV = 3.5%). (*Unpublished data*, Cereal Quality Lab, Texas A&M Univ.)

Efforts by breeders, agronomists, and food technologists have produced tan white food-type sorghums with significantly improved food-quality attributes. These sorghums can be processed into whole grain products easily because most have a thin pericarp and, when grown under good environmental conditions, produce excellent grain quality. For high quality, the white tan sorghums should be grown in environments with low humidity and low risk of grain mold or weathering. Experimental red tan plant hybrids also have significantly better milling properties than the red purple sorghum hybrids. The red tan plant sorghums are more useful in high-rainfall or high-humidity areas such as the Coastal Bend area of Texas.

Grain Molds and Staining

The environmental conditions during caryopsis development and maturation greatly affect the appearance of sorghum because the panicle or head is exposed to biotic and abiotic stress. A hot, humid environment during maturation negatively affects sorghum quality. Deterioration results from insects, molds, moisture, and sunshine. Physical damage resulting from insect attack causes the plant to secrete phenolic compounds that produces discolored spots in the pericarp and endosperm. Mold colonization discolors the pericarp surface, breaks down the endosperm structure, and adversely affects processing quality (Waniska et al 1989). Sorghums that have an open panicle structure and caryopses with thin pericarp, condensed tannins, corneous endosperm, and large, tight glumes are generally considered more resistant to molding and weathering. Grain molds are a major limitation preventing more widespread use of sorghum in foods around the world.

Food-Type Sorghums Around the World

White food sorghums grown in the *Rabbi* season are used extensively in India, where they sell at prices higher than those for wheat. The *Rabbi* sorghums are preferred for food because of their light color, sweet taste, and functional properties for *roti*, a flatbread. Sorghum of good quality is necessary for value-added products. The products are acceptable and purchased by consumers, provided convenience, good taste, appearance, and consistent quality are available at competitive prices. In South Africa, significant quantities of Mabella (sorghum) meal for thick porridges are consumed, even though the price is significantly higher than for mealy meal (maize). Botswana is an example where maize consumption is decreasing while sorghum consumption is increasing, even though red or brown sorghum must be imported from South Africa. The white sorghums are preferred for *injera* in Ethiopia, according to recent studies (Yetneberk 2004).

In Mali, white tan-plant, photoperiod-sensitive, guinea sorghums have been developed to replace white purple-plant guineas. The grain yields of the new tan-plant guineas are equal to or better than those they are replacing, and both farmers and processors like the improved taste and color of the food products made from these grains. Contract production with identity preservation of the tan varieties is now beginning, and processors are making improved-quality food products.

A similar situation exists in Central America, where sorghum is used alone or in mixtures with maize for tortillas, *pan dulce*, muffins, bread, *rosquettes*, *rosquillos*, and other variations of these products (Almeida-Dominguez et al 1991). The new white tan-plant sorghum varieties Sureno, Dorado, Soberano, RCV, SV-3, and others are preferred by farmers because the grain yields are equal to or better than those of the old varieties (Maicillo Criollos), and the forage and food quality is significantly improved. Many small farmers produce the white tan varieties, store the grain, and market it in baked products over the following year as value-added marketing. This illustrates the value of the tan plant color because the old varieties (Maicillo Criollos) with white kernels and purple plant color often produced dark purple tortillas and off-color bread because of the anthocyanin pigments.

Significant interest exists in the use of sorghum flour in blends and alone for baked products (Gordon 2001). Thus, whole grain white sorghum flours can be utilized in a wide variety of food systems in baking as a partial or complete substitute for wheat flour. The bland flavor of sorghum is particularly important, as it allows a greater percentage of substitution without loss of flavor or taste. For example, because of its strong taste, maize meal cannot be substituted for more than 5–10% wheat flour. Sorghum can go to very high levels if it is a white food type.

The white food sorghums can be used as whole ground grains for the brewing of beer and for production of extracts for nonalcoholic beverages because of their light color, thin pericarp, and reduced oil compared to maize. New technologies for filtration of the commercial enzyme-converted sorghum mash allow practical industrial application. Thus, it is likely that, in most African areas, sorghum malting will be replaced by conversion with commercial enzymes since dry matter losses during conventional malting are up to 20% of the original weight. The white sorghums provide excellent raw materials. The beer produced has acceptable properties although it differs from barley beer. In addition, other sources of color and flavor can be added to the beverages more economically. This practice is increasing, especially in Nigeria.

Extrusion Processing

Several extruded salty snacks and milled products based on identity-preserved U.S. white food sorghums are sold by Japanese food companies. Other countries are interested in using white food sorghums. It is possible to produce an array of expanded sorghum products directly from whole and ground, undecorticated white or brown sorghum grains, using low-cost friction extruders (Acosta 2003, Maranphal 2003). These smaller extruders are often used in areas where infrastructure does not permit the use of more costly, sophisticated extruders and processes. The ability to produce snacks directly from whole clean grain is a distinct advantage for sorghum. Extrudates of 100% whole tannin sorghums have acceptable texture that can be used to produce whole grain snacks and ready-to-eat breakfast foods.

Whole or milled sorghums can be expanded directly by using low-cost friction extruders (Figure 4). Sorghum extrudates compared favorably with extrudates from rice and corn, depending upon the decortication levels, particle size distribution, and moisture content. As the decortication level increased, the extrudates became whiter, more expanded, less dense, and more crisp. The extrudates made from coarse-particle-size materials had the most desirable characteristics compared to the other particle sizes used. Some sorghum products had a higher expansion ratio than both rice and corn with similar bulk density and texture characteristics. White sorghum had excellent extrusion properties and could compete with rice and corn for expansion ratio. Different varieties of sorghum differ in expansion ratio. Heterowaxy and waxy varieties expanded more than normal, nonwaxy varieties (Gomez et al 1988).

Sorghum has been extruded with single- and twin-screw extruders to produce bland-flavored, light-colored, highly expanded extrudates that carry mild flavors and seasonings similar to rice, at lower cost. For example, in some applications, rice does not expand properly without the use of potato starch or other expensive ingredients, but sorghum can expand properly without additives, and the cost of the sorghum is often lower than that of rice. Obviously, cost depends upon the kind of rice and the quality of the sorghum as well. Experience around the world consistently indicates that sorghum can be

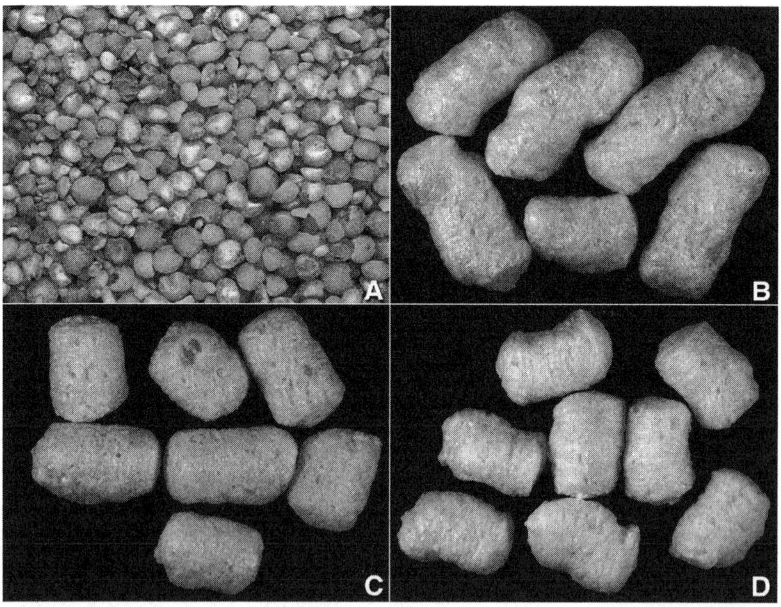

Fig. 4. Extrudates of decorticated food sorghum **(A),** direct-expanded sorghum **(B),** corn meal **(C),** and rice **(D)**. Samples were extruded through a short barrel, high friction type Maddox extruder. (Adapted from Acosta, 2003)

extruded into a wide variety of products quite efficiently. Extrusion appears to significantly reduce the degree of polymerization (DP) of sorghum tannins, which may be beneficial in human foods (see the section entitled "Antioxidants in Special Sorghums").

Sorghum Flour and Grain in Specialty Products

Sorghum flour can be substituted for 100% of the wheat flour in a variety of products that are used in gluten-free diets for celiac-sprue patients who are intolerant of wheat and some other cool-season cereals. Sorghum flour produces acceptable baked products with additives to substitute for its lack of gluten. Various prepared mixes, flours, and other products containing sorghum have been introduced into specialty markets recently. Sorghum has excellent ethnic appeal for many African and Asian immigrants and can be increasingly found in specialty shops in the United States and Europe.

Sorghum can be used to produce couscous and other ricelike products. Whole grain can be cooked and added to soups to improve texture. An excellent whole grain salad can be made using cooked grain, with olive oil, lemon juice, feta cheese, and fresh basil or parsley. Whole grain can be popped and added to salads as a croutonlike product (Suhendro et al 1998).

Special Black and Tannin Sorghums

The tannin sorghums have high levels of proanthocyanidins (condensed tannins) that are known to be powerful antioxidants. The black sorghums are especially a rich source of anthocyanins that possess several therapeutic benefits and are also useful natural food pigments. These specialty sorghum varieties are generating a lot interest because of increasing demand for natural therapeutic agents and functional foods.

Antioxidants in Special Sorghums

Antioxidant activities of specialty sorghums and their bran are equal to or higher than those of common high-antioxidant fruits like blueberries and plums (Figure 5). The high oxygen radical absorbance capacity levels in sorghum brans demonstrate their potential compared to fruits as a source of natural antioxidants and related phytochemicals.

Specialty sorghums and their products have high antioxidant activity when measured by different methods (Table 2). The tannin and black sorghums and their brans had the highest levels of antioxidant activity (Awika et al 2003b). Since the phenols are concentrated in the outer layers of the sorghum kernel, the bran obtained by abrasive decortication or roller milling has three to four times the antioxidant activity of the whole grains.

The grain and bran fractions of the tannin and black sorghums make excellent-quality breads that contain high levels of antioxidants, dietary fiber, and a natural dark brown color (Gordon 2001). A blend of tannin sorghum bran, barley flour, flaxseed, and gluten produced an excellent-quality, healthful bread (Rudiger 2003). Direct friction-type extrusion produces whole grain snacks and ready-to-eat breakfast foods from these tannin or black sorghums. Cookies, tortilla chips, and many other foods have been produced (Leon-Chapa 1999, Zelaya 2001).

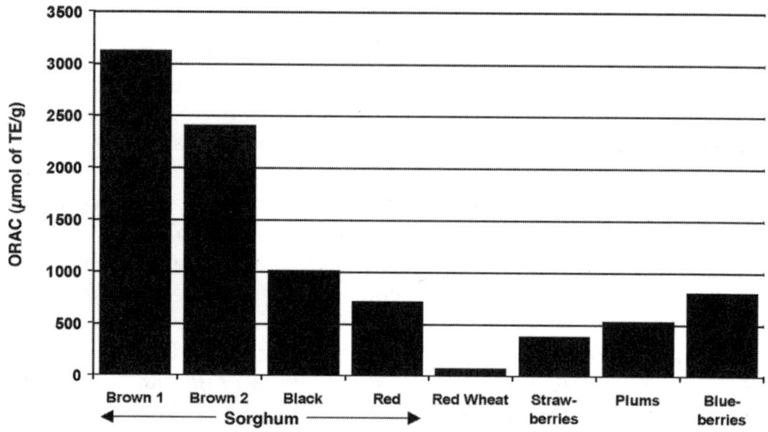

Fig. 5. Oxygen radical absorbance capacity (ORAC) levels in different sorghum brans compared to those in wheat bran and fruits (dry basis). TE = Trolox equivalent. (Adapted from Awika et al 2003a)

TABLE 2
Phenol Contents and Antioxidants (μmol Trolox equiv./g sample, dry wt) in Sorghum and Sorghum Products Measured by Three Methods[a,b]

Sorghum	ORAC[c]	ABTS[d]	DPPH[e]	Phenols[f]
White grain	22	6	6	0.8
White bran	64	28	21	4.8
Red grain	140	53	28	6.6
Red bran	710	230	71	19.9
Black grain	220	57	41	6.4
Black bran	1,000	250	184	26.0
High-tannin grain	450	108	118	12.3
High-tannin bran	2,400	512	495	54.9
Sumac grain, brown	870	226	202	19.8
Sumac bran, brown	3,100	768	716	66.3
CV,%	6.8	3.5	5.3	5.97

[a] Adapted from Awika et al (2003b).
[b] Samples were extracted in 70% aqueous acetone.
[c] ORAC = oxygen radical absorbance capacity, fluorescein used as a probe.
[d] ABTS = 2,2′-azinobis (3-ethyl-benzothiazoline-6-sulfonic acid); activity was measured in pH 7.4 phosphate buffer saline.
[e] DPPH = 2,2-diphenyl-1-picrylhydrazyl; activity was measured in methanol.
[f] Phenols, mg gallic acid equivalents per gram (Folin-Ciocalteu method).

High-temperature, high-pressure extrusion and expansion change the molecular weight (MW) distribution of the tannins in sorghum significantly (Figure 6). It causes the higher-MW polymers of the proanthocyanidins to break down into lower-MW constituents (monomers to tetramers) that are presumably more readily available for direct absorption. Other wet processes such as baking and cooking did not produce a net increase in the lower-MW proanthocyanidins, as observed in the extrudates (Awika et al 2003a). This information should be confirmed by additional experiments, but extrusion seems to alter the MW distribution of the proanthocyanidins and potentially improves their bioavailability.

Levels of Tannins in Sorghum

Deshpande et al (1985) summarized methods used to quantify tannins and discussed limitations. The methods broadly fall under colorimetric (most common) and chromatography-based assays (more recent). Gravimetric methods and techniques based on the ability of tannins to precipitate proteins have also been used (Hagerman and Butler 1978, 1980; Reed et al 1985; Makkar 1989).

Quantification of tannins from any source is complicated by the lack of appropriate standards and difficulty in extraction; changes occurring during extractions are often time and solvent dependent. Many researchers fail to recognize that they are measuring total phenols and not just condensed tannins. The standards used (e.g., catechin) vary significantly and are valid for comparisons only in a given laboratory. Thus, many tannin-free sorghums are erroneously reported to contain significant levels of tannins.

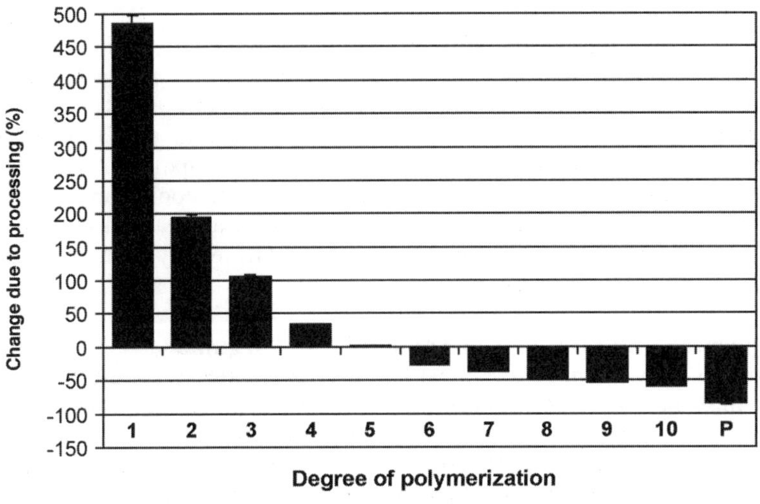

Fig. 6. Change in tannin sorghum procyanidin distribution due to extrusion. "P" represents polymers with DP > 10. A normal-phase HPLC method was used to quantify proanthocyanidins. (Adapted from Awika et al 2003b)

The vanillin-HCl method originally reported by Burns (1971) and later modified (Maxson and Rooney 1972, Price et al 1978) is widely used for sorghums. The corrected vanillin-HCl method is generally more appropriate for tannins than the redox assays like the Folin-Denis or Prussian blue methods. With the vanillin-HCl method, tannin levels of up to 68 mg/g have been reported for sorghum grains. However, factors like particle size, type of solvent, extraction time, temperature, and standards significantly influence the measured tannin content. For example, Price et al (1978) reported, and we confirmed (Awika 2003), that extraction for 2–24 hr with 1% HCl in methanol gave a 40–70% reduction in assayable tannins compared to a 20-min extraction time. The tannins react with other components in the extract to form products that do not react positively in the vanillin-HCl test.

Modern Analysis of Tannins

Quantitative assays of tannins based on HPLC to separate and analyze the high MW proanthocyanidins, which are the most abundant forms of the tannins in sorghum, are promising (Hammerstone et al 1999, Gu et al 2002). The advantage of the HPLC assay is that it determines the relative proportions of the various MW polymers present in condensed tannins. This provides useful information, since polymer chain length affects organoleptic, antioxidant, and other properties of the tannins (Rigaud et al 1993, Tebib et al 1997, Lotito et al 2000). Hence, information on the relative proportions of the different proanthocyanidin oligomers and polymers may help predict their overall effectiveness as functional components of diet.

The HPLC analysis of sorghum proanthocyanidins (condensed tannins) indicated that more than 60% of the polymers had a degree of polymerization greater than 10 (Awika et al 2003a), as shown in Table 3. Different sorghum varieties show significant differences in MW distribution. The direct extrusion of tannin sorghums significantly reduced the polymer size of the proanthocyanidins and increased the percentages of oligomers with less than five units, which may positively affect the biological significance of the antioxidants (Fig. 6). The type of processing is important, since similar changes did not occur when the brans were baked into cookie and breads. It is likely that the high pressure and friction of extrusion caused fission of the tannin polymers. These findings must be confirmed by additional experiments, which are under way.

Composition and Structure of Tannins from Sorghum

Tannins of sorghum are almost exclusively of the condensed type. They are mainly polymerized products of flavan-3-ols or flavan-3,4-diols. Glycosylated and nonglycosylated polymers of flavan-4-ols with various substitution patterns were also reported in sorghum (Gujer et al 1986). No tannic acid or hydrolyzable tannins have been detected in sorghum. Krueger et al (2003) observed the presence of DP2–DP7 mixtures of proluteolinidin and proapigeninidin polyflavans, with eriodictoyl or eriodictoyl-*O*-β-glucoside as the terminal units in sorghum. Significant heterogeneity also occurs in the poly-

TABLE 3
Proanthocyanidin Content[a] of Brown Sorghums Compared to Those of Freeze-Dried Cocoa and Blueberry[b]

DP[c]	Sumac Grain	Sumac Bran	Cocoa	Blueberry
1	0.18	0.33	14.24	0.18
2	0.40	1.33	8.57	0.46
3	0.51	1.61	8.10	0.38
4	0.69	2.32	8.89	0.50
5	0.74	2.51	8.86	0.47
6	1.10	3.61	9.99	0.69
7	0.79	2.56	6.38	0.48
8	0.74	2.29	5.97	0.61
9	1.17	3.48	7.36	0.93
10	0.55	1.52	3.22	ND[d]
P[e]	15.09	36.87	16.17	15.28
Total	21.97	58.44	97.76	19.99
% oligo[f]	31.31	36.33	83.45	23.51
CV (%)	2.0	10.2	5.4	2.1

[a] In milligrams per gram, obtained by normal-phase HPLC with fluorescence detection.
[b] Adapted from Awika et al (2003a).
[c] Degree of polymerization.
[d] Not detected.
[e] Mixture of polymers with DP >10.
[f] Oligomers (DP <10) as a percent of total.

flavans (proanthocyanidin) polymers in terms of interflavan linkages (A or B type) and the presence of gallocatechin/epigallocatechin hydroxylation patterns (Krueger et al 2003). HPLC analysis also suggested the presence of epicatechin gallate as a significant component of the lower-MW procyanidins of tannin sorghums (Awika 2003). Some of the tannins found in sorghum have been identified in other common foods (e.g., cocoa and blueberries) (Hammerstone et al 1999, Gu et al 2002).

High-Anthocyanin Sorghums

Special varieties of sorghum exist that have very high levels of anthocyanins. These sorghums have a thick pericarp with intense red pigments that turn deep black or purple when exposed to the sun during maturation. The genetics of the black pericarp are recessive. Gous (1989) reported the 3-deoxyanthocyanidins, luteolinidin, and apigeninidin as the major anthocyanidins from a black sorghum variety. These special black sorghums have very high levels of anthocyanins (3-deoxyanthocyanidins) that are relatively rare in nature (Clifford 2000). They lack an OH group at the C–3 position. These 3-deoxyanthocyanidins are more stable in acidic solutions compared to the other anthocyanidins commonly found in fruits and vegetables (Sweeny and Iacobucci 1981). This suggests a potential advantage of sorghum as a viable commercial source of unique anthocyanins.

The black sorghums have been used to produce tortillas and tortilla chips, extruded snacks, and baked products with dark purple or blue colors and high levels of phenols and antioxidants as measured by *in vitro* tests (Gordon 2001, Zelaya 2001). The black sorghum can be decorticated to yield bran that is high in anthocyanins because the pericarp is easily removed (Awika 2000).

Like tannins, effective quantification of anthocyanins is hampered by lack of appropriate standards, efficient extracting solvents, and separation techniques. Awika (2003) showed that acidified methanol extraction gave higher anthocyanin values than aqueous acetone extraction for sorghum anthocyanins. Lu and Foo (2001) demonstrated that acetone, when used as a solvent, reacts with anthocyanins in a time-dependent manner to form pyranoanthocyanins, which are spectrally different from anthocyanins. Anthocyanins are also pH sensitive and polymerize with other phenols to form structures that are hard to isolate or characterize (Remy et al 2000). The anthocyanins normally isolated may be mostly solvent-modified derivatives.

The pH differential method is still the most common spectroscopy method for crude anthocyanin estimation. The method is rapid and estimates both monomeric as well as polymerized anthocyanins. However, the values are greatly affected by the standard used.

HPLC analysis has revolutionized anthocyanin analysis. The anthocyanin levels in black sorghums (2.3–2.8 mg/g in grain and 8.9–11.0 mg/g in bran) compare well to those of fruits and vegetables commonly used as commercial anthocyanin sources.

Phenolic Acids of Sorghum

In general, sorghums have levels of phenolic acids comparable to those of other cereals (Hahn et al 1983, Adom and Liu 2002). The phenolic acids of sorghum exist largely as benzoic or cinnamic acid derivatives. Like other cereals, the sorghum phenolic acids are mostly concentrated in the bran and are esterified to cell wall polymers. Ferulic acid is the most abundant bound phenolic acids in sorghum (Hahn et al 1983) and other cereals (Adom and Liu 2002). The phenolic acids have good antioxidant activity *in vitro* and thus may contribute significantly to the health benefits associated with whole grain consumption. However, sorghum does not have any advantages over other cereals in terms of phenolic acid content.

Antioxidants in Sorghum Syrup or Molasses

Sorghum syrup is composed of sucrose, glucose, and fructose and contains significant quantities of phenolic acids, organic acids, and other components that are present in the sap (Kwon and Kim 2003). The high oxygen radical absorbance capacity values of sorghum syrups range from 35.0 to 81.3 μmol of Trolox equivalents per gram, which means that they are a significant source of antioxidants (Forberg 2003). The antioxidant activity is likely due to the extraction and concentration of phenolic acids and their derivatives from the stalks. More information is required to determine the potential of sorghum syrup as a source of antioxidants.

The stalks of special sweet sorghum varieties are crushed and the sap is concentrated by boiling to produce sorghum syrup, or molasses, as it is sometimes called. The syrup is a light amber, viscous liquid with a strong, unique flavor. The flavor, color, and viscosity are developed during boiling of the sap to concentrate the solids.

Other Phenolic Compounds from Sorghum

Several other phenolic compounds have been isolated from sorghum. Naringenin (a flavanone) was identified and quantified in our laboratory as a major phenolic component of a bright red sorghum (TX 2911) variety (0.95 mg/g of bran) (Rooney et al 2000, Awika 2003). The bright red sorghums have reported resistance to molds; naringenin could play a role in this resistance. Naringenin and its glucoside were previously reported in sorghum by Gujer et al (1986). Monomeric forms of proapigeninidin, apiforol, proluteolinidin, and luteoforol were identified in sorghum leaves and grain (Watterson and Butler 1983). Gujer et al (1986) also reported taxifolin and eriodictoyl and their glucosides in sorghum grain. No information on the role of these compounds in sorghum quality or properties is available.

Bioavailability of Sorghum Phenols

Currently, antioxidant activity is the most common *in vitro* parameter used to assess or predict potential benefits of plant phytochemical compounds. However, correlations and relationships between *in vitro* antioxidant activity and actual health benefits are largely unknown. Additionally, antioxidant activity measured *in vitro* tells us nothing about release and uptake of the compounds, as well as their distribution and metabolism in the body. However, antioxidant activity provides useful information for screening plant materials and products with desirable compounds and properties that can be used for further biological testing. In sorghum, phenol content correlates strongly with antioxidant activity (Awika 2003, Awika et al 2003b).

Condensed Tannins

Tannins from sorghum show powerful antioxidant activity *in vitro* (Hagerman et al 1998, Riedl and Hagerman 2001). However, because of their large molecular size and binding with proteins and carbohydrates to form insoluble complexes, their bioavailability is greatly compromised. However, Riedl and Hagerman (2001) demonstrated that even when complexed with proteins, sorghum tannins retained at least 50% of their antioxidant activity. The protein-complexed tannins may serve as free-radical sinks in the digestive system, thus sparing other antioxidants. Available data indicate that the lower-MW tannins (monomers, dimers, and to a limited extent, trimers) can be directly absorbed in the small intestine (Deprez et al 2001, Ross and Kasum 2002). Additionally, Spencer et al (2000) reported that the interflavan bond in the procyanidins was unstable in a simulated gastric juice (pH 2), which degraded the higher-MW polymers to monomers and dimers. However, Rios et al (2002) reported that the procyanidins were actually stable during gastric transit in humans. Part of the nonabsorbed tannins is degraded by colon microflora into phenolic acids that may be absorbed to provide additional benefits (Deprez et al 2000, Tapiero et al 2002).

Anthocyanins

We have not found any work reporting bioavailability of the 3-deoxyanthocyanidins commonly found in sorghum. This is probably because these relatively rare anthocyanins have not been considered of economic interest. The high antioxidant capacity of black sorghums and their brans was correlated with their anthocyanin contents. Hence anthocyanins may contribute significantly to any potential health benefits of these sorghums. Boveris et al (2001) demonstrated that a 3-deoxyanthocyanidin (apigeninidin) isolated from soybean had strong dose-dependent quenching ability against ascorbyl and lipid radicals. Anthocyanins from fruits possess several therapeutic benefits, including vasoprotective and anticancer properties (Lietti et al 1976, Karaivanova et al 1990). The sorghum anthocyanins should be investigated for health properties.

Other Compounds

Phenolic acids are more readily absorbed than other phenols from food because of their small molecular sizes (Scalbert et al 2002). The bound forms of phenolic acids were, until recently, considered unavailable for absorption. However, Andreasen et al (2001a,b) demonstrated that human colonic esterases (mostly of microbial origin) are capable of releasing esterified diferulates and other hydroxycinnamic acids from cereal brans. This suggests that the bound phenolic acids are potentially bioavailable and the actual contribution of phenolic acids to health benefits associated with consumption of whole grains may be greater than previously assumed.

Phytosterols

Phytosterols are cholesterol-like compounds that are structural components of plant cell membranes. In grains, they are extracted in the bran oil. These compounds promote cardiovascular health because they reduce serum cholesterol levels. Singh et al (2003) reported total phytosterol levels of 0.5 mg/g for sorghum grain, compared to 0.9 mg/g for corn. The fiber fraction isolated from sorghum by a corn wet-milling procedure had 0.7–0.8 mg/g phytosterols. However, Singh et al (2003) reported that the wet-milling procedure they used resulted in a loss of 53–73% of the phytosterols in the isolated sorghum fractions relative to whole grain. Additionally, the values they reported were only for the hexane-extractable (nonbound) forms of the compounds. Actual phytosterol values for sorghum may be higher with hydrolytic or otherwise optimized extraction procedures. The phytosterols exist in free forms and as esters of fatty acids or hydroxycinnamic acids or conjugated with sugars (primarily glucose). In sorghum, the free phytosterols include campesterol, stigmasterol, and sitosterol (Avato et al 1990). Sorghum contains esterified forms, with fatty acid chains of C14–C24 (Avato et al 1990) and ferulates (Singh et al 2003).

Policosanols

Policosanols are a mixture of high-MW aliphatic alcohols (fatty alcohols) that are part of plant waxes. These alcohols have 24–34 C atoms with the general chemical formula of CH_3-$(CH_2)_n$-CH_2OH. The compounds are currently commercially obtained from sugarcane wax by hydrolytic cleavage and further purification (Gouni-Berthold and Berthold 2002, Pepping 2003). In sorghum, wax comprises about 0.2–0.3% of the grain, generally higher than in other cereals. The policosanols represent 19–46% of the sorghum wax (Avato et al 1990). This translates to 38–92 mg of policosanols per 100 g sorghum grain.

The policosanols may be the most valuable components of sorghum grain based on their current market value (Weller and Hwang 2003). They exist in high levels in distiller's dry grains, a coproduct of ethanol production (Weller and Hwang 2003). The bloom types of sorghum have high levels of wax covering the leaves and stems, which may be another source of these compounds. The policosanols are gaining popularity because they reduce cholesterol levels as effectively as statins (Gouni-Berthold and Berthold 2002). The policosanols are destined to gain importance as natural, safe, and effective dietary alternatives to statin medication. The efficacy and economic potential of the sorghum policosanols should be investigated.

Dietary Fiber and Other Components

Most of the fiber is present in the pericarp and cell walls. Sorghum contains 6.5–7.9% insoluble fiber, hemicellulose, and cellulose and 1.1–1.2% soluble fiber, composed primarily of β-glucans and pentosans. Sorghum contains approximately 1.3% total pentosans, located mainly in the pericarp. Approximately 70% of these pentosans are alkali soluble, and some 30% are water soluble. Dietary fiber in cell walls of the aleurone and endosperm are associated with ferulic and caffeic acid. Dietary fiber in the pericarp provides structural and protective functions; therefore, the fiber content of sorghum products depends on the extent of pericarp removal during milling. Abrasive decortication of 10–15% of the initial weight of the kernel produces bran with a dietary fiber content of 41–48%, depending upon the sorghum (Table 4).

TABLE 4
Composition of Special Sorghum[a] Brans (%, dry matter basis)

Bran	Crude Protein	Crude Fat	Ash	NFE[b]	Crude Fiber	Dietary Fiber
Wheat	17.2	4.7	6.4	71.6	...	47.5
White sorghum	13.2	8.3	3.5	65.0	9.9	41.3
Tannin sorghum	12.7	10.4	5.1	63.8	8.0	45.0
Black sorghum	15.0	4.4	3.8	68.3	9.7	43.4

[a] Sorghum brans obtained using an abrasive decorticator at 12–15% yield. Adapted from Gordon (2001).

[b] Nitrogen-free extract.

Sorghum dietary fiber contains more associated proteins than dietary fiber from other cereals. Insoluble dietary fiber increases during food processing due to increased levels of bound protein (mainly kafirins) and enzyme-resistant starch (Knudsen and Munck 1985). In tannin sorghum, cooking also forms insoluble polyphenol-protein complexes, which increase dietary fiber.

Sorghum bran fed to human subjects increased stool weight, decreased intestinal transit time, and increased the frequency of evacuation. Klopfenstein et al (1981) compared several sources of cereal fibers and found that sorghum bran was effective in lowering serum and liver cholesterol levels in guinea pigs. Rooney et al (1992) decorticated white and brown sorghums to remove approximately 7.5% of the caryopsis. The resulting pericarp-rich tissue (bran) contained 47.8 and 35.1% insoluble dietary fiber and 1.6 and 1.0% soluble fiber, respectively. Sorghum brans were excellent bulking agents in rats. Brown sorghum bran (containing tannins) had better bulking ability than white sorghum bran.

The bran of tannin sorghum is also high in phytates and natural brown or black pigments that impart attractive colors to baked products such as cookies and multigrain breads. A healthful bread that contains modest levels of high-tannin sorghums as a source of antioxidants is currently being sold by a commercial bakery in Wisconsin. A bread mix containing brown or black sorghum bran with flaxseed, gluten, barley, and wheat flour was developed (Rudiger 2003). The bread has excellent flavor and texture, and high levels of dietary fiber, antioxidants, lignans, and omega-3 fatty acids with a natural brown color. Black sorghum bran in breads resulted in appearance, texture, color, and specific volume (cm^3/g) similar to those of commercial specialty or dark rye breads.

Sorghum Phytochemicals and Human Health

Cardiovascular Disease (CVD)

Various epidemiological data indicate that whole grain consumption significantly lowers mortality from CVD (Kushi et al 1999, Slavin et al 2000, Anderson 2003). The phytosterols in the cereal brans are believed to contribute to these beneficial effects. Other components of the whole grains, including polyphenols and fiber, also play a role in CVD prevention.

Klopfenstein et al (1981) reported a cholesterol-lowering effect of low-tannin sorghum grain fed to guinea pigs at 58% of the diet. This effect was greater than that produced by wheat, rolled oats, or pearl millet. More recently, Cho et al (2000) found that sorghum and proso millet hexane extracts inhibited rat liver microsomal 3-hydroxy-3-methylglutaryl CoA (HMG-CoA) reductase in a dose-dependent manner. They observed that fecal bile acid excretion and high-density lipoprotein cholesterol levels were increased, without a change in total cholesterol, when whole sorghum, proso millet, or buckwheat was fed to rats at 30% of diet. Lee and Pan (2003) demonstrated that tannin-sorghum distillery residues inhibited 63–97% of hemoglobin-catalyzed oxidation of linoleic acid in cultured mullet fish compared to soybean (13%) and rice bran

(78%). The sorghum residues significantly improved blood-thinning and erythrocyte membrane integrity of the fish blood cells during winter; they attributed the prevention of red blood cell hemolysis to the antioxidant activity of the tannins and other polyphenols present in the sorghum residue.

In general, several epidemiological studies show that red wine and tea consumption correlate with reduced risk of CVD (Chung et al 1998, Higdon and Frei 2003). The effects are largely attributed to the tannins and other polyphenols in these food products. There is no epidemiological data on tannin-sorghum consumption and CVD in humans, probably because CVD is not a major problem in populations that consume high levels of sorghum. The unique tannins and anthocyanins in sorghum (discussed earlier) are likely to produce beneficial effects. A hypoglycemic effect of sorghum has also been demonstrated (Lakshmi and Vimala 1996), which might contribute to lower risk of CVD. This and the above animal data suggest that a controlled clinical trial is warranted.

Obesity

Tannin sorghums may help depress weight gain in humans as has been observed in animals. Most of the negative press about sorghum originated from the fact that the high-tannin sorghums have reduced calorie value relative to corn and thus leads to depressed livestock growth and weight gain compared to corn and other cereals.

Tannin sorghums reduce nutritive value by binding food proteins and carbohydrates into insoluble complexes that cannot be easily broken down by digestive enzymes. Another mechanism involves the direct binding of digestive enzymes, including sucrase, amylases, trypsin, chymotrypsin, and lipases (Al-Mamary et al 2001), thus inhibiting their activity. Inhibition of intestinal brush-border bound amino acid transporters by sorghum tannins has been reported (King et al 2000). There is evidence that the higher-DP tannins are more involved in these interactions than the low-DP ones (Sarni-Manchado et al 1999).

Effects of the sorghum tannins on animal weight gain depend on levels fed as well as animal species. Numerous reports on reduced weight gain of rats, pigs, rabbits, and poultry fed high-tannin sorghum are available (Cousins et al 1981, Lizardo et al 1995, Al-Mamary et al 2001, Muriu et al 2002). Al-Mamary et al (2001) found that a high-tannin (3.5% CE) sorghum diet markedly decreased live weight gain and feed-conversion ratio in rabbits, whereas a 1.4% CE sorghum had no effect. Cousins et al (1981) reported a 10% reduction in feed efficiency (relative to corn) when high-tannin (3.1–3.4% CE) sorghums were fed to pigs. A low-tannin sorghum had feed efficiency similar to that of corn. Lizardo et al (1995) also observed a 10% reduction in weight gain when pigs were fed a tannin-sorghum diet compared to corn. Broiler chicks fed low-tannin sorghums (0.6–0.9% CE) had weight gain and feed efficiency similar to that from corn (Ambula et al 2001). However, tannin sorghums (2.7–3.5% CE) significantly reduced the weight gain of broilers.

The differential response of animals to sorghums with different tannin levels may be due to adaptation of animals to dietary tannins by release of proline-rich salivary proteins (Mehansho et al 1983, Mole et al 1990). Hence, there appears to be a tannin-level threshold for every animal species. No reports exist on how tannin-sorghums might be used to lower calorie intake in human diets. Epidemiological data on humans are lacking, probably because obesity is not common in locations where tannin sorghums are consumed. With the growing problem of obesity in certain parts of the world, the potential of tannin sorghums to control weight should be explored.

Cancer

Beneficial effects of sorghum and or millet consumption on cancer have been documented. Van Rensburg (1981) reported that sorghum consumption consistently correlated with low incidences of esophageal cancer in various parts of the world (including several parts of Africa, Russia, India, China, and Iran), whereas wheat and corn consumption correlated with elevated levels. These regions also had deficiencies of certain minerals and vitamins in their diets. In attempting to explain this phenomenon, the author proposed that nutrient deficiencies were responsible for the high esophageal cancer incidences, and that sorghum and millet consumption promoted resistance to esophageal cancer. Chen et al (1993) reported similar results for epidemiological data from Sachxi Province, China. These authors studied 21 communities within the province over a period of six years. The regions that consumed the highest amounts of sorghum, and to a lesser extent millet, had 1.4–3.2 times lower mortality from esophageal cancer than areas that mainly consumed wheat flour or corn. Consumption of other foods like alcohol, tea, meats, and vegetables did not contribute significantly to esophageal cancer mortality. These findings suggest the presence of anticarcinogenic compounds in sorghum that are either lacking or are not present in significant quantities in wheat or corn.

In vitro studies have also demonstrated the anticarcinogenic properties of sorghum. Grimmer et al (1992) found antimutagenicity to be associated with sorghum polyphenol extracts. The high-MW procyanidins (tannins) had higher antimutagenic activity compared to the lower-MW tannins. Gomez-Cordovez et al (2001) showed that sorghum tannins had anticarcinogenic activity against human melanoma cells, as well as positive melanogenic activity. Similar melanogenic activity in red wine extracts was not detected. On the other hand, Parbhoo et al (1995) reported that sorghum procyanidin extracts may induce cytochrome P-450, a protein capable of converting certain promutagens to mutagenic derivatives in rat liver. These conflicting findings are typical of these endeavors. More work on sorghum is required to validate these reported anticarcinogenic properties.

Plenty of literature (often conflicting) is available on properties of various polyphenol-rich foods, especially tea and red wine and grapes in relation to various types of cancer in humans (reviewed by Chung et al 1998, Higdon and Frei 2003). The overall trend suggests that polyphenol-rich products are anticarcinogenic, but a consensus on their efficacy is currently lacking. For example, even though tea is reported as anticarcinogenic in many *in vitro* and epidemiological studies, Higdon and Frei (2003) concluded that available data do not support the notion that tea is protective against cancer. Yang et al (2001) also provided useful insight on the limitations of various cancer-related studies.

For sorghum, available data on cancer are too limited to draw meaningful conclusions. However, the corroborative epidemiological evidences reported by Van Rensburg (1981) and Chen et al (1993) against esophageal cancer warrant further investigation. Additional *in vitro* data as well as controlled animal studies are necessary to understand how the levels and composition of polyphenols in sorghum affect cancer, and which specific components are responsible.

Summary

Sorghum types vary from the white food hybrids that have excellent properties for use in a wide variety of processed foods to brown high-tannin and black high-anthocyanin types containing high levels of antioxidants. The white food types have functionality similar to rice with a bland flavor and light color, and they can be extruded, flaked, and made into a wide variety of food products. Moreover, these new hybrids have excellent yields and are widely adapted.

Tannin and black sorghums have a diversity of phytochemicals with potential significant impact on human health. The sorghum phytochemicals show high antioxidant activities against different free radicals *in vitro* that compare favorably with high-antioxidant fruits and vegetables. The tannin sorghums can be processed into bran that can be used to produce foods rich in antioxidants and desirable phenolic compounds. The sorghum brans are also rich in phytosterols and policosanols, which are known to promote cardiovascular health. More information on how sorghum phytochemicals affect human health is required. However, current overall epidemiological evidence suggests that special sorghums have anticarcinogenic properties, promote cardiovascular health, and may reduce caloric availability of foods.

The brown (tannin) sorghum brans produce baked products with dark natural color, acceptable flavor, and improved levels of antioxidants and dietary fiber. The protein complexed with condensed tannins has the potential to slow digestion and reduce caloric content of foods. These special sorghums are available in high-yielding cultivars and hybrids. The grain can be stored indefinitely and processed into brans and extracts to produce an array of useful products for health foods and related products. Knowledge of sorghum genetics permits designing special types of sorghum with even greater variation in phenol type and contents. The combination of high anthocyanins and tannins is a promising option.

Acknowledgments

We thank all of our colleagues, former colleagues, and graduate students who have contributed much to our improved understanding of factors that affect the utilization of sorghum and millets and how to define quality in breeding and improvement programs. The long-term financial support through the USAID Title XII INTSORMIL Collaborate Research Support Program has been a key factor in our program.

References

Acosta, D. 2003. White food-type sorghum in direct-expansion extrusion applications. M.S. thesis, Texas A&M University, College Station, TX.

Adom, K. K., and Liu, R. H. 2002. Antioxidant activity of grains. J. Agric. Food Chem. 50:6182-6187.

Al-Mamary, M., Al-Habori, M., Al-Aghbari, A., and Al-Obeidi, A. 2001. *In vivo* effects of dietary sorghum tannins on rabbit digestive enzymes and mineral absorption. Nutr. Res. 21:1393-1401.

Almeida-Dominguez, H. D., Serna-Saldivar, S. O., and Rooney, L. W. 1991. Properties of new and commercial sorghum hybrids for utilization in alkaline cooked foods. Cereal Chem. 68:25-30.

Ambula, M. K., Oguho, G. W., and Tuitoek, J. K. 2001. Effects of sorghum tannins, a tannin binder (polyvinylpyrrolidone) and sorghum inclusion level on the performance of broiler chicks. Asian Aust. J. Anim. 14:1276-1281.

Anderson, J. W. 2003. Whole grain protects against atherosclerotic cardiovascular disease. Proc. Nutr. Soc. 62:135-142.

Andreasen, M. F., Kroon, P. A., Williamson, G., and Garcia-Conesa, M. 2001a. Esterase activity able to hydrolyze dietary antioxidant hydroxycinnamates is distributed along the intestine of mammals. J. Agric. Food Chem. 49:5679-5684.

Andreasen, M. F., Kroon, P. A., Williamson, G., and Garcia-Conesa, M. 2001b. Intestinal release and uptake of phenolic antioxidant diferulic acid. Free Rad. Biol. Med. 31:304-314.

Avato, P., Bianchi, G., and Murelli, C. 1990. Aliphatic and cyclic lipid components of Sorghum plant organs. Phytochemistry 29:1073-1078.

Awika, J. M. 2000. Sorghum phenols as antioxidants. M.S. thesis, Texas A&M University, College Station, TX.

Awika, J. M. 2003. Antioxidant properties of sorghum. Ph.D. dissertation, Texas A&M University, College Station, TX.

Awika, J. M., Suhendro, E. L., and Rooney, L. W. 2002. Milling value of sorghums compared by adjusting yields to a constant product color. Cereal Chem. 79:249-251.

Awika, J. M., Dykes, L., Gu, L., Rooney, L. W., and Prior, R. L. 2003a. Processing of sorghum (*Sorghum bicolor*) and sorghum products alters procyanidin oligomer and polymer distribution and content. J. Agric. Food Chem. 51:5516-5521.

Awika, J. M., Rooney, L. W., Wu, X., Prior, R. L., and Cisneros-Zevallos, L. 2003b. Screening methods to measure antioxidant activity of sorghum (*Sorghum bicolor*) and sorghum products. J. Agric. Food Chem. 51:6657-6662.

Boveris, A. D., Galatro, A., Sambrotta, L., Ricco, R., Gurni, A. A., and Puntarulo, S. 2001. Antioxidant capacity of 3-deoxyanthocyanidin from soybean. Phytochemistry 58:1097-1105.

Burns, R. E. 1971. Methods for estimation of tannin in grain sorghum. Agron. J. 63:511-514.

Chen, F., Cole, P., Mi, Z. B., and Xing, L. Y. 1993. Corn and wheat consumption and mortality from esophageal cancer in Shanxi, China. Int. J. Cancer 53:902-906.

Cho, S.-H., Choi, Y., and Ha, T.-Y. 2000. In vitro and in vivo effects of prosomillet, buckwheat and sorghum on cholesterol metabolism. FASEB J. 14:A249.

Chung, K.-T., Tit, Y. W., Cheng, I. W., Yao-Wen, H., and Yuan, L. 1998. Tannins and human health: A review. Crit. Rev. Food Sci. Nutr. 38:421-464.

Clifford, M. N. 2000. Anthocyanins—Nature, occurrence and dietary burden. J. Sci. Food Agric. 80:1063-1072.

Cousins, B. W., Tanksley, T. D., Knabe, D. A., and Zebrowska, T. 1981. Nutrient digestibility and performance of pigs fed sorghums varying in tannin concentration. J. Anim. Sci. 53:1524-1529.

Cruz-Celis, L. P., Rooney, L. W., and McDonough, C. M. 1996. A ready-to-eat breakfast cereal from food-grade sorghum. Cereal Chem. 73:108-114.

Deprez, S., Brezillon, C., Rabot, S., Philippe, C., Mila, I., LaPierre, C., and Scalbert, A. 2000. Polymeric proanthocyanidins are catabolized by human colonic microflora into low-molecular weight phenolic acids. J. Nutr. 130:2733-2738.

Deprez, S., Mila, I., Huneau, J. F., Tome, D., and Scalbert, A. 2001. Transport of proanthocyanidin dimer, trimer, and polymer across monolayers of human intestinal epithelial Caco-2 cells. Antioxid. Redox. Signal 3:957-967.

Deshpande, S. S., and Cheryan, M. 1985. Tannin analysis of food products. CRC Crit. Rev. Food Sci. Nutr. 24:401-449.

Dykes, L., Awika, J., McDonough, C. M., Rooney, L. W., and Waniska, R. D. 2002. False positives for tannin sorghum in non-tannin sorghum using the bleach test. Online: http://www.aaccnet.org/meetings/2002/abstracts/a02ma286.asp

Earp, C. F., Doherty, C. A., and Rooney, L. W. 1983. Fluorescence microscopy of the pericarp, aleurone layer and endosperm cell walls of three sorghum cultivars. Cereal Chem. 60:408-410.

Earp, C. F., McDonough, C. M., Awika, J. M., and Rooney, L. W. 2004. Microscopic changes during development of sorghums with and without pigmented testa. J. Cereal Sci. 39:153-161.

Forberg, C. 2003. Stop the Clock Cooking. Avery, Penguin Putnam, Inc., New York.

Gomez, M. H., Rooney, L. W., Waniska, R. D., and Lusas, E. 1988. Extrusion cooking of sorghum containing different amounts of amylose. J. Food Sci. 53:1818-1822.

Gomez-Cordovez , C., Bartolomez, B., Vieira, W., and Viradir, V. M. 2001. Effects of wine phenolics and sorghum tannins on tyrosinase activity and growth of melanoma cells. J. Agric. Food Chem. 49:1620-1624.

Gordon, L. A. 2001. Utilization of sorghum brans and barley flour in bread. M.S. thesis, Texas A&M University, College Station, TX.

Gouni-Berthold, I., and Berthold, H. K. 2002. Policosanol: Clinical pharmacology and therapeutic significance of a new lipid-lowering agent. Am. Heart J. 143:356-365.

Gous, F. 1989. Tannins and phenols in black sorghum. Ph.D. dissertation, Texas A&M University, College Station, TX.

Grimmer, H. R., Parbhoo, V., and McGarth, R. M. 1992. Antimutagenicity of polyphenol-rich fractions from *Sorghum bicolo*r grain. J. Sci. Food Agric. 59:251-256.

Gu, L., Kelm, M., Hammerstone, J. F., Beecher, G., Cunnigham, D., Vannozzi, S., and Prior, L. 2002. Fractionation of polymeric procyanidins from lowbush blueberry and quantification of procyanidins in selected foods with an optimized normal-phase HPLC-MS fluorescent detection method. J. Agric. Food Chem. 50:4852-4860.

Gujer, R., Magnolato, D., and Self, R. 1986. Glucosylated flavonoids and other phenolic compounds from sorghum. Phytochemistry 25:1431-1436.

Hagerman, A. E., and Butler, L. G. 1978. Protein precipitation method for the quantitative determination of tannins. J. Agric. Food Chem. 26:809-812.

Hagerman, A. E., and Butler, L. G. 1980. Condensed tannin purification and characterization of tannin-associated proteins. J. Agric. Food Chem. 28:947-952.

Hagerman, A. E., Riedl, K. M., Jones, G. A., Sovik, K. N., Ritchard, N. T., Hartzfeld, P. W., and Riechel, T. K. 1998. High molecular weight plant polyphenolics (tannins) as biological antioxidants. J. Agric. Food Chem. 46:1887-1892.

Hahn, D. H., and Rooney, L. W. 1986. Effects of genotype on tannins and phenols of sorghum. Cereal Chem. 63:4-8.

Hahn, D. H., Rooney, L. W., and Faubion, J. M. 1983. Sorghum phenolic acids, their HPLC separation and their relation to fungal resistance. Cereal Chem. 60:255-259.

Hammerstone, J. F., Lazarus, S. A., Mitchel, A. E., Rucker, R., and Schmitz, H. H. 1999. Identification of procyanidins in cocoa (*Theobroma cocoa*) and chocolate using high-performance liquid chromatography/mass spectrophotometry. J. Agric. Food Chem. 47:490-496.

Higdon, J. V., and Frei, B. 2003. Tea catechins and polyphenols: Health effects, metabolism, and antioxidant functions. Crit. Rev. Food Sci. Nutr. 43:89-143.

Karaivanova, M., Drenska, D., and Ovcharov, R. 1990. A modification of the toxic effects of platinum complexes with anthocyanins. Eksp. Med. Morfol. 29:19-24.

King, D., Fan, M. Z., Ejeta, G., Asem, E. K., and Adeola, O. 2000. The effects of tannins on nutrient utilization in the White Pekin duck. Br. Poult. Sci. 41:629-630.

Klopfenstein, C. F., Varriano-Marston, E., and Hoseney, R. C. 1981. Cholesterol-lowering effect of sorghum diet in guinea pigs. Nutr. Rep. Int. 24:621-626.

Knudsen, K. F., and Munck, L. 1985. Dietary fiber content and composition of sorghum and sorghum based foods. J. Cereal Sci. 3:153-164.

Krueger, C. G., Vestling, M. A., and Reed, J. D. 2003. Matrix-assisted laser desorption/ionization time-of-flight mass spectrometry of heteropolyflavan-3-ols and glucosylated heteropolyflavans in sorghum (*Sorghum bicolor* (L.) Moench). J. Agric. Food Chem. 51:538-543.

Kushi, L. H., Meyer, K. A., and Jacobs, D. R. 1999. Cereals, legumes, and chronic disease risk reduction: evidence from epidemiologic studies. Am. J. Clin. Nutr. 70(Suppl.):451S-458S.

Kwon, Y. S., and Kim, C. M. 2003. Antioxidant constituents from the stem of *Sorghum bicolor*. Arch. Pharm. Res. 26:535-539.

Lakshmi, K. B., and Vimala, V. 1996. Hypoglycemic effect of selected sorghum recipes. Nutr. Res. 16:1651-1658.

Lee, S. M., and Pan, B. S. 2003. Effects of dietary sorghum distillery residue on hematological characteristics of cultured grey mullet (*Mugil cephalus*)—An animal model for prescreening antioxidant and blood thinning activities. J. Food Biochem. 27:1-18.

Leon-Chapa, M. 1999. Methods to improve and measure texture of sorghum cookies. M.S. thesis, Texas A&M University, College Station, TX.

Lietti, A., Cristoni, A., and Picci, M. 1976. Studies of *Vaccinium myrtillus* anthocyanosides. I. Vasoprotective and anti-inflammatory activity. Arzneim. Forsch 26:829-832.

Lizardo, R., Peiniau, J., and Aumaitre, A. 1995. Effect of sorghum on performance, digestibility of dietary-components and activities of pancreatic and intestinal enzymes in the weaned piglet. Anim. Feed Sci. Technol. 56:67-82.

Lotito, S. B., Actis-Goretta, L., Renart, M. L., Caligiuri, M., Rein, D., Schmitz, H. H., Steinberg, F. M., Keen, C. L., and Fraga, C. G. 2000. Influence of oligomer chain length on antioxidant activity of procyanidins. Biochem. Biophys. Res. Comm. 276:945-951.

Lu, Y., and Foo, L. Y. 2001. Unusual anthocyanin reactions with acetone leading to proanthocyanin formation. Tetrahedron Lett. 42:1371-1373.

Makkar, H. P. S. 1989. Protein precipitation methods for quantitation of tannins: A review. J. Agric. Food Chem. 37:1197-1202.

Maranphal, N. 2003. Direct expanded snacks from sorghum. M.S. thesis, Texas A&M University, College Station, TX.

Maxson, E. D., and Rooney, L. W. 1972. Evaluation of methods for tannin analysis in sorghum grain. Cereal Chem. 49:719-729.

McDonough, C., Anderson, B. J., Acosta-Zuleta, H., and Rooney, L. W. 1998. Steam flaking characteristics of sorghum hybrids and lines with differing endosperm characteristics. Cereal Chem.75:634-638.

Mehansho, H., Hagerman, A., Clements, S., Butler, L., Rogler, J., and Carlson, D. M. 1983. Modulation of proline-rich protein-biosynthesis in rat parotid glands by sorghums with high tannin levels. Proc. Natl. Acad. Sci. U.S.A., Biol. Sci. 80:3948-3952.

Miller, F. R., Clova, R., and Guiragossian, V. 1992. Registration of A/BTx635 sorghum. Crop Sci. 32:1517-1518.

Mole, S., Butler, L. G., and Iason, G. 1990. Defense against dietary tannin in herbivore—A survey for proline rich salivary proteins in mammals. Biochem. Syst. Ecol. 18:287-293.

Muriu, J. I., Njoka-Njiru, E. N., Tuitoek, J. K., and Nanua, J. N. 2002. Evaluation of sorghum (*Sorghum bicolor*) as replacement for maize in the diet of growing rabbits (*Oryctolagus cuniculus*). Asian Aust. J. Anim. Sci. 15:565-569.

Parbhoo, V., Grimmer, H. R., Cameron-Clarke, A., and McGarth, R. M. 1995. Induction of cytochrome P-450 in rat liver by a polyphenol-rich extract from a bird-resistant sorghum grain. J. Sci. Food Agric. 69:247-252.

Pepping, J. 2003. Policosanol. Am. J. Health-Syst. Pharm. 60:1112-1114.

Price, M. L., Van Scoyoc, S., and Butler, L. G. 1978. A critical evaluation of vanillin reaction as an assay for tannin in sorghum. J. Agric. Food Chem. 26:1214-1218.

Reed, J. D., Horvath, P. J., Allen, M. S., and Vansoest, P. J. 1985. Gravimetric-determination of soluble phenolics including tannins from leaves by precipitation with trivalent ytterbium. J. Sci. Food Agric. 36:255-261.

Remy, S., Fulcrand, H., Labarbe, B., Cheynier, V., and Moutounet, M. 2000. First confirmation in red wine of products resulting from direct anthocyanin-tannin reactions. J. Sci. Food Agric. 80:745-751.

Riedl, K. M., and Hagerman, A. E. 2001. Tannin-protein complexes as radical scavengers and radical sinks. J. Agric. Food Chem. 49:4917-4923.

Rigaud, J., Escribano-Bailon, M. T., Prieur, C., Souquet, J. M., and Cheynier, V. 1993. Normal-phase high-performance liquid chromatography separation of procyanidins from cacao beans and grape seeds. J. Chromatagr. A 654:255-260.

Rios, L. Y., Bennett, R. N., Lazarus, S. A., Remesey, C., Scalbert, A., and Williamson, G. 2002. Cocoa procyanidins are stable during gastric transit in humans. Am. J. Clin. Nutr. 76:1106-1110.

Rooney, L. W., and Miller, F. R. 1982. Variation in structure and kernel characteristics of sorghum. Pages 143-162 in: International Symposium on Sorghum Grain Quality. International Crops Research Institute of the Semi-arid Tropics,, Patancheru, India.

Rooney, L. W., and Pflugfelder, R. L. 1986. Factors affecting starch digestibility with special emphasis on sorghum and corn. J. Anim. Sci. 63:1607-1623.

Rooney, L. W., and Waniska, R. D. 2000. Sorghum food and industrial utilization. Pages 689-729 in: Sorghum: Origin, History, Technology, and Production. C. W. Smith and R. A. Frederiksen, Eds. Wiley, Hoboken, NJ.

Rooney, T. K., Rooney, L. W., and Lupton, J. R. 1992. Physiological characteristics of sorghum and millet brans in the rat model. Cereal Foods World 37:782-786.

Rooney, W. L., Miller, F. R., and Frederiksen, R. A. 2000. Registration of Tx2911 sorghum germplasm. Crop Sci. 40:584-585.

Ross, J. A., and Kasum, C. M. 2002. Dietary flavonoids: Bioavailability, metabolic effects, and safety. Annu. Rev. Nutr. 22:19-22.

Rudiger, C. 2003. The formulation of a nutraceutical bread mix using sorghum, barley, and flaxseed. M.S. thesis, Texas A&M University, College Station, TX.

Rusnak, B. A., Chou, C., and Rooney, L. W. 1980. Effect of micronizing on kernel characteristics of sorghum varieties with different endosperm type. J. Food Sci. 45:1529-1532.

Sarni-Manchado, P., Cheynier, V., and Mountounet, M. 1999. Interactions of grape seed tannins with salivary proteins. J. Agric. Food Chem. 47:42-47.

Scalbert, A., Morand, C., Manach, C., and Remesy, C. 2002. Absorption and metabolism of polyphenols in the gut and impact on health. Biomed. Pharmacother. 56:276-282.

Singh, V., Moreau, R. A., and Hicks, K. B. 2003. Yield and phytosterol composition of oil extracted from grain sorghum and its wet-milled fractions. Cereal Chem. 80:126-129.

Slavin, J. L., Jacobs, D., and Marquart, L. 2000. Grain processing and nutrition. Crit. Rev. Food Sci. Nutr. 40:309-326.

Spencer, J., Chaudry, F., Pannala, A., Srai, S., Debnam, E., and Rice-Evans, C. 2000. Decomposition of cocoa procyanidins in the gastric milieu. Biochem. Biophys. Res. Commun. 272:236-241.

Suhendro, E. L., McDonough, C. M., Rooney, L. W., Waniska, R. D., and Yetneberk, S. 1998. Effects of processing conditions and sorghum cultivar on alkaline-processed snacks. Cereal Chem. 75:187-193.

Sweeny, J. G., and Iacobucci, G. A., 1981. Synthesis of anthocyanidins-III: Total synthesis of apigeninidin and luteolinidin chlorides. Tetrahedron 37:1481-1483.

Tapiero, H., Tew, K. D., Nguyen, G. B., and Mathe, G. 2002. Polyphenols: Do they play a role in prevention of human pathologies? Biomed. Phamacother. 56:200-207.

Taylor, J. R. N., and Dewar, J. 2000. Fermented products: Beverages and porridges. Pages 689-729 in: Sorghum: Origin, History, Technology, and Production. C. W. Smith and R. A. Frederiksen, Eds. Wiley, Hoboken, NJ.

Tebib, K., Rouanet, J. M., and Besancon, P. 1997. Antioxidant effects of dietary polymeric grape seed tannins in tissue of rats fed a high cholesterol-vitamin E-deficient diet. Food Chem. 59:135-141.

USDA, Foreign Agricultural Services. 2004. World sorghum production, consumption and stocks. Online: www.fas.usda.gov/psd. (Search: Grains.)

Van Rensburg, S. J. 1981. Epidemiological and dietary evidence for a specific nutritional predisposition to esophageal cancer. J. Natl. Cancer Inst. 67:243-251.

Waniska, R. D., and Rooney, L. W. 2000. Structure and chemistry of the sorghum caryopsis. Pages 649-688 in: Sorghum: Origin, History, Technology, and Production. C. W. Smith and R. A. Frederiksen, Eds. Wiley, Hoboken, NJ.

Waniska, R. D., Poe, J. H., and Bandyopadhyay, R. 1989. Effects of growth conditions on grain molding and phenols in sorghum caryopsis. J. Cereal Sci. 10:217-225.

Watterson, J. J., and Butler, L. 1983. Occurrence of an unusual leucoanthocyanidin and absence of proanthocyanidin in sorghum leaves. J. Agric. Food Chem. 31:41-45.

Weaver, C. A., Hamaker, B. R., and Axtell, J. D. 1998. Discovery of grain sorghum germ plasm with high uncooked and cooked *in vitro* protein digestibilities. Cereal Chem. 75:665-670.

Weller, C. L., and Hwang, K. T. 2003. Recoverable lipids from grain sorghum dry distiller's grain. Proc. Biennial Grain Sorghum Res. and Util. Conf., 23rd. J. A. Dahlberg, R. Kochenower, R. Klein, B. Rooney, S. Bean, B. Pendleton, J. Stack, and B. Maunder, Eds. National Grain Sorghum Producers Association, Lubbock, TX.

Yang, C. S., Landau, J. M., Huang, M.-T., and Newmark, H. L. 2001. Inhibition of carcinogenesis by dietary polyphenolic compounds. Annu. Rev. Nutr. 21:381-406.

Yetneberk, S. 2004. Sorghum *injera* quality improvement through processing and development of cultivar selection criteria. Ph.D. dissertation, University of Pretoria, Pretoria, S. Africa.

Zelaya, N. May 2001. Characterization of tortillas and tortilla chips from sorghum varieties high in phenolic compounds. M.S. thesis, Texas A&M University, College Station, TX.

CHAPTER 12

Blue and Purple Grains

G. Mazza[1] and L. Gao[2]

[1]Agriculture and Agri-Food Canada, Pacific Agri-Food Research Centre, Summerland, BC, Canada V0H 1Z0; [2]PEI Food Technology Centre, Charlottetown, PEI, Canada C1A 7N8

Cereal grains are the most important crops in the world, as most of the world's population depends on one or more of them as staple foods. However, blue and purple grains are only a small proportion of these since breeding programs do not usually select for these color features or, indeed, may attempt to eliminate them. Breeders have usually selected for high yield, high protein, desirable agronomic performance, and storage and processing properties. Colored strains have usually received little or no attention and are mostly in wild or semiwild status.

In recent years, there has been a renewed interest in grains and grain-based foods that are recognized as health-promoting. This development has resulted from recent epidemiological and clinical studies that have linked the consumption of grains with reduced risk of chronic and aging-related diseases. Also, consumption of foods rich in phytochemicals, such as anthocyanins and other phenolics, has been associated with a reduced risk of such diseases (Mazza 2000a). Colored grains are perceived by consumers to be rich in these phytonutrients. Although this does not establish the link between colored grains and their health benefits, they are receiving increased attention by both scientists and technologists for potential new products.

The appearance of the purple and the blue colors of grains is mainly a result of phenolic compounds on the surface of the grains, particularly anthocyanins, a group of reddish to purple flavonoids. However, the myriad shades of the colors are a result of virtually unlimited combinations of the anthocyanins and their interactions with other phenolic compounds through copigmentation (Mazza and Miniati 1993). These other phenolics, including the groups of flavans, proanthocyanidins, flavones, flavonols, and phenolic acids, are extensively documented (e.g., Harborne 1988). They are also included here wherever the information is available. This chapter reviews the genetics and breeding, grain and flour characteristics, pigment composition, and current and potential uses of blue and/or purple barley, buckwheat, corn/maize, oats, rice, rye, triticale, sorghum, millet, quinoa, amaranth, wheat, and wild rice. Wherever appropriate, the properties of these grains are discussed relative to the regular grains.

Barley

Barley can be of many different colors: white, blue, purple, black, and red. Cultivated barley (*Hordeum vulgare*) is in the family Poaceae, tribe Triticeae, and genus *Hordeum* and is one of 31 *Hordeum* species, among which 30 are wild. The wild species are mostly diploid ($2n = 14$) with the remaining being about equally divided into tetraploid ($2n = 28$) and hexaploid ($2n = 42$), with seven, 14, or 21 pairs of chromosomes, respectively (Nilan and Ullrich 1993). Only the varieties of blue and white kernels are extensively grown, and the white varieties dominate.

Genetics and Breeding

The pigmentation of various parts of the barley plant can be black, which is generally due to the presence of melanins, or blue, red, or purple due to anthocyanins (Takahashi 1955). The purple color of the barley kernel is located in the pericarp, while the blue is localized in the aleurone layer of the kernel.

According to Woodward and Thieret (1953), the presence of anthocyanin pigmentation in seeds and ears of barley is controlled by two complementary genes, *P* and *C*. The origin of these genes is believed to be the purple forms of a wild species, *H. agriocrithon* var. *dawoense*, native to the region of Tibet. The blue-colored aleurone is governed by the complementary genes *B1* and *B12* (Mayler and Stanford 1942). The pigmentation is present in almost all wild species and in many cultivated ones. It is a dominant character over white and is inherited monofactorily (Litzenberger and Green 1951). Other plant parts containing anthocyanins are the auricle, node, and stem (Takahashi et al 1953, Murty and Jain 1959). Gonzalez-Ceniceros and Franckowiak (1990) found that mutants of *Ant* genes at the *ant* 13, *ant* 17, and *ant* 18 loci in barley, which suppress expression of some or all of the colored pigments in the plant, also suppress the expression of blue aleurone in barley.

Pigmentation Characteristics

Anthocyanins occur in pigmented varieties of barley and in plants subjected to nutritional or pathological stresses. In the purple-seeded varieties, the spermoderm and aleurone may be strongly pigmented and the diffusion of the anthocyanins may obscure the cell walls; the pigmentation of the aleurone is genetically independent, while that of the lemma and palea is linked to that of the caryopsis (Mullick and Brink 1966, Mullick 1967). Accumulation of anthocyanins following nitrogen deficiency was reported by Gassner and Straib (1937), and production of anthocyanins due to phosphorous deficiency was observed by Hamy (1983). Takahashi and Yamamoto (1950) reported on the distribution of anthocyanin and melanin pigmentation in the beard, glume, seed, auricle, and ligule of barley grown in different areas. According to Narula and Mathur (1966), the purple pigmentation of the auricle is controlled by a single dominant gene and is associated with the genes that control pigment accumulation in straw, lemma, and pericarp.

Mullick et al (1958) found glycosides of cyanidin and delphinidin in three blue and two purple varieties of barley and in the lemma and caryopsis of one black variety. The purple varieties also contained pelargonidin derivatives. In all, Mullick et al (1958) provided evidence for the presence of six anthocyanins in barley: two cyanidin, two delphinidin, and two pelargonidin derivatives. In barley malt, McFarlane et al (1955) found cyanidin, delphinidin, and several unidentified anthocyanins. More recently, Jende-Strid (1978) found that the yellow, blue, and black varieties of barley seeds contained delphinidin and cyanidin, while the purple varieties also contained pelargonidin. Metche and Urion (1961) however, found cyanidin-3-arabinoside in the seed coat of barley. These early results were based on paper chromatography, and the exact identity of the anthocyanins should be established by modern analytical techniques.

TABLE 1
Anthocyanins and Other Phenolics of Barley (*Hordeum vulgare* L.)[a]

Compound	Plant Part	Reference
Anthocyanins		
Pelargonidin	Pericarp and aleurone	Mullick et al (1958)
Pelargonidin glycosides	Pericarp and aleurone	Mullick et al (1958)
Cyanidin	Pericarp and aleurone	Mullick et al (1958)
Cyanidin glycosides	Pericarp and aleurone	Mullick et al (1958)
Delphinidin	Pericarp and aleurone	Mullick et al (1958)
Delphinidin glycosides	Pericarp and aleurone	Mullick et al (1958)
Proanthocyanins		
Procyanidin B-3 dimer	Aleurone cells	Jende-Strid (1981)
(+)-Catechin	Aleurone cells	Jende-Strid (1981)
Leucocyanidin	Whole grains	Metche and Urion (1961)
Leucodelphinidin	Aleurone cells	Jende-Strid (1981)
Flavonols		
Chrysoeriol	Whole grains	Bhatia et al (1972)
Phenolic acids		
p-Hydroxybenzoic acid	Whole grains	Van Sumere et al (1972)
Salicylic acid	Whole grains	Slominski (1980)
Protocatechuic acid	Whole grains	Slominski (1980)
Vanillic acid	Whole grains	Slominski (1980)
Syringic acid	Flour	Sosulski et al (1982)
p-Coumaric acid	Whole grains	Slominski (1980)
m-Coumaric acid	Whole grains	Slominski (1980)
o-Coumaric acid	Whole grains	Van Sumere et al (1972)
Ferulic acid	Whole grains	Van Sumere et al (1972)
Sinapic acid	Flour	Sosulski et al (1982)
	Whole grain	Slominski (1980)
Phenol glucosides		
p-Hydroxybenzoic acid 4-*O*-β-glucoside	Whole grain	Van Sumere et al (1972)
Vanillic acid 4-*O*-β-glucoside	Whole grain	Van Sumere et al (1972)
o-Coumaric acid 2-*O*-β-glucoside	Whole grain	Van Sumere et al (1972)
Ferulic acid 4-*O*-β-glucoside	Whole grain	Van Sumere et al (1972)

[a] Adapted from Mazza and Miniati (1993).

Uses and Products

An economically important use of barley is in the brewing industry. Traditionally, however, anthocyanin is not desired in beer in significant quantities (Devreux 1961). In addition to anthocyanins, barley contains several other flavonoids, phenolic acids, and phenol glucosides (Bhatia et al 1972, Van Sumere et al 1972, Slominski 1980, Jende-Strid 1981, Sosulski et al 1982) (Table 1) that may contribute to formation of turbidity in beer (Jende-Strid and Lundqvist 1978). However, blue barley varieties are acceptable for beer production as some varieties are accepted for use in North America.

Purple hulless barley, also referred to as "black barley," is cultivated on a limited scale in North America, but the yield of this grain is low. Purple barley for food use is available with the bran layer attached to the kernel as edible grain without being further polished. It may be used in soups and stuffings or alone as an exotic alternative to rice, although it has a chewier texture than rice. The whole grain resembles a coffee bean in shape and cooks to a glossy purplish mahogany color in recipes.

Buckwheat

Buckwheat, *Fagopyrum esculentum*, is commonly grown for its black or gray triangular seeds. Buckwheat is technically a pseudocereal since it is not from the grass family but is an annual related to rhubarb. There are three known species of buckwheat: common buckwheat, *F. esculentum* Moench; tartary buckwheat, *F. tataricum* Gaertn.; and perennial buckwheat, *F. cymosum* L. Common buckwheat is also known as *F. sagittatum* Gilib. and is by far the most important species, accounting for over 90% of the world buckwheat production (Mazza 1993, 2000b; Mazza and Oomah 2005).

The biosynthesis of anthocyanins in *F. sagittatum* depends on light intensity (Troyer 1964). According to Harraschain and Mohr (1963), the light-induced synthesis of anthocyanins in buckwheat depends on the phytochrome and the high-energy photomorphogenetic system and not on photosynthesis. The biosynthesis of flavonoid precursors is inhibited by aminooxyacetate (Amrhein 1979) and stimulated by nitrogen deficiency (Margna et al 1974). Extensive studies have dealt with flavonoid metabolism in buckwheat, utilizing anthocyanins as markers (Shropshire and Mohr 1970, Tohver 1976, Margna and Vainjarv 1981, Tohver 1987), and it has been established that dihydrokaempferol (aromadendrin) is a very efficient precursor for cyanidin and quercetin in buckwheat seedlings.

Pigmentation Characteristics

Kaerstens (1939) found red pigments in the epidermis, the subepidermal layer, and the cells of the cortex of the hypocotyl of common buckwheat. Later, Inoue et al (1982) identified cyanidin-3-glucoside, cyanidin-3-galactoside, and at least two other biosides, one of which is believed to be cyanidin-3-rhamnosylgalactoside, in the hypocotyls of common buckwheat. Troyer (1958) characterized the anthocyanins in buckwheat hypocotyls as derivatives of cyanidin.

Buckwheat contains many phenolic compounds, including rutin, quercetin, hyperin, vitexin, isovitexin, orientin, and isoorientin. In addition, the phenolic acids of buckwheat seeds include hydroxybenzoic acids such as syringic, *p*-hydroxybenzoic, vanillic, and *p*-coumaric acids. Also in buckwheat seed are found soluble oligomeric condensed tannins, which, along with the phenolic acids, provide astringency and affect the color and nutritive value of buckwheat products (Troyer 1955, 1956; Durkee 1977; Margna et al 1990).

Uses and Products

Buckwheat is a valuable food crop for humans, although it can be grown for other purposes (Marshall and Pomeranz 1982). Buckwheat is gaining popularity because of its potential health benefits as human food. In Eastern Europe, buckwheat is a basic food item in porridges and soups. In North America, it is marketed primarily in pancake mixes, which may contain buckwheat mixed with other grain products. In Japan, buckwheat is marketed primarily as flour for manufacturing a variety of noodles (*soba*) and as groats. Groats from dehulling, and farina from groats, are used for breakfast food, porridge, and thickening materials in soups, gravies, and dressings. Buckwheat is also used with vegetables and spices in *kasha* and with wheat, maize, or rice in bread and pasta products (Marshall and Pomeranz 1982, Mazza 1993, Mazza and Oomah 2005).

Corn

Corn, or maize, is perhaps the most domesticated of all field crops. Many of the native people of North and South America still maintain varieties that produce a colorful mixture of red, purple, yellow, and white kernels (collectively called "blue corn" as a commodity), mostly of the flint and flour types. Blue corn has important roles both in history and in future specialty-grain crop development. Blue corn continues to serve the Southwestern American native people as a staple and as a religious symbol.

Genetics and Breeding

Corn, which is classified into a single botanical species, *Zea mays*, may have descended from a wild perennial teosinte plant. Cultured corn appears to have been first selected by Native Americans between 3400 and 2300 B.C., with continued improvement until 1500 A.D. (Martin et al 1976). Corn has 10 pairs of chromosomes, the same number found in teosinte, which crosses readily with corn. Because corn is normally open pollinated, varietal names of corn mean less than those of almost any other crop. Even so, native tribes maintained their own strains of corn, to a large degree, for many years. Corn is among the best-characterized food crop, and considerable information on its genetics is available (Coe at al 1988).

Emerson (1921) showed that the *R* locus is responsible for anthocyanin pigmentation in both aleurone and plant tissues. He designated four classes of pigmentation patterns: *R-r* (pigment in both aleurone and plant), *R-g* (pigmented aleurone and green plant), *r-r* (nonpigmented aleurone and pigment in plant), and *r-g* (nonpigmented aleurone and green plant). Stadler (1946, 1948) confirmed that the locus consists of two elements that can independently change from pigment-producing (dominant) to nonpigmented (recessive). The element S (*R*, dominant; *r*, recessive) is the seed component that functions in the aleurone and embryo, and the element P (*–r*, dominant; *–g*, recessive) is the plant component that determines color in seedlings and certain mature tissues, notably anthers. The genetic model of complexity was further studied by Rhoades (1945). Pigment production in the aleurone is controlled by five complementary genes, distributed among different chromosomes and symbolized as *A1, A2, C1, C2*, and *R*. Other genes, *Pr, Bz1*, and *Bz2*, are known to exert their control upon the kind of pigment that is synthesized (Harborne and Gavazzi 1969). The gene *Bh* controls the aleurone color pattern, and *In* controls the concentration. Anthocyanin production in the pericarp and other tissues is controlled by members of the *R* and *A1* series along with others, and McClintock (1965) confirmed this at the molecular level by correlating the presence of distinctive cross-hybridizing DNA restriction fragments with the genetic determination of plant (*P*) and seed (*S*) function in the *R-r* standard allele (Dellaporta et al 1987). Two other regulatory genes, *B* and *Pl*, function in both the seed and plant, but there is no evidence for complexity at either locus (Taylor and Briggs 1990). Some *B* and *R* alleles can substitute for each other in regulating kernel pigmentation, which is not true for anthocyanin accumulation in plant tissues.

Recently, several genes controlling the synthesis of anthocyanins in corn have been identified and cloned. These include the structural genes for chalcone synthase (*C2*) (Wienand et al 1986), dihydroquercetin reductase (*A1*) (O'Reilly et al 1985), uridine 5′-diphosphate-glucose-flavonol glucosyltransferase (bronze, *Bz1*) (Fedoroff et al 1984), and *Bz2* (bronze-2) (McLaughlin and Walbot 1987), and the regulatory genes, *C1, R, Pl*, and *B*, which control the expression of the unlinked structural genes (Dellaporta et al 1987). Table 2 illustrates the expression of purple color in the corn kernel (Coe et al 1988).

Pigmentation Characteristics

Despite the significant advances in the genetic regulation of anthocyanin biosynthesis, surprisingly, the exact structures of the maize anthocyanins have not been fully clarified (Table 3). Straus (1959) identified cyanidin- and pelargonidin-3-glucosides in endosperm tissue of the cultivar Black Mexican Sweet Corn. Harborne and Gavazzi (1969) found the same pigments in the seed coat or aleurone layer of the endosperm of *PrPr prpr* corn, but they were accompanied by two unstable aliphatic acylated derivatives of each. In the shoots of maize seedlings, Lawanson and Osude (1972) found cyanidin-3-galactoside, rather than 3-glucoside, accompanying pelargonidin-3-glucoside. Cyanidin-3-galactoside was also found in Peruvian dark-seeded corn, where it may be acylated with *p*-coumaric acid (Baraud et al 1974). Nakatani et al (1979) identified cyanidin-3-glucoside as the major anthocyanin in cobs and kernels of the Bolivian purple corn variety Maize Morado. Pelargonidin- and peonidin-3-glucosides were minor components, and more than seven other anthocyanins were detected.

Seah and Styles (1969) isolated seven pigments by chromatography of *PrPr* strains of the W22 selection. Two of these pigments were cyanidin and pelargonidin derivatives; the third was a peonidin glycoside. Later, Styles and Ceska (1972) identified 3-deoxyanthocyanidin luteolinidin as well as the glycosides of cyanidin, pelargonidin, and peonidin and five additional pigments. According to Reddy and Reddy (1973), the 3-deoxyanthocyanidin is present in the form of luteoforol, which is the precursor of the "bronze" pigment. More recently, Harborne and Self (1987) identified two acylated pigments as cyanidin 3-(6″-malonylglucoside) and cyanidin 3-dimalonylglucoside in reddened corn. Pascual-Teresa et al (2002) reported the identity of the anthocyanins from the corncob as cyanidin-3-glucoside, pelargonidin-3-glucoside, peonidin-3-glucoside, and their respective malonyl derivatives.

TABLE 2
Expression of Anthocyanins in Aleurone and Pericarp of Blue and Purple Kernels with Specific Genotypes of Corn[a]

	Tissue[b]		
Genotype	**Aleurone**	**Pericarp**	**Husk**
A1 A2 A3 Anl B bh bn Brn Bz1 Bz2 C1 C2 ch Da Dek1 In lc orp1 orp2 P-rr Pl Pr R-r Sm sn Ufo Vp1 Whp	P	L	P
a3 B-b	P	L	P
a3 b	P	L	MP
b	P	L	MP
b pl	P	L	G
B-b R-g	P	L	MP
B-Peru R-g	P	L	MP
brn	P		
c2 in	MP	ML	MP
c2 su	MP	ML	MP
Ch b P-ww	P	B	MP
da	MP	L	
In-D	MP	O	P
orp1 orp2 P-wr	P	C	X
P-wr b	P	L	MP
P-rw b	P	MR	MP
P-ww b	P	L	MP
pl	P	L	S
R-g	P	L	P
R-g b	P	L	G
sm	P	L	P
sm P-ww	P	C	
Ufo b P-ww	P	C	MP
whp	P	L	P

[a] Adapted from Coe et al (1988).
[b] P = purple; L = lacquer-red; O = orange; M = medium color; C = colorless; X = dies; B = brown; R = red; S = sun-dependent red; G = green (not P or R).

TABLE 3
Anthocyanins of Maize (*Zea mays* L.)[a]

Anthocyanin	Plant Part	Reference
Cyanidin-3-glucoside	Seed coat	Straus (1959), Harborne and Gavazzi (1969)
	Throughout plant	Styles and Ceska (1972)
	Seed coat and cobs	Nakatani et al (1979)
	Leaves	Harborne and Self (1987)
Cyanidin-3-galactoside	Shoot tissues and seed	Lawanson and Osude (1972), Baraud et al (1974)
Cyanidin-3-(6"-malonylglucoside)	Leaves	Harborne and Self (1987)
Cyanidin-3-dimalonylglucoside	Leaves	Harborne and Self (1987)
Pelargonidin-3-glucoside	Seed coat	Straus (1959), Harborne and Gavazzi (1969)
Pelargonidin-glycoside	Throughout plant	Styles and Ceska (1972)

[a] Adapted from Mazza and Miniati (1993).

Environmental factors, particularly light, influence the concentration and perhaps the composition of anthocyanin in maize. This is generally contrary to what has been found in most fruits (Mazza and Miniati 1993) and is likely due to differences in the physiology of the tissues examined. Knoll et al (1964) noted that a low phosphorus level together with low temperature in the root zone were probably two elements that stimulated anthocyanin production in corn.

Uses and Products

In the past, multicolored corn has been used in mainstream culture primarily for decoration. In recent years, however, it has gained popularity for specialty food and functional food products. The colorful appearance of corn kernels provides eye appeal, and the colored corn adds a unique flavor to many finished foods. Blue tortillas made from blue corn have appeared on the market in North America. In home cooking, blue corn is used to produce thick Mexican stews, often flavored with pork, and in tomato soups and rice dishes containing spices. Blue or purple corns, commercially called Posole (Woodland Foods Inc., Gurnee, IL), for example, have a deep blue or deep purple color and, when cooked, a soft, coherent texture. Ground corn is used in products such as corn meal, corn starch, masa farina, and corn flour. Corn flour, in turn, is used in manufacturing food products such as tortillas, pancake mixes, cornbread mixes, corn chips, and cereal, as well as in home cooking for stews, soups, and casseroles.

The anthocyanins in corn have a very long history of use as colorants and were apparently used by the Incas (Paris and Pereira-Alarcon 1968). Recently, interest in corn anthocyanins has resurged, and several patents describing various preparation and application processes for colorants from purple corn have been granted. Most processes use the red Morado and Kulli corn varieties and an aqueous solvent extraction to obtain an anthocyanin extract, which is then used to color candies and sugared syrups. A process patented by the Sugiyama Chemical Institute of Tokyo also uses Morado corn as the raw material but obtains the pigments by enzymatic digestion of the ground corn followed by spray drying.

Recently, a purple corn color extract was found to have strong inhibitory effects on the induction of cancer by a carcinogen (Hagiwara et al 2001). In this study, the color extract inhibited colorectal carcinogenesis in young male F344 rats and caused no detectable adverse effects up to the 5% level in the diet.

Oats

Oats, one of the five major grains, is used extensively by the world's population. The crop seems to have been first cultivated by Europeans (Martin et al 1976) and is particularly popular for food use in Europe. Despite its food use, oats is grown mainly for feed. Like barley, the cultivated oat is covered by a hull that is removed before direct food use.

Genetics and Breeding

The cultivated oat, *Avena sativa* L., belongs to the *A. sativa* subsection that contains all the hexaploid species with the AACCDD chromosomes (Baum 1997). A total of 27 recognized species of oats is classified into seven sections. These contain wild oats species, each with seven or 14 haploid chromosomes. Cultivated oat varieties are believed to have been derived mainly from two species, the common wild oat (*A. fatua*) and the wild red oat (*A. sterilis*). However, both *A. sativa* and *A. fatua* may have derived from *A. byzantina* or *A. sterilis*.

In cultivated oats, the formation of anthocyanins is genetically regulated by a single recessive gene, *P*, which requires red light for its activation (Tegenkamp 1962). Nittler (1968) reported that phosphate deficiency caused anthocyanins to develop in seedlings of Russell oats. To our knowledge, no free or glycosylated anthocyanidins have been characterized in oats. However, they contain many phenolic compounds, including kaempferol, quercetin, luteolin, tricin, vitexin, isovitexin, the flavonone homoeriodictyol and its related chalcone, and a variety of phenolic acids. The structure, occurrence, and function of oat phenolics have been thoroughly reviewed by Collins (1986, 1989).

Uses and Products

Oats is a traditional food crop in North America and Europe, and many existing products are derived from this grain. Oats was the first food that obtained official recognition (in 1997) by the U.S. Food and Drug Administration (FDA) for its specific health benefits—before the other grains that were later recognized as a group for their functional properties. The development of blue or purple oats may eventually provide an additional attraction to the consumer for its health benefits, and the grains may be produced for niche markets.

Rice

About half of the world population relies on rice, *Oryza* spp., of the tribe Oryzaea, as their main food. Normally, the color of the seed coat is white, but in some varieties it is red, purplish red, purple, or dark purple. Rice may be pigmented in the pericarp and essentially all other parts of the plant, including the root. The pigmentation in the pericarp provides the color of the grain. The red and/or purple color of the rice kernel is due mainly to the presence of anthocyanins. The presence of a blue protein in rice bran was reported (Morita et al 1971), but this should not significantly contribute to the color of rice due to its low concentration.

Genetics and Breeding

Rice, *O. sativa,* probably originated in India or southeastern Asia from a wild form that no longer exists. Another rice species, *O. glaberrima*, which is restricted to western and central Africa, probably originated there as a derivative of *O. breviligulata. O. sativa*, the most important cultivated species, is divided into the varieties indica (widespread throughout the tropical and subtropical regions), japonica, and javanica. *O. sativa* behaves like and is generally considered to be a diploid species. It has 24 somatic chromosomes, and tetraploid species have 48.

The first studies on the inheritance of anthocyanins in rice were conducted in the first decades of this century (Van der Stok 1908, Hector 1916, Parnell et al 1917, Jones 1930). In the 1940s and 1950s, several studies dealt with the distribution of anthocyanin pigments in various parts of the rice plant (Dave 1948, Ramiah 1953, Ghose et al 1956), and several authors identified the different genes that control the anthocyanin pigmentation. In 1959, under the direction of the International Rice Research Institute, new genetic symbols were developed to accommodate the need for naming the new information (Anonymous 1959).

Variations in color intensity observed in various parts of the plant suggest the existence of different genes that control the pigmentation in those different organs. Ramiah (1945) and Misro et al (1960) observed in extensive varietal collections that the pigment distribution was never uniform and, in some, appeared to be an independent characteristic. In segregating progenies, the ratio between colored and uncolored is different in different parts (Nair 1958, Iyer 1959).

According to Nagao et al (1962), two complementary allele series at the *C* and *A* loci determine the anthocyanin formation. The base gene for "chromogene" production is *C*; the conversion of chromogene into anthocyanin is controlled by *A*. There is a series of multiple alleles at the two loci: six alleles at locus *C* and four at locus *A*. Five other loci control the anthocyanin distribution in the other plant parts: *P* controls the distribution of anthocyanin precursors in the apiculate; *Pr* controls the color in the glume and rachilla; *Pl*, with three alleles, controls the distribution of the pigment in the leaf lamina, leaf sheath, pulvinus, auricle, ligule, node, internode, and rachilla; *Pn* governs the color in the leaf apex and margins; and *Ps* controls the localization of the pigment in the stigma. The genes for anthocyanin pigmentation in the different plant organs are found on seven chromosomes (Shafi and Aziz 1959, D'Cruz and Dhulappanavar 1963, Misro 1981).

Recent studies have revealed the presence of a greater number of genes than previously reported. In Group III, the total number of genes has reached

16. The genetics of anthocyanin pigmentation has been studied in rice (Kinoshita and Takahashi 1991). However, a reliable relationship between identified genes and their specific role in the anthocyanin biosynthesis pathway is still lacking (Reddy et al 1995). A summary of the known genes is presented in Table 4. The presence of *C* and *A* genes are mandatory for pigment production in any rice tissues. The different combinations of the genes determine the phenotype of the rice genotype. For example, the Pl^w allele, in addition to *C* and *A*, contributes to the pigmentation in the pericarp.

Hayashi (1944, 1946) identified the pigment in *O. sativa* var. *atropurpurea* as a monoglucoside of cyanidin. Sharma and Seshadri (1955) identified cyanidin diglucoside and delphinidin monoglucoside in different types of rice. According to Nagai et al (1960, 1962), the anthocyanin composition of rice is made up of four pigments: cyanidin-3-glucoside, cyanidin-3-rhamnoglucoside, cyanidin-3,5-diglucoside, and malvidin-3-galactoside. These pigments were distributed differently in the various cultivars examined and were not found in all plant parts. Cyanidin-3-glucoside and cyanidin-3-rutinoside are the most

TABLE 4
Description of Known Genes of the Anthocyanin Pigmentation System and Their Phenotype Effects in Kernel Pericarp and Other Parts of Rice[a]

Gene	Status	Phenotype Effect
C (chromogen)	Mandatory	Essential for anthocyanin synthesis
	Structural genes	Alleles: C^B, C^{Br}, C^+ (null), etc.
A (activator)	Mandatory	Activation of C gene; essential for anthocyanin synthesis
	Structural genes	Alleles: A^o, A^E, *A*, and A^+ (null), etc.
Pl (purple leaf)	Pericarp and other tissues	Localizer of anthocyanin in leaf
	Tissues	Alleles Pl^W: leaf blade, leaf sheath, auricles, ligule, and pericarp *Pl*: leaf blade, leaf sheath, collar, auricles, ligule, node, and internode Pl^l: leaf blade, leaf sheath, ligule, and internode Pl^+: null allele resulting into colorless phenotype tissue
Prp (purple pericarp)	Pericarp	Localizer of anthocyanin in pericarp
Rc (brown pericarp)	Pericarp	Synthesis of brown pigments in pericarp
Rc and *Rd* (brown pericarp)	Pericarp	Synthesis of brown pigments in pericarp
Pn (purple node)	Node	Localizer of anthocyanin in node
P (purple)	Apiculus	Distributor of anthocyanin in apiculus
I-Pl (inhibitor to purple leaf)	Inhibitory	Dominant inhibitor of purple anthocyanin pigments
I-Pl-1, *I-Pl*-2, *I-Pl*-3	Inhibitory	Inhibit action of both Pl^W and Pl^l alleles
I-Pl-4, *I-Pl*-5	Inhibitory	Inhibit action of *Prp* locus
I-Pl-6	Inhibitory	Inhibit action of *Pli* allele

[a] Adapted from Reddy et al (1995), based on Chang and Jordan (1963), Takahashi (1982), and Kinoshita and Takahashi (1991).

diffuse, while malvidin-3-galactoside is found particularly in the multicolored seed coats (Table 5). Nagai et al (1962) characterized cyanidin-3-glucoside and malvidin-3-galactoside as the predominant red pigments of the rice grains, with other glycosylated cyanidins in other parts of the plant. Reddy et al (1995) confirmed that the major anthocyanins occurring in rice tissues are cyanidin and peonidin derivatives. Recent analyses of "colorful" rice grains showed that the anthocyanin pattern of rice includes the 3-glucosides of cyanidin and peonidin and trace amounts of cyanidin-3-gentiobioside (Fossen et al 2002). No acylated anthocyanins have thus far been found in rice, although cyanidin-3-(6″-malonylglucoside) and minor amounts of cyanidin-3-(6″-succinyl-β-glucopyranoside) have been found in the related species *Phragmites australis* (Arundineae) (Fossen and Andersen 1998).

Pigmentation Characteristics

In a recent study, six rice cultivars (two red, two purple, and two white) were compared for their antioxidant activities and differential distribution of active components (Itani et al 2002a). Ethanol extracts prepared from red- and purple-hulled rice exhibited remarkably high superoxide- and free radical-scavenging activities as compared with those from the white-hulled rice. The activities were found to be mostly localized in pericarp and testa, namely in the rice bran. Colored rice contained polyphenols much more abundantly than white rice, and the polyphenol contents were related to their antioxidant activities. The major antioxidant substances in the purple and red rice were shown to be anthocyanins and tannins, respectively (Itani et al 2002a). Ryu et al (2000) compared the antioxidant activities of eight cultivars and found that the scavenging activity by the 1,1-diphenyl-2-picrylhydrazyl (DPPH) radical method, using methanol extract of rice, varied with rice cultivars. The activity of the purple cultivars was twice that of the white cultivar. One purple cultivar of rice was four times stronger than the white rice. The researchers concluded

TABLE 5
Anthocyanins of Rice (*Oryza sativa* L.)[a]

Anthocyanin	Plant Part	Relative Concentration
Cyanidin-3-glucoside	Seed	++++
	Leaves	++++
	Internode	++++
	Flower (stigma)	++++
Cyanidin-3-rhamnoside	Seed	+
	Leaves	+++
	Internodes	+++
	Flower	+++
Cyanidin-3,5-diglucoside	Leaves	+
	Internodes	+
Malvidin-3-galactoside	Seed	+++

[a] Adapted from Mazza and Miniati (1993).

that the scavenging effect of rice extracts was related to the total anthocyanin content of the extract. Ichikawa et al (2001) compared the antioxidant activity of purple rice with that of blueberry extract. The rice extract had a slightly lower superoxide-scavenging activity than the blueberry extract. Both the rice and the blueberry extracts showed 10–25 times higher activity than that of Trolox (α-tocopherol analogue) at the same concentration. The hydroxyl-radical-scavenging activities of both extracts were several times lower than that of Trolox, but the rice extract was twice as strong as that of blueberry extract. It was further noted that the purified anthocyanin from the rice retained approximately 74% of the antioxidant activity of the original raw extract.

Park et al (1998) surveyed the anthocyanin contents of several hundred rice cultivars, including 140 pigmented and 186 white cultivars. The authors found by reverse-phase-HPLC analysis that the major anthocyanin in rice, cyanidin-3-glucoside, was present at levels ranging from trace amounts to 552 mg/100 g of rice. Ryu et al (2000) found that the contents of cyanidin-3-glucoside and peonidin-3-glucoside from 591 rice cultivars ranged from zero to 452 mg/100 g of unpolished rice, while peonidin-3-glucoside ranged from zero to 42.7 mg/100 g. However, the total anthocyanin content of purple rice was reported to be as high as 1,300 mg/100 g of rice (Kim et al 2000).

The color of blue and purple-black rice is only on the surface of the dehulled rice. The anatomical structure and composition of this characteristic were investigated by abrasive milling from the outer layer to the inner portions of dehulled rice (Itani et al 2002b). The color of the flour samples became pure white when the outside layer was removed from purple rice. In addition to color, the levels of amylose, nitrogen, and several minerals (P, K, Mg, Ca, and Mn) tested in the rice kernels of 11 cultivars were found to vary greatly, from extremely rich in the outer layer to a few times lower in the center of the rice. This characteristic provides opportunities in processing and utilization, such as in the production of a pigment-enriched product. Table 6 illustrates the disproportionate distribution of these characteristics (Itani et al 2002b).

Glahn et al (2002), however, found that iron availabilities were noticeably lower for the more brown to purple rice cultivars using an *in vitro* bioavailability model. No correlation was observed between availability of Fe and its concentration in rice. The results suggested that certain unknown factors related to the color of rice may limit Fe availability (Glahn et al 2002). In a different study of a limited number of rice cultivars, the purple rice was found to have the highest free fatty acid content (Singh et al 1999).

Uses and Products

Purple rice is a major rice product in South Asia and China and is commonly used in China as a functional food, alone or with other dark-colored grains and oilseeds. The rice is locally regarded as an enriched rice with medicinal effects, and the purple pigment is widely used as a food colorant in bread, ice cream, and liquor (Yoshinaga 1986, Takahashi and Yoshizawa 1987, Cho et al 1996, Park et al 1998). In recent times, rice

TABLE 6
Amylose, N, and Mineral Content and the Mg/K Ratio of Different Layers of an Indica-Type Purple Rice (cv. Kuromai) Compared with Regular Rice

	Content, db (relative to hulled rice, %)							
Cultivar and Fraction	Amylose, % (% initial)	N, % (% initial)	P, mg/100 g (% initial)	Mg, mg/100 g (% initial)	K, mg/100 g (% initial)	Ca, mg/100 g (% initial)	Mn, mg/100 g (% initial)	Mg/K Ratio
Kuromai[a]								
F0	0.7 (91)	3.17 (155)	2,092.3 (465)	893.3 (520)	1,712.4 (485)	25.1 (152)	20.63 (530)	1.68
F1	1.0 (130)	3.40 (167)	1,852.2 (412)	731.5 (426)	1,396.6 (396)	21.5 (131)	11.23 (289)	1.68
F2	0.7 (90)	3.31 (162)	1,249.2 (278)	502.2 (292)	938.8 (266)	22.4 (136)	6.43 (165)	1.72
F3	0.7 (86)	3.16 (155)	795.2 (177)	303.5 (177)	582.7 (165)	17.3 (105)	3.58 (92)	1.68
F4	0.7 (81)	2.99 (147)	489.1 (109)	173.1 (101)	336.9 (95)	12.2 (74)	2.20 (57)	1.65
F5	0.7 (84)	2.67 (131)	243.4 (54)	79.1 (46)	167.5 (47)	8.4 (51)	1.35 (35)	1.52
F6	0.7 (91)	1.52 (74)	42.9 (10)	8.2 (5)	51.1 (14)	4.6 (28)	0.71 (18)	0.52
Akamochi[b]								
F0	0.6 (78)	3.02 (173)	2,184.7 (554)	894.4 (633)	1,911.2 (566)	24.6 (157)	22.18 (516)	1.51
F1	0.7 (81)	3.35 (192)	1,528.8 (388)	587.6 (416)	1,220.2 (361)	27.0 (173)	11.35 (264)	1.55
F2	0.7 (84)	3.10 (178)	848.7 (215)	312.4 (221)	670.8 (199)	27.0 (173)	6.82 (159)	1.5
F3	0.7 (85)	2.85 (163)	388.1 (98)	111.2 (79)	276.5 (82)	14.7 (94)	3.56 (83)	1.29
F4	0.7 (85)	2.41 (138)	178.9 (45)	41.3 (29)	137.7 (41)	9.9 (63)	2.29 (53)	0.96
F5	0.7 (91)	2.02 (115)	101.5 (26)	17.2 (12)	89.1 (26)	8.3 (53)	1.78 (41)	0.62
F6	0.8 (103)	1.22 (70)	41.3 (10)	2.3 (2)	53.0 (16)	5.7 (37)	1.17 (27)	0.14
Koshihikari[c]								
F0	2.4 (13)	3.02 (196)	2,519.3 (697)	1,192.1 (789)	1,946.1 (726)	18.0 (170)	17.69 (634)	1.97
F1	8.2 (45)	3.34 (216)	1,598.8 (442)	741.6 (491)	1,143.8 (427)	14.9 (141)	8.66 (310)	2.09
F2	11.8 (66)	3.24 (210)	637.8 (176)	276.4 (183)	447.8 (167)	14.6 (137)	4.18 (150)	1.99
F3	14.4 (80)	2.64 (171)	242.1 (67)	90.2 (60)	168.2 (63)	8.2 (77)	1.97 (71)	1.72
F4	16.0 (89)	2.07 (134)	164.0 (45)	43.1 (29)	100.1 (37)	6.5 (61)	1.33 (48)	1.39
F5	17.4 (97)	1.76 (114)	115.0 (32)	23.6 (16)	70.5 (26)	5.6 (53)	1.00 (36)	1.08
F6	20.4 (113)	0.99 (64)	60.7 (17)	6.2 (4)	42.7 (16)	4.5 (43)	0.73 (26)	0.47

[a] A glutinous indica type of rice originated from China, with length/width = 2.59, 1,000 grain weight = 19, and thickness = 1.5 mm. (Adapted from Itani et al 2002b)

[b] Red glutinous.

[c] A major regular Japanese rice.

anthocyanins were extracted from the kernels of various red-pigmented *Oryza* spp. and from the anthocyanin-containing husks and used in the production of colored sake and *daikon* (Katayama et al 1986). The process patented by Katayama et al (1986) uses red leaves and stems as the raw material for production of anthocyanins, while the process of Fukui and Wagi (1990) uses red rice bran for the extraction of the anthocyanins. Purification of the extract is by ion exchange.

Several purple rice cultivars are available commercially in North America. Purple sticky rice with a typical rice shape, said to have originated in Thailand, is now also grown in California. Purple sticky rice has a charred appearance when uncooked, but when cooked, it imparts a shiny indigo color in dishes with a sweet flavor and a sticky texture. Most colored rice is used in specialty cooking and niche products. Purple sticky rice is often cooked as a dessert rice and is commonly used in stuffings, puddings, and rice balls in Southeast Asia. Another purple rice, described by wholesalers as Chinese black rice, is similar to the purple sticky rice in color and is used as a dessert ingredient alone or is mixed with regular white rice for color and texture in stuffings, desserts, rice molds, pudding, and rice balls. This rice is now used in North America and most often found served with main courses to give an exotic appearance.

Rye and Triticale

Rye

Rye, *Secale cereale* L., native to Southwest Asia, is an important cereal crop in the cool climates of northern Europe, Asia, and North America. Rye is now a very popular bread grain, especially in Europe.

Genetics and Breeding

The genus *Secale* L. (cultivated and wild ryes) is classified in the subtribe Triticinae of the tribe Triticeae within the grass family Graminaeae. Members of the Triticeae have a basic chromosome number of $n = 7$, and, in the case of *Secale*, all species are characterized by a diploid chromosome number of $2n = 14$ (Evans and Scoles 1976). Rye is a cross-pollinated species, and inbred lines usually lack vigor.

The presence of anthocyanins in rye has been used as an aid in understanding the genetics of this plant. Thus, several authors have reported on the heritability of anthocyanins in rye. According to Watkins (1966) and Watkins and White (1964), the occurrence of anthocyanins in the rye cultivar Prolific is genetically controlled by the complementation of two genes, *A* and *B* for the seed color and *A* and *R* for the red color in the coleoptile. In the plant type *virescens*, two independent, dominant genes, *A1* and *A2*, control the anthocyanin production.

Melz et al (1984) isolated the gene for the lack of anthocyanins in chromosome 7R while the gene for pigmented grain, coleoptile, and aleurone is on chromosome 3 (Sturm et al 1981a) and is controlled by either a single dominant gene or by multiple, closely linked genes (Sturm et al 1981b).

Pigmentation Characteristics

Anthocyanin pigmentation may occur in the aleurone layer of the grain and other tissues. The seed color of rye has been described as either green due to blue anthocyanin pigmentation or yellow due to the lack of it (Dedio et al 1969) in the presence of chlorophyll and carotenoids. In seeds of Prolific rye, Dedio et al (1969) identified delphinidin-3-rutinoside as the aleurone anthocyanin. In the pericarp of purple-seeded rye cultivars, Dedio et al (1972) found cyanidin-3-glucoside, peonidin-3-glucoside, and the acylated forms of these glycosides as the major anthocyanins, as well as trace amounts of cyanidin-3-rutinoside, peonidin-3-rutinoside, and their acylated derivatives. The proportion of the acylated forms and the ratio of the aglycones vary among cultivars. More recently, Busch et al (1986) identified cyanidin-3-gentiobioside in the primary leaves of *S. cereale*.

Uses and Products

Because rye is a grain similar to wheat, many product formulations utilize rye in place of wheat to take advantage of the high protein and B vitamin contents of rye. Rye also produces a mild nutty flavor in final products. Rye does not contain typical gluten as wheat does and thus has limited performance in the traditional pan bread type of breadmaking. However, rye is still widely used in the specialty bread market, traditionally in Europe and more recently in North America. In the United States and Canada, rye is currently used in soups, breads, stews, stuffings, pilafs and casseroles, breakfast porridge, and as a substitute for rice.

Triticale

Triticale (*Triticosecale* Widdmark), a cereal from the hybridization of wheat and rye, was the first serious effort at engineering a new crop, performed at the University of Manitoba in 1954. In the 1970s, triticale production was expanded for use as a fodder crop and as a supplement to bread flour. Since both wheat and rye have purple and blue varieties, it is possible to have purple and blue triticale kernels. However, reports on the colored kernels are rare, and future development of purple cultivars will depend on the need for and uses of the colored kernels.

Characteristics

Triticales were examined for the quality parameters required for traditional applications of wheat (Johnson 1990). They were found to be similar to hexaploid wheats in grain hardness (Williams 1986), an indicator of grain quality in milling and baking. Protein, ash, and fat levels are frequently found to be higher than those of wheat (Vaidehi 1984). The protein was also found to be high in biological value. Boldajaj et al (1986) found no difference in metabolized energy values among maize, triticale, wheat, and barley when these grains were fed to white leghorn chickens. Certain triticale cultivars may be useful for breads, white rye rolls, and noodles, and extrusion has produced acceptable breakfast cereals and pancake mixes. Improved cultivars and renewed market interest in whole grain and multigrain breads have continued to provide interest in triticale.

As a flour, triticale differs from wheat flour. A hybrid of rye and wheat, it has more protein and less gluten than wheat. Lorenz et al (1972) found the flour to be deficient in gluten quality and quantity and to have high proteolytic activity. Such enzyme activity weakens the dough by protein hydrolysis. Triticale flour is also weaker because of its high sulfhydryl content, varying from 1.2–16 μmol/g for seven triticales as compared with only about 1.0 μmol/g for wheat (Tsen 1974).

Uses and Products

Initial interest in triticale was focused on its use in breadmaking and other uses in place of wheat. Triticale closely resembles soft wheat in terms of breadmaking characteristics. Its flour is suitable for making noodles, cakes, cookies, crackers, waffles, tortillas, and whole-meal breads. Many uses now take advantage of its high protein and low gluten. In domestic recipes, triticale can be readily used in specialty bakery products, cereals, and casseroles.

Triticale is finding its market niche based upon its adaptability in specialty bakery products and for animal feed. Its adaptability to marginal environments has led to the expansion of its production in Eastern Europe. As a specialized use crop, it will not replace other common grains. It will be interesting to see whether blue or purple colored triticale varieties will give this grain any edge in niche markets.

Sorghum and Millet

Sorghum

The cultivated type of sorghum, *Sorghum bicolor* (L.) Moench., is a major staple grain crop on the African and Asian continents, used for food, feed, and other uses (Creelman et al 1982). The several colors of sorghum range from gray and brown to purple. The color of the sorghum kernel results from the color of the pericarp, the thickness of the mesocarp, and the presence or absence of a colored testa. The pigmentation in sorghum grain is due to the presence of polyphenols in the seed coat, where they accumulate to form a continuous pigmented layer (Earp 1984).

Genetics and Breeding

Sorghum belongs to the family Gramineae and the tribe Andropogonneae and is a native of Africa in the zone south of the Sahara Desert. The cultivated species are very diverse, and several closely related wild species are found in the growing areas. *S. bicolor* includes the annual sorghum with 10 pairs of chromosomes, namely "grain sorghum," and a few other species (Martin et al 1976).

Pigments are found in the pericarp, testa, and endosperm of the sorghum kernel. The presence or absence of the testa is genetically determined. If present, the testa is either brown or purple at maturity. The grain color is determined largely by eight genes. The genes *R*, *Y*, and *I* influence pericarp color; the genes *Z* and *S* determine the thickness and chalkiness of the mesocarp; and the genes B_1 and B_2 determine the presence or absence of a testa. The gene *Tp* determines the testa color. Golmirzaie and York (1992) found that *Tp* produced a testa with brown color and *tptp* produced a purple testa color. However, they did not find a linkage between the genes controlling the testa color and the genes controlling pericarp colors or the presence of a testa (*B1* and *B2*), spreader (*S*), or mesocarp (*Z*). They also found that testa color genes *Tp* and *tp* did not affect the inheritance of pericarp and other testa genes. In brown, high-tannins sorghum with a dominant *spreader* gene, polyphenols are also present in the epicarp (Rooney and Miller 1982).

The major polyphenol components of sorghum grain are the flavonoids and their polymers, condensed tannins; their concentration varies widely in different cultivars (Creelman et al 1982, Butler 1989). Cultivars with increased levels of these and other phenolic compounds exhibit resistance to disease, insects, mold, birds, and postharvest sprouting but show nutrient deficiencies (Rooney and Miller 1982, Earp 1984, Butler 1989).

The genes, *R, Y, B1, B2,* and *S* control the color and quality and quantity of polyphenols in the pericarp and testa of sorghum seed. The dominant genes, *R* and *Y*, strongly increase the degree of anthocyanin pigmentation (Hahn 1984). In white sorghum, the pigment is made up of three chromogenes (I, II, and III), which give eriodictyol and pelargonidin by hydrolysis, and polymers are also present (Yasumatsu et al 1965). Kambal and Bate-Smith (1976) identified the yellow pigment as eriodictyol chalcone, while luteolinidin was obtained from the red seeds by hydrolysis. This deoxyanthocyanidin was derived from a pentahydroxyflavone, luteoforol, a reduction product of eriodictyol, by the gene *R*. Flavonoids were formed by the action of gene *Y*, which regulates biosynthesis.

Pigmentation Characteristics

The anthocyanins of sorghum are derivatives of cyanidin, pelargonidin, apigeninidin, luteolinidin, and fisetinidin. The unidentified orange pigment observed in whole kernels of red varieties of grain sorghum (Nip and Burns 1971) is believed to be luteolinidin, since both luteolinidin and apigeninidin were subsequently found even in the seed of white varieties (Nip and Burns 1969). Seed and leaf tissue of some cultivars have relatively high levels of the flavan-4-ols apiforol and luteoforol (Table 7), which have hydroxylation patterns similar to those of apigeninidin and luteolinidin; these tissues have no detectable flavan-3-ols, catechin, or epicatechin, which correspond to the hydroxylation pattern of cyanidin (Watterson and Butler 1983, Butler 1989). The proanthocyanidins or polymeric flavonoids of sorghum, on the other hand, have been found to have the hydroxylation pattern of cyanidin, not that of the 3-deoxyanthocyanidins.

TABLE 7
Anthocyanins and Other Flavonoids of Sorghum (*Sorghum bicolor* (L.) Moench.)

Compound	Plant Part	Reference
Cyanidin	Mesocotyl	Stafford (1965)
Cyanidin glycosides	Mesocotyl, roots and shoots	McGrath et al (1982)
Apigeninidin	Mesocotyl, glumes	Stafford (1965)
Apigeninidin glycoside	Mesocotyl, roots, shoots, grain	McGrath et al (1982)
	Glumes	Misra and Seshadri (1967), Bate-Smith (1969)
Luteolinidin	Mesocotyl, glumes	Stafford (1965)
Luteolinidin glycoside	Mesocotyl, roots, shoots, seed coat and cobs	Misra and Seshadri (1967), Bate-Smith (1969)
	Grain and glumes	McGrath et al (1982), Gupta and Haslam (1978)
Pelargonidin glycoside	Grain	Misra and Seshadri (1967)
Fisetinidin	Grain	Blessin et al (1963)
Apigenin glycoside	Shoots	Stafford (1969)
Luteolin	Mesocotyl	Stafford (1965)
Luteolin glycoside	Shoots	Stafford (1969)
Luteolin-7-*O*-methyl	Glumes	Misra and Seshadri (1967)
Naringenin	Grain	Gujer et al (1986)
Eriodictyol	Grain	Gujer et al (1986), Yasumatsu et al (1965)
(+)-Catechin	Grain	Gujer et al (1986)
Luteoforol	Grain	Bate-Smith and Rasper (1969)
	Several	Bate-Smith (1969)
Apiforol	Grain, leaf	Watterson and Butler (1983)
	Leaf	Haskins and Gorz (1986)
Kaemperol	Grain	Nip and Burns (1969)
(+)-Taxifolin	Grain	Gujer et al (1986)
Naringeninchalcone	Grain	Gujer et al (1986)

The presence of anthocyanins in sorghum is linked to its susceptibility to rust *(Puccinia purpurea)* (Indira et al 1983) and to its resistance to downy mildew (*Peronosclerospora sorghi*) (Bhat et al 1982). The herbicide Alachlor inhibits the formation of anthocyanin in etiolated sorghum mesocotyls by interfering with the synthesis of phenylpropionic acid (Molin et al 1986).

Uses and Products

Flour made from seeds of sorghum contains 11% protein, 3% lipids, and 71% starch (Hulse et al 1980). The presence of polyphenols, however, makes the flour astringent and reduces its palatability and digestibility. Traditionally, pigment-free cultivars, which have a higher carotenoid content in the endosperm and fewer tannins, are most suited for processing into food products. The bran produced from the grain of a sweet sorghum contains cyanidin and pelargonidin glycosides and has been suggested for use as a food colorant for cookies, candies, gelatins, and other products (Olifson et al 1978). According to Olifson et al (1978), this colorant is nontoxic and, when fed to guinea pigs for six months, produced no morphological changes in the liver, pancreas, kidneys, or thyroid, and no glycogens were found in the blood. In China, sorghum has been traditionally used for food; the current major food use is to produce specialty alcoholic beverages. It is also commonly used as a feed grain.

Millet

Pearl millet or cattail millet, *Pennisetum americanum* (L.) Leeke (syn. *P. typhoides* or *P. glaucum*), is a very important food crop in many countries; it is widely grown in most semiarid regions of Africa and Asia (Reichert et al 1980), as well as in North America. The origin of pearl millet is probably in the Africa savannah zone, and it has been grown in Africa and Asia since ancient times.

The color of the pearl millet kernel varies from white, yellow, or brown to purple, which is due to the combined effects of pigmentation in the pericarp, aleurone, and endosperm, as well as to the pericarp thickness. Purple kernels have pigments in the epicarp, aleurone, and endosperm but have a thin pericarp. White kernels have few pigmented areas; yellow kernels have pigments primarily in the epicarp and endosperm; and brown kernels have pigments in the epicarp, aleurone, and endosperm. The majority of white, yellow, and brown kernels have a thick pericarp (McDonough and Rooney 1989). Gray kernels have pigments in the aleurone and endosperm and have a thin pericarp.

Foxtail millet, or Italian millet, *Setaria italica*, is one of the oldest cultivated crops, grown in China as early as 2700 B.C. The crop probably has its origin in southern Asia and is still grown mostly in eastern Asia. The small, convex seeds are enclosed in the hulls (the lemma and palea). The color of the hulls differs with variety and may be creamy, pale yellow, orange, reddish, green, dark purple, or a mixture of various colors.

Characteristics

Analysis of colored pearl millets has revealed the presence of polyphenols in all the colored samples tested (McDonough and Rooney 1989). A purple variety was found to contain polyphenols up to 0.33 g/100 g of sample, while the gray and yellow varieties averaged 0.22 and 0.19 g/100 g, respectively. None of the varieties tested contained tannins, which agrees with earlier reports (Reichert 1979). HPLC analysis of purple, gray, and yellow varieties revealed high levels of ferulic, coumaric, cinnamic, and genistic acids for all colored varieties. While total phenolic acid levels were similar, the purple variety had higher levels of genistic acid and lower levels of cinnamic acid (McDonough and Rooney 1989).

Polyphenols in the grain are responsible for a gray pigmentation that some populations in the world find undesirable. Traditionally, the bluish gray color of milled grain is removed by soaking overnight in water containing sour milk or tamarind pods, which decrease the pH and remove pH-dependent pigments. Reichert et al (1980) suggested that *C*-glycosylflavonoids are responsible for the natural gray color. In the leaves of 109 pure lines from a world collection of cultivated foxtail millet (*S. italica* (L.) Beauv.), Gluchoff-Fiasson et al (1990) identified 30 vitexin (8-*C*-glucosylapigenin) and 24 orientin (8-*C*-glucosylluteolin) derivatives.

In purple and sun-red varieties of *P. americanum*, Raju et al (1985) identified derivatives of cyanidin, delphinidin, and pelargonidin, with the proportion of aglycones varying among the cultivars. In *P. japonicum*, Shibata and Sakai (1958) identified cyanidin-3-glucoside, and in a related species, *Panicum melinis*, originating from Brazil, Bobbio et al (1988) found peonidin-3-arabinosylglucoside.

Uses and Products

In the major millet-producing areas in Africa, light-colored millets are generally preferred. As for other products, the use of colored millets in food depends on the economic and technical factors affecting the development and consumer acceptance of new products. Current use in North America seems to be limited to bird feed.

Quinoa and Amaranth

Quinoa

Quinoa or quinua (*Chenopodium quinoa* Willd.) is native to the Andes Mountains of Bolivia, Chile, and Peru. It was a staple food of the Inca people (Johnson 1990), means "mother grain" in the Inca language, and is referred to as a pseudocereal, similar in this respect to buckwheat. Two closely related species, *canihua (C. pallidacuale*) and *huazontle* (*C. nuttaliae*), are also utilized for food. Quinoa seeds range in color from pink and orange to blue-black, purple, and red. The pigments are localized in the seed coats together with saponin. The grain size of quinoa measures about 1.0 mm thick and ranges in diameter from 1.0 to 2.5 mm; the seed weight ranges from 1.9 to 4.3 g/1,000 seeds (Alvarez et al 1990).

Genetics and Breeding

Quinoa (*C. quinoa* Willd.) is an annual broadleaf, nongrassy plant species in the goosefoot family, which also includes sugar beet, table beet, and spinach. Quinoa is generally considered to be a single species within the Chenopodiaceae, and over 120 species have been found within the genus *Chenopodium* (Wilson 1990). Quinoa is primarily an inbreeding species, with plants bearing hermaphroditic flowers. Two species, *C. berlandieri* and *C. hircinum*, contain the same chromosome number as quinoa ($2n = 36$).

Based upon the geographic location or elevation of cultivation, quinoa has been classified into four main types: valley, altipiano, salar, and sea level types (Galwey 1989). Wilson (1990) has proposed a division of quinoa into two distinct groups: northern and southern. The northern group, being less diverse than the southern, may be derived from the southern group. Evaluation of germ plasm can be difficult, given the array of accessions available. Significant differences in agronomic value in the United States were observed among 15 cultivars for protein, seed size, and yield, with no significant location effects (Johnson and Ward 1993).

Uses and Products

Excellent nutritional qualities, adaptation to cold and dry climates, ease of processing, and similarity to rice make quinoa a crop of considerable value to highland areas around the world. The nutritional quality has been compared to that of dried whole milk by the Food and Agriculture Organization (FAO) of the United Nations. The protein quality and quantity in quinoa seed are superior to those of the more common cereal grains. Quinoa is higher in lysine than wheat is, and the amino acid content of quinoa seed is considered well balanced for human and animal nutrition, being similar to that of casein.

Another important nutritional characteristic of the grain, when compared with other cereals, is a relatively high oil content (Koziol 1992). On a fresh-weight basis, quinoa has an oil content ranging from 1.8 to 9.5%, with a global calculated mean of 5.8%, which is higher than the 3–4% oil in normal corn. As with corn, the oil is concentrated in the germ, which in quinoa represents 25–30% of the weight of the grain (Fuentes 1972). Because the quinoa germ encircles the endosperm, it can easily be removed by a modified polishing procedure to give a fraction containing 19% oil.

A major antinutritional factor of quinoa is the saponins, which are glycosides of a steroid or a triterpene (Burnouf-Radosevich et al 1985; Mizui et al 1988, 1990; Ma et al 1989; Ridout et al 1991; Koziol 1992). Most of these are concentrated in the outer layers of the grain (perianth, pericarp, seed coat, and a cuticlelike layer), which facilitates their removal industrially by abrasive dehulling (Reichert et al 1986) or, traditionally, by washing the grains with water. Quinoa as a product can be classified according to its saponin concentrations as either "sweet" (saponin free or having less than 0.11% saponins on a fresh-weight basis) or "bitter" (containing more than 0.11% saponins).

Other potential uses of quinoa include using the oil press cake as a dietary supplement and the starch granules (mostly less than 3 μm in diameter) for their special pasting behavior (Singer et al 1990). Besides its potential for processing to components, quinoa is gaining popularity in North America because of its unique texture, peanutlike flavor, and nutritional quality. The versatility of black quinoa allows it to be used in Western cooking and as a substitute for couscous, bulgur, or rice. In addition, quinoa can be sprouted to produce a delicate, nutty-flavored sprout for salads.

Amaranth

Amaranth (*Amaranthus cruentus* and other *Amaranth* spp.) is an annual ancient grain crop. It was traditional and sacred to the Aztecs, Mayans, and Incas and was used to make statues of their deities. Several species produce colored seeds, among them *A. edulis*, with red heads and purple to black seeds, and *A. hypochondriacus*, with purple and purple-green seeds. Amaranth is extremely hardy, drought tolerant, and requires virtually no cultivation. It is another pseudocereal because it is a seed from a broadleaf herbaceous plant.

Uses and Products

Amaranth seeds are round and tiny, smaller than mustard seeds, and gold with flecks of black. The grain of amaranth has a protein content of 16%, higher than those of corn, rice, and wheat. Amaranth seeds can be boiled or milled into flour. They have a crunchy texture and a pleasant fresh cornlike aroma and woody peppery flavor. Amaranth is very versatile and can be used as a substitute for wheat for gluten-intolerant individuals, but of course, since it is gluten free, it lacks wheat's breadmaking characteristics. It can be consumed as a hot breakfast cereal, added to cold salads, or used in place of rice in recipes.

Wheat

Wheat is among the world's most important grain crops since it provides the main food for hundreds of millions of people worldwide. Among the wheat types, common wheat (*Triticum* spp.) and durum wheat (*T. durum*) are probably the most economically important ones. Most of the cultivated wheat species, however, do not usually have blue and purple varieties because production is determined by agronomic, milling, and end-use requirements. Wheat with blue and purple kernels may occur in nature in diploid, tetraploid, and hexaploid wheats. These are either wild or are currently used in certain areas as a specialty crop.

Genetics and Breeding

Breeding of colored wheat species relies on the available germ plasm pool. The general path of evolution in the wheat group is characterized by a group of diploid species in which there are eight distinct genomes (A, S, Mt, D, M, Un, C, and U) and a group of polyploids (tetra- and hexaploid) in which seven of the eight diploid genomes plus two more (B and G) are found (Kimber and Sears 1987). The commonly known durum wheat is a tetraploid (AABB), and the common wheat is a hexaploid (AABBDD).

The evolutionary development of the demonstrably successful cultivated forms of this group may well be based on several events involving introgression from related forms (Kimber and Sears 1987). Nine diploid species are recognized, some of which are thought to carry genes somewhat modified from other closely related diploids. The 17 polyploid species, subspecies, and ploidy forms in the genus contain a total of 40 genomes. Only 21 of these have been identified on the basis of classic genome analysis and 17 more by numerical genome analysis. The remaining ones have been identified on the basis of morphological comparison.

According to Tusnjakova (1956), the cultivars with red-pigmented seeds are better adapted to the rigid conditions of the northern regions. The presence of anthocyanins in the stele is a characteristic associated with rust resistance (Priilinn 1972). Jonard (1933) observed that red-pigmented cultivars germinate more slowly than the white ones. Tandon et al (1970) found that in *T. aestivum* the red pigmentation in the seeds is associated with a higher protein content. The red-seeded cultivars had about 1.8% more protein than the amber types. In the dark-red, light-red, and white cultivars, a relationship exists between the catechin and tannin contents and the degree of pigmentation. The pigment is contained almost exclusively in the seed coat (Miyamoto and Everson 1958).

Accessions of diploid wheat are known to possess blue aleurone, and no hexaploid wheat with blue grains was described before the artificial introgression of genes from diploid wheat and *Agropyron* species (the latter commonly called "wheat grass"). There are a number of reports on blue and purple kernels of wheat, and the breeding history of these grain accessions is described by Zeven (1991). The blue color is due to the coloring of the aleurone layer and is controlled by the gene *Ba* on chromosome 4A of diploid wheat. The purple color is from the pericarp of the kernel and is therefore the color of the mother plant since the pericarp consists of maternal tissue. The purple color has different shades, ranging from deep purple to black. Cermeno and Zeller (1988) surveyed several European strains and one Chinese blue-grained strain of common wheat and found that the chromosome 4A or 4B was completely alien in these wheats; in one strain, a segment of the alien chromosome conferring the blue aleurone color was involved in translocation. However, it was unknown at that point from which alien species the chromosome pair conferring blue aleurone color had originated from these European wheat strains. Zeven (1991) concluded that an array of gene alleles was responsible for the pigmentation of the grains.

In *Triticum* spp., different organs of the plant are subject to anthocyanin pigmentation. In *T. durum*, the purple pigmentation of the pericarp and the red color of the auricle are inherited as dominant monogenic characters (Villanueva 1956, Sharman 1958). The pigmentation intensity in *T. durum* is determined by genetic factors as well as environmental conditions such as light intensity and temperature. Paquet (1956) observed that the intensity of red pigment depended also on the physical composition of the endosperm—lighter for fleshy endosperms and darker for vitreous ones.

Pigmentation Characteristics

The first studies on anthocyanin pigmentation in wheat were conducted by Nillson-Ehle (1911, 1914). Recent reviews provide much information about the flavones, carotenoids, and xanthophylls in wheat, but almost nothing is reported on anthocyanins (Fortmann and Joiner 1971). Recent interest in these wheats has resulted in some attempts to rectify this situation (Abdel-Aal and Hucl 1999, 2003).

The anthocyanins of wheat, which have been reasonably well characterized, are listed in Table 8. These results apparently need to be validated with regard to wheat types and growing conditions. The data are specific for the wheat source and may not be predicative of composition in other strains since different genes may control the synthesis of anthocyanins. In addition, the blue-aleuroned and purple-pericarped grains may contain different anthocyanins caused by tissue-specific genes. Abdel-Aal and Hucl (2003) found different anthocyanin profiles between a purple-kerneled and a blue-kerneled bread wheat by HPLC analysis. Van Bragt et al (1967) found cyanidin and peonidin in coleoptiles from irradiation of wheat sprouts. Gale and Flavell (1971) reported the presence of cyanidin and peonidin glucosides and at least three other derivatives of the two aglycones, with two of them being acylated. In the coleoptiles of 13 cultivars of winter and summer wheat from Switzerland, Vogel (1970) found peonidin-3-glucoside (the most abundant), cyanidin-3-gentiobioside, and cyanidin-3-glucoside. This author also showed that it was impossible to characterize cultivars based on the qualitative composition of these three anthocyanins, as all cultivars analyzed contained the same three pigments.

In the pericarp of purple-seeded wheat, *T. aestivum*, cv. UM606a (Hard Federation/Chinese Spring/Nero/3/3* Pitic 62), Dedio et al (1972) identified cyanidin-3-glucoside, peonidin-3-glucoside, and trace amounts of the corresponding rutinosides. Acylated derivatives of cyanidin and peonidin glucosides were also detected. The coleoptiles contained mostly cyanidin-3-rutinoside, acylated cyanidin glucoside, and acylated cyanidin rutinoside, with smaller amounts of the corresponding peonidin derivatives. There were also two acylated glycosides of cyanidin that were not characterized. The acyl groups of the acylated pigments were not aromatic in character. In experimental lines of two wheat cultivars, a blue-kerneled wheat (cv. Purendo) contained an average of 155 and 458 mg of anthocyanin per kilogram of wheat and bran (Udy Cyclone sample mill), respectively, while a purple wheat (cv. Konini) had 104 and 251 mg/kg of wheat and bran (Abdel-Aal and Hucl 2003). These contents showed great variations in wheats over a three-year growing period.

Bolton (1968) found cyanidin and delphinidin derivatives in the grains of lines Blue A and PBB, whereas purple grains of NY1 and NY3 had malvidin derivatives and those of ND2, delphinidin and malvidin derivatives. According to Zeven (1991), purple grain color is caused by anthocyanins in the peri-

TABLE 8
Anthocyanins of Wheat (*Triticum* spp.)[a]

	Relative Concentration		
	Grain	Coleoptile	
Anthocyanin	**a**	**a**	**b**
Cyanidin-3-glucoside	++++	+	+++
Peonidin-3-glucoside	+++	–	++++
Acylated cyanidin glucoside	++	+++	–
Acylated peonidin glucoside	++	–	–
Cyanidin-3-rutinoside	+	++++	–
Peonidin-3-rutinoside	+	++	–
Acylated cyanidin rutinoside	–	++	–
Acylated peonidin rutinoside	–	+	–
Cyanidin-3-gentiobioside	–	–	++

[a] Column a from Dedio (1972); b from Vogel (1970). (Adapted from Mazza and Miniati 1993)

carp, whereas blue color is caused by anthocyanins in the aleurone layer. Purple grains occur in tetraploid wheats from Ethiopia and in one bread wheat accession apparently native to China. Purple pericarp and blue aleurone grains have been studied primarily for their use as markers for special purple (feed) wheats to enable their distinction from those used for human consumption (Gilchrist and Sorrells 1982, Zeven 1991). Both purple and blue grains, however, have also been suggested for use as markers in the production of hybrid seeds and in studies to measure the degree of natural cross pollination and of gamete transmission (Zeven 1991). The genetics of purple pericarp and blue aleurone characteristics is discussed in detail in the review of Zeven (1991).

In addition to anthocyanins, wheat contains a variety of other flavonoids that probably contribute relatively little to the purple or blue color of the kernel but whose presence may have significant effects on the physiological and technological properties of the grain and its processed products. Commercial wheat bran has been found to contain low levels of catechin and di-, tri-, and oligomeric proanthocyanidins (McCallum and Walker 1990) in addition to 6,8-di-*C*-glycosylapigenins and their sinapic and ferulic acid esters (Feng and McDonald 1989).

Uses and Products

Blue and purple grains are used as markers in breeding, but these types of wheat have not found practical applications in end-use products for food and feed. In Canada and other countries, the selection and release of a new wheat variety must meet stringent requirements. One requirement is the easy visual distinction between these kernels and wheat kernels from existing cultivars. The color of wheat kernels would have good potential to be used for grain segregation and cleaning.

Purple grains occur in tetraploid wheats from Ethiopia. These are apparently grown for agronomical advantages and used as food locally. Purple-colored bread wheat accessions were also reported in China (Zeven, 1991). A purple-kerneled bread wheat was also reported in New Zealand (Bezar, 1982), where it was used mainly for whole-meal loaves and as a kibbled wheat for decorating loaves. However, use of these grains as a staple or by a large population has not been reported.

Myer and Barnett (1987) evaluated the use of purple-seeded soft wheat in diets for young swine and found that the wheat satisfactorily replaced all the corn, and even part of the soybean meal, because of its higher lysine content. In a similar study, a different purple-seeded wheat line sample successfully replaced up to 100% of corn in diets for broiler chickens (Bowyer and Waldroup 1987).

Wild Rice

Wild rice, *Zizania* spp., of the grass tribe Zizanieae, is genetically remote from ordinary rice (*Oryza* spp.), although both species belong to the Oryzaceae family. From a botanical point of view, wild rice, sometimes called

Indian rice, is not really rice but a seed from an aquatic grass. Wild rice was originally consumed by Native Americans as a staple food (Lorenz 1981) and is also recorded as a folk remedy for burns and heart and stomach ailments. It occurs naturally over a large portion of eastern North America, extending from New Brunswick westward across Canada to Eastern Manitoba and southward to Massachusetts and Nebraska, but it is grown mainly in the northern United States and southern Canada along lake shores around the Great Lakes region. It is called "wild rice" because it is not cultivated, but it is used in the same manner as ordinary rice.

Genetics and Taxonomy

Zizania, the genus to which all wild rice belongs, has several species. Two annuals native to North America are 1) *Z. aquatica*, var. *aquatica* (Southern wild rice) and var. *brevis* (Estuarine wild rice) and 2) *Z. palustris* var. *palustris* (Northern wild rice) and var. *interior* (interior wild rice). There are differing opinions to whether these should be treated as separate species (Aiken et al 1988). Two species of wild rice are perennial: 1) *Z. Texana* (Texas wild rice), localized along the San Marcos River in Texas, and 2) *Z. latifolia* (Manchuria water rice), native to Asia, occurring from the northeast (Manchuria) region of China to Northeast India (Dore 1969, Aiken et al 1988). These species differ from each other in shape and size, among other characteristics.

Recognized techniques of breeding and selection have not been applied to the improvement of wild rice. If artificial breeding were attempted, the wild rice plant should prove a favorable subject for experimentation. The individual florets are unsexual, making the need for emasculation unnecessary; the sexes are segregated, making the control of pollination by bagging almost as simple as with corn. The florets are large, single, and easy to measure and count. For those wild rice species that are annual, a new generation can be obtained in a year (Dore 1969). Seeds fully ripened on the stalk have a definite dormancy of long duration. However, it is known that when seed is stored dry, the ability to germinate is lost rather rapidly. The germination percentage of wild rice is high when the seed is allowed to lie naturally in the bottom of a river over winter or is stored in containers under conditions of similar saturation and low temperature.

The most common variety of wild rice in Canada is Northern wild rice. This is a variety of great economic importance. It grows in extensive beds in the shallow brown waters of rivers or lakelike expansions. This variety has the largest kernel of all varieties and therefore is the most desirable in the market (Dore 1969). Southern wild rice is widely distributed and is the chief species in the United States (Dore 1969).

Pigmentation Characteristics

Wild rice is very dark brown to black in color. Reports on the pigments are scarce. The anthocyanins of the leaf sheath and staminate florets of wild rice from Manitoba were identified by Gutek et al (1981) as cyanidin-3-glucoside and cyanidin-3-rhamnoglucoside, which account for 75 and 25% of the total anthocyanin, respectively. At least a simple dominant gene (designated *A*) has been shown to control the anthocyanin production in wild rice. However, the occurrence of red progeny from a self-pollinated white plant suggests the presence of a more complex control mechanism that remains to be elucidated.

Wang et al (2002) reviewed the literature on wild rice and examined the structure and physicochemical properties of wild rice starches as compared with those of a long-grain rice. The starches of six wild rice cultivars were similar in morphological appearance, X-ray diffraction pattern, and water solubility index, but they were different in amylose content, β-amylosis limit, branch-chain-length distribution, and thermal and pasting properties. The structure of wild rice amylopectins was similar to that of waxy rice amylopectins, with more branching and a larger proportion of short branch chains of DP 6–12 as compared with amylopectin from rice with a similar amylose content.

Uses and Products

Wild rice was important to the survival of many native tribes around the Great Lakes when hunting and fishing became difficult in the harsh winters. Presently, wild rice is mainly used in gourmet food products, such as soup, stuffings, desserts, and meat dishes because of its unique color, flavor, and texture. Wild rice has a chewy, nutty flavor. It is often served with game meat, such as venison or pheasant, and used in special recipes such as wild rice with wild mushrooms in soups or pilafs and wild rice cooked with cranberries as an exotic side dish. Oelke and Boedicker (1991) reviewed the processing and utilization of wild rice in more detail.

Conclusion

The last decade has witnessed the tremendous growth of knowledge about the functional properties of phytonutrients in health maintenance and disease prevention. The U.S. FDA has officially recognized the health benefits of grain consumption. The colored grains provide visual appeal and suggest the presence of phytonutrients in the grains. The unique composition of phytonutrients in specialty grains is probably the central reason for the adoption of these grains in our diets. These grains offer many opportunities for cultivar development, although in the past they have received little scientific attention, especially with respect to their health benefits.

Breeding programs for these specialty grains can be anticipated to become more active than in the past. The characteristics of the grains and products will be better studied, and health benefits will gradually be elucidated. As a result, the demand for these grains will increase. However, success for these grains will greatly depend on the avenues for utilization, either through commercially processed foods or widely accepted household uses. In either case, the development of new food products and formulations will be the key to the breeding and growing of these crops. Equally important will be characterization of the health-promoting properties of these grains to stimulate interest in them.

In order for blue and purple grains to increase in popularity, they need to offer consumers visual attractiveness, good taste, and health benefits. However, these colored grains may not necessarily provide higher efficacy than normally colored grains in terms of their health benefits. This is because many constituents in grains are likely to collectively contribute to the benefits, and the pigments, although of desirable visual appeal, are only one of the groups of phytonutrients in grains with positive health effects.

References

Abdel-Aal, E-S. M., and Hucl, P. 1999. A rapid method for quantifying total anthocyanins in blue aleurone and purple pericarp wheats. Cereal Chem. 76:350-354.

Abdel-Aal, E-S. M., and Hucl, P. 2003. Composition and stability of anthocyanins in blue-grained wheat. J. Agric. Food Chem. 51:2174-2180.

Aiken, S. G., Lee, P. F., Punter, D., and Stewart, J. M. 1988. Wild Rice in Canada. NC Press, Ltd., Toronto, ON, Canada.

Alvarez, M., Pavón, J., and von Rütte, S. 1990. Caracterización. Pages 5-30 in: Quinua: Hacia su cultivo comercial. C. Wahli, Ed. Latinreco S.A., Quito, Ecuador.

Amrhein, N. 1979. Biosynthesis of cyanidin in buckwheat hypocotyls. Phytochemistry 18:585.

Anonymous. 1959. Genetic symbols for rice recommended by the International Rice Commission. Int. Rice Comm. Newsl. 8:1-10.

Baraud, J., Genevois, L., and Panart, J. P. 1974. Anthocyanins of corn. J. Agric. Trop. Bot. Appl. 11:55. (CA 62:3062c.)

Bate-Smith, E. C. 1969. Luteoforol (3′,4,4′,5,7-pentahydroxyflavan) in *Sorghum vulgare*. Phytochemistry 8:1803-1806.

Bate-Smith, E. C., and Rasper, V. 1969. Tannins of grain sorghum: Luteoforol (leucoluteolinidin), 3′,4,4′,5,7-pentahydroxyflavan. J. Food Sci. 34:203-207.

Baum, B. R. 1997. Oats: Wild and Cultivated: A Monograph of the Genus *Avena* L. (Poaceae). Supply and Services Canada, Ottawa, ON.

Bezar, H. J. 1982. Konini, specialty bread wheat. N.Z. Wheat Rev. 15:62-63.

Bhat, M. G., Gowda, B. T. S., Anahosur, K. H., and Goud, J. V. 1982. Inheritance of plant pigmentation and downy mildew resistance in sorghum. SABRAO J. 14:53, 1982. (PBA 1984:5085.)

Bhatia, I. S., Kanshal, G. P., and Bajaj, K. L. 1972. Chrysoeriol from barley seeds. Phytochemistry 11:1867.

Blessin, G. W., VanEtten, C. H., and Dimler, R. J. 1963. An examination of anthocyanogens in grain sorghum. Cereal Chem. 40:201-205.

Bobbio, F. O., Bobbio, P. A., and De Souza, S. C. 1988. Comparative stability of anthocyanins from *Panicum melinis* and *Solanum americanum*. Bull. Liaison Groupe Polyphenol 14:138-142.

Boldajaj, F., Goeger, M. P., Nakaue, H. S., Arscott, G. H., and Savage, T. F. 1986. Apparent true and nitrogen corrected metabolized energy values of different varieties of triticale, wheat and barley in poultry. Nutr. Rep. Int. 33:499-503.

Bolton, F. E. 1968. Inheritance of blue aleurone and purple pericarp in hexaploid wheat. Diss. Abstr. Int. 844B:19. (PBA 1970:2684.)

Bowyer, B. L., and Waldroup, P. W. 1987. An evaluation of high lysine purple-seeded wheat in diets for broiler chickens. Nutr. Rep. Int. 35:825-830.

Burnouf-Radosevich, M., Delfel, N. E., and England, R. E. 1985. Gas chromatography-mass spectrometry of oleanane- and ursane-type triterpenes—Application to *Chenopodium quinoa* triterpenes. Phytochemistry 24:2063-2066.

Busch, E., Strack, D., and Weissenböck, G. 1986. Cyanidin 3-gentiobioside from primary leaves of rye (*Secale cereale* L.), Z. Naturforsch. C (Biosci.) 41(1/2):485. (FCA 1986:4940.)

Butler, L. G. 1989. Sorghum polyphenols. Page 95 in: Toxicants of Plant Origin, Vol. IV, Phenolics. P. R. Cheeke, Ed. CRC Press, Inc., Boca Raton, FL.

Cermeno, M. C., and Zeller, F. J. 1988. Cytological investigation on the identity of the alien chromosome pair in several European blue-grained common wheat strains. Pages 227-230 in: Proc. Int. Wheat Genetics Symp., 7th. Vol 1. Institute for Population and Social Research, Cambridge, U.K.

Chang, T. T., and Jordan, N. E. 1963. Monitoring of gene symbols in rice. Int. Rice Commun. Newsl. 12(4):18-29.

Cho, M.-H., Yoon, H.-H., and Hahn, T.-R. 1996. Thermal stability of the major color component, cyanidin 3-glucoside, from a Korean pigmented rice variety in aqueous solution. Agric. Chem. Biotech. 39:245-248.

Coe, E. H., Jr., Neuffer, M. G., and Hoisington, D. A. 1988. The genetics of corn. Pages 81-258 in: Corn and Corn Improvement, 3rd ed. G. F. Sprague and J. W. Dudley, Eds. American Society of Agronomy, Inc., Madison, WI.

Collins, F. W. 1986. Oat phenolics: Structure, occurrence and function. Pages 227-295 in: Oats: Chemistry and Technology. F. H. Webster, Ed. Am. Assoc. Cereal Chem., St. Paul, MN.

Collins, F. W. 1989. Oat phenolics: Avenanthramides, novel substituted *N*-cinnamoylanthranilate alkaloids from oat groats and hulls. J. Agric. Food Chem. 37:60.

Creelman, R. A., Rooney, L. W., and Miller, F. R. 1982. Sorghum. Pages 395-426 in: Cereals: A Renewable Resource—Theory and Practice. Y. Pomeranz, and L. Munck, Eds. Am. Assoc. Cereal Chem., St. Paul, MN.

D'Cruz, R., and Dhulappanavar, C. V. 1963. Inheritance of pigmentation in rice. Indian J. Genet. 23:3. (PBA 1964:2260.)

Dave, B. B. 1948. Inheritance of colour in Central Province's rice. Nagpur Agric. Coll. Mag. 23:20.

Dedio, W., Kaltisikes, P. J., and Larter, E. N. 1969. The anthocyanins of *Secale cereale*. Phytochemistry 8:2351-2352.

Dedio, W., Hill, R. D., and Evans, L. E. 1972. Anthocyanin in the pericarp and coleoptiles of purple wheat. Can. J. Plant Sci. 52:977.

Dellaporta, S. L., Greenblatt, I., Kermicle, J. L., Hicks, J. B., and Wessler, S. R. 1987. Molecular cloning of the maize *R-nj* allele by transposon tagging with *Ac*. Page 263 in: Chromosome Structure and Function: Impact of New Concepts, 18th Stadler Genetics Symposium. J. P. Gustafson and R. Appels, Eds. Plenum Press, New York.

Devreux, A. 1961. Development of anthocyanins during brewing. Brass. Malt. Belge 11:137.

Dore, W. G. 1969. Wild-rice. Information Canada, Ottawa, ON.

Durkee, A. B. 1977. Polyphenols of the bran-aleurone fraction of buckwheat seed *Fagopyrum sagittatum* Gilib. J. Agric. Food Chem. 25:287.

Earp, C. F. 1984. Microscopy of the mature and developing caryopsis of *Sorghum bicolor* (L.) Moench. Diss. Abstr. Int., B 45:3673.

Emerson, R. A. 1921. The genetic relations of plant colors in maize. Cornell Univ. Agric. Exp. Stn. 39:3.

Evans, L. E., and Scoles, G. J. 1976. Cytogenetics, plant breading and agronomy. Pages 13-26 in: Rye: Production, Chemistry, and Technology, 1st ed. W. Bushuk, Ed. Am. Assoc. Cereal Chem., St. Paul, MN.

Fedoroff, N. V., Furtek, D. B., and Nelson, O. E., Jr. 1984. Cloning of the *bronze* locus in maize by a simple and generalizable procedure using the transposable controlling element *Activator* (*Ac*). Proc. Natl. Acad. Sci. U.S.A. 81:3825.

Feng, Y., and McDonald, C. E. 1989. Comparison of flavonoids in bran of flour classes of wheat. Cereal Chem. 66:516.

Fortmann, K. L., and Joiner, R. R. 1971. Wheat pigments and flour color. Pages 493-522 in: Wheat: Chemistry and Technology, 2nd ed. Y. Pomeranz, Ed. Am. Assoc. Cereal Chem. Inc., St. Paul, MN.

Fossen, T., Andersen, Ø. M. 1998. Cyanidin-(6″-succinyl-β-glucopyranoside) and other anthocyanins from *Phragmites australis*. Phytochemistry 49:1065–1068.

Fossen, T., Slimestad, R., Øvstedal, D. O., and Andersen, Ø. M. 2002. Anthocyanins of grasses. Biochem. Syst. Ecol. 30:855–864.

Fuentes P., E. J. 1972. Importancia de la quinua (*Chenopodium quinoa* Willd.) en la solución del problema de las proteínas en la alimentación chilena. Simiente 42:15-20.

Fukui, K., and Wagi, M. 1990. Anthocyanin-type red food color and its manufacture from red rice, Japanese patent 2,248,465. (CA 114:246180.)

Gale, M. D., and Flavell, R. B. 1971. The genetic control of anthocyanin biosynthesis by homoeologous chromosomes in wheat. Genet. Res. 18:237.

Galwey, N.W. 1989. Exploited plants—Quinoa. Biologist 36:267-274.

Gassner, G., and Straib, W. 1937. Untersuchungen ueber den Einfluss der Mineralsalzernaehrung auf die Anthocyanbildung an jugen Gerstenpflanzen, Angew. Bot. 19:225.

Ghose, R. L. M., Ghadge, M. B., and Subrahmanyan, V. 1956. Rice in India. Indian Council for Agricultural Research (I.C.A.R.), New Delhi, India.

Gilchrist, J. A., and Sorrells, M. E. 1982. Inheritance of kernel colour in 'Charcoal' wheat, J. Hered. 73:457.

Glahn, R. P., Cheng, Z., and Welch, R. M. 2002. Comparison of iron bioavailability from 15 rice genotypes: Studies using an in vitro digestion/Caco-2 cell culture model. J. Agric. Food Chem. 50:3586-3591.

Gluchoff-Fiasson, K., Jay, M., and Viricel, M.-R. 1990. Detection of new flavonoid patterns in foxtail millet (*Setaria italica* (L.) Beauv.): Comparison between pure lines and hybrids. Biochem. Syst. Ecol. 18:221.

Golmirzaie, A. M,. and York, J. O. 1992. Interrelationship of brown and purple testa genes with pericarp and other testa genes in *Sorghum bicolor*. Heredity 83:330-334.

Gonzalez-Ceniceros, F., and Franckowiak, J. D. 1990. Effect of Ant genes on aleurone color. Barley Genet. Newsl. 19:20-22.

Gujer, R., Magnolato, D., and Self, R. 1986. Glycosylated flavonoids and other phenolic compounds from sorghum. Phytochemistry 25:1431-1434.

Gupta, R. K., and Haslam, E. 1978. Plant proanthocyanidins. V. Sorghum polyphenols. J. Chem. Soc. Perkin Trans. 1:892.

Gutek, L. H., Woods, D. L., and Clark, K. W. 1981. Identification and inheritance of pigments of wild rice. Crop Sci. 21:79, 1981.

Hagiwara, A., Miyashita, K., Nakanishi, T., Sano, M., Tamano, S., Kadota, T., Koda, T., Nakamura, M., Imaida, K., Ito, N., and Shirai, T. 2001. Pronounced inhibition by a natural anthocyanin, purple corn color, of 2-amino-1-methyl-6-phenylimidazo [4,5-b]pyridine (PhIP)-associated colorectal carcinogenesis in male F44 rats pretreated with 1,2-dimethylhydrazine. Cancer Lett. 171:17-25.

Hahn, D. H. 1984. Phenols of sorghum and maize: The effect of genotype and alkali processing, Diss. Abstr. Int., B 45:3674.

Hamy, A. 1983. Effect of phosphorous deficiency on barley leaf pigments. C.R. Sci. Acad. Agric. Fr. 69:935.

Harborne, J. B. 1988. The Flavonoids: Advances in Research Since 1980. Chapman and Hall, New York.

Harborne, J. B., and Self, R. 1987. Malonated cyanidin 3-glucosides in *Zea mays* and other grasses. Phytochemistry 26:2417.

Harborne, J. B., and Gavazzi, G. 1969. Effect of *Pr* and *pr* alleles on anthocyanin biosynthesis in *Zea mays*. Phytochemistry 8:999.

Harraschain, H., and Mohr, H. 1963. Effect of visible light on the flavonoid synthesis and morphogenesis of buckwheat seedlings (*Fagopyrum esculentum*). II. Flavonol synthesis and hypocotyl growth. Z. Bot. 51:277.

Haskins, F. A., and Gorz, H. J. 1986. Inheritance of leucoanthocyanidin content in sorghum leaves. Crop. Sci. 26:286-292.

Hayashi, K. 1944. Anthocyanins. XIII. Several anthocyanins containing cyanidin as the aglycone. Acta Phytochim. 14:55. (CA 45:4786.)

Hayashi, K. 1946. Pigment of purple rice. Misc. Rep. Res. Inst. Natl. Resources, Jpn. 9:1. (CA 44:9012i.)

Hector, G. P. 1916. Observations on the inheritance of anthocyanin pigment in paddy varieties. Mem. Dep. Agric. India Bot. Ser. 8(2):89.

Hulse, J. H. 1980. Polyphenols in Cereals and Legumes. International Development Research Centre, Ottawa, ON, Canada.

Hulse, J. H., Laing, E. M., and Pearson, O. E. 1980. Sorghum and the Millets: Their Composition and Nutritive Value. Academic Press, London.

Ichikawa, H., Ichiyanagi, T, Xu, B., Yoshi, Y., Nakajima, M., and Koishi, T. 2001. Antioxidant activity of anthocyanin extract from purple black rice. J. Med. Food 4:211-218.

Indira, S., Rana, B. S., Rao, V. J. M., and Rao, N. G. P. 1983. Host plant resistance to rust in sorghum. Indian J. Genet. Plant Breed. 43:193. (PBA 1985:3487.)

Inoue, K., Hosokama, Y., and Shimadate, T. 1982. Anthocyanin pigments of buckwheat hypocotyls. Kenkyu Kiyo Nihon Daigaku Bunrigakubu Shizen Kagaku Kenkyusho, 17:26. (CA 97:88690m.)

Itani, T., Tatemoto, H., Okamoto, M., Fijii, K., and Muto, N. 2002a. A comparative study on antioxidative activity and polyphenol content of colored kernel rice. Nippon Shokuhin Kagaku Kogaku Kaishi 49:540-543. (In Japanese)

Itani, T., Tamaki, M., Arai, E., and Horino, T. 2002b. Distribution of amylose, nitrogen, and minerals in rice kernels with various characters. J. Agric. Food Chem. 50:5326-5332.

Iyer, K. N. 1959. Genetics of rice (*Oryza sativa* L.). The inheritance of awning, auricle, ligule, and junctura and anthocyanin pigmentation and the interrelationship of genes governing these characters. (Res. rep.) Indian Agricultural Research Institute, New Delhi, India.

Jende-Strid, B. 1978. Mutation affecting flavonoid synthesis in barley. Carlsberg Res. Commun. 43:265.

Jende-Strid, B. 1981. Characterization of mutants in barley affecting flavonoid synthesis. Hoppe-Seyler's Z. Physiol. Chem. 362:12.

Jende-Strid, B., and Lundqvist, U. 1978. Diallelic tests of anthocyanin-deficient mutants. Barley Genet. Newsl. 8:57.

Johnson, D. L. 1990. New grains and pseudograins. Pages 122-127 in: Advances in New Crops. J. Janick and J. E. Simon, Eds. Timber Press, Portland, OR.

Johnson, D. L., and Ward, S. M. 1993. Quinoa. Pages 219-221 in: New Crops. J. Janick and J. E. Simon, Eds. Wiley, New York.

Jonard, P. 1933. Relation entre la couleur du grain de diverses varietes de blé et leur aptitude a germer en moyettes. Selectioneur 2:41.

Jones, J. W. 1930. Inheritance of anthocyanin pigments in rice. J. Agric. Res. 40:1105.

Kaerstens, W. K. H. 1939. Anthocyanin and anthocyanin formation in seedlings of *Fagopyrum esculentum* Moench. Rec. Trav. Bot. Neerl. 36:85. (CA 33:8687.)

Kambal, A. E., and Bate-Smith, E. C. 1976. A genetic and biochemical study on pericarp pigments in a cross between two cultivars of grain sorghum, *Sorghum bicolor*. Heredity 37:413.

Katayama, M., Onoe, A., Egawa, H., Imaki, T., and Nakano, J. 1986. Red colors for acidic foods. Japanese patent 61:158,762. (CA 105:207826.)

Kim, S. L., Hwang, J. J., Song, J., Song, J. C., and Jung, K. H. 2000. Extraction, purification, and quantification of anthocyanins in colored rice, black soybean, and black waxy corn. Korean J. Breed. 32:146-152.

Kimber, G., and Sears, E. R. 1987. Evolution in the genus *Triticum* and the origin of cultivated wheat. Pages 154-164 in: Wheat and Wheat Improvement, 2nd ed. E. G. Heyne, Ed. American Society of Agronomy, Madison, WI.

Kinoshita, T., and Takahashi, M. 1991. The one-hundredth report of genetical studies on rice plant. Linkage studies and future prospects. J. Fac. Agric. Hokkaido Univ. 65:1-61.

Knoll, H. A., Lathwell, D. J., and Brady, N. C. 1964. Influence of root zone temperature on the growth and contents of phosphorous and anthocyanin in maize. Proc. Soil Sci. Soc. Am. 28:400.

Koziol, M. J. 1992. Chemical composition and nutritional evaluation of quinoa (*Chenopodium quinoa* Willd.). J. Food Comp. Anal. 5:36-68.

Lawanson, A. O., and Osude, B. A. 1972. Identification of the anthocyanin pigments of *Zea mays* var. E.S.I. Z. Pflanzenphysiol. 67:460.

Litzenberger, S. C., and Green, J. M. 1951. Inheritance of awns in barley. Agron. J. 43:117.

Lorenz, K. 1981. Wild rice: The Indian's staple and the white man's delicacy. CRC Crit. Rev. Food Sci. Nutr. 15:281-319.

Lorenz, K., Welsh, J., Norman, R., and Maga, J. 1972. Composition, mixing and baking properties of wheat and triticale flours. Cereal Chem. 49:187-193.

Ma, W.-W., Heinstein, P. F., and McLaughlin, J. L. 1989. Additional toxic, bitter saponins from the seeds of *Chenopodium quinoa*. J. Nat. Prod. 52:1132-1135.

Margna, U., and Vainjarv, T. 1981. Buckwheat seedlings flavonoid do not undergo rapid turnover. Biochem. Physiol. Pflanz. 176(1):44.

Margna, U., Laanest, L., Margna, E., Otter, M., and Vainjarv, T. 1974. Nitrogen-induced changes in the accumulation of buckwheat seedling flavonoids. Eesti NSV Tead. Akad. Toim., Biol. Seer. 23(4):298. (CA 82:72078.)

Margna, U., Margna, E., and Paluteder, A. 1990. Localization and distribution of flavonoids in buckwheat seedling cotyledons. J. Plant Physiol. 136:166.

Marshall, H. G., and Pomeranz, Y. 1982. Buckwheat: Description, breeding, production, and utilization. Pages 157-169 in: Advances in Cereal Science and Technology, Vol. 5. Y. Pomeranz, Ed. Am. Assoc. Cereal Chem., St. Paul, MN.

Martin, W., Leonard, W., and Stamp, D. L. 1976. Indian corn or maize. Pages 323-382 in: Principles of Field Crop Production, 3rd ed. J. A. Macmillan Publishing Co. Inc., New York.

Mayler, J. L., and Stanford, E. H. 1942. Color inheritance in barley. J. Am. Soc. Agric. 34:427.

Mazza, G. 1993. Buckwheat (*Fagopyrum esculentum*), the crop and its importance. Pages 516-521 in: Encyclopedia of Food Science, Food Technology and Nutrition. R. MacRae, Ed. Academic Press Ltd., London, UK.

Mazza, G. 2000a. Health aspects of natural colors. Pages 289-314 in: Natural Colors. G. J. Lauro and F. J. Francis, Eds. Marcel Dekker, Inc., New York.

Mazza, G. 2000b. Buckwheat. Pages 90-97 in: Cambridge History and Culture of Food and Nutrition. K. F. Kiple, Ed. Cambridge University Press, Cambridge, U.K.

Mazza, G., and Miniati, E. 1993. Anthocyanins in fruits, vegetables, and grains. CRC Press, Boca Raton, FL.

Mazza, G., and Oomah, B. D. 2005. Buckwheat. Pages 375-393 in: Specialty Grains for Food and Feed. E. Abdel-Aal and P. Wood, Eds. Am. Assoc. Cereal Chem., St. Paul, MN.

McClintock, B. 1965. The control of gene action in maize. Brookhaven Symp. Biol. 18:162.

McCallum, J. A., and Walker, J. R. L. 1990. Proanthocyanidins in wheat bran. Cereal Chem. 67:282.

McDonough, C. M., and Rooney, L. W. 1989. Structural characteristics of *Pennisetum americanum* (pearl millet) using scanning electron and fluorescence microscopy. Food Microstruct. 8:137-149.

McFarlane, W. D., Wye, E., and Grant, H. L. 1955. Proc. Congr. Eur. Brew. Conv., 5:298.

McGrath, R. M., Kaluza, W. Z., Daiber, K. H., van der Riet, W. B., and Glennie, C. W. 1982. Polyphenols of sorghum grain, their changes during malting, and their inhibitory nature. J. Agric. Food Chem. 30:450-454.

McLaughlin, M., and Walbot, V. 1987. Cloning of a mutable *bz2* allele of maize by transposon tagging and differential hybridization. Genetics 117:771.

Melz, G., Neumann, H., Muller, H. W., and Sturm, W. 1984. Genetical analysis of rye (*Secale cereale* L.). I. Results of gene localization on rye chromosomes using primary trisomics. Genet. Polon. 25:111. (PBA 1985:7692.)

Metche, M., and Urion, E. 1961. Isolation and identification of anthocyanin derivatives in the husk of barley. C.R. Acad. Sci. France 252:356.

Misra, K., and Seshadri, T. R. 1967. Chemical components of *Sorghum durra* glumes. Indian J. Chem. 5:409. (CA 68:51145.)

Misro, B. R. H. 1981. Linkage studies in rice (*Oryza sativa* L.). Oryza 18:185. (PBA 1983:438.)

Misro, B., Seetharaman, R., and Richharia, R. H. 1960. World genetic stock of rice. I. Pattern of anthocyanin pigment distribution. Indian J. Genet. Plant Breed. 20:113. (CA 58:12868d.)

Miyamoto, T., and Everson, E. H. 1958. Wheat seed pigmentation. Agron. J. 50:733.

Mizui, F., Kasai, R., Ohtani, K., and Tanaka, O. 1988. Saponins from brans of quinoa, *Chenopodium quinoa* Willd., I. Chem. Pharm. Bull. 36:1415-1418.

Mizui, F., Kasai, R., Ohtani, K., and Tanaka, O. 1990. Saponins from brans of quinoa, *Chenopodium quinoa* Willd., II. Chem. Pharm. Bull. 38:375-377.

Molin, W. T., Anderson, E. J., and Porter, C. A. 1986. Effects of alachlor on anthocyanin and lignin synthesis in etiolated sorghum (*Sorghum bicolor* (L.) Moench.) mesocotyles. Pestic. Biochem. Physiol. 25:105.

Morita, Y., Wadano, A., and Ida, S. 1971. Studies on respiratory enzymes in rice kernel. Part VI. Characterization of blue protein of rice bran. Agric. Biol. Chem. 35:255-260.

Mullick, D. B. 1967. Biochemical genetics of the anthocyanins of barley (*Hordeum vulgare* L.). Diss. Abstr. B 27:2247.

Mullick, D. B., and Brink, V. C. 1966. Localization of anthocyanins by peeling the investments of the barley pericarp. Crop Sci. 6:204.

Mullick, D. B., Faris, D. G., Brink, D. G., and Acheson, R. M. 1958. Anthocyanins and anthocyanidins of the barley pericarp and aleurone tissues. Can. J. Plant Sci. 38:445.

Murty, G. S., and Jain, K. B. L. 1959. Genetic studies in barley. I. Inheritance of pigmentation in various plant parts. J. Indian Bot. Soc. 38:561.

Myer, R. O., and Barnett, R. D. 1987. Evaluation of purple-seeded, high protein, soft wheats in diets for young, growing swine. Nutr. Rep. Int. 35:819-824.

Nagai, I., Suzushino, G., and Suzuki, Y. 1960. Anthoxanthins and anthocyanins in *Oryzaceae*. Jpn. J. Breed. 10:247. (CA 61:11007.)

Nagai, I., Suzushino, G., and Tsuboki, Y. 1962. Genetic variation of anthocyanins in *Oryza sativa*. Idengaku Zasshi 31:441. (PBA 1965:518.)

Nagao, S., Takahashi, M., and Kinoshita, T. 1962. Genetical studies on rice plant. XXVI. Mode of inheritance and causal genes for one type of anthocyanin color character in foreign rice varieties. J. Fac. Agric. Hokkaido Univ. 52:20. (PBA 1963:4545.)

Nair, N. R. 1958. Genetics of rice (*Oryza sativa* L.). The inheritance of hairiness, clustering, beaked habit, anthocyanin pigmentation and interrelationship of genes governing these characters. (Res. rep.) Indian Agricultural Research Institute, New Delhi, India.

Nakatani, N., Fukuda, H., and Fuwa, H. 1979. Major anthocyanin of Bolivian purple corn (*Zea mays* L.). Agric. Biol. Chem. 43:389.

Narula, P. N., and Mathur, V. S. 1966. Genetic studies in barley. II. Inheritance of pigmentation. J. Indian Bot. Soc. 45:24. (PBA 1967:4113.)

Nilan, R. A, and Ullrich, S. E. 1993. Barley: Taxonomy, origin, distribution, production, genetics and breeding. Pages 1-29 in: Barley: Chemistry and Technology. A. W. MacGregor and R. S. Bhatty, Eds. Am. Assoc. Cereal Chem., St. Paul, MN.

Nillson-Ehle, H. 1911. Kreuzungsuntersuchung an Hafer und Weizen. Lunds Univ. Arsskr., Afd. 2, Bd. 7(6):3.

Nillson-Ehle, H. 1914. Zur Kenntnis der mit der Keimungsphysiologie des Weizens in Zusammenhang stehenden inneren Faktorn. Pflanzenzuechtung 2:153.

Nip, W. K. and Burns, E. E. 1969. Pigment characterization in grain sorghum. I. Red varieties. Cereal Chem. 46:490.

Nip, W. K. and Burns, E. E. 1971. Pigment characterization in grain sorghum. II. White varieties. Cereal Chem. 48:74.

Nittler, L. W. 1968. Varietal differences among phosphorous-deficient oat seedlings, Crop Sci. 8:393.

O'Reilly, C., Shepherd, N. S., Pereira, A., Schwartz-Sommer, Z., Bertram, I., Robertson, D. S., Peterson, P. A., and Saedler, H. 1985. Molecular cloning of the *a1* locus of *Zea mays* using the transposable elements *En* and *Mu1*. EMBO J. 4:877.

Oelke, E. A., and Boedicker, J. J. 1991. Wild rice: Processing and utilization. Pages 401-439 in: Handbook of Cereal Science and Technology. K. J. Lorenz and K. Kulp, Eds. Marcel Dekker, Inc., New York.

Olifson, L. E., Nechaev, A. P., Osadchaya, N. L., and Mikhailova, L. F. 1978. A new food dye made from sorghum grain and its toxicological characteristics. Vopr. Pitan. 1:76. (CA 88:119568.)

Paquet, J. 1956. Interaction de la coloration du tegument et de la texture de l'albumine dans la determination de l'intensité de la couleur du grain de blé. Ann. Inst. Natl. Rech. Agron., Paris Ser. B. 6:27.

Paris, R., and Pereira-Alarcon, A. 1968. Flavonoids of some Peruvian dye plants. Plant. Med. Phytother. 2:90. (CA 69:74492.)

Park, S-Z, Lee, J.-H., Han, S-J, Kim, H-Y, and Ryu, S-N. 1998. Quantitative analysis and varietal difference of cyanidin 3-glucoside in pigmented rice. Korean J. Crop Sci. 43:179-183. (In Korean)

Parnell, F. R., Ayyangar, G. N. R., and Ramiah, K. 1917. Inheritance of characters in rice. Mem. Dept. Agric. India Bot. Ser. 9:75.

Pascual-Teresa, S., Santos-Buelga, C., and Rivas-Gonzalo, J. C. 2002. LC-MS analysis of anthocyanins from purple corn cob. J. Sci. Food Agric. 82:1003-1006.

Priilinn, O. 1972. A study of mutation variability in spring wheat on using chemical mutagens. Industirov. Mutagenez Rast. Tallin, Estonia. 1972:284. (PBA 1973:3444.)

Raju, N. S. N., Rao, Y. S., Subba Rao, M. V., and Manga, V. 1985. Anthocyanidins of purple and sun-red pigmentation in pearl millet (*Pennisetum americanum*). Indian J. Bot. 8:185. (CA 105:187656.)

Ramiah, K. 1945. Anthocyanin genetics of cotton and rice. Indian J. Genet. Plant Breed. 5:1.

Ramiah, K. 1953. Rice Breeding and Genetics. Indian Council for Agricultural Research, New Delhi, India.

Reddy, G. M., and Reddy, A. R. 1973. Action of *bronze-I* locus in anthocyanin synthesis in maize. Proc. Symp. Contr. Mech. Cell Processes 1973:397-102.

Reddy, V. S., Dash, S., and Reddy, A. R. 1995. Anthocyanin pathway in rice (Oryza sativa L.): Identification of a mutant showing dominant inhibition of anthocyanins in leaf and accumulation of proanthocyanidins in pericarp. Theor. Appl. Genet. 91:301-312.

Reichert, R. D. 1979. The pH-sensitive pigments in pearl millet. Cereal Chem. 56:291-294.

Reichert, R. D., Tatarynovich, J. T., and Tyler, R. T. 1986. Abrasive dehulling of quinoa (*Chenopodium quinoa*): Effect on saponin content determined by an adapted hemolytic assay. Cereal Chem. 63:471-475.

Reichert, R. D., Young, C. G., and Christensen, D. A. 1980. Polyphenols in *Pennisetum* millet. Cited in Hulse (1980).

Rhoades, M. M. 1945. Effect of the bronze locus on the anthocyanin formation in maize. Proc. Natl. Acad. Sci. U.S.A. 31:91.

Ridout, C. L., Price, K. R., DuPont, M. S., Parker, M. L., and Fenwick, G. R. 1991. Quinoa saponins—Analysis and preliminary investigations into the effects of reduction by processing. J. Sci. Food Agric. 54:165-176.

Rooney, L. W., and Miller, F. R. 1982. Variation in the structure and kernel characteristics of sorghum. Page 143 in: Proc. Int. Symp. Sorghum Grain Quality. L. W. Rooney. and D. S. Murty, Eds. International Crops Research Institute of the Semi-arid Tropics, Andhra Pradesh, India.

Ryu, S. N., Han, S. J., Park, S. Z., and Kim, H. Y. 2000. Antioxidative activity and varietal difference of cyanidin 3-glucoside and peonidin 3-glucoside contents in pigmented rice. Korean J. Crop Sci. 45:257-260.

Seah, K. T., and Styles, E. D. 1969. Anthocyanins in maize. Can. J. Genet. Cytol. 11:482.

Shafi, M., and Aziz, M. A. 1959. The inheritance of anthocyanin pigment in the outer glume and apiculus of rice. Agric. Pak. 10:217. (PBA 1960:420.)

Sharma, J. N., and Seshadri, T. R. 1955. Survey of anthocyanins from Indian sources. J. Sci. Ind. Res. 14B:211. (CA 50:5846g.)

Sharman, B. C. 1958. Purple pericarp: A monofactorial dominant in tetraploid wheats. Nature 181:929.

Shibata, M., and Sakai, E. 1958. Anthocyanin in the hair of spike or Japanese pearl millet (*Pennisetum japonicum*). Bot. Mag. Tokyo 71:193.

Shropshire, W., Jr., and Mohr, H. 1970. Gradient formation of anthocyanin in seedlings of *Fagopyrum* and *Sinapis* unilaterally exposed to red and far red light. Photochem. Photobiol. 12:145-149.

Singer, N. S., Tang, P., Chang, H.-H., and Dunn, J. M. 1990. Carbohydrate cream substitute. European patent 0 403 696 A1, Office Européen des Brevets, Paris.

Singh, S., Kalia, M., and Malhotra, S. R. 1999. Effect of parboiling, hand-pounding and machine-milling on chemical composition of rice. J. Food Sci. Technol. 36:434-435.

Slominski, B. A. 1980. Phenolic acids in the meal of developing and stored barley seeds. J. Sci. Food Agric. 31:1007.

Sosulski, F., Krygier, K., and Hogge, L. 1982. Free, esterified and insoluble-bound phenolic acids. III. Composition of phenolic acids in cereal and potato flours. J. Agric. Food Chem. 30:337.

Stadler, L. J. 1946. Spontaneous mutation of the *R* locus in maize. I. The aleurone-color and plant-color effects. Genetics 31:377.

Stadler, L. J. 1948. Spontaneous mutation at the *R* locus in maize. II. Race differences in mutation rate. Am. Nat. 82:289.

Stafford, H. A. 1965. Flavonoids and related phenolic compounds produced in the first internode of *Sorghum vulgare* Pers. in darkness and in light. Plant Physiol. 40:130-134.

Stafford, H. A.1969. Changes in phenolic compounds and related enzymes in young plants of sorghum. Phytochemistry 8:743-747.

Straus, J. 1959. Anthocyanin synthesis in maize endosperm tissue cultures. I. Identity of pigments and general factors. Plant Physiol. 34:536.

Sturm, W., Muller, H. W., and Neumann, H. 1981a. Preliminary results on the use of primary trisomics to locate genes in rye. Tagungsber. Akad. Landwirt.-Wiss. Deut. Demokr. Rep. N. 198:153. (PBA 1982:10221.)

Sturm, W., Neumann, H., and Melz, G. 1981b. Trisomic analysis for the trait anthocyanin coloration in *Secale cereale* L. Ark. Zuechtungsforsch. 11:49. (PBA 1981:7016.)

Styles, E. D., and Ceska, O. 1972. Flavonoid pigments in genetic strains of maize, Phytochemistry 11:3019.

Takahashi, K., and Yoshizawa, K. 1987. Red rice pigments and brewing of alcoholic beverages containing them. J. Brew. Soc. Jpn. 82:740-747.

Takahashi, M. 1982. Genetical studies on rice plants. LXXX. Gene analysis and its related problems. J. Fac. Agric. Kokkaido Univ. 61:91-142.

Takahashi, R. 1955. The origin and evolution of cultivated barley. Adv. Genet. 7:227.

Takahashi, R., and Yamamoto, J. 1950. Studies on the classification and geographical distribution of barley varieties. XII. On the pigmentation of the plant parts. Rep. Ohara Agric. Res. 39:25. (PBA 1957:1758.)

Takahashi, R., Yamamoto, J., Yasuda, S., and Itano, Y., 1953. Inheritance and linkage studies in barley. Ber. Ohara Inst. Landwirt. Forsch. 10:29.

Tandon, J. P., Dhillon, S. S., and Goswami, A. K. 1970. An association between locus for grain colour and protein content in wheat (*Triticum aestivum*). Can. J. Genet. Cytol. 12:28.

Taylor, L. P. and Briggs, W. R. 1990. Genetic regulation and photocontrol of anthocyanin accumulation in maize seedlings. Plant Cell 2:115.

Tegenkamp, T. R. 1962. Phenomena associated with hereditary albinism in *Avena*. Diss. Abstr. 22:3824. (PBA 1963:1332.)

Tohver, A. 1976. Effect of exogenous phenylalanine on the light sensitivity of anthocyanin accumulation in buckwheat seedlings. Regul. Rosta Pitan. Rast. 1976:33. (CA 87:16465.)

Tohver, A. 1987. Anthocyanin accumulation in buckwheat hypocotyl under intermittent red and far red light. Fiziol. Rast. 34:742. (CA 107:131053v.)

Troyer, J. 1964. Anthocyanin formation in excised segments of buckwheat seedling hypocotyls. Plant Physiol. 39:907-912.

Troyer, J. R. 1955. The distribution of rutin and other flavonoid substances in buckwheat seedlings. Plant Physiol. 30:68-172.

Troyer, J. R. 1956. Distribution of rutin and other flavonoid substances in mature buckwheat plants. Lloydia 19:216-221.

Troyer, J. R. 1958. Anthocyanin pigments of buckwheat hypocotyls. Ohio J. Sci. 58:187. (CA 52:12090h.)

Tsen, C. C. 1974. Triticale: First Man-Made Cereal. Am. Assoc. Cereal Chem., St. Paul, MN.

Tusnjakova, M. M. 1956. Red-grained and red-eared forms of some wheat varieties. Tr. Inst. Genet. N. 23:145. (PBA 1957:2786.)

Vaidehi, M. P. 1984. Nutritional and rheological properties of triticale varieties. Mysore J. Agric. Sci. 18:70-74.

Van Bragt, J., Brouner, J. B., and Zeven, A. C. 1967. The colour of the coleoptile of wheat. I. Anthocyanins of the coleoptiles of some Triticinae. Wheat Inf. Serv. 25:2.

Van der Stok, J. E. 1908. On the inheritance of grain color in rice. Teysmannia 65:5.

Van Sumere, C. F., Cottenie, J., de Greef, J., and Kint, J. 1972. Biochemical studies in relation to the possible germination regulatory role of naturally occurring coumarin and phenolics. Recent Adv. Phytochem. 4:166.

Villanueva, N. R. 1956. Inheritance of colour of auricles in wheat. Bol. Trimestr. Exp. Agropec., Progr. Coop. Exp. Agropec., Lima 5(2):25. (PBA 1957:3918.)

Vogel, F. 1970. Identification of anthocyanin pigments in wheat coleoptiles. Schweiz. Landw. Forsch. 9:97. (FCA 1971:127.)

Wang, L., Wang, Y.-J., and Porter, R. 2002. Structure and physicochemical properties of six wild rice starches. J. Agric. Food Chem. 50:2695-2699.
Watkins, R. 1966. The inheritance of anthocyanin pigments in rye (*Secale cereale* L.), Diss. Abstr. Int. 26:4986. (PBA 1967:4080.)
Watkins, R., and White, W. J. 1964. The inheritance of anthocyanins in rye (*Secale cereale* L.). Can. J. Genet. Cytol. 6:403-407.
Watterson, J. J., and Butler, L. G. 1983. Occurrence of an unusual leucoanthocyanidin and absence of proanthocyanidins in sorghum leaves. J. Agric. Food Chem. 31:41.
Wienand, U., Weydemann, U., Niesbach-Klösgen, U., Peterson, P. A., and Saedler, H. 1986. Molecular cloning of the *c2* locus of *Zea mays*, the gene coding for chalcone synthase. Mol. Gen. Genet. 203:202.
Williams, P. C. 1986. The influence of chromosome number and species on wheat hardness. Cereal Chem. 63:56-58.
Wilson, H. D. 1990. Quinoa and relatives (*Chenopodium* sect. *Chenopodium* subsect. Cellulata). Econ. Bot. 44:92-110.
Woodward, R. W., and Thieret, J. W. 1953. A genetic study of complementary genes for purple lemma, palea, and pericarp in barley (*Hordeum vulgare* L.). Agron. J. 45:182.
Yasumatsu, K., Nakayama, T. O. M., and Chichester, C. O. 1965. Flavonoids of sorghum. J. Food Sci. 30:663-667.
Yoshinaga, K. 1986. Liquor with pigments of red rice. J. Brew. Soc. Jpn. 81:337-342.
Zeven, A. C. 1991. Wheats with purple and blue grains: A review. Euphytica 56:243-258.

CHAPTER 13

Amaranth

Massimo F. Marcone

Department of Food Science, Ontario Agricultural College, University of Guelph, Guelph, ON, Canada N1G 2W1

Plants make up 95% of the earth's food supply, with the common cereal grains such as wheat, rye, barley, rice, corn, sorghum, and millet providing more than 75% of basic human protein requirements. Consumption trends show increased use of nonconventional, noncereal grains (Shewry and Miflin 1985). This increased interest in noncereal grains exists not only because these grains commonly possess two to four times more protein than traditionally used cereal grains, but because their proteins are often of higher nutritional quality (Lambert and Yarwood 1992). One such alternative grain, amaranth, from the Amaranthaceae family, has been shown to possess great economic potential as well as high nutritional value, especially for use in processed foods (Bejosano and Corke 1998).

Few edible plants of economic importance today have had a historical, cultural, or spiritual origin comparable to those of the Amaranthaceae family (Saunders and Becker 1984). Archaeological studies conducted in Peru, Mexico, and the United States have shown that the production of amaranth grain was important as early as 8000 B.C. Production of amaranth grain peaked in Central America during the Mayan and Aztec periods and then declined catastrophically because of a legislative ban placed on its production in 1519 by the Spanish conqueror Cortez (Saunders and Becker 1984, Bressani 1989). With this ban, amaranth grain gained the rare distinction of being one of the very few plant species in recorded history to be eliminated from popular cultivation as a result of a legislative act (Saunders and Becker 1984). After that time, there was virtually no production or consumption of amaranth until a recent resurgence driven in part by its agronomic and nutritional properties (Saunders and Becker 1984, Coimbra and Salema 1994, Lehmann 1996). *Amaranthus* species (which are dicotyledonous C_4 plants) are successfully grown worldwide from the tropics to semiarid regions because of their environmental hardiness and their ability to grow in places where other, more conventional grains such as cereals cannot (Saunders and Becker 1984, Bressani 1989, Fadel et al 1996, Lehmann 1996). Nutritionally, based on essential amino acid composition, amaranth grain has been assigned an exceptionally high chemical score of 73 in the recommended FAO/WHO scoring patterns (Bressani 1989). Indeed, when amaranth grain is processed under conditions that do not damage the availability of essential amino acids, its protein quality is very close to that of casein (Mendoza and Bressani 1987, Bressani 1989). Additionally, the protein quality (protein efficiency ratio [PER]) of amaranth grain increases significantly on wet cooking as compared to the raw grain (Bejosano and Corke 1998, Bressani 1989). Nutritional improvement of a variety of baked goods such as breads, pastries, and cookies and extrusion products such as cereal flakes, tortillas, and pasta has been achieved by incorporation of amaranth (Sanchez-Marroquin 1984). Amaranth starch is suitable for enrichment of hypoallergenic baby foods (containing 18% protein) because of the absence of gluten and lactose (Sanchez-Marroquin 1984). Other studies have demonstrated a variety of potential health benefits from amaranth consumption, including its ability to lower blood glucose response in noninsulin-dependent diabetics, and to lower serum cholesterol levels (Dunz and Lupton 1992, Lehmann 1996, Chanturvedi et al 1997).

Amaranth Cultivation and Grain Production

Amaranth belongs to a family of dicotyledonous plants known as Amaranthaceae and is an annual broad-leaved plant that varies in height from 0.5 to 3 m (Kigel 1994, Berghofer and Schoenlechner 2002) (Fig. 1). Amaranth grain is lenticular in shape, usually measures approximately 0.8–1.0 mm in diameter, and weighs approximately 1 mg (1,000 seeds = 1 g) (Fig. 1).

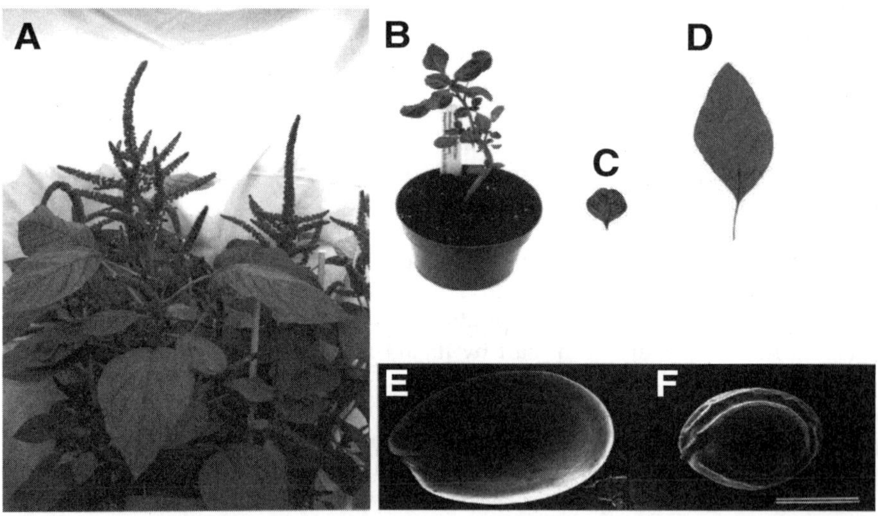

Fig. 1. A, Grain amaranth *Amaranthus hypochondriacus* K343 (*A. hypochondriacus* × *A. hybridus*) plant. **B,** *A. pumilus* (seabeach amaranth) plant; **C,** *A. pumilus* leaf; **D,** *A. hypochondriacus* leaf; **E,** scanning electron micrographs of *A. pumilus* seed and, **F,** *A. hypochondriacus* seed. (Bar represents 720 μm.)

Amaranth's dramatic revival today as a favorable food crop can be ascribed to its C_4 photosynthetic metabolic capacity, which endows it with a number of agronomic attributes, including environmental hardiness and a capacity for efficient water utilization. These qualities enable successful competition for the limited farmable lands and diminishing water supplies in many countries worldwide. Amaranth is cultivated in all climatic regions, from the true tropics to the semiarid regions, but it is commonly grown within 30° latitude of the equator.

The yield of amaranth grain per hectare varies from 2,100 to 2,500 kg ha^{-1}, as shown in cultivation trials in Germany. In China, where 40,000 ha are currently under cultivation to amaranth, grain yield varies from 2,200 to as high as 5,500 kg ha^{-1}. In North America, 1,800 kg ha^{-1} was achieved in Pennsylvania and 4,000 kg ha^{-1} in Montana.

Mechanical harvesting of amaranth grain may pose a problem, depending on the particular variety, because its seeds drop easily out of the spikes. Nevertheless, equipment similar to that used for harvesting more common cereal grains is used in harvesting amaranth grain.

Genetic Diversity in Amaranth

The development of grain amaranth as a new field crop has been aided by the availability of considerable genetic variation within the cultivated species (Amaranth Institute 1990). This provides readily accessible genetic resources for plant breeders to develop improved lines and has been paramount in the assembly of the 1,374 entries of amaranth by the Rodale Research Station in Pennsylvania and by the USDA Collection housed at Ames, Iowa (Amaranth Institute 1990). Commercialization of grain

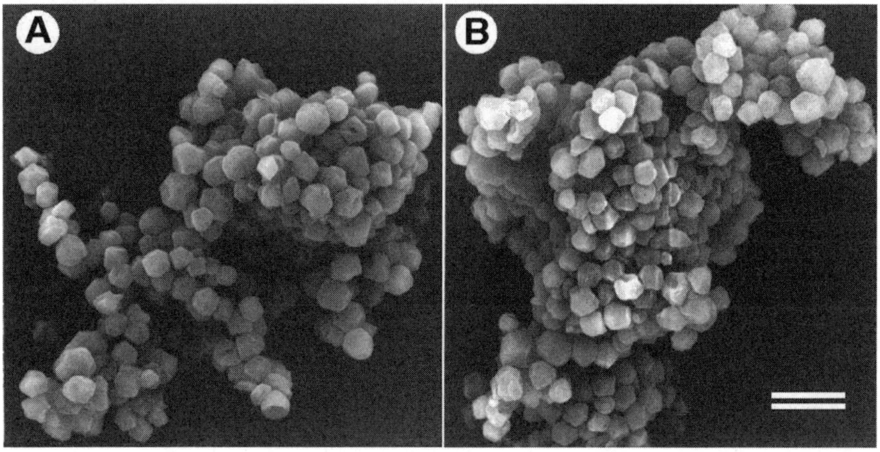

Fig. 2. Scanning electron micrographs of starch isolates from *Amaranthus pumilus* (**A**) and *A. hypochondriacus* (**B**). (Bar represents 3.0 µm.)

amaranth has required genetic improvements and selection of species with cold tolerance and shorter growing seasons suitable for areas of the southwestern United States and southern Canada (Saunders and Becker 1984). One such species, Plainsman (*Amaranthus hypochondriacus* K343), a *A. hypochondriacus* × *A. hybridus* L. cross (Figs. 1 and 2), was developed and selected for commercial grain production in western Nebraska, where the largest concentration of U.S. amaranth production presently occurs. It is favored because it matures earlier, has a light seed color, and produces a shorter plant height, which facilitates mechanized harvesting. Early-maturing grain amaranth lines (i.e., 110 days to maturity) have also been developed and can be grown from North Dakota to Missouri and in other regions where an annual precipitation of 350–500 mm rain occurs. Breeding programs focus on selecting plants with desirable attributes such as high yield, insect resistance, reduced seed shattering, light seed color, and suitability for mechanical harvesting.

Not only has the broad genetic diversity found within amaranth led to the selection of amaranth cultivars with desirable agronomic attributes, but it has also led to noteworthy differences in the phytochemical composition of the grain.

Proteins—Genetic Diversity

Subunit Composition of Main Storage Protein (11S Globulin—Amaranthin)

In a recent survey of seven currently available amaranth hybrid lines grown in the United States—namely K436, MT-3, K433, K432, K266, K283, and K343—Marcone and Yada (1998) found major differences in the molar ratio of individual subunits composing their main protein storage protein, the 11S salt-soluble globulin (amaranthin). This is important because the relative ratio of basic to acidic-type subunits varies among various plant species as well as within individual plant cultivars (Mori et al 1981). For example, the relative ratio of basic to acidic-type subunits of the 11S soybean globulin was found to have a profound effect on functional properties such as gelation and emulsification (Mori et al 1981, 1982, Nakamura et al 1984, 1985, Nishinari et al 1991, Kang et al 1994, Ma et al 1996). Similarly, a particular subunit of wheat glutenin can be correlated with specific functional properties (i.e., particularly breadmaking quality) (Payne et al 1979). The variable subunit ratios observed in the amaranth globulin by Marcone and Yada (1998) are likely to affect the functional properties listed above. Determination of these effects could allow the determination of the most desirable subunit ratios for various amaranth food applications. The variability in subunit ratio could then facilitate the genetic breeding of superior amaranth lines with enhanced functional and nutritional properties.

7S Amaranth Storage Globulin

Because a substantial degree of genetic variability was noted in the 11S globulin between species, other seed components (particularly other proteins) have been examined to determine whether a similar degree of variability was shown. Marcone (1999) reported the presence of another important storage protein within the seed, the 7S globulin, and found it to possess different molecular weight, subunit composition, amino acid composition, and thermal properties compared to the more abundant 11S globulin. Therefore, differences in functional as well as nutritional properties within the finished food product, can be expected. Variations in the 7S:11S globulin ratio could affect the nutritional and rheological properties of the grain. Marcone (1999) evaluated the 7S:11S globulin ratio of seven currently available *Amaranthus* hybrid lines grown in the United States to determine whether the variation occurring could potentially affect the nutritional and functional properties of the grain. Of seven *Amaranthus* lines investigated, four lines—K343, K436, K432, and K433—had 7S:11S globulin ratios ranging from 0.47 to 0.81, and three lines—*Amaranthus* MT-3, K266, and K283—contained only the 11S globulin form. Thus, varietal differences appeared to play a substantial role in the observed 7S:11S globulin ratios. Similar varietal variation in 7S:11S globulin ratios have also been observed in soybean (Hughes and Murphy 1983, Kitamura 1995, Ma et al 1996, Murphy et al 1997, Pazdernik et al 1996). The observed difference in amaranth 7S:11S globulin ratios occurred despite a lack of difference in total seed protein content in these varieties (Marcone and Yada 1998).

Amaranth 7S globulins contained substantially lower levels of important essential amino acids, particularly tryptophan and methionine, compared to the 11S globulin. This is also the case for 7S globulins from other plants such as the 7S soybean globulin (Derbyshire et al 1976). The amaranth 7S globulins were also found to contain substantially lower levels of other major essential amino acids (lysine, histidine, phenylalanine, valine, and isoleucine) compared to the 11S globulin. Arginine, an essential amino acid for children, was also found to be substantially lower in the 7S globulin, which may be of nutritional significance when amaranth grain is used in the manufacture of infant food formulations. Varieties with lower 7S:11S ratios or those containing the 11S globulin exclusively may be of superior nutritional value because it is unknown whether environmental conditions alter 7S:11S globulin ratios, as observed in soybeans (Kitamura 1995, Pazdernik et al 1996).

Lipids and Fat-Soluble Components

Fatty Acid-Triacylglycerol Composition

The fatty acid composition of the oils of various *Amaranthus* species (Budin et al 1996) and similarities to corn (*Zea mays*), buckwheat (*Fagopyrum esculentum*), and cottonseed (*Gossypium hirsutum*) have been reported. Recent studies (Marcone 2000) have confirmed these observations and helped elucidate the extent to which genetic differences in amaranth species affect these lipid components.

The fatty acid compositions of amaranth oil from five *Amaranthus* accessions were found to be similar in overall composition (Marcone et al 2000) (Table 1). More specifically, the major fatty acids were linoleic acid (39.4–

TABLE 1
Fatty Acid Composition (%) of Five Amaranthus Accessions[a]

Fatty Acid	Group I[b]			Group II[b]	
	A. hypochondriacus × *A. hybridus*, K343	*A. hypochondriacus* × *A. hybridus*, K433	*A. hypochondriacus* × *A. hybridus*, K432	*A. cruentus*, R149	*A. cruentus*, RRC1011
14:0	0.29	0.28	0.21	0.26	0.27
16:0	23.8	23.8	21.4	23.4	22.2
16:1	0.11	0.19	0.10	0.15	0.11
18:0	3.11	3.65	3.98	3.68	3.57
18:1	23.0	23.7	22.8	31.5	30.1
18:2	47.9	46.7	49.1	39.4	42.2
18:3	0.88	0.83	0.93	0.65	0.69
20:0	0.56	0.62	0.89	0.60	0.68
20:1	0.18	...	0.23	0.24	...
22:0	0.14	0.22	0.32	0.19	0.24
S/U[c]	0.39	0.4	0.37	0.39	0.37

[a] Representing two species (*A. hypochondriacus* and *A. cruentus*), Group I, and a cross between *A. hypochondriacus* and *A. hybridus*, Group II.
[b] Groups are based on fatty acid compositions.
[c] Saturated/unsaturated ratio.

49.1%), oleic acid (22.8–31.5%), and palmitic acid (21.4–23.8%). These oils were high in total unsaturates (71.4–73.2%). Thus it appears that the genetic variation in five accessions of two *Amaranthus* species and a cross between one of these and a third species did not dramatically alter fatty acid composition. A small difference was noticed with amaranth R149 and amaranth RRC1011. These two accessions had higher oleic acid and lower linoleic acid levels compared to K343, K433, and K432.

The fatty acid composition of oils extracted from grains and oilseed samples with petroleum ether were also determined for comparison (Table 2). The fatty acid composition of amaranth species (Table 1) were all within the range of published results (Przybylski et al 1979). The major fatty acids were linoleic acid (34.8–56.5%), oleic acid (17.7–42.4%), and palmitic acid (9.51–25.7%). The total unsaturated fatty acid content ranged from 70.6 to 86.9%, and the total saturated fatty acid content ranged from 13.1 to 29.4%. As expected, there were more variations in the composition in these oil samples than between *Amaranthus* species. A comparison of the average fatty acid composition of the amaranth oil with other grain and seed oils (Table 2) identified cottonseed and buckwheat oils as having similar profiles. Lyon and Becker (1987) reported similar fatty acid compositional data for amaranth, cottonseed, and corn oils. The other four seed oils in that study differed from amaranth in only one or two fatty acids. Soybean and quinoa contained substantial amounts of linolenic acid (7.0–7.2%) compared to amaranth (0.65–0.93%). Sesame and rice bran oil had higher levels of oleic acid (40.0–42.4%) compared to amaranth (22.8–31.5%), and three oils (quinoa, sesame, and corn) had lower palmitic acid (9.5–11.6%) levels compared to amaranth (21.4–23.8).

Comparison of saturated-to-unsaturated (S/U) fatty acid ratios showed cottonseed and buckwheat oil having ratios very close to those of amaranth

TABLE 2
Fatty Acid Composition (%) of Grain, Oilseed, and Bran Oils

Fatty Acid	Buckwheat	Corn	Rice Bran	Soybean	Sesame	Quinoa	Cottonseed
14:0	0.24	...	0.51	0.12	0.02	0.32	1.00
16:0	19.5	11.6	18.6	12.7	9.51	11.4	25.7
16:1	0.25	0.14	0.23	0.11	0.11	0.07	0.53
18:0	2.18	1.91	1.75	3.96	5.41	0.79	2.45
18:1	37.1	27.8	42.4	21.7	40.0	25.6	17.7
18:2	35.5	56.5	34.8	53.9	43.5	52.8	52.1
18:3	1.93	1.65	1.10	7.23	0.33	7.00	0.22
20:0	1.49	0.40	0.49	0.28	0.60	0.29	0.25
20:1	...	0.05	...	0.04	0.18	1.00	0.05
22:0	1.31	0.05	...	0.05	0.14	0.24	0.05
22:1	...	0.05	...	...	...	0.52	0.05
24:0	0.51	0.05	...	...	0.09	...	...
S/U[a]	0.34	0.16	0.27	0.2	0.19	0.15	0.41

[a] Saturated/unsaturated ratio.

(Tables 1 and 2). Corn, soybean, sesame, and quinoa, on the other hand, had higher levels of unsaturated fatty acids (>82%) compared to amaranth (<74%), resulting in much smaller S/U ratios.

Although the fatty acid composition can be used to evaluate the stability and nutritional quality of fats and oils, it cannot always predict their func-

TABLE 3
Triacylglycerol (TAG) Composition (%) of Five *Amaranthus* Accessions[a]

	Group I[b]				Group II[b]	
TAG profile	***A. hypochondriacus* K343**	***A. hypochondriacus* K433**	***A. hypochondriacus* K432**		***A. cruentus* R149**	***A. cruentus* RRC1011**
Mono- and acylglycorol and unknown	1.92	1.84	2.00		2.72	2.19
LnLnL	0.34	0.65	0.91		0.31	1.11
LnLL	1.06	1.68	1.85		1.27	2.40
LLL	8.03	7.87	8.66		5.44	5.94
PLnL	0.98	1.10	1.34		0.85	1.10
OLL, OOLn	11.60	10.73	10.40		11.23	10.97
PLL, PLnO	20.33	18.33	18.65		14.08	14.48
OOL, PoOO	7.96	7.16	6.72		10.94	10.95
POL	17.21	16.87	16.47		18.67	16.69
PPL	8.84	8.76	9.00		7.42	7.01
MPO	0.70	0.51	0.83		0.35	0.58
OOO, MSO, OOP, PSL	15.62	16.86	17.23	OOO, MSO	6.13	4.82
				OOP, PSL	13.30	11.80
POP	...	...	...		3.13	3.27
PPO	1.05	1.07	0.86		0.56	0.64
PPP	...	0.95	...		...	...
OOS	1.01	1.23	1.70		0.73	1.27
POS	0.77	...	1.49		0.86	0.49
PSS	0.15	...	...		...	...
SOS, SSO	0.55	...	...		...	...
UUU[c]	33.6	33.0	34.2		34.3	35.7
UUS	50.2	48.1	46.8		46.1	43.4
USS	11.9	10.6	11.3		13.2	12.5

[a] Representing two species (*A. hypochondriacus* and *A. cruentus*), Group I, and a cross between *A. hypochondriacus* and *A. hybridus*, Group II.

[b] Groups are based on TAG composition: S, stearic acid; P, palmitic acid; O, oleic acid; L, linoleic acid; Ln, linolenic acid; Po, palmitoleic acid; M, myristic acid.

[c] UUU (triunsaturates), UUS (diunsaturates), USS (monounsaturates). The UUU and USS compositions in multiple bands were calculated on the basis of the fatty acid/TAG balance.

tional properties. The type and the amounts of the various triacylglycerol (TAG) species in the oil is important in determining the final physical and functional properties of the oils. Table 3 shows the TAG composition of the oil from five *Amaranthus* accessions (Marcone et al 2000), using reversed-phase high performance liquid chromatography (RP-HPLC). Overall, the TAG compositions were found to be similar, but much greater similarities were found among species K343, K433, and K432 (Group I) and between species R149 and RRC1011 (Group II). The main differences between the two groups were in the TAG LLL, PLL, and OOL (where L is linoleic, P is palmitic, and O is oleic). It appears that the amaranth accessions can be split into two groups by fatty acid composition or by TAG composition. The predominant TAG in the three *Amaranthus* species were PLL (14.1–20.3%), POL (16.5–18.7%), OLL (10.4–10.9%), OOL+PoOO (6.7–10.9%), and LLL (5.4–8.6%). A large, unresolved chromatographic peak containing a mixture of OOO/MSO/OOP/PSL/POP (3.1–17.2%) was also detected (Table 3) (Marcone et al 2000).

As with fatty acid composition, the TAG compositions of the grain, bran, and seed oils were very diverse (Table 4). The predominant TAGs were diverse (Table 4) and were PLL (8.54–28.08%), OLL (9.42–20.4%), OOL (3.1–16.3%), LLL (2–20.5%), and POL (9.5–15.6%). A broad, unresolved chromatographic peak contained mixtures of OOO+MSO (1.99–11.3), OOP+PSL (1.7–10.94), and POP (0.02–2.31%) (Table 4).

Differences in TAG compositions were much greater between the grain and seed oils than between the *Amaranthus* accessions (Tables 3 and 4). Although cottonseed oil shows some similarity in fatty acid composition to that of amaranth, the low-melting TAG compositions (i.e., LLL, PLL, OOL, PPL) were different in amaranth and cottonseed oil. The LLL in corn, soybean, and quinoa oils were higher (19.83, 20.5, and 19.22%, respectively) compared to the *Amaranthus* species (5.44–8.66%). The PPL, OLL, POL, OOO, and OOP levels in corn, soybean, and quinoa oils also showed dramatic differences from *Amaranthus* oil. The OOL and PLL in rice bran and sesame oil were also different from those in *Amaranthus* accessions (Table 4).

By recalculating the data on the basis of triunsaturates (UUU), diunsaturates (UUS), and monounsaturates (USS), general similarities and differences between the five *Amaranthus* accessions and the seven grain and oilseed oils become apparent (Tables 3 and 4). The *Amaranthus* accessions contained slightly more diunsaturates (43.4–50.2%) than triunsaturates (33–35.7%). The majority of the grain and seed oils were the reverse, with substantially more UUU than UUS. The exceptions were buckwheat and cottonseed, which had TAG (UUU, UUS, and USS) compositions very close to those of the *Amaranthus* accessions. On the basis of tri-, di-, and monounsaturates in the TAG composition, one would expect the amaranth oils to have functional properties similar to those of buckwheat and cottonseed.

The very polar materials, which were soluble in acetone, appeared at retention times almost below the void volume. These compounds have been reported to be monoglycerides, diglycerides, phospholipids, and terpenoids (i.e., squalene) (Bondioli et al 1993, Sun et al 1997). Squalene is an unsaturated hydrocarbon with a higher polarity than TAG except for trilinolenin. Under the RP-HPLC conditions used to separate TAG, the squalene in all *Amaranthus* accessions, rice bran, and quinoa eluded near the void volume. Based on the peak area, the percentages of squalene in the TAG samples were calculated to be 8.0% in K343, 11.1% in K433, 11.2% in K432, 10.0% in R149, 9.2% in RRC1011, 3.4% in quinoa, and 3.1% in rice bran. The amount

TABLE 4
Triacylglycerol (TAG) Composition (%) of Grain, Oilseed, and Bran Oils[a]

TAG Profile	Buckwheat	Corn	Rice Bran	Soybean	Sesame	Quinoa	Cottonseed
Mono- and acylglycorol and unknown	4.91	7.29	8.4	1.59	1.37	4.23	2.94
LnLnLn	...	0.91	...	0.38	...	...	0.32
LnLnL	1.13	0.47	0.26	1.58	...	1.09	...
LnLL	1.03	2.07	0.60	7.45	0.52	6.04	...
LLL	2.08	19.83	6.61	20.50	11.94	19.22	16.17
PLnL	1.15	0.70	0.50	3.98	...	2.86	1.66
OLL OOLn	9.42	20.45	13.91	14.95	17.89	21.09	9.95
PLL PLnO	11.75	12.09	9.71	14.94	8.54	11.34	28.08
OOL PoOO	13.83	11.37	16.21	7.37	16.29	12.78	3.08
POL	15.63	10.70	15.12	11.97	14.59	9.47	15.09
PPL	3.24	1.42	3.14	2.22	...	1.54	12.99
MPO	2.61	0.63	...	1.02	...	...	...
OOO MSO	9.27	3.28	11.32	4.33	8.88	1.99	5.08
OOP PSL	7.83	6.14	10.94	1.70	13.09	3.88	3.51
POP	0.96	2.10	2.31	...	0.02	1.97	...
PPO	3.19	...	...	...	0.24	0.61	...
PPP	...	...	...	...	...	0.34	...
OOS	2.61	...	...	2.93	4.10	0.41	1.02
POS	4.63	...	...	...	2.52	...	...
PSS	...	...	...	...	...	...	...
SOS SSO	...	...	...	...	...	...	...
UUU[c]	35.3	58.8	46.2	54.2	46.6	62.15	30.1
UUS	37.1	24.9	37.0	33.3	27.0	26.6	49.8
USS	17.1	3.1	7.7	3.9	6.2	5.68	16.9

[a] Groups are based on TAG composition: S, stearic acid; P, palmitic acid; O, oleic acid; L, linoleic acid; Ln, linolenic acid; Po, palmitoleic acid; M, myristic acid; UUU (triunsaturates), UUS (diunsaturates), USS (monounsaturates). The UUU and USS compositions in multiple bands were calculated on the basis of the fatty acid/TAG balance.

of squalene in 11 *Amaranthus* seed oil has been reported to be approximately 4.9–8.1% (Saunders and Becker 1984, Sun et al 1997). Squalene is a terpenoid derived primarily from shark (*Cantrophorus squarmosus*) and whale liver (*Physeter macrocephalus*) oils and is expensive. It is an ingredient in cosmetics, skin penetrates, pharmaceuticals, and lubricants for computer disks (Sun et al 1995, Budin et al 1996). Because all squalene used in the United States is imported (200–300 metric tons per year) and because of the concern for marine animal protection, attention has been focused on identifying crop sources of squalene (Sun et al 1997). Therefore, amaranth may potentially serve as a rich vegetable source of squalene as well as provide edible oil and protein for various specialized purposes.

Although previous studies have shown that *Amaranthus* may potentially be a rich vegetable source of squalene as well as provide edible oil, Marcone et al (2000) indicated that genetic differences exist between various *Amaranthus* accessions, which may be exploited for various specialized purposes.

Phytosterols

Epidemiological studies have consistently shown a positive correlation between high levels of serum total cholesterol and LDL cholesterol with coronary heart and peripheral arterial disease (Qureshi et al 1996, Maier et al 2000).

Because of health benefits from lowering the serum cholesterol levels of hypercholesterolemic people, nonpharmaceutical approaches are desirable (Moghadasian and Frohlich 1999). Dietary intervention is effective and safe and can be achieved by consuming plant-soluble fibers such as β-glucans from oats and by restricting the intake of saturated fats and cholesterol (Lehmann 1996, Qureshi et al 1996).

It has also been clearly shown that consumption of phytosterols or plant sterols significantly reduces plasma cholesterol levels without causing noticeable side effects (Anonymous 1999). Phytosterols are encountered mainly in the unsaponifiable portion of plant oils and are structurally related to cholesterol found in animals (Awad et al 2000). Although structurally related to animal sterols, they are absorbed at a much lower rate (Pegel 1997) but are still found in appreciable amounts within the blood as well as in the breast milk of lactating women (Anonymous 1999).

In amaranth, several potentially important cholesterol-lowering agents have been postulated, including dietary fibers, squalene, tocotrienols, isoprenoid compounds, and other unknown factors (Lehmann 1996). Several of these compounds have been identified and studied, but the possible presence of phytosterols had not been investigated until recently. Therefore, Marcone et al (2001) determined the types, quantities, and varietal differences of phytosterols in amaranth seed.

Table 5 shows the phytosterol content of selected vegetable oils and foods. The most common phytosterols found in higher plants are β-sitosterol, campesterol, and stigmasterol (Awad et al 2000). Analysis of four commonly available amaranth varieties similarly revealed the presence of all three major

TABLE 5
Major Sterols of Selected Foods (μg/100 g)[a]

Food	Total Sterol	β-Sitosterol	Campesterol	Stigmosterol
Vegetable				
Cabbage	11	7	2	...
Carrot	12	7	1	3
Cauliflower	18	12	3	2
Legumes				
Broad bean	124	95	8	9
Kidney bean	127	91	3	31
Pea	135	106	10	10
Fruit				
Apple	12	11	1	...
Peach	10	6	1	3
Pear	8	7	...	...
Nuts				
Almond	143	122	5	3
Cashew	158	130	13	tr[b]
Walnut	108	87	6	...
Vegetable oil				
Coconut	91	53	6	14
Palm	49	30	10	6
Cottonseed	327	303	20	tr
Peanut	206	131	31	19
Olive	176	153	6	2
Soybean	221	123	47	47

[a] Data from Kritchevsky (1997).
[b] Trace.

phytosterols, with total content being significantly higher than those found in other studied plants (Marcone et al 2001). As with vegetables, nuts, and vegetable oils (Table 5), β-sitosterol was the principal phytosterol present in all four amaranth varieties and was significantly higher than the levels found in other plants (Table 6).

Previous research has shown that animal diets supplemented with amaranth oil (source of phytosterols) significantly lowered total serum cholesterol and LDL cholesterol levels while increasing HDL cholesterol (Qureshi et al 1996). This study revealed a lack of a marked inhibition of the HMG-CoA reductase enzyme (the rate-limiting enzyme for cholesterol biosynthesis), which indicated the presence of a potent, lipid-soluble, cholesterol-lowering component other than the commonly accepted active components tocotrienols and squalene. This conclusion was very interesting in light of the present data (Table 6) showing very high levels of phytosterols (i.e., compounds known to induce hypocholesterolemic effects in animals and humans) in the oil portion of amaranth. It is also worth noting that Qureshi et al (1996) also found that the level of cholesterol reduction was affected by the variety of the amaranth tested. This can be explained by the data of Table 6, which show significant differences ($P \leq 0.05$) in total phytosterol and β-sitosterol content between

TABLE 6
Major Sterols Determined in Amaranth Grain (μg/100 g)[a,b]

Amaranth Oil[c]	Total Sterol	β-Sitosterol	Campesterol	Stigmosterol
Amaranthus K343	834 a (±21)	811 a (±20)	9 a (±2)	14 a (±3)
A. RRC1011	543 b (±7)	508 b (±7)	8 a (±3)	27 b (±5)
A. K433	561 c (±8)	531 c (±7)	9 a (±3)	21 c (±4)
A. K432	611 d (±11)	578 b (±10)	9 a (±4)	24 b (±5)

[a] Adapted from Marcone et al (2000).
[b] Values with different letters (within each column) are significantly different ($P = 0.05$).
[c] K343 = *A. hypochondriacus* × *A. hybridus*; K433 = *A. hypochondriacus* × *A. hybridus*; K432 = *A. hypochondriacus* × *A. hybridus*; RRC1011 = *A. cruentus.*

amaranth varieties. *Amaranthus*-K343 had by far the highest levels of phytosterols and is the most commonly cultivated variety within the United States, accounting for 60% of the commercial market.

Future studies should examine the effects of amaranth varieties of known phytosterol content on their ability to lower serum cholesterol in people and establish a definitive link. This may lead to the development of screening for superior amaranth varieties with enhanced ability to lower cholesterol. Antibacterial, anti-inflammatory, and anticancer activities are also reported to be associated with the consumption of phytosterols (Wachter et al 1995, Awad et al 1997, Salvador et al 1997, Anonymous 1999).

Starch

Research into starches with novel properties may lead to applications in foods and nonfood products. Amaranth starch has received attention because of its small and uniform granules with diameters of 1–2 μm (Uriyapongson and Rayas-Duarte 1994, Baker and Rayas-Duarte 1998, Radosavljevic et al 1998) compared to the 3–8 μm of rice starch, the smallest granule of the commercially produced starches. The extremely small starch granules of amaranth provide unique functional properties for food and nonfood applications, including food thickeners, paper coatings, laundry starch, dusting powders, cosmetics, fat replacers, and thickeners in the printing of textiles and biodegradable plastics (Breene 1991, Lehmann 1992, Ahamed et al 1996). Marcone (2000) examined the starch of the threatened *A. pumilus* species compared to the starch of the more common, commercially cultivated *A. hypochondriacus*, grown under the identical controlled-environmental conditions. No significant difference ($P \leq 0.05$) was observed in the total seed starch content (approx. 60%) of these lines, a value within the range reported in the literature for other studied *Amaranthus* species (Uriyapongson and Rayas-Duarte 1994). The proximate composition and starch characteristics of the two lines are shown in Table 7. The starches showed no significant difference ($P \leq 0.05$) in moisture, ash, protein, fat, or color and were comparable to those of other studied *Amaranthus* species (Uriyapongson and Rayas-Duarte 1994). However, *A. pumilus* starch had significantly higher (*P*

TABLE 7
Comparison of the Chemical, Physical, and Thermal Properties of the Isolated Starch and Flour from the Seeds of *Amaranthus hypochondriacus* K343 (Plainsman) and *A. pumilus* (Seabeach amaranth)[a,b]

	A. hypochondriacus (Plainsman)	*A. pumilus* (Seabeach amaranth)
Chemical analysis of starch (%)		
Total starch (in seed)	61.0 a	61.4 a
Moisture	11.1 a	10.3 b
Ash	1.3 a	1.0 a
Protein	0.05 a	0.07 a
Fat	0.87 a	1.1 a
Amylose content of starch	4.17 a	8.20 b
Morphological properties of starch granules		
Starch granule size by SEM (μm)	1.1 a	1.1 a
Starch granule size by light scattering (μm)	1.09 a	1.07 a
Specific surface area (m^2/cm^3)	5.5282 a	5.5977 a
Starch color		
L (color)	93.20 a	93.85 a
a (color)	0.85 a	0.83 a
b (color)	3.07 a	2.97 a
Thermal properties of starch/flour[c]		
To (°C) (starch/flour)	(62.0/64.2) a	(63.4/66.2) b
Tp (°C) (starch/flour)	(70.6/73.2) a	(71.6/74.3) b
Te (°C) (starch/flour)	(78.9/77.5) a	(80.0/82.8) b
ΔH (J/g) (starch/flour)	(13.0/6.6) a	(12.2/6.3) a

[a] Adapted from Marcone et al (2000).
[b] Means followed by the same letter within each row are not significantly different (P = 0.05), $n = 3$.
[c] *To*, *Tp*, and *Te* = onset, peak, and ending temperature, respectively. ΔH = enthalpy change.

≤ 0.05) amylose content (8.2%) compared to *A. hypochondriacus* starch (4.2%) (Table 7). Because low levels of amylose typically found in amaranth starch (as in this study) cause amaranth starch to perform poorly in bread and cake formulations (Stone and Lorenz 1984), the higher levels of amylose of *A. pumilus* starch indicate a potential to improve its performance in the above products.

Scanning electron microscopy (SEM) of *A. pumilus* and *A. hypochondriacus* starch granules showed that both had a uniform average diameter of 1 μm (Fig. 3, Table 7). Integrated laser light scattering analyses confirmed the SEM and showed an average diameter (1.1 μm) with a very narrow size distribution (Table 7). SEM showed that the starch granules were polygonal with smooth surfaces, and there was no evidence of fissures. The smooth granule surfaces of both starch isolates indicate a relatively low level of amylase activity within the seed and resistance to mechanical shear during isolation (Quian and Kuhn 1999). These morphological characteristics are

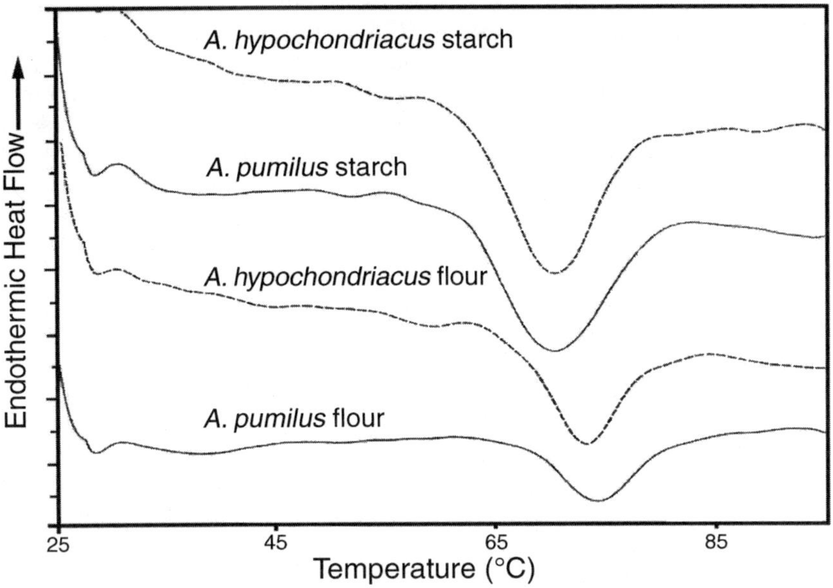

Fig. 3. Differential scanning calorimetric thermograms of starches and flours from *Amaranthus pumilus* and *A. hypochondriacus.*

in agreement with the findings of other investigators (Hoover et al 1998, Radosavljevic et al 1998).

Gelatinization and melting-transition properties of starches were also studied, using differential scanning calorimetry (DSC), and typical curves are shown in Figure 3. The starch and flour of *A. pumilus* seed showed small but significantly higher ($P \leq 0.05$) onset temperatures (*T*o) compared to those of *A. hypochondriacus* starch and flour. This might indicate that *A. pumilus* starch possesses amorphous regions that are thermally and structurally more stable than *A. hypochondriacus* (Leszkowiat 1988) (Table 7). The corresponding peak temperature (*T*p) values were also slightly higher in both *A. pumilus* starch and flour compared to *A. hypochondriacus* samples, suggesting that starch from the former has a greater resistance to gelatinization (Hoover and Sosulski 1985). The significantly higher *T*p of *A. pumilus* starch suggests either a more highly ordered crystalline structure (Hoover and Sosulski 1985) or possibly less amorphous regions. The end temperature (*T*e) is thought to be indicative of the true melting of crystallites undisturbed by amorphous regions (Maurice et al 1985). The significantly higher *T*e of *A. pumilus* would suggest a more stable or more highly ordered crystalline region. The higher content of amylose found in *A. pumilus* starch correlates well with DSC data, since the lower amylose-higher amylopectin content of *A. hypochondriacus* and, therefore, the overall higher degree of chain branching in the starch would disrupt the organization of crystalline regions and decrease the amount of intra- and intermolecular hydrogen bonds required for stability (Biliaderis et al 1985). Despite these temperature differences, no significant difference ($P \leq 0.05$) between the enthalpy of gelatinization of *A. pumilus* flour or starch and that of *A. hypochondriacus* flour was noted. Starch interactions with other seed components may affect the overall properties of the starch when used as part of a whole grain formulation. Although further studies of starch properties are needed, it is clear that *A. pumilus* may have benefit in breeding programs.

Novel Amaranth Species for the Amelioration of Currently Cultivated Amaranth

Although considerable genetic variation is available within the species (Chan and Sun 1997), a few wild species, including *A. brownii* and *A. pumilus*, are quickly being extirpated from their native habitats, potentially reducing the biodiversity available to plant breeders for improving amaranth cultivars (Weakley et al 1996). Many of the species that are presently disappearing are those that possess desirable genetic traits such as ability to grow in arid or high-saline environments.

Currently, a pressing global challenge is to find adequate amounts of water and agricultural land to support the world's increasing food requirements. Studies conducted by the United Nations Food and Agriculture Organization (FAO) conservatively estimate that an additional 200 million hectares of agricultural land will be required over the next 30 years just to keep pace with feeding the world's growing population at current levels. Unfortunately, compounding this problem is present irrigation rates and practices that are significantly increasing soil salinity, in turn resulting in reduced crop yield. Lu et al (2000) estimated that, in the United States alone, more than 20 million hectares annually of crop and pastureland is being affected by salinity, resulting in an estimated crop yield loss of approximately 9%. Globally this problem becomes more prevalent as more and more land is claimed and irrigated for agricultural production. Ultimately, soil salinity increases. Approximately 130 million hectares (of the required 200) have the potential for cultivation, provided that an appropriate halophytic food crop becomes available. Of the 130 million ha presently available, about 50 million hectares are in tropical coastal deserts that have easy accessibility to seawater irrigation. In this context, several salt-tolerant, wild (halophytic) plants have been screened for their potential use for future human or animal consumption, and wild halophytes with the requisite salt tolerance have been identified for their high biomass or seed yields under seawater or standard irrigation practices (Glenn et al 1991, 1997). One of the promising halophytes identified is *A. pumilus*.

A. pumilus (seabeach amaranth) is a halophyte with no apparent close relatives, is an annual endemic to the barrier island beaches of the Atlantic coast, and is historically recorded in 31 counties in nine states from Massachusetts to South Carolina (Weakley et al 1996) (Fig. 1). Over the past decade, the species has been completely extirpated from six of the nine states of its original range. By 1993, with fewer than 55 remaining populations left in the wild (or approximately 1,000 individuals known), this plant species was given a global rank of G2, or "globally imperiled" and received federal protection as a threatened plant under the United States Endangered Species Act (Weakley et al 1996). By all current accounts, the most recent hurricanes of 1999 (Dennis and Floyd) have almost completely destroyed all remaining populations and put the survival of the species in imminent danger.

If not driven to extinction, the seabeach amaranth may potentially serve as a useful plant resource in future breeding programs. Favorable genetic traits include its tolerance to high soil salinity and ability to grow in poor soil containing nearly pure silica sand substrate; these factors may expand the geographic range for the cultivation of amaranth grain (U.S. Fish and Wildlife Service 1996). Other useful characteristics include the ability to reduce wind-induced erosion, and large seed size (the largest of all studied amaranth species), which should make harvesting easier and permit more biomass production (Weakley et al 1996).

In consideration of the imminent danger posed to the survival of the seabeach amaranth in its native environment and the almost complete lack of any scientific literature about the species, Marcone (2000) studied the chemical components and composition of its seed compared to the more commonly cultivated *A. hypochondriacus.*

Characterization of *Amaranthus pumilus*

Physical characterization of the seeds of *A. hypochondriacus* (AH) and *A. pumilus* (AP) showed major differences between them in shape, size, and overall color (Table 8, Fig. 1). AP seeds were larger than AH (by 1.6-fold) and possessed more of an elongated lenticular shape than those of AH (Fig. 1C and D). These observed morphological differences were reflected in the almost threefold higher seed weight of AP, making these the largest amaranth seed ever studied and therefore of potentially valuable higher biomass content. AP seeds were sufficiently darker (lower L^* values) and more reddish brown than those of AH. Although pale-colored seeds are generally more desirable for food use (Lehman 1996), examination of AP seed meal revealed that the darker pigment was confined to the seed coat, and the overall meal color was substantially lighter.

The total carbohydrate content of AP and AH seeds was similar and was the major component (Table 8). There were significant differences in the content of sucrose, glucose, and fructose. The levels of sucrose found in AP were more consistent with those normally reported in common cereals such as wheat, rye, and millet (Saunders and Becker 1984); the amount of total soluble sugar found in AH fell within the range reported for 63 accessions of amaranth (Saunders and Becker 1984).

The total mineral (ash) content in both species was higher than in conventional grains, and AP was lower than AH, as previously reported (Saunders and Becker 1984). This result is consistent with the larger seed size of AP, which would lead to more endo- and perisperm and less seed coat and bran,

TABLE 8
Compositional Analysis of the Seeds of *Amaranthus hypochondriacus* K343 (AH) and *Amaranthus pumilus* (Seabeach amaranth) (AP)[a,b]

	AH	AP		AH	AP
Proximate analysis (%)[c]			Triacylglycerol (%)		
Moisture	7.30 a	11.60 b	Mono-, diglycerides	1.16	...
Ash	3.32 a	2.10 b	Ln Ln Ln	...	...
Protein	17.90 a	10.22 b	L L L	8.26 a	14.18 b
Fat	7.87 a	12.73 b	OLL + OOLn	13.43 a	26.81 b
Carbohydrate (by difference)	63.61 a	63.35 a	PLL + PLnO	21.40 a	12.20 b
Seed characteristics			OOL + PoOO	10.35 a	18.42 b
Color			POL	17.78 a	11.51 b
L (seed/seed meal)	66.57 a/83.02 b	25.57 c/61.35 d	PPL + MPO	10.46 a	2.59 b
a (seed/seed meal)	5.79 a/1.71 b	4.34 a/2.42 c	OOO + MSO + OOP + PSL + POP	11.45 a	12.97 a
b (seed/seed meal)	27.25 a/15.99 b	2.41 c/10.90 d	PPO + PPP + OOS + POS + SOS + SSO	5.77 a	1.31 b
Average seed weight (mg)	0.8 a	2.1 b	LM/MM (low melting/medium melting)	4.80 a	6.00 b
Average seed size (mm)	1.2 a	1.9 b	Squalene (% in oil)		
Mineral (ppm)			Squalene	9.26 a	10.34 b
Phosphorous (P)	1,700 a	4,500 b	Squalene (% in seed)	0.73 a	1.32 b
Potassium (K)	6,720 a	4,340 b	Tocopherols (μg/g seed)		
Calcium (Ca)	3,270 a	2,250 b	α-Tocopherol	18.37 a	34.95 b
Magnesium (Mg)	3,000 a	1,450 b	β-Tocopherol	32.90 a	65.43 b
Iron (Fe)	65.1 a	241 b	γ-Tocopherol	9.18 a	22.05 b
Free carbohydrate (%)			Total tocopherol (per g of seed)	60.45 a	122.43 b
Fructose	0.05 a	0.01 b	Protein (%)		
Glucose	0.76 a	0.05 b	Albumins	17.73 a	22.08 b
Sucrose	1.63 a	0.69 b	Globulin	29.58 a	20.10 b
Fatty acid (%)			Prolamines	1.20 a	1.60 a
Palmitic (C16:0)	21.26 a	9.12 b	Glutelins (contains globulin fraction)	51.49 a	56.21 a
Palmitoleic (C16:1)	4.11 a	1.41 b	Nitrogen Solubility Index (%)	26.06 a	29.26 b
Stearic (C18:0)	3.39 a	1.96 b	Globulin/albumin ratio	1.67 a	0.91 b
Oleic (C18:1)	22.70 a	31.48 b	Trypsin inhibitor activity/mg		
Linoleic (C18:2)	40.83 a	48.31 b	TUI/mg	3.5 a	3.6 a
Linolenic (C18:3)	7.72 a	7.71 a			
Saturated/unsaturated (S/U)	0.327 a	0.125 b			

[a] Adapted from Marcone et al (2000).
[b] Means followed by the same letter within each row are not significantly different ($P = 0.05$).
[c] On dry seed weight basis.

where higher levels of minerals are usually located. Both AP and AH are much richer sources of phosphorus, potassium, calcium, magnesium, and iron than the more common cereal grains (Saunders and Becker 1984); AP was found to be a much richer (3.7 and 2.6 times) source of iron and phosphorus, respectively, compared to AH.

The second most abundant component of each seed meal was protein, but AH had a significantly higher level than AP (Table 8). Differences were also noted in the composition of the total seed proteins as evidenced by a slight difference in the electrophoretic fingerprint patterns of their respective total seed proteins. To determine the types and quantities of proteins responsible for those observed differences, a modified Osborne protein fractionation scheme was employed to classify them in terms of selective solubility in various types of solvents, following defatting. Aqueous soluble proteins (i.e., albumins and globulins) were extracted together from each seed meal; AH had a slightly higher level (47.3%) of this fraction than AP (42.2%). Further separation of these proteins by dialysis revealed significant differences in the globulin-to-albumin ratios. Electrophoretic fingerprinting of crude albumin and globulin fractions separately showed that the differences in the total seed proteins resulted from differences in the composition in both the albumin and globulin fractions. The next sequential extraction of the seed meals of each species with organic solvents revealed extremely low levels of prolaminlike proteins. Although the final extraction with alkali, for glutelins, indicated very high levels of this type of protein, examination of the electrophoretic patterns revealed considerable contamination with globulins. Extraction of salt-soluble proteins (globulins) from various plant sources have been reported to be substantially reduced when the meal is defatted before extraction (Byers et al 1983, Fu and Sapirstein 1996) and the residual globulins appear in the glutelin fraction. Therefore, the 47.31 and 42.12% total albumin plus globulin for AH and AP, respectively, may be underestimations, and amounts may be as high as 85% (Fu and Sapirstein 1996). Despite this, a few unique subunit bands were distinctly visible in the glutelin fraction from each species, and differences were also observable in these bands between the species, indicating additional differences in the types of glutelinlike proteins in each. Slight differences were also observed in the amino acid compositions of total seed proteins between species (particularly in the globulin fraction), but the overall amino acid composition (Table 9) was comparable to that observed for other amaranth species (Saunders and Becker 1984).

There was no difference in trypsin inhibitor activities between species, with values well below those known to affect weight gain in laboratory animals. A value of 104.7 trypsin inhibitor unit/mg (TIU/mg) was noted for a raw soybean reference sample, well within expected values.

AP was not only substantially higher in crude fat content than AH (Table 8), but was also substantially higher (by 29%) than 21 *amaranthus* accessions as reported by Budin et al (1996). Differences were also observed in the fatty acid composition of AP and AH, and those of the 21 *amaranthus* species studied by Budin et al (1996). AP was significantly lower in saturated fatty acids such as palmitic (C16:0) and stearic (C18:0), but significantly higher in mono- and polyunsaturates such as oleic (C18:1) and linoleic (C18:2) (Table 8). These differences resulted in a much lower S/U ratio in AP than in AH, or in the other studied species (Budin et al 1996) and indicates that AP is potentially a nutritionally better source of oil. Although fatty acid compositions and ratios are important indicators in determining whether an oil is edible and has nutritional and functional value, these are not the sole indicators for comparing oil qualities, and therefore oils were further analyzed for TAG composition. Major differences were observed in the position of fatty acids in the triacylglycerol backbone between AP and AH, as indicated by differences in the amounts of LLL, 00Ln, and PLn0 (Table 8). The differences in the distribution of low-melting (LM) and medium-melting (MM) TAGS in each species leads to differences in their LM/MM ratios, which ultimately determines the oil's thermal behavior, stable polymorphism when crystallized, and functional properties. Although the lipid composition of AP may suggest a nutritionally superior oil, the higher LM/MM ratio would result in an overall lower melting range, oxidative stability, and functionality if a plastic fat is required.

Further analysis of the lipid material from both species revealed that AP was substantially higher in both vitamin E and squalene. Both species contained α-, β-, and γ-tocopherols, but AP contained more of each, with twice the total tocopherol content (Table 8). The total tocopherol content of AP is the highest in amaranth species studied to date (Budin et al 1996). Although

TABLE 9
Amino Acid Composition of the Seeds and Globulin Fractions of *Amaranthus hypochondriacus* K343 and *A. pumilus* (Seabeach amaranth)

	***A. hypochondriacus* K343**		***A. pumilus* (Seabeach amaranth)**	
	Whole Seed	**Globulin**	**Whole Seed**	**Globulin**
Aspartic + asparagine	8.1	7.8	9.6	8.2
Threonine	3.4	2.9	4.0	2.8
Serine	8.3	5.6	7.1	5.7
Glutamic + glutamine	17.3	20.9	16.5	23.3
Glycine	14.0	9.8	11.0	9.4
Alanine	7.2	5.8	7.3	6.3
Valine	5.1	5.2	6.2	4.8
Methionine	2.0	3.3	2.3	2.7
Isoleucine	3.5	4.0	4.3	3.4
Leucine	5.8	6.3	7.0	5.6
Tyrosine	2.6	3.3	2.6	3.0
Phenylalanine	4.0	5.2	4.9	4.8
Lysine	7.8	7.1	7.0	6.8
Histidine	3.5	3.8	3.6	3.1
Arginine	7.4	9.0	6.5	10.2

the low S/U and high LM/MM TAGS ratios of AP oil would indicate a lower oxidative stability compared to AH, the higher content of tocopherols should help stabilize the oil against oxidation during heating. AP was also higher (10.3%) in squalene content than AH (9.3%) and the other amaranth varieties (6–8%) (Sun et al 1997). In light of the importance and high demand for squalene in cosmetics and skin penetrates and as an oxidation-resistant industrial lubricant and the concern for marine animal protection (the primary industrial source of squalene), AP may one day serve as a valuable source of this compound.

In conclusion, the genetic diversity described here between AP and AH indicates that breeding improvements into commonly cultivated amaranth lines exist. *A. pumilus* offers a much larger and more desirable seed size and weight for improved biomass production. In addition to the higher edible oil content found in *A. pumilus*, its lower S/U ratio—one of the lowest measured so far—makes it a potentially better source of oil nutritionally. Differences in both fatty acid and triacylglycerol composition offer great potential for *A. pumilus* use in breeding programs for the manipulation of oil composition for various food end uses. Further added value may be realized from the higher level of vitamin E and squalene.

Conclusion

Amaranth's resurgence today as a food crop can be ascribed to its C_4 photosynthetic metabolic capacity, which endows it with a number of agronomic attributes, including environmental hardiness and a capacity for efficient water utilization, qualities essential for a plant to successfully compete for the limited farmable lands and diminishing water supplies experienced worldwide. In addition, the successful development of grain amaranth as a new field crop has been aided by the great deal of genetic variation available within the cultivated species, which has allowed the development of early-maturing, high-yielding lines, insect resistance, reduced seed scattering, and light-colored seed. More recent studies have also shown that the genetic diversity in these lines is expressed in varied levels of components, including protein types, lipid, squalene, and lipid-soluble compounds. All of these components could have value to particular industrial, nutraceutical, and pharmaceutical end uses. Exploitation of the available genetic diversity could lead to improved varieties tailor-made for specific uses and applications.

References

Ahamed, N. T., Singhal, R. S., Kulkarni, P. R., Kale, D. D., and Pal, M. 1996. Studies on *Chenopodium quinoa* and *Amaranthus paniculatas* starch as biodegradable filters in LDPE films. Carbohydr. Polym. 31:157-160.

Amaranth Institute. 1990. Proceedings of the Fourth National Amaranth Symposium: Perspectives on Production Processing and Marketing. University of Minnesota Extension, St. Paul, MN.

Anonymous. 1999. Phytosterols. Crit. Rev. Food Sci. Nutr. 39:275-283.

Awad, A. B., Garcia, M. D., and Fink, C. S. 1997. Effect of dietary phytosterols on rat tissue lipid. Nutr. Cancer 29:212-216.

Awad, A. B., Chan, K. C., Downie, A. C., and Fink, C. S. 2000. Peanuts as a source of β-sitosterol, a sterol with anticancer properties. Nutr. Cancer 36:238-241.

Baker, L. A., and Rayas-Duarte, P. 1998. Retrogradation of amaranth starch at different storage temperatures and the effects of salts and sugars. Cereal Chem. 75:308-314.

Bejosano, F. P., and Corke, H. 1998. Protein quality evaluation of *Amaranthus* wholemeal flours and protein concentrates. J. Sci. Food Agric. 76:100-106.

Berghofer, E., and Schoenlechner, R. 2002. Grain amaranth. Pages 12-16 in: Pseudocereals and Less Common Cereals—Grain Properties and Utilization Potential. P. S. Belton and P. S. Taylor, Eds. Springer, New York.

Biliaderis, C. G., Page, C. M., Slade, L., and Sirett, R. R. 1985. Thermal behaviour of amylose-lipid complexes. Carbohydr. Polym. 5:367-389.

Bondioli, P., Mariana, C., Lanzani, A., Fedeli, E., and Muller, A. 1993. Squalene recovery from olive oil deodorizer distillates. J. Am. Oil Chem. Soc. 70:763-766.

Breene, W. M. 1991. Food uses for grain amaranth. Cereal Foods World 36:426-430.

Bressani, R. 1989. The proteins of grain amaranth. Food Rev. Int. 5:13-38.

Budin J. T., Breene, W. M., and Putnam, D. H. 1996. Some compositional properties of seeds and oils of eight *Amaranthus* species. J. Am. Oil Chem. Soc. 73:475-481.

Byers, M., Miflin, B. J., and Smith, S. J. 1983. A quantitative comparison of the extraction of protein fractions from wheat grain by different solvents and of polypeptide and amino acid composition of alcohol-soluble proteins. J. Sci. Food Agric. 34:447-467.

Chan, K. F., and Sun, M. 1997. Genetic diversity and relationships detected by isozyme and rapid analysis of crop and wild species of Amaranthus. Theor. Appl. Genet. 95:865-873.

Chanturvedi, A., Sarojini, G., Nirmala, G., Nirmalammay, N., and Satyanarayana, D. 1997. Glycemic index of amaranth grain, wheat and rice in NIDDM subjects. Plant Foods Hum. Nutr. 50:171-178.

Coimbra, S., and Salema, R. 1994. *Amaranthus hyochondriacus*: Seed structure and localization of seed reserves. Ann. Bot. 74:373-379.

Derbyshire, E., Wright, D. J., and Boulter, D. 1976. Legumin and vicilin, storage proteins of legume seeds. Phytochemistry 15:3-24.

Dunz, R. A., and Lupton, J. R. 1992. Physiological effects of dietary amaranth (*Amaranthus cruentus*) on rats. 1997. Cereal Foods World 37:489.

Fadel, J. G., Pond, W. G., Harrold, R. L., Cavert, C. C., and Lewis, B. A. 1996. Nutritive value of three amaranth grains fed either processed or raw to growing rats. Can. J. Anim. Sci. 76:253-257.

Fu, B. X., and Sapirstein, H. D. 1996. Procedure for the isolating monomeric protein and polymoric glutellin of wheat flour. Cereal Chem. 73:143-152.

Glenn, E., O'Leary, J., Watson, M., Tompson, T. L., and Kuehl, R. 1991. *Salicornia bigelovii* Torr. with seawater-irrigation on sand in a coastal desert environment. Science 251:1065-1067.

Glenn, E., Miyamoto, S., Moore, D., Brown, J. J., Thompson, T. T., and Brown, P. 1997. Water requirements for cultivating *Salicernia Bigelovii* Torr with seawater on sand in a coastal desert environment. J. Arid Environ. 36:711-730.

Hoover, R., and Sosulski, F. 1985. Studies on the functional characteristics and digestibility of starches from *Phaseolus vulgaris* biotypes. Starch/Stærke 37:181-191.

Hoover, R., Sinnott, W., and Perera, C. 1998. Physicochemical characterization of starches from *Amaranthus cruentus* grains. Starch/Stærke 50:456-463.

Hughes, S. A., and Murphy, P. A. 1983. Varietal influence on the quantity of glycinin in soybeans. J. Agric. Chem. 31:376-379.

Kang, I., Matsumura, Y., and Mori, T. 1994. Characterization of texture and mechanical properties of heat induced soy protein gels. J. Am. Oil Chem. Soc. 68:339-345.

Kigerl, J. 1994. Development of ecophysiology of amaranthus. Pages 39-73 in: Amaranth Biology, Chemistry and Technology. O. Paredes-Lopez, Ed. CRC Press, Boca Raton, FL.

Kitamura, K. 1995. Genetic improvement of nutritional and food processing quality in soybean. JARQ 29:1-8.

Kritchevsky, D. 1997. Phytosterols. Adv. Exp. Med. Biol. 427:235-243.

Lambert, N., and Yarwood, J. N. 1992. Engineering legume seed storage proteins. Pages 167-187 in: Plant Protein Engineering. P. R. Shewry and S. Guteridge, Eds. Cambridge University Press, London, UK.

Lehmann, J. W. 1996. Case history of grain amaranth as an alternative crop. Cereal Foods World 41:399-403, 406-441.

Lehmann, J. W. 1992. Grain amaranth: Developing 21st century product from the legendary sister crop of maize. Int. Food Ingred. 3:26-35.

Leszkowiat, M. J. 1988. Biochemical-physical characteristics and processing quality of field and storage type potatoes. M.S. thesis, University of Guelph, Ontario, Canada.

Lu, Z., Glenn, E. P., and John, M. M. 2000. *Saliconia Biyelovii*, an overview. Inform. 11:418-423.

Lyon, C. K., and Becker, R. 1987. Extraction and refining of oil from amaranth seed. J. Am. Oil Chem. Soc. 64:233.

Ma, C. Y., Buzzell, R. I., Jessop, D. B., and Buttery, B. R. 1996. Technical Bulletin: The Expert Newsletter Technical Bulletin by the Ontario Soybean Growers' Marketing Board 1:1-2.

Maier, S. M., Turner, N. D., and Lupton, J. R. 2000. Serum lipid in hypercholesterolemic men and women consuming oat bran and amaranth product. Cereal Chem. 77:297-302.

Marcone, M. F. 1999. First report of the characterization of the threatened plant species *Amaranthus pumilus* (seabeach amaranth). J. Agric. Food Chem. 48:378-382.

Marcone, M. F. 2000. Starch properties of *Amaranthus pumilus* (seabeach amaranth): A threatened plant species with potential benefits for the breeding/amelioration of present *Amaranthus* cultivars. Food Chem. 73:61-66.

Marcone, M. F., and Yada, R. Y. 1998. Structural analysis of globulin isolated from genetically different *Amaranthus* hybrid lines. Food Chem. 61:319-326.

Marcone, M. F., Jahaniaval, F., and Kakuda, Y. 2000. Fatty acid and triacylglycerol compositions of seed oils of five *Amaranthus* accessions and their comparison to other oils. J. Am. Oil Chem. Soc. 77:847-852.

Marcone, M. F., Kakuda, Y., and Yada, R. Y. 2001. Amaranth as a rich dietary source of β-sitosterol and other phytosterols. Plant Foods Hum. Nutr. 2:1-6.

Maurice, T. J., Slade, L., Sinett, R. R., and Page, C. M. 1985. Polysaccharide-water interactions. Thermal behavior of rice starch. Pages 211-227 in: Properties of Water in Foods. D. Simatos and J. L. Multon, Eds. Martinus Nijhoff Publishers, Dordrecht, Holland.

Mendoza, C. M., and Bressani, R. 1987. Nutritional and functional characteristics of extrusion-cooked amaranth flour. Cereal Chem. 64:218-222.

Moghadasian, M. H., and Frohlich, J. J. 1999 Effects of dietary phytosterols on cholesterol metabolism and atherosclerosis: Clinical and experimental evidence. Am. J. Med. 107: 588-596.

Mori, T., Nakamura, T., and Utsumi, S. 1982. Formation of pseudoglycinins and their gel hardness. J. Agric Food Chem. 30:828-831.

Mori, T., Utsumi, S., Inaba, H., Kitamura, K., and Harada, K. 1981. Differences in subunit composition of glycinin among soybean cultivars. J. Agric. Food Chem. 29:20-23.

Murphy, P. A., Chen, H-P., Hauck, C., and Wilson, L.A. 1997. Soybean protein composition and tofu quality. Food Technol. 51(3):86-88.

Nakamura, T., Utsumi, K., Kitamura, K., Harada, K., and Mori, T. 1984. Cultivar differences in gelling characteristics of soybean glycinin. J. Agric. Food Chem. 32:647-650.

Nakamura, T., Utsumi, K., and Mori, T. 1985. Formation of pseudoglycinins from intermediary subunits of glycinin and their gel properties and network structure. J. Agric. Biol. Chem. 49:2733-2740.

Nishinari, K., Kohyama, K., Zlang, Y., Kitamura, K., Sugimoto, T., Saio, K., and Kawamura, Y. 1991. Rheological study on the effect of the subunit on the gelation characteristics of soybean proteins. J. Agric. Biol. Chem. 55:351-355.

Payne, P. I., Carfield, K. G., and Blackman, J. A. 1979. Wheat proteins. Theor. Appl. Genet. 55:153-156.

Pazdernik, D. L., Plehn, S. J., Halgerson, J. L., and Orf, J. H. 1996. Effect of temperature and genotype on the crude glycinin fraction (11S) of soybean and its analysis by near-infrared reflectance spectroscopy (near-IRS). J. Agric. Food Chem. 44:2278-2281.

Pegel, K. H. 1997 The importance of sitosterol and sitosterolin in human and animal nutrition. S. Afr. J. Sci. 93:263-268.

Przybylski, R., Chauhan, G. S., and Esin, N. A. M. 1994. Characterization of quinoa (*Chenopedium quinoa*) lipids. Food Chem. 51:187-192.

Quian, J. Y., and Kuhn, M. 1999. Characterization of *Amaranthus cruentus* and *Chenopodium quinoa* starch. Starch/Starke 51:116-120.

Qureshi, A. A., Lehmann, J. W., and Peterson, D. M. 1996. Amaranth and its oil inhibit cholesterol biosynthesis in 6-week-old female chickens. J. Nutr. 126:1972-1977.

Radosavljevic, M., Jane, J., and Johnson, I. A. 1998. Isolation of amaranth starch by diluted alkaline-protease treatment. Cereal Chem. 75:571-577.

Salvador, M. J., Ito, I. Y., and Dians, D. A. 1997. Evaluation of the antibacterial activity of crude extracts and sterols (stigmasterol, β-sitosterol and campesterol) from *Alternathera maritima*. Bol. Chim. Farma. 138:66.

Sanchez-Marroquin, 1984. Amaranth as an enriching product in staple foods. Pages 20-45 in: Proceedings of the Third Amaranth Conference: Grain Amaranth: Expanding Consumption Through Improved Cropping, Marketing and Crop Development. Rodale Press, Emmaus, PA.

Saunders, R. M., and Becker, R. 1984. *Amaranthus*: A potential food and feed resource. Pages 357-396 in: Advances in Cereal Science and Technology, Vol. 6. Y. Pomeranz, Ed. Am. Assoc. Cereal Chem., St. Paul, MN.

Shewry, P. R., and Miflin, B. J. 1985. Seed storage proteins of economically important cereals. Pages 1-83 in: Advances in Cereal Science and Technology, Vol. 7. Y. Pomeranz, Ed. Am. Assoc. Cereal Chem., St. Paul, MN.

Stone, L. A., and Lorenz, K. 1984. The starch of amaranthus-physico-chemical properties of functional characteristics. Starch/Stærke 36:232-237.

Sun, H., Wiesenborn, D., Rayas-Duarte, P., Mohamed, A., and Hagen, K. 1995. Bench-scale processing of amaranth seed for oil. J. Am. Oil Chem. Soc. 72:1551-1555.

Sun, H., Wiesenborn, D., Tostenson, K., Gillespie, J., and Rayas-Duarte, P. 1997. Fractionation of squalene from amaranth seed oil. J. Am. Oil Chem. Soc. 74:413-418.

Uriyapongson, J., and Rayas-Duarte, P. 1994. Comparison of yield and properties of amaranth starches using wet and dry-wet milling processes. Cereal Chem. 71:571-577.

U.S. Fish and Wildlife Service. Seabeach Amaranth Species Fact Sheet, 1996. U.S. Fish Wildlife Serv., Cortland, NY. pp. 1-2.

Wachter, R., Salka, B., and Magnet, A. 1995. Phytosterol. Cosmet. Toiletries 110:72-82.

Weakley, A., Bucher, M., and Murdock, N. 1996. Recovery plan for seabeach amaranth (*Amaranthus pumilus*). (Technical release.) U.S. Fish Wildlife Serv., Southeast Region, Atlanta, GA.

CHAPTER 14

Buckwheat as a Food and Feed

G. Mazza and B. Dave Oomah

Agriculture and Agri-Food Canada, Pacific Agri-Food Research Centre, Summerland, British Columbia, Canada V0H 1Z0

Buckwheat is a crop commonly grown for its black or gray triangular seeds. It can also be grown as a green manure crop, a companion crop, a cover crop, a source of buckwheat honey, and as a pharmaceutical plant yielding rutin. Buckwheat belongs to the Polygonaceae family and is not a true cereal. However, like cereals such as wheat, corn, and rice, which belong to the grass family, the grain of buckwheat is a dry fruit.

Buckwheat is believed to have originated in central and northeastern Asia and was probably cultivated in China during the fifth and sixth centuries. It was introduced into Europe through Turkey and Russia during the fourteenth and fifteenth centuries and into North America in the seventeenth century (Marshall and Pomeranz 1982, Mazza 2000). World production of buckwheat peaked in the early nineteenth century and has declined since then. During the past five years, it has averaged about 3 million metric tons, with China and the former Soviet Union accounting for 58 and 34% of the global production, respectively. Other major producing countries are Brazil, Poland, the United States, Japan, Canada, France, Bhutan, the Republic of Korea, and South Africa.

Types and Cultivars

Although the genus *Fagopyrum* contains at least 15 species of buckwheat, only two are utilized as food or feed, and wild buckwheat (*Fagopyrum cymosum*), mainly found as tetraploid, is used sporadically as a green vegetable or as cattle forage. There are three major species of buckwheat: common buckwheat, *F. esculentum*; tartary buckwheat, *F. tataricum*; and perennial buckwheat, *F. cymosum*. Common buckwheat is also known as *F. saggitatum,* and a form of tartary buckwheat may be called *F. kashmirianum*. However, perennial buckwheat, particularly the diploid type, is generally believed to be the ancestral form of both tartary and common buckwheat (Marshall and Pomeranz 1982).

Tartary buckwheat is cultivated in the Himalayan region of India and China, in eastern Canada, and occasionally in mountain areas of the eastern

United States. It has some frost tolerance and is therefore grown at higher altitudes, where risk of frost damage is greater. The seeds and products made from them are greenish and somewhat bitter. Tartary buckwheat is used primarily as feed or as a mixture of wheat and buckwheat flour and is often used as a source of rutin.

Common buckwheat is by far the most economically important species of buckwheat, accounting for more than 90% of the world production. Many types, strains, and cultivars of common buckwheat exist. There are late- and early-maturing types, Japanese and European types, and summer and fall types. Within a given type, there may be strains or varieties with tall or short plants, gray or black seeds, and white or pink flowers. In general, however, common buckwheat varieties from different parts of the world may be divided into two major groups. The first group includes tall, vigorous, late-maturing, photoperiod-sensitive varieties found in Japan, Korea, southern China, Nepal, and India. The second group is rather insensitive to photoperiod and is small and early maturing. All of the varieties in Europe and northern China belong to this type.

Before 1950, producers of buckwheat planted unnamed strains of buckwheat harvested from their own fields or obtained from their neighbors or local stores. Named varieties developed through plant breeding were first released in the 1950s. Tokyo, the oldest of the named cultivars introduced into North America, was licensed by Agriculture and Agri-Food Canada, Ottawa, in 1955. Other cultivars licensed for production in Canada are Tempest, Mancan, and Manor, all developed at Agriculture and Agri-Food Canada, Morden, Manitoba, since 1965. Mancan, which has large, dark brown seeds, thick stems, and large leaves, is the Canadian cultivar preferred in the Japanese market because of its large seed, desirable flavor and color, and high yield of groats in the milling process. Recently, these older cultivars have been supplanted by newer cultivars such as AC Manisoba, Koban, and Koto. These new cultivars produce larger seeds and have an increased seed yield.

Cultivars licensed in the United States are Pennquad, released by the Pennsylvania Agricultural Experimental Station and the USDA in 1968, and Giant American, a Japanese-type cultivar apparently selected by a Minnesota farmer.

Cultivars developed in the USSR since the 1950s include Victoria, Galleya, Eneida, Podolyaka, Diadema, Aelita, and Aestoria. Representative cultivars from other areas of the world include Pulawska, Emka, and Hruszowska from Poland; Bednja 4n from Yugoslavia; and Botan-Soba, Shinano No. 1, Kyushu-Akisoba Shinshu, and Miyazaki Oosoba from Japan.

Plant and Seed Morphology and Microstructure

Buckwheat is a broad-leaved, erect, herbaceous plant that grows to a height of 0.70–1.5 m. It has a main stem and several branches and can reach full maturity in fewer than 90 days. The stem is usually grooved, succulent, and hollow, except for the nodes. Before maturity, the stems and branches are green to red and turn brown after maturity. The plant has a shallow taproot from which branched, lateral roots arise. Its root system is less extensive than that of cereals and constitutes only 3–4% of the dry weight of the total plant.

Buckwheat has an indeterminate flowering habit, with perfect but incomplete flowers. They have no petals, but the calyx is composed of five petal-like sepals that are usually white but may also be pink or red. The flowers are arranged in dense clusters at the ends of branches or on short pedicels arising from the axils of the leaves. Common buckwheat has plants bearing one of two types of flowers. The pin-type flower has long styles, or female parts, and short stamens, or male parts, and the thrum-type has long styles and short pistils. The pistil consists of a one-celled superior ovary and a three-part style with knoblike stigmas and is surrounded by eight stamens. Nectar-secreting glands are located at the base of the ovary. The plants of common buckwheat are generally self-infertile, as self-fertilization is prevented by self-incompatibility. Seed production is usually dependant on cross-pollination between the pin and thrum flowers. Honeybees and leaf-cutter bees are effective pollinators. They increase seed set and seed yield.

The buckwheat kernel is a triangular, dry fruit (achene) 4–9 mm long, consisting of a hull or pericarp, spermoderm, endosperm, and embryo. Large seeds tend to be concave-sided, and small seeds are usually convex-sided. The hull may be glossy, gray, brown, or black, and it may be solid or mottled. It may be either smooth or rough with lateral furrows. The hulls represent 17–26% (in tartary buckwheat 30–35%) of the kernel weight. Diploid varieties usually have less hull than tetraploids.

Scanning electron microscopy of the buckwheat kernel has revealed that the hull, spermoderm, endosperm, and embryo are each composed of several layers. For the hull, these are, in order from the outside toward the inside, epicarp, fiber layers, parenchyma cells, and endocarp. The spermoderm is composed of the outer epiderm, the spongy parenchyma, and the inner epiderm. The endosperm is composed of an aleurone layer 10–5 μm thick, and subaleurone endosperm containing starch granules surrounded by proteinaceous matrix. The embryo, with its two cotyledons, extends through the starchy endosperm. The terminal parts of cotyledons are often parallel under the kernel surface (Pomeranz 1983).

Grading, Handling, and Storage

Grading

In most countries, buckwheat grain is priced according to its physical condition in terms of size, soundness, and general appearance. In Canada, buckwheat is marketed according to grades established under the Canada Grain Act. Grades are No. 1, No. 2, and No. 3 Canada, and Sample. Grade determinants are minimum test weight, degree of soundness, and maximum limits of foreign material (Table 1). Grades No. 1 and 2 Canada must be free from objectionable odors; No. 3 Canada may have a ground or grassy odor but should not be musty or sour. Test weight, seed size, and foreign material are determined on a dock-

TABLE 1
Primary Grade Determinants of Buckwheat (Canada)

Grade	Minimum Seed Density (kg hl^{-1})	Degree of Soundness	Maximum Limits of Foreign Material (%)				
			Stones[a]	Ergot	*Sclerotinia*	Cereal Grains	Total Foreign Material
No. 1	58	Well matured, cool and sweet	3.0	0.0	0.0	1.0	1.0
No. 2	55	Reasonably well matured, cool and sweet	3.0	0.05	0.05	2.5	3.0
No. 3	None	May have a ground or grassy odor, but shall not be musty or sour	3.0	0.25	0.25	5.0	5.0

[a] Number of kernel-size stones in 500 g.

age-free sample. Seed size is determined with a No. 8 slotted sieve (3.18 × 19.05 mm) and is added to and becomes part of the grade name (e.g., buckwheat, No. 1 Canada large). Foreign material refers to cereal grains (wheat, rye, barley, oats, and triticale), weed seeds, and other grains that are not readily removable by mechanical cleaners and may include peas, beans, corn, and other domestic or wild weeds. Samples containing in excess of 5% are graded buckwheat, sample Canada (size) account admixture. Damaged seeds include frosted, moldy, distinctly green, or otherwise unsound and dehulled seeds.

In the United States, buckwheat is not marketed under official grades established by the USDA. However, some states (e.g., Minnesota) have Official Grain Standards that specify the use of Grades 1, 2, 3 and Sample. The grade determinants are similar to those of the Canadian grading system. The Soviet standards for food buckwheat are moisture ≤14.5%, extraneous matter ≤3% (including 0.2% mineral admixture of which 0.1% may be stones), pernicious admixtures ≤0.2%, and spoiled grain ≤0.5%. The Japanese Buckwheat Millers Association prefers buckwheat that has large and uniform seeds with black hulls and greenish groats.

Handling

Handling methods vary among production areas. However, losses and quality changes of the grain occur mostly at various postharvest stages. During harvest, shattering and losses from germination, animals such as birds and rodents, and infection by molds occur in all countries. Threshing is done with combines or by beating the dried plants against stones or wooden bars, or by trampling the plants under bullock feet, carts, or tractor wheels. Transportation of grain from the field to market results in losses and quality deterioration. Losses during transportation are mainly from spillage. However, exposure of the grain to rain or frost during transit leads to subsequent spoilage through infection by microorganisms.

Storage

Like other grain crops, buckwheat is stored to ensure an even supply through time, to preserve the surplus grain for sale to deficit areas, and to be used as seed in the next planting season. Storage of the seeds may be at the farm, trader, market, government, retail, or consumer levels. Storage containers range from sacks to straw huts to bulk storage bins. In developing countries, traditional storage structures include granaries of gunny, cotton, or jute bags, or manufactured from reed, bamboo, or wood and plastered with mud and cow dung. In North America, storage structures include metal, concrete, or wooden bins at the farm level; elevators and annex at centralized receiving, storage, and shipping points; and concrete silos at grain terminals. Bagged buckwheat is highly susceptible to attack by insects and rodents. Bulk storage in bins, elevators, and silos is recommended.

A moisture content of 16% or less is required for safe storage of buckwheat. If the seed requires drying, the maximum temperature should not exceed 43°C. This temperature limit applies to seed for both seeding and processing. During storage at ambient temperature and relative humidity, the color of the aleurone layer changes from a desirable light green to the undesirable reddish brown. This undesirable quality change can be reduced by storing the seed at a lower temperature and at a relative humidity below 45%. Seeds can also be stored under controlled atmospheres (97% N_2, 1.5% O_2, and 1.5% CO_2). However, concentration of the major volatiles decreases, while the content of odor-active volatiles such as hexyl acetate and 1-hexanol increases in seeds stored under controlled atmosphere for 60 weeks (Mazza et al 1999).

Primary Processing

Primary processing of buckwheat includes cleaning, dehulling, and milling. The aim of seed cleaning is to remove other plant parts, soil, stones, weed seeds, chaff, dust, seeds of other crops, metallic particles, and small and immature buckwheat seeds. The extent and sophistication of the cleaning equipment depends largely on the size of the operation and the requirements for the finished product. Buckwheat seed can be milled by nearly any equipment capable of milling cereal grains. Hammer mills, stone mills, pin mills, disk mills, and roller mills have been used to mill buckwheat, but stone mills and roller mills are probably used most extensively today.

The milling process may be of two types. In the first and most common type, the whole seeds are first dehulled and then milled. In the second type, the seeds are milled and then screened to remove the hulls. When dehulling and milling are separate operations, the seeds are segregated according to size and may be steamed and dried before dehulling. Dehulling is done by impact or abrasion against emery stones or steel, followed by air or screen separation of groats and hulls. A widely used buckwheat dehuller is built on the principle of the stone-milling, with emery stones set to crack the hull without breaking the groat. The effectiveness of this type of dehuller depends on the clearance between the seed-cracking surfaces and the optimum setting for seed size. The ease of dehulling and yield of undamaged groats depend on variety and moisture content. From the dehuller, the groats are separated by sieving into whole groats and two or more sizes of broken groats. Flour is produced by passing the groats through stone or roller grinders.

When buckwheat seed is to be processed only into flour, and production of groats is not a requirement, the seeds are ground on break rolls or stone mills and then screened to separate the coarse flour from the hulls. The coarse flour is further reduced by a series of size-reduction rolls, each grinding operation followed by sifting to fractionate the mixture of particles according to size. The flour yield ranges from 50 to 75% depending on the size, shape, and condition of the seeds and the efficiency of the dehulling and milling operations.

Composition

The proximate composition and selected mineral profiles of Mancan, Manor, and Tokyo buckwheat groats are shown in Table 2.

TABLE 2
Proximate Composition, on a Dry Weight Basis (dwb), and Selected Mineral Profile of Three Dehulled Buckwheat Cultivars[a]

	Cultivar		
Assay	Mancan (±SD)	Manor (±SD)	Tokyo (±SD)
Moisture %	16.2 ± 0.9	10.1 ± 0.2	10.9 ± 0.1
Protein[b] (%)	14.2 ± 0.6	14.6 ± 0.3	11.9 ± 0.4
Crude fiber (%)	1.57 ± 0.30	1.21 ± 0.03	1.57 ± 0.10
Ash (%)	1.85 ± 0.01	1.66 ± 0.01	1.39 ± 0.01
Lipids[c] (%)	2.6 ± 0.3	2.2 ± 0.3	2.1 ± 0.2
Carbohydrates[d] (%)	79.8 ± 1.6	80.3 ± 0.8	83.0 ± 1.1
K (%)	0.440 ± 0.005	0.419 ± 0.009	0.407 ± 0.005
P (%)	0.359 ± 0.018	0.347 ± 0.003	0.262 ± 0.016
Mg (%)	0.214 ± 0.002	0.201 ± 0.012	0.195 ± 0.010
Ca (ppm)	180.5 ± 7.4	180.5 ± 10.6	220.5 ± 6.5
Fe (ppm)	24.8 ± 1.8	21.4 ± 0.3	21.2 ± 0.9
Zn (ppm)	23.4 ± 0.4	22.0 ± 1.6	22.8 ± 1.1
Mn (ppm)	10.2 ± 0.2	10.0 ± 0.5	10.2 ± 0.4
Cu (ppm)	4.6 ± 0.3	3.7 ± 0.1	4.3 ± 0.2

[a] Data from Mazza (1988).
[b] N × 6.25.
[c] Soxhlet, petroleum ether for 8 hr.
[d] By difference.

Carbohydrates

Starch is quantitatively the major component of buckwheat seed, and its concentration varies with the method of extraction and between cultivars. In whole grain (i.e., with hull) of common buckwheat, the starch content ranges from 59 to 70% of the dry matter. The composition of starch isolated from buckwheat grains is different from that of cereal starches, with the amylose having a degree of polymerization varying from 12 to 45 and varying in content from 15 to 52%. Buckwheat starch granules are irregular, 1–11 μm in size, with noticeable flat areas from compact packing in the endosperm (Kim et al 1977, Soral-Smietana et al 1984). The starch has a water-binding capacity of 79–104%, a blue value of 0.35, a swelling power and solubility at 60°C of 2.35 and 0.5%, respectively, an amylograph viscosity at 92°C of 640 Brabender Units (BU), an enzyme susceptibility (percentage of solubilized starch) of 2.63%, and initial and final gelatinization temperatures of 61.5°C and 76.0°C, respectively. Scanning electron microscopy studies by Lorenz and Dilsaver (1982) showed granules of buckwheat starch to be round or polygonal and smaller than wheat starch granules in average particle size.

There were significant differences in the physicochemical properties of three common and three tartary buckwheat starches grown in China compared to wheat starch (Li et al 1997). Differences between Italian buckwheat starches depending on region of growth were also reported (Acquistucci and Fornal 1997). Buckwheat starch has a higher swelling power than wheat starch, probably as a consequence of the weaker but more extensive bonding forces in the granule structure. Buckwheat starch granules are polygonal and have a smaller diameter than wheat starch granules. There were significant differences in the digestibility of starch from the Italian buckwheats.

Whole groats also contain 2% soluble carbohydrates, 7% total dietary fiber (TDF), and 2% ash. Bran, with little central endosperm, contains 18% starch, 6% soluble carbohydrates, 15% TDF, 7% ash, and 7% other components (Steadman et al 2001). Sucrose is the major component among the low-molecular-weight sugars. There is a small amount of arabinose, xylose, glucose, and probably the disaccharide melibiose.

Proteins

Protein content in buckwheat varies from 7 to 21%, depending on variety and environmental factors during growth. Most currently grown cultivars yield seeds with 11–15% protein. The major protein fractions are globulins, which represent almost half of all proteins. The globulins consist of a major 13S leguminlike and a minor 8S vicilinlike protein (Ikeda et al 1991). The 13S protein consists of eight subunits with molecular weights between 43 and 68 kDa. The 8S protein consists mainly of 57 kDa polypeptides with a few subunits in the 26–36 kDa range. The albumin represents about 25% of the total seed proteins and consists mainly of low-molecular-mass single-chain polypeptide of 8–16 kDa. Glutelin represents only 4% of the total seed protein. Prolamin has been fractioned into at least two peaks by gel filtration on Sephacryl S-200, and into three major and several minor components by sodium dodecyl sulfate-polyacrylamide gel electrophoresis (SDS-PAGE). Comparisons of buckwheat and wheat proteins according to amino acid composition, electrophoresis, and immunological reaction show little or no similarities. Whereas most of the material extracted from wheat flour by 70% ethanol (following salt extraction) is protein in nature, similar extracts from buckwheat contained only 2.4% nitrogen (Skerritt 1986). Also, buckwheat proteins are particularly rich in lysine. They contain less glutamic acid and proline, and more arginine, aspartic acid, and tryptophan, than cereal proteins. The amino acid composition changes markedly in maturing cereals (e.g., wheat, barley, and oats) and legumes (e.g., peas) but is very stable in maturing buckwheat. For limiting amino acids (e.g., lysine) and amino acids of storage proteins (e.g., glutamic acid), changes in buckwheat are intermediate between those of true cereals and legumes (Pomeranz et al 1975, Pomeranz 1983).

Due to the high lysine content, buckwheat proteins have a higher biological value than cereal proteins such as those of wheat, barley, rye, and corn. Also, buckwheat proteins have a higher solubility than soy protein isolates at pH 2–10, but lower than that of casein at pH 7–10. The emulsifying stability and water-holding capacity of buckwheat proteins are lower than those of soy protein and casein at high pH levels (Tomotake et al 2002).

Digestibility of buckwheat protein, however, is rather low, probably because of the high phenolics contents. Recently, a considerable interaction between polyphenols and proteins was reported to occur during the hydrothermal treatment of buckwheat groat proteins, and this interaction may reduce the digestion of proteins through the small intestine; microbial processes in the large intestine enhance the digestibility of the protein (Skrabanja et al 2000).

Lipids

Whole buckwheat seeds contain 1.5–3.7% total lipids. The highest concentration is in the embryo and the lowest in the hull, each containing 7–14% and 0.4–0.9%, respectively. Groats or dehulled seeds of Mancan, Tokyo, and Manor buckwheat contain 2.1–2.6% total lipids (Table 2), of which 81–85% are neutral lipids, 8–11% phospholipids, and 3–5% glycolipids. The major fatty acids of buckwheat lipids are palmitic (16:0), oleic (18:1), linoleic (18:2), stearic (18:0), linolenic (18:3), arachidic (20:0), behenic (22:0), and lignoceric (24:0). Of these, the 16 and 18 carbon acids are commonly found in all cereals. The long-chain acids—arachidic, behenic, and lignoceric—which represent, on average, 8% of the total acids in buckwheat, are only minor components or are not present in cereals (Mazza 1988).

Phenolic Compounds

The content of phenolics in hulls and groats of common buckwheat is about 1.9 and 1.3%, and that of tartary buckwheat 2.0 and 1.5%. Common buckwheat grown in Canada contains 1.2–1.6% of total phenolics with 70–79% of the phenolic acids being etherified. The total flavonoid concentration in common buckwheat seed and hulls varies with cultivar and location and ranges from 19 to 387 and 74 to 1,314 mg/100 g, respectively (Oomah and Mazza 1996). Six flavonoids—rutin, orientin, vitexin, quercetrin, isovitexin, and isoorientin—have been isolated and identified in buckwheat. Rutin and isovitexin are the only flavonoid components of buckwheat seed, while the hulls contain all six compounds. Rutin (quercetin 3-rutinoside), a well-known flavonol diglucoside used as a drug for treatment of vascular disorders caused by abnormally fragile or permeable capillaries, occurs in leaves, stems, flowers, and fruit of buckwheat. On average, about 300, 1,000, and 46,000 ppm of rutin is found in leaves, stems, and flowers, respectively, of common buckwheats. Other reported flavonols are quercitin (quercetin 3-rhamnoside) and hyperin (quercetin 3-galactoside). At least three red pigments have been found in hypocotyls of buckwheat seedlings (Mazza and Miniati 1993). One of these is cyanidin, the other two are presumed to be glycosides of cyanidin. The phenolic acids of buckwheat seed are the hydroxybenzoic acids, syringic, *p*-hydroxybenzoic, vanillic, and *p*-coumaric acids. Also in seed are soluble oligomeric condensed tannins, which, along with the phenolic acids, provide astringency and affect color and nutritive value of buckwheat products.

End Products

Traditional Products

Buckwheat has multiple uses. It is used to make alcoholic drinks, the liquor prepared from tartary buckwheat being ascribed medicinal qualities. In China, it is used in the production of vinegar. Common buckwheat is also used as a source of nectar for honey production in many countries. Buckwheat is useful as a green manure crop for renovation of low-productivity land. The plant has been used as a smother crop, as it germinates rapidly and produces a dense canopy that controls broadleaf weeds. It also acts as a feed and cover crop for wildlife, including deer, wild turkeys, and other birds.

The color of buckwheat flour is generally dark because of the presence of hull fragments. In North America, buckwheat flour is used primarily for making buckwheat pancakes and is commonly marketed in the form of prepared mixes. These mixes generally contain buckwheat flour, wheat, corn, rice, oat, or soybean flours, and a leavening agent. Buckwheat is also used with vegetables and spices in kasha and soup mixes, and with wheat, corn, or rice in ready-to-eat breakfast products, porridge, and bread and pasta products (Pomeranz 1983, Mazza 2000).

In Japan, buckwheat flour is used primarily for making *soba* or *sobakiri* (buckwheat noodles) and *Teuchi Soba* (handmade buckwheat noodles) (Shiratori and Nagata 1986). These products are prepared at *soba* shops or at home from a mixture of buckwheat and wheat flours. The wheat flour is used because of its binding properties and availability. *Soba* is made by hand or mechanically. In both methods, buckwheat and wheat flours are mixed together and then with water to form a stiff dough that is kneaded, rolled into a thin sheet (1.4 mm) with a rolling pin or passed between sheeting rolls, and cut into long strips. The product may be cooked immediately, sold fresh, or dried.

In Europe, most buckwheat is milled into groats, which are used in porridge, cabbage rolls, or meat products (especially hamburger), or consumed with fresh or sour milk. Buckwheat groats with cottage cheese, sugar, peppermint, and eggs are used as stuffing in a variety of dumplings. Buckwheat flour is used with wheat or rye flour and yeast to make fried specialty products such as bread, pasta, biscuits, and other confectioneries (Bonafaccia and Kreft 1994). An extruded, ready-to-eat corn-buckwheat breakfast product of high nutritional value is being produced and marketed in western Europe. This product contains more than 14% protein and 8% soluble fiber. Similar products have been developed in Poland and the USSR.

In most countries, the quality of buckwheat end products is controlled by law. According to Canadian Government Specifications, buckwheat flour must have ≤1.5% ash, ≥11% protein nitrogen on a 14% moisture basis, and contain ≤12% moisture when delivered. Class B Pancake Mix should contain more than 40% and less than 50% buckwheat flour with admixtures of 50% wheat, corn, rice, or soybean flour.

Buckwheat as a Functional Food and Nutraceutical

Some reported therapeutic uses of buckwheat are based on the possible pharmacological actions of several active compounds, especially polyphenols, fagopyritols (D-chiro-inositol) (D-CI), and proteins (Table 3).

Buckwheat has significant antioxidant activity (AOA) mainly associated with the presence of its polyphenolics, fagopyritols, and other phytochemicals. Oomah and Mazza (1996) examined the relationship between phenolics and antioxidant activity and indicated that flavonoid content was weakly correlated with AOA. However, purified flavonoid fractions exhibit radical scavenging activity, despite a low AOA of crude extracts (Watanabe et al 1997). In buckwheat hull, the active components include protocatechuic acid, 3,4-dihydroxybenzaldehyde, hyperin, rutin, and quercetin (13.4, 6.1, 5, 4.3, and 2.5 mg/100 g dried hull, respectively). Proanthocyanins also contribute to the radical-scavenging activity, while vitexin and isovitexin (4.6 and 3.3 mg/100 g, respectively) are inactive. The fractionation of buckwheat groat extracts results in four catechin compounds, namely (–)-epicatechin, (–)-epicatechin 3-*O*-*p*-hydroxybenzoate, (–)-epicatechin 3-*O*-(3,4-di-*O*-methyl)-gallate, and (+)-catechin 7-*O*-β-D-glucopyranoside, that have better radical scavenging activity than rutin. These differences in phenolic composition of the milled fractions of buckwheat seed are reflected in their antioxidant activity.

Methanolic extracts of groats are more effective in protecting against lipid oxidation than the extracts from hulls (Przybylski et al 1998). Ethyl acetate and acetone extracts have superior radical-scavenging activity as assessed by 2,2-diphenyl-1-picrylhydrazyl (DPPH). Antioxidant activity of buckwheat leaves is more than triple that of the seeds, dehulled seeds, straws, and hulls in model samples containing 20% of tested material (Holasova et al 2002). Buckwheat flour has higher antioxidant efficiency against reactive oxygen species, hydrogen peroxide, hypochlorous acid, and superoxide anion com-

TABLE 3
Buckwheat Constituents and Their Pharmacological Effects[a]

Constituents	Activities
Fagopyritols (D-chiro-inositol)	Antioxidant, hydroxyl radical scavenger, improves postprandial glycemic control and increases insulin action, effectively manages prediabetes and non-insulin-dependent diabetes in animal models.
Flavonoids	Apoptosis of human acute myelogenous leukemia HL-60 cells.
Flavonols	Anti-inflammatory activity in mice and rats.
Polyphenolics	Antioxidant in vitro and in vivo, protects against in vitro oxidative stress, reduces blood glucose level, improves brain activity and inhibits progression of renal failure in rats, inhibits histamine release and cytokine gene expression in mast cells, increases bacterial degradation of flavonoid in the human digestive system, anti-tumor activity.
Protein products	Inhibit Angiotensin I-convertmg enzyme (ACE) activity in hypertensive rats, improve cholesterol metabolism, reduce cell proliferation and protect against colon and mammary carcinogenesis in rats, reduce hepatic triglyceride concentration and body fat, suppress gallstone formation in hamsters, activate lymphocyte and cytokine production in humans.

[a] Sources: Wang et al (1992); Oomah and Mazza (1996); Watanabe et al (1997); Quettier-Deleu et al (2000); Tomotake et al (2001); Pei et al (2002); Simmering et al (2002); Kosuna (2003); Kawa et al (2003a), Liu et al (1998).

pared to the hull because of its higher flavanolic content (220 vs. 159 mg/100 g, respectively), and higher total flavonols and proanthocyanidins, respecttively (Quettier-Deleu et al 2000).

An aqueous extract rich in phenolic compounds, from buckwheat hull, exhibits strong *in vitro* and *in vivo* scavenging effect and protection against lipid peroxidation (Mukoda et al 2001). The hull extract almost equaled green tea extract in antioxidant activity, superoxide dismutase (SOD) scavenging activity, and inhibitory effect on oxidation of low-density lipoprotein (LDL) (lipid peroxidation) in blood and other organs when administered to mice (0.75% of hull extract, mixed with standard diet for 14 days). The extract's strong inhibition of linoleic acid and LDL oxidation was probably due to the high concentration of the efficient radical-scavengers rutin and quercetin. Since buckwheat hull extract strongly inhibited LDL oxidation (complete suppression of LDL oxidation at 200 μg/L hull extract, similar to green tea extract), it might prevent atherosclerosis, since oxidation is an early event in the buildup of atherosclerotic plaque. The significant-free-radical scavenging activities and antilipid peroxidation effects of the hull extracts might protect organs susceptible to oxidative stress such as blood, liver, and brain. Li and Zhang (2001) also reviewed the literature on recent advances in the development of functional foods from buckwheat.

Buckwheat seeds contain relatively high amounts of free D-CI and galactosyl derivatives of D-CI known as fagopyritols (Horbowicz et al 1998), which may reduce serum glucose concentrations in diabetes patients. A recent study (Kawa et al 2003b) evaluated the effects of a buckwheat concentrate containing D-CI on hyperglycemia and glucose tolerance in streptozotocin (STZ)-induced diabetic rats. In STZ rats, two doses of the buckwheat concentrate (containing 10 and 20 mg of D-CI per kilogram of body weight) were both effective in lowering serum glucose concentrations by 12–19% at 90 and 120 min after administration. These animal data indicate that a buckwheat concentrate containing D-CI may be useful in treatment to lower serum glucose levels in people with noninsulin-dependent diabetes mellitus (NIDDM).

A buckwheat protein product (61.9% protein, 11.3% lipids, 11.3% starch, and 10.1% water), when fed to hamsters for two weeks, markedly suppressed gallstone formation and reduced cholesterol concentration in gallbladder, plasma, and liver (Tomotake et al 2000). The suppression of gallstone formation by this buckwheat protein product is believed to be due to alterations in biliary cholesterol and bile acids and effects on fecal steroids by up-regulation of bile acid synthesis and higher fecal excretion of steroids. Buckwheat protein seems to exert gallstone-suppressive effects similar to that of dietary fiber. Thus, buckwheat may be beneficial in the treatment of both hypercholesterolemia and gallstones. A protein-rich product also reduced plasma cholesterol and adipose tissue weight when fed to rats for three weeks (Kayashita et al 1996). These alterations were reported as associated with reduced hepatic activities of lipogenic enzymes and reduced digestibility of dietary fat and protein.

Kayashita et al (1997) reported that buckwheat protein has a strong hypocholesterolemic activity in rats fed a cholesterol-enriched diet containing 5 g/kg cholesterol and 1.25 g/kg sodium cholate. In one experiment, rats fed buckwheat protein for three weeks had significantly lower concentrations of plasma cholesterol and enhanced excretion of fecal total neutral sterols and nitrogen compared with rats fed casein. There was a significant correlation between fecal total neutral sterols and nitrogen ($r = 0.89$, $P < 0.01$). Fecal excretion of acidic sterols was unaffected by buckwheat protein. In a second experiment, plasma cholesterol in rats fed trypsin-digested buckwheat protein for two weeks was significantly higher than in rats fed intact buckwheat protein. In a third experiment, rats were fed buckwheat protein, a low-molecular-weight fraction of the digest of buckwheat protein, or a high-molecular-weight fraction of the digest of buckwheat protein for three weeks. Plasma cholesterol levels were lower in the buckwheat protein group than in the low-molecular-weight-fraction group ($P < 0.05$), whereas levels in the high-molecular-weight-fraction group were intermediate. The *in vitro* digestibility of low-molecular-weight fractions by pepsin and pancreatin was significantly lower than that of casein.

Comparison of the effects of a buckwheat protein product, soy protein isolate, and casein on plasma cholesterol level and fecal steroid excretion in rats fed on a cholesterol-free diet (Tomotake et al 2001), showed that the consumption of buckwheat protein suppressed plasma cholesterol by enhancing the fecal excretion of both neutral and acidic steroids. These effects of the buckwheat protein product were stronger than those of soy protein isolate.

Despite the traditional and herbal medicinal uses of buckwheat, only a few human studies have been done to evaluate the therapeutic value of buckwheat preparations.

The potential for buckwheat to reduce the incidence of cardiovascular disease was investigated in a study by He et al (1995). The study examined the effect of buckwheat intake in 850 Yi people (an ethnic minority in southwest China) using a questionnaire, measurement of blood pressure on three consecutive days, and measurement of serum total cholesterol, high-density lipoprotein (HDL) cholesterol, and triglyceride after a 14-hr fast. Buckwheat intake (100 g/day) was associated with lower serum total cholesterol and LDL cholesterol and a higher HDL-to-total-cholesterol ratio.

A buckwheat herbal tea, standardized to a total flavonoid content of 5% (w/v) prevented edema in patients with chronic venous insufficiency (CVI). This positive pharmacological effect is thought to arise from the action of rutin on the capillaries, resulting in improved venous microcirculation (Ihme et al 1996).

A fraction of buckwheat, extracted by 100% methanol, had an antiallergic action that may be due to the inhibition of histamine release and cytokine gene expression in mast cells (Kim et al 2003). The extract dose dependently inhibited histamine-induced vascular permeability, interleukin-4 (IL-4), and induction of tumor necrosis factor-α (TNF-α) messenger ribonucleic acid (mRNA).

Prebiotic activity of buckwheat was demonstrated in rats in which cooked buckwheat (1:2 w/v in water for 20 min) fed for 30 days increased lactic and bifido bacteria and decreased enterobacteria (Préstamo et al 2003). In a human study, Simmering et al (2002) investigated the influence of different dietary flavonoids on the fecal population of the flavonoid-degrading bacterium *Eubacterium ramulus*. Dried buckwheat leaves (corresponding to 28 mg of rutin per kilogram of body mass) were fed to subjects and found to stimulate the growth of the *E. ramulus* population in the gastrointestinal tract, resulting in the formation of flavonoid degradation products in the fecal flora of healthy subjects. On day 7 following the ingestion of flavonoids, the cell counts of *E. ramulus* in the buckwheat group increased 60-fold, from 5.3×10^7 cells per gram of dry mass to 3.5×10^9 cells per gram of dry mass, corresponding to 6.9% (±5.9%) of the total flora.

Buckwheat flour has been proposed to have value in the treatment of diabetes, which may be related to the effects of D-CI, discussed above. A brief report was made about a decrease in blood sugar levels in 75 diabetic patients fed tartary buckwheat biscuits (Wang et al 1992). In a very small clinical trial (Bok et al 2000), three men in their fifties were treated for two months with daily oral doses of 5 mg/kg, 10 mg/kg, and 5 mg/kg of naringin, hesperidin, and rutin, respectively. Blood glucose levels determined before and after administration showed reductions of 17% for naringin, 23% for hesperidin, and 33% for rutin. The value of buckwheat for treating elevated glucose levels may therefore be related to rutin content rather than, or in addition to, D-CI.

Two patents have recently claimed specific beneficial, therapeutic effects for buckwheat extracts (Table 4). Animal, cell culture, and human studies are described. These data are not from peer-reviewed journals, but the results indicate potential value and merit consideration.

One patent claimed that an aqueous extract of buckwheat seed composed of material of molecular weight from about 1 kDa to about 10 kDa improved brain function in rats and humans (Kosuna 2003). The extract was administered in capsules (250 mg of dry powder, four capsules per day for 14 days) to 31 healthy volunteers, and resulted in an apparent improvement in memorization ability, decreased blood lipid peroxidation, and enhanced SOD activity. When administered for two months to eight healthy volunteers, the buckwheat seed extract increased the ability of the subjects to concentrate, and reduced irritation and insomnia. There was no placebo or control phase, and thus the reported beneficial effects on the functioning of the brain and nervous systems of the subjects (Kosuna 2003) solely related to a before-and-after comparison. Such comparisons must be treated with caution, since effects may arise simply from inclusion in a study.

In another patent, Pei et al (2002) reported that an ethanolic buckwheat extract containing 63% total tannin and 0.4% epicatechin inhibited the growth of Lewis lung carcinoma and cervical carcinoma U14 in mice, and also inhibited colony formation of a human gastric carcinoma cell line SGC-7901. The extract also alleviated xylene-induced ear inflammation in the mouse and protected against gamma ray irradiation.

TABLE 4
Patent Reports of Clinical Trials of Buckwheat

Author	Subject Description	Dosage and Duration	Outcome
Kosuna (2003)	20 males and 11 females; healthy volunteers, ages 20–69	250 mg dry powder (catechin polymer of an aqueous extract of buckwheat seed) 4 capsules per day for 14 days	Improvement in brain function and memorization ability
Kosuna (2003)	6 females and 2 males; healthy volunteers, ages 14–68	250 mg dry powder 4 capsules per day for 2 months	Improvement in nervous system, calmness and ability to concentrate and reduction in irritability and insomnia
Pei et al (2002)	102 males and 34 females; patients with intermediate- and late-stage of lung cancer, ages 31–80	1.2- to 1.6-g capsules containing 200 mg of the active components (buckwheat tannin 58.6% + 0.98% epicatechin) 3 times a day for 2 months	Improvement in blood picture (hemoglobin, leucocyte and platelet counts), kidney function, weight gain and appetite, partial remission rate and clinical symptoms
Pei et al (2002)	35 males and 25 females; patients with lung cancer, ages 35–76; 48 patients received radiotherapy or chemotherapy 6 or 3 months before	1.6-g capsules 8 capsules 3 times a day for 2 months	Improvement in Karnofsky performance scores and safety reduction in toxic reaction and debility
Pei et al (2002)	68 males and 12 females; patients with small cell lung carcinoma, ages 41–70	20 patients treated with active component, 20 with chemotherapy and 30 patients treated with combination of active component + chemotherapy	Synergistic effect with chemotherapy and reduction in toxic effect of single chemotherapy
Pei et al (2002)	60 males and 10 females; patients with lung cancer, ages 28–77	40 patients treated with 1.2- to 1.6-g capsules 3 times per day for 2 months + radiotherapy 150–200 cGy ^{60}Co 5 times weekly and 30 patients treated with radiotherapy alone	Improvement in sample remission rate, reduction in adverse effects of radiotherapy due to the synergistic effect of buckwheat polyphenolics with radiotherapy

The same patent described a reduction of the toxic and adverse effects of chemotherapy and radiotherapy in four separate clinical trials with lung cancer patients. In the first trial, the ethanol extract (containing 200 mg of tannin and epicatechin, 1.2–1.6 g each time, three times daily for two months) administered to 136 patients diagnosed with intermediate and late stages of lung cancer, apparently alleviated major clinical symptoms, specifically by increasing the hemoglobin, leucocyte, and platelet counts of the subjects, but no control was used and no statistics reported.

In the second study, 60 lung cancer patients were randomly divided into a treatment group and a control group. Patients in the treatment group were administered the extract orally (1.6 g, i.e., eight capsules) three times a day. The control group was treated by standard chemotherapy. Therapeutic effectiveness of the pharmaceutical composition of buckwheat extract was evaluated according to "the established criteria of four grades": complete remission, partial remission, stableness, and tumor progression. Two months after medication, no complete remission was observed. The partial remission rate in the control group was higher than in the treatment group. The stableness rate in the treatment group was significantly higher than the control group. The combined rate of partial remission and stableness in the treatment group (83.3%) was higher than that in the control group (63.3%). The number of patients with progression of tumor in the control group was about twice that in the treatment group. Again, no statistical analysis was provided.

In the third study, 80 patients diagnosed with small cell lung carcinoma received the buckwheat extract alone (20 patients), extract combined with chemotherapy (30 patients) or, as the control group, the chemotherapeutic agent alone (30 patients). The extract showed some statistically significant synergistic effects with chemotherapy in improving partial remission and stability of disease and also had some statistically significant effects in reducing the toxic and unwanted side effects of chemotherapy alone.

In the last clinical study, 70 patients with lung cancer were used. Forty patients with intermediate and late-stage lung cancer treated with the extract (1.2–1.6 g each time, three times daily for two months) combined with radiotherapy (150–200 cGy ^{60}Co, five times a week) were compared with 30 patients treated with radiotherapy alone. The extract showed statistically significant synergistic effects with radiotherapy, in improving partial and complete remission, and stabilization, and reducing progression of disease. Administration of the extract with the radiotherapy also brought about a statistically significant improvement in measures of the toxic and adverse side-effects of radiotherapy alone.

A commercial buckwheat (*F. cymosum)* product (WeiMaiNing) based on the patented ethanol extract of Pei et al (2002) has apparently been manufactured in China and is being further evaluated for the treatment of lung and other cancers (Chan 2003).

Conclusions

Buckwheat has been grown for about 2,000 years in China, 600 years in Europe, and almost 300 years in North America. Hence, it is not surprising that China produced 50% of the world's buckwheat during the past five years,

Russia about 25%, and Ukraine about 15%. Buckwheat is rated as one of the best sources of high biological value protein in the plant kingdom. The potential for buckwheat to reduce the risk of disease is beginning to be recognized. Limited animal tests and clinical trials in China have indicated that tartary buckwheat flour may prevent or treat diabetes, hypertension, cerebral atherosclerosis, and cardiovascular disease. It may also aid digestion, enhance the immune system, and alleviate inflammation. A U.S. patent claims that *F. cymosum* root extracts may help with the treatment of lung cancer.

It is imperative to more firmly establish the therapeutic or risk-reduction applications of the various species and extracts of buckwheat, and in particular to follow up the patent reports with peer-reviewed studies. These data would enable the exploitation of each of these species for the manufacture of functional foods and nutraceutical and pharmaceutical products of high value. Different management strategies would be needed for each of these species, such as greenhouse-based hydroponic systems for *F. cymosum* roots exposed to elicitors capable of stabilizing the production of the bioflavonoids that may have therapeutic value, or alternatively devising synthetic routes.

Despite long and widespread use, epidemiological and clinical studies on buckwheat and its constituents are limited and very recent. The association of buckwheat consumption with reduced risk of cardiovascular disease has been documented in one epidemiological study. The possible therapeutic benefits of buckwheat consumption in other degenerative diseases common in developed, industrialized nations, warrants further investigations.

References

Acquistucci, R., and Fornal, J. 1997. Italian buckwheat (*Fagopyrum esculentum*) starch: Physicochemical and functional characterization and in vitro digestibility. Nahrung 41:281-284.

Bonafaccia, G., and Kreft, I. 1994. Technological and qualitative characteristics of food products made with buckwheat. Fagopyrum 14:35-42.

Bok, S-H., Jeong, T-S., Bae, K-H., Park, Y-B., Choi, M-S., Moon, S-S., Kwon, Y-K., Lee, E-S., Hyun, B-H., Choi, Y-K., Lee, C-H., Ahn, B-T., and Lee, S-B. 2000. Method for lowering blood glucose level by the administration of bioflavonoid. U.S. patent 6,096,364.

Chan, P-K. 2003. Inhibition of tumor growth in vitro by the extract of fagopyrum cymosum (fago-c). Life Sci. 72:1851-1858.

Horbowicz, M., Brenac, P., and Obendorf, R. L. 1998. Fagopyritol Bl, O-α-D-galactopyranosyl-(1-2)D-chiro-inositol, a galactosyl cyclitol in maturing buckwheat seeds associated with desiccation tolerance. Planta 205:1-11.

He, J., Klag, M. J., Whelton, P. K., Mo, J. P., Chen, J. Y., Quian, M. C., Mo, P. S., and He, G. Q. 1995. Oats and buckwheat intakes and cardiovascular disease risk factors in an ethnic minority of China. Am. J. Clin. Nutr. 61:366-372.

Holasova, M., Fiedlerova, V., Smrcinova, H., Orsak, M., Lachman, J., and Vavrreinova, S. 2002. Buckwheat—The source of antioxidant activity in functional foods. Food Res. Int. 35:207-211.

Ihme, N., Kiesewetter, H., Jung, F., Hoffmann, K. H., Birk, A., Muller, A., and Grützner, K. I. 1996. Leg oedema protection from a buckwheat herb tea in patients with chronic venous insufficiency: A single-centre, randomised, double-blind, placebo-controlled clinical trial. Eur. J. Clin. Pharmacol. 50:443-447.

Ikeda, K., Sakaguchi, T., Kusano, T., and Yasumoto, K. 1991. Endogenous factors affecting protein digestibility in buckwheat. Cereal Chem. 68:424-427.

Kawa, J. M., Przybylski, R., and Taylor, E. G. 2003a. Urinary chiro-inositol and myo-inositol excretion is elevated in the diabetic db/db mouse and streptozotocin diabetic rat. Ex. Biol. Med. 228:907-914.

Kawa, J. M., Taylor, C. G., and Przybylski, R. 2003b. Buckwheat concentrate reduces serum glucose in streptozotocin-diabetic rats. J. Agric. Food Chem. 51:7287-7291.

Kayashita, J., Shimaoka, I., Nakajoh, M., and Kato, N. 1996. Feeding of buckwheat protein extract reduces hepatic triglyceride concentration, adipose tissue weight, and hepatic lipogenesis in rats. J. Nutr. Biochem. 7:555-559.

Kayashita, J., Shimaoka, I., Nakajoh, M., Yamazaki, M., and Kato, N. 1997. Consumption of buckwheat protein lowers plasma cholesterol and raises fecal neutral sterols in cholesterol-fed rats because of its low digestibility. J. Nutr. 127:1395-1400.

Kim, S. K., Hahn, T. R., Kwon, T. W., and D'Appolonia, B. L. 1977. Physicochemical properties of buckwheat starch. Korean J. Food Sci. Technol. 9:138-143.

Kim, C. D., Lee, W-K., No, K-O., Park, S-K., Lee, M-H., Lim, S. R., and Roh, S-S. 2003. Anti-allergic action of buckwheat *(Fagopyrum esculentum* Moench) grain extract. Int. Immunopharmacol. 3:129-136.

Kosuna, K-I. 2003. Composition for the treatment of symptoms and conditions associated with aging. U.S. patent 2003054057.

Li, W., Lin, R., and Corke, H. 1997. Physicochemical properties of common and tartary buckwheat starch. Cereal Chem. 74:79-82.

Li, S. Q., and Zhang, O. H. 2001. Advances in the development of functional foods from buckwheat. Crit. Rev. Food Sci. Nutr. 41:451-464.

Liu, J., Wang, S., Qi, J., Wang, X., and Song, Y. 1998. The immunostimulatory effect of bio-active peptides from pollen on murine and human lymphocytes. Mech. Aging Dev. 104:125-132.

Lorenz, K., and Dilsaver W. 1982. Buckwheat (*Fagopyrum esculentum*) starch physicochemical properties and functional characteristics. Starch/Stærke 34:217-220.

Marshall, H. G., and Pomeranz, Y. 1982. Buckwheat: Description, breeding, production, and utilization. Pages 201-217 in: Cereals '78: Better Nutrition for the World's Millions. Y. Pomeranz, Ed. Am. Assoc. Cereal Chem., St. Paul, MN.

Mazza, G. 1988. Lipid content and fatty acid composition of buckwheat seed. Cereal Chem. 65:122-126.

Mazza, G. 2000. Buckwheat. Pages 90-97 in: Cambridge History and Culture of Food and Nutrition. K. F. Kiple, Ed. Cambridge University Press, Cambridge, U.K.

Mazza, G., T. Cottrell, L., Malcomson, B., Girard, B. D., Oomah, D., and Eskin, N. A. M. 1999. Headspace gas chromatography and sensory analyses of buckwheat stored under controlled atmosphere. J. Food Qual. 22:341-352.

Mazza, G., and Miniati, E. 1993. Buckwheat. Pages 226-227 in: Anthocyanins in Fruits, Vegetables and Grains. G. Mazza and E. Miniati, Eds. CRC Press Inc., Boca Raton, FL.

Mukoda, T., Sun, B., and Ishiguro, A. 2001. Antioxidant activities of buckwheat hull extract toward various oxidative stress *in vitro* and *in vivo*. Biol. Pharm. Bull. 24:209-213.

Oomah, B., and Mazza, G. 1996. Flavonoids and antioxidant activities in buckwheat. J. Agric. Food Chem. 44:1746-1750.

Pei, H., Qlyu, G., Bo, C., and Hongwu, Z. 2002. *Fagopyrum cymosum* (Trev.) Meisn composition, method to prepare and analyze the same and uses thereof. U.S. patent 6,451,353 Bl.

Pomeranz, Y. 1983. Buckwheat: Structure, composition and utilization. CRC Crit. Rev. Food Sci. Technol. 19:213-258.

Pomeranz, Y., Marshall, H. G., Robbins, G. S., and Gilbertson, J. T. 1975. Protein content and amino acid composition of maturing buckwheat (*Fagopyrum esculentum* Moench). Cereal Chem. 52:479-484.

Préstamo, G., Pedrazuela, A., Peñas, E., Lasunción, M. A., and Arroyo, G. 2003. Role of buckwheat diet on rats as prebiotic and healthy food. Nutr. Res. 23:803-814.

Przybylski, R., Lee, Y., and Eskin, N. 1998. Antioxidant and radical-scavenging activities of buckwheat seed components. J. Am. Oil Chem. Soc. 75:1595-1601.

Quettier-Deleu, C., Gressier, B., Vasseur, J., Dine, T., Brunet, C., Luyckx, M., Cazin, M., Cazin, J-C., Bailleul, F., and Trotin, F. 2000. Phenolic compounds and antioxidant activities of buckwheat *(Fagopyrum esculentum* Moench) hulls and flour. J. Ethnopharmacol. 72:35-42.

Shiratori, R., and Nagata, Y. 1986. Utilization of buckwheat in modem Japan. Fagopyrum 6:23-46.

Skerritt, J. H. 1986. Molecular comparison of alcohol-soluble wheat and buckwheat proteins. Cereal Chem. 63:365-369.

Simmering, R., Pforte, H., Jacobasch, G., and Blaut, M. 2002. The growth of the flavonoid-degrading intestinal bacterium, *Eubacterium ramulus,* is stimulated by dietary flavonoids in vivo. FEMS Microbiol. Ecol. 40:243-248.

Skrabanja V., Laerke H. N., and Kreft, I. 2000. Protein-polyphenol interactions and in vivo digestibility of buckwheat groat proteins. Pflug. Arch. 440 (5 Suppl):R129-131.

Soral-Smietana, M., Fornal, L., and Fornal, J. 1984. Characteristics of buckwheat grain starch and the effect of hydrothermal processing upon its chemical composition, properties and structure. Starch/Stærke 36:153-158.

Steadman, K. J., Burgoon, M. S., Lewis, B. A., Edwardson, S. E., and Obendorf, R. L. 2001. Buckwheat seed milling fractions: Description, macronutrient composition and dietary fibre. J. Cereal Sci. 33:271-278.

Tomotake, H., Shimaoka, I., Kayashita, J., Nakajoh, M., and Kato, N. 2002. Physicochemical and functional properties of buckwheat protein product. J. Agric. Food Chem. 50:2125-2129.

Tomotake, H., Shimaoka, I., Kayashita, J., Yokoyama, F., Nakajoh, M., Kato, N. 2001. Stronger suppression of plasma cholesterol and enhancement of the fecal excretion of steroids by a buckwheat protein product than by a soy protein isolate in rats fed on a cholesterol-free diet. Biosci. Biotech. Biochem. 65:1412-1414.

Tomotake, H., Shimaoka, I., Kayashita, J., Yokoyama, F., Nakajoh, M., and Kato, N. 2000. A buckwheat protein product suppresses gallstone formation and plasma cholesterol more strongly than soy protein isolate in hamsters. J. Nutr. 130:1670-1674.

Wang, J., Liu, Z., Fu, X., and Run, M. 1992. A clinical observation on the hypoglycemic effect of Xinjiang buckwheat. Pages 465-467 in: Proc. 5th Int. Symp. on Buckwheat. L. Rufa, Z. Ming-De, T. Yongru, L. Jianying, and Z. Zongwen, Eds. Agricultural Publishing House, Taipei, Taiwan.

Watanabe, M., Osshita, Y., and Tsushida, T. 1997. Antioxidant compounds from buckwheat *(Fagopyrum esculentum* Moench) hulls. J. Agric. Food Chem. 45:1039-1044.

CHAPTER 15

Specialty Grains and Health

P. J. Wood

Food Research Program, Agriculture and Agri-Food Canada, Guelph, Ontario Canada[1]

Many of the grains and agricultural and food practices described in this book can be considered "alternative" in that, for some consumers and suppliers, production and consumption are part of a lifestyle that excludes the use of mainstream produce from agri-food businesses. Both personally and environmentally, healthy living is of paramount importance to persons who adhere to this lifestyle. Some specialty uses described in this book, such as producing unusual and attractively colored food using pigmented grains, may have no immediately apparent health benefit. However, a thread of potential value to health runs throughout this book. Arguments support these potential health benefits in a general way, but no clearly established relationships using currently accepted criteria of clinical research specifically identify benefits peculiar to the grain or agricultural practice described. This question requires more research because, to date, there are too few sufficiently well-controlled studies to make valid comparisons (Bourn and Prescott 2002).

Dealing first with safety rather than positive benefits, this topic is chiefly addressed in the chapter on organic grains (Chapter 2). In organic production, pesticides (including herbicides and fungicides) are not used, and, not unexpectedly, a lower pesticide residue may sometimes be found in organic produce than in conventionally grown produce (Baker et al 2002). However, this does not mean that the levels detected pose a danger and does not suggest that organically grown produce is safer than mainstream produce as a result. There are some reports of higher levels of mycotoxins and other contaminants such as heavy metals in organically produced foods (Malmauret et al 2002), which might lead to consumption exceeding suggested maximum tolerable limits (Leblanc et al 2002), but conversely, there is no evidence that conventional produce is safer in regard to contaminants. Nevertheless, the fact that data have been published showing differences in potentially harmful residues, in either direction, suggests that such analyses should be expanded to obtain a

[1] For the Department of Agriculture and Agri-Food Canada, Food Research Program, Government of Canada. Publication number M013.

clearer overall quantitative picture. Data from such analyses will vary widely with geography and jurisdiction. Both the individual exposures to natural or artificial toxins and the individual responses to these will similarly vary, and more study is needed to evaluate these complex issues.

Canary seed is the one grain included in this book that does not have a history of human consumption, and it will require safety testing, as discussed in Chapter 8. In Canada, canary seed would be treated as a novel food, a classification that can lead to lively debate and disagreement. For example, at what point or by what criteria should unusual cultivars be considered sufficiently different to be a "novel" food as defined by Health Canada, meaning, in general terms, a food or a composition of food for which there is no history of consumption and therefore no long-term evidence of safety? Although it might seem reasonable to say that, in canary seed, the hazard (siliceous hair) is absent from the new cultivars, this focuses on the known hazard, whereas regulatory agencies must also concern themselves with the unknown because of the lack of history of human consumption.

The possibility that there may be components or combinations of components in specialty grains that enhance health or reduce risk of disease is of considerable interest. Dietary fiber is one of the most well-established functional components of foods with specific health benefits, and whole grains tend to be a primary source of dietary fiber. None of the grains discussed in this book, however, have a dietary fiber level or component that contrasts strongly with the more usual sources of fiber. Differences from mainstream produce may arise in part from a tendency toward less refining, which means that there is a greater proportion of the fiber- and mineral-rich outer layers of the grain in flours produced for this specialty market. The health benefits of consuming whole or less-refined grain or cereal are apparent from many prospective studies (Rimm et al 1996, Salmeron et al 1997, Hill 1998, Wolk et al 1999, Steffen et al 2003). In many of these studies, the effect is correlated with the dietary fiber intake as well as with whole grain intake. Phenolics and antioxidant activity are also believed to play a role, although these effects are less clearly documented.

Between specialty and conventional grains, there are, of course, some differences in fiber composition, just as there are differences in phenolics, minerals, vitamins, and protein and amino acid composition. No specific health benefit can be clearly attached to these differences, although health benefits must be considered in terms of the target population. High protein content and good amino acid balance may be of critical importance to some populations, but these are not usually considerations for most persons living in developed industrial societies, in which chronic, age-associated diseases are of greatest concern. As an example, the similarities in the lysine and arginine compositions of canary seed protein and soy protein, which may indicate the potential to lower serum cholesterol levels, may be more relevant than the content of limiting amino acids. Bioactive peptides, or amino acid sequences, may have health effects that have nothing to do with overall protein composition. While some of these effects may be harmful, as discussed in Chapter 5 in relation to celiac disease, they may also have beneficial properties (Kitts 1994, Gibbs et al 2004). Similarly, the loss of micronutrients during refining may lead to deficiency diseases in some communities, but this loss is of less concern in developed nations.

Producers, manufacturers, and consumers of specialty grains are often vigorous advocates of health benefits, especially as associated with organic production, despite the fact that most scientific and clinical evidence for such benefits is weak. Obviously, financial motivations exist for producers and manufacturers to promote their products, but consumer motivation is less easily identified. As already suggested, consumer motivation is probably associated with an interest in health promotion and environmentally "friendly" behavior (Williams and Hammitt 2001). Williams and Hammitt (2001) also reported that buyers of organic foods have a greater belief that conventional foods are more hazardous than organic foods, and they are more suspicious of regulatory agencies than are buyers of conventional foods. Many people also view large corporations with suspicion. Although there are likely to be geographic variations in attitude not accounted for, to the extent that such beliefs drive the market, the development of ancient and other specialty grains and organic foods into large, financially successful operations, and the development of such product lines by the major corporations, may be self-limiting. One consequence of the food supply being delivered en masse by large corporations is that, when something goes wrong, many people might be affected, and considerable adverse publicity may result. Smaller, geographically limited operations are as likely to have occasional problems, but their consequences are more limited. Finally, if the majority of consumers embraced diets based on organic foods and specialty grains, the grains and practices described in these chapters might be insufficient to meet the total demand for them.

Despite government campaigns and other publicity, most people have great difficulty modifying their diets over the long term, even when problems such as high serum cholesterol levels or obesity are present. The growing specialty market would seem to be a route by which many are able to make a decisive change in their diet, leading perhaps serendipitously to adoption of the dietary advice given to the public. The overall changes associated with a change in diet to specialty products or organic food are usually so numerous that studies of population differences are inevitably confounded, and conclusions are likely to be flawed (Williams 2002). Nevertheless, through research and development, specific functional values, including health benefits, of specialty crops will become better accepted and will lead to improved and diverse food products. In a general sense, increased diversity in agricultural production and diet is worthwhile whether or not specific benefits can be immediately identified as long as there are no attendant risks. Consumers do not seem to demand that healthful foods and diets be supported by regulated health claims. However, the typical requirements for such guidelines are worth reviewing in terms of what the industry and interested groups should be considering if health benefits are to feature as a prominent functionality and if health claims are to gain in credence.

Both Canada and the United States provide guidelines and standards to be followed for any health claims made for foods. (Relevant websites are, for the

United States, http://www.cfsan.fda.gov/~dms/lab-hlth.html; for Canada, http://www.hc-sc.gc.ca/food-aliment/ns-sc/ne-en/health_claims-allegations_sante/e_health_canada_policy.html). The strength of evidence and the relation of this to the strength of claim are important in generating such regulations. Claims for reduction of disease risk[2] require a greater weight of evidence than claims of structure or function.[3] General statements about health and well-being (for instance, that a product promotes regularity) are allowed by many jurisdictions, without specific regulations. Although consumers can judge claims like these for themselves, the vagueness of terms such as "well-being" have been criticized, for example in the European Union.

Human studies are essential. In clinical trials, a double-blind, placebo-controlled design is best. Such clinical trials cannot be conducted with the manifestation of disease as the end point, however, because the studies are designed to predict the occurrence of chronic illnesses, which take many years to develop. Accordingly, clinical studies are feasible only when there is a biomarker, and few of these exist at present. Recent possible heart disease biomarkers are C-reactive peptide and homocysteine levels, but serum cholesterol level—specifically, low-density lipoprotein cholesterol—is perhaps the best or longest-established biomarker. Interestingly, however, it is well recognized that elevated circulating cholesterol is only part of the chronic condition that leads to atherosclerotic plaque; there is good evidence that oxidative changes are also involved, which may be modified by antioxidant intake. The grains covered in this book all have components with antioxidant properties, and indeed the chapter on pigmented grains (Chapter 12) deals specifically with phenolics that possess this activity. As knowledge of mechanisms involved in diet-health relationships become better understood, suitable biomarkers will be established and generally accepted, allowing demonstration of the benefits and efficacy of many materials, including the grains discussed in this book. Where antioxidant activity is concerned, any reactive oxygen and nitrogen species are believed to be potentially harmful, and thus any demonstrable effect of antioxidants against these is desirable (Astley 2003). A randomized, controlled clinical study reported that people consuming organic foods had greater urinary excretion of some flavonoids compared to those consuming conventional foods (Grinder-Pedersen et al 2003). However, the results may have been confounded by the different varieties of grain used in the organic foods.

Both Canada and the United States now allow some health claims for foods. Health Canada has allowed five claims to date, under a classification referred to as "generic claims." None of these include grains. This surprising omission may relate to wording, since the initial approach was to review the first 10 claims allowed by the U.S. Food and Drug Administration (FDA) under the Nutrition and Labeling Education Act (NLEA). The FDA claims

[2] For example, consumption of whole grain cereals might lower the risk of heart disease.

[3] For example, consumption of oats might lower serum cholesterol levels.

that specified grains included reference to dietary fiber. Health Canada was evidently not convinced by the use of dietary fiber in the claims as allowed by the FDA and suggested that further review was needed. In the case of oat products, the first specific food to be identified by the FDA as meriting a health claim, Health Canada again decided that further review was needed to "determine the direction that this claim should take." Although this may relate to a question as to whether such a claim is generic or product-specific, some controversy does remain over the ability of oats and oat products to lower serum cholesterol levels sufficiently to be physiologically significant. The message from this is perhaps simply that it is difficult to establish relationships between food consumption and physiological benefit with complete scientific agreement. This area of nutritional science is in its infancy, and much research will be needed to identify mechanisms and the role of genetics and other factors that contribute to these relationships. The health claims allowed in Canada and the United States are shown in Table 1. At this time, few countries have a regulatory structure dealing with health claims for foods. Japan has the FOSHU system—foods for specified health use—which are

TABLE 1
A List of Health Claims Allowed for Foods and Food Ingredients in the United States and Canada

United States		
Miscellaneous	**Grains and Oilseeds**	**Canada**
Calcium and osteoporosis	Fiber-containing grain products, fruits and vegetables and cancer	Sodium and hypertension
Sodium and hypertension	Fruits, vegetables and grain products that contain fiber, particularly soluble fiber, and risk of coronary heart disease	Calcium and osteoporosis
Folate and neural tube defects	Soluble fiber from certain foods and risk of coronary heart disease (whole oats and oatrim, psyllium)	Dietary fat and heart disease
Dietary fat and cancer	Soy protein and risk of coronary heart disease	Fruits and vegetables and cancer
Dietary saturated fat and cholesterol and risk of coronary heart disease	Whole grain foods and the risk of heart disease and certain cancers (FDAMA)	Dietary sugar alcohols and dental caries
Dietary sugar alcohol and dental caries		
Fruits and vegetables and cancer		
Plant sterol/stanol esters and risk of coronary heart		
Potassium and the risk of high blood pressure and stroke (FDAMA)		

foods that may improve specific health conditions. The subject is under debate in the European Union and other jurisdictions. Some European countries individually allow claims. The claims in Table 1 are disease risk reduction claims.

Although most authorities emphasize the need for human studies, at least when the purpose is to obtain government-sanctioned health claims, strong evidence can be accumulated through cell culture and animal studies. It is important, however, when reviewing evidence, to make a clear distinction between these and human trials. Such distinction is a well-established practice for promising new drugs but is sometimes emphasized less for functional foods and nutraceuticals. It is certainly of interest when, for example, a compound or a food suppresses growth of a chemically induced tumor in a rat, but it needs to be clearly indicated that this is the circumstance and that human response may be different. Although overstating the benefits of an established food carries little risk, overstatement may lead vulnerable people to overconsume these products or, worse, reject established drug therapies. Conversely, the reporting of associations of lifestyle and diet with chronic and life-threatening illness can place an inappropriate burden of guilt on those suffering from the illnesses. The diseases are multifactorial. Finally, the assessment of risk and benefit for a food is different than that for a therapeutic drug; unless a prescribed medical use or condition is involved, no hazard (side effect) should be attached to food consumption.

Much of the recognition of diet-health relationships has arisen initially from epidemiological or population comparisons. This includes, for example, the observations of Dennis Burkitt and others (Burkitt 1995) relating differences in dietary fiber intake and fecal output of rural populations in Africa compared to the populations of developed industrial societies. The most powerful of the human population studies are prospective, in which a large cohort is entered into the study, diet and other lifestyle records are kept, and disease development in the population is related to patterns of intake. Of particular note, and receiving perhaps the greatest attention in North America, has been the Health Professionals Follow-up Study of Walter Willett and colleagues. The study indicated a number of relationships that have become generally accepted, such as between fiber and cereal intake and the reduced risk of coronary heart disease and noninsulin-dependent diabetes mellitus (Rimm et al 1996, Salmeron et al 1997, Wolk et al 1999, Fung et al 2002). Whole grain products and fiber consumption have also been associated with reduced weight gain in the studies of Willett and colleagues (Liu et al 2003).

Results from different observational studies may come to different conclusions and (unfortunately, since significant media attention is given to them) recommendations on what constitutes healthy or protective diets seem to vary. For example, the Health Professionals Study reported that fiber intake did not reduce risk of colon cancer (Fuchs et al 1999), whereas a similar observational study in Europe (Bingham et al 2003) did find that grain and fruit fiber protected against colon cancer. The reasons for such disagreements (Hill 1998) are not clear but tell us that great care must be taken before a hypothesis is accepted or dismissed, since there may be difficulties with methodology. For example, estimates of soluble and insoluble dietary fiber intake from food tables and diet diaries may have errors; unknown confounding factors may be involved; and, despite the very large population base, very few people might actually be consuming much of the item of interest. A relatively small number of people consume any of the individual grains covered in this book. Collectively, however, with the growth that is reported for some products, such as ancient and organically grown grains, an adequate population to evaluate may be available. To our knowledge, no attempt to evaluate these grains has yet been made in any major population study presently in progress. Such a study might give some very valuable leads as to benefits of the grains, but the expense might be prohibitive. A case control study, in which a population with a particular disease is matched retrospectively with an equivalent disease-free group, might be more readily done. As discussed earlier, such a study might be difficult to control because of the many confounding lifestyle factors that will inevitably be found in the group consuming organic and specialty grains.

No food is generally accepted unless it has the appealing organoleptic qualities expected of a food. The perception of what is appealing differs with culture and history, and modern mass production and marketing have unquestionably influenced taste. Possibly the move to ancient or different grains and organic foods reflects, in part, a revolt against the mass market but this does not mean that organoleptic appeal does not also apply to the use of these specialty grains as food ingredients. Indeed, a specific taste or texture might be developed for the mass market that cannot be obtained with conventional material. These qualities must, of course, be available at reasonable cost. Mainstream supermarket goods do not succeed unless they are competitively priced, and, despite the fact that many consumers name nutrition as a primary purchasing consideration, cost, taste, and texture can all be barriers to acceptance. As outlined in Chapter 2, the organic grains market appears not to follow the norm where price is concerned. However, the produce clearly must have some specific appeals, and as noted in Chapter 5, consumers of baked goods made from spelt enjoy a flavor that differs from that of common wheat and also describe a psychological response—a feeling of well-being. Mass production tries to appeal to the maximum number of consumers but also has a tendency to aim at the lowest common denominator, the product least likely to give offense, which may result in blandness. Thus, specialty grains and their products appeal to the need for diversity of texture and flavor, as well as providing agricultural diversity.

Despite the cautionary notes, there seems little doubt that many who use organic foods and related specialty grains enjoy improvements in their general sense of well-being. As documented in this book, there are numerous ingredients and compositions that are bioactive and that individually or synergistically could have specific health benefits. Investigation of these grains and their composition and effects is likely to lead to a better understanding of diet-health relationships and to the development of new, healthful food products.

References

Astley, S. B. 2003. Dietary antioxidants—Past, present and future? Trends Food Sci. Technol. 14:93-98.

Baker, B. P., Benbrook, C. M., Groth E., and Benbrook, K. L. 2002. Pesticide residues in conventional, integrated pest management (IPM)-grown and organic foods: Insights from three U.S. data sets. Food Addit. Contam. 19:427-446.

Bingham, S. A., Day, N. E., Luben, R., Ferrari, P., Slimani, N., Norat, T., Clavel-Chapelon, F., Kesse, E., Nieters, A., Boeing, H., Tjonneland, A., Overvad, K., Martinez, C., Dorronsoro, M., Gonzalez, C. A., Key, T. J., Trichopoulou, A., Naska, A., Vineis, P., Tumino, R., Krogh, V., Bueno-de-Mesquita, H. B., Peeters, P. H., Berglund, G., Hallmans, G., Lund, E., Skeie, G., Kaaks, R., and Riboli, E. 2003. Dietary fibre in food and protection against colorectal cancer in the European Prospective Investigation into Cancer and Nutrition (EPIC): An observational study. Lancet 361:1496-501.

Bourn, D., and Prescott, J. 2002. A comparison of the nutritional value, sensory qualities, and food safety of organically and conventionally produced foods. Crit. Rev. Food Sci. Nutr. 42:1-34.

Burkitt, D. 1995. Historical aspects. Pages 3-10 in: Dietary Fiber in Health and Disease. D. Kritchevsky and C. Bonfield, Eds. Am. Assoc. Cereal Chem., St. Paul, MN.

Fuchs, C. S., Giovannucci, E. L., Colditz, G. A., Hunter, D. J., Stampfer, M. J., Rosner, B., Speozer, F. E., and Willett, W. C. 1999. Dietary fiber and the risk of colorectal cancer and adenoma in women. N. Engl. J. Med. 340:169-176.

Fung, T. T., Hu, F. B., Pereira, M. A., Liu, S. M., Stampfer, M. J., Colditz, G. A., and Willett, W. C. 2002. Whole grain intake and the risk of type 2 diabetes: A prospective study in men. Am. J. Clin. Nutr. 76:535-540.

Gibbs, B. F., Zougman, A., Masse, R., and Mulligan, C. 2004. Production and characterization of bioactive peptides from soy hydrolysate and soy-fermented food. Food Res. Int. 37:123-131.

Grinder-Pedersen, L., Rasmussen, S. E., Bugel, S., Jorgensen, L. V., Dragsted L. O., Gunderson, V., and Sandstrom, B. 2003. Effects of diets based on foods from conventional versus organic production on intake and excretion of flavonoids and markers of antioxidative defense in humans. J. Agric. Food Chem. 51:5671-5676.

Hill, M. J. 1998. Cereals, cereal fiber and colorectal cancer risk: A review of the epidemiological literature. Eur. J. Cancer Prev. 7(Suppl. 2):S5-S10.

Kitts, D. D. 1994. Bioactive substances in food: Identification and potential uses. Can. J. Physiol. Pharmacol. 72:423-434.

Leblanc, J. C., Malmauret, L., Delobel, D., and Verger P. 2002. Simulation of the exposure to deoxynivalenol of French consumers of organic and conventional foodstuffs. Regul. Toxicol. Pharmacol. 36:149-154.

Liu, S., Willett, W. C., Manson, J. E., Hu, F. B., Rossner B., and Colditz, G. 2003. Relation between changes in intakes of dietary fiber and grain products and changes in weight and development of obesity among middle-aged women. Am. J. Clin. Nutr. 78:920-927.

Malmauret, L., Parent-Massin, D., Hardy, J. L., and Verger, P. 2002. Contaminants in organic and conventional foodstuffs in France. Food Addit. Contam. 19:524-532.

Rimm, E. B., Ascherio, A., Giovannucci, E., Spiegelman, D., Stampfer M. J., and Willett, W. C. 1996. Vegetable, fruit and cereal fiber intake and risk of coronary heart disease among men. J. Am. Med. Assoc. 275:447-451.

Salmeron, J., Manson, J. E., Stampfer, M. J., Colditz, G. A., Wing, A. L., and Willett, W. C. 1997. Dietary fiber, glycemic load and risk of non-insulin dependent diabetes mellitus in women. J. Am. Med. Assoc. 277:472-477.

Steffen, L. M., Jacobs, D. R., Stevens, J., Shahar, E., Carithers, T., and Folsom, A. R.

2003. Associations of whole-grain, refined grain, and fruits and vegetable consumption with risks of all-cause mortality and incident coronary artery disease and ischemic stroke: The Atherosclerosis Risk in Communities (ARIC) Study. Am. J. Clin. Nutr. 78:383-390.

Williams, C. M. 2002. Nutritional qualities of organic foods: Shades of grey or shades of green? Proc. Nutr. Soc. 61:19-24.

Williams, P. R., and Hammitt, J. K. 2001. Perceived risks of conventional and organic produce: Pesticides, pathogens and natural toxins. Risk Anal. 21:319-330.

Wolk, A., Manson, J. E., Stampfer, M. J., Colditz, G. A., Hu, F. B., Speizer, F. E., Hennekens, C. H., and Willett, W. C. 1999. Long-term intake of dietary fiber and decreased risk of coronary heart disease among women. J. Am. Med. Assoc. 281:1998-2004.

Index